Therapeutics in

Rheumatology

Therapeutics in
Rheumatology

Edited by

J. M. H. MOLL
BSc DM PhD FRCP

Consultant physician in Rheumatology and Head, Sheffield Centre for Rheumatic Diseases, Nether Edge Hospital, Sheffield; Honorary Clinical Lecturer in Rheumatic Diseases, University of Sheffield.

H. A. BIRD
MA MD FRCP

Lecturer in Rheumatology, University Department of Medicine, General Infirmary at Leeds; Honorary Consultant Rheumatologist, General Infirmary at Leeds, and Royal Bath Hospital, Harrogate.

A. RUSHTON
MB ChB MRCP

Drug team leader, Clinical Research Department, Imperial Chemical Industries PLC, Pharmaceuticals Division, Alderley Park, Macclesfield.

Springer-Science+Business Media, B.V.

British Library Cataloguing in Publication Data

Therapeutics in rheumatology.
1. Rheumatism—Chemotherapy
I. Moll, J.M.H. II. Bird,
H.A. III. Rushton, A.
616.7'23061   RC927

ISBN 978-0-412-24540-4   ISBN 978-1-4899-2883-2 (eBook)
DOI 10.1007/978-1-4899-2883-2
Softcover reprint of the hardcover 1st edition 1986

Contents

SECTION III

Clinical applications and implications

Contributors

H. Berry
MA, DM, FRCP

Consultant in Rheumatology and Rehabilitation, King's College Hospital, London, England.

H. A. Bird
MA, MD, FRCP

Senior lecturer in Rheumatology, University Department of Medicine, General Infirmary at Leeds; Honorary Consultant Rheumatologist, General Infirmary at Leeds, and Royal Bath Hospital, Harrogate, England.

H. A. Capell
MB, BCh, FRCP

Consultant Physician, The Centre for Rheumatic Diseases, University Department of Medicine, The Royal Infirmary, Glasgow, Scotland.

D. E. Caughey
MB, FRCP(Ed.),
FRACP

Clinical Reader in Medicine, Auckland Medical School; Consultant Rheumatologist, Auckland Hospital, Auckland, New Zealand.

D. M. Grennan
MD, PhD,
FRCP(Glasg.)

Consultant and Senior Lecturer, University of Manchester Rheumatic Diseases Centre, Hope Hospital, Salford, England.

N. D. Hall
MA, PhD

Lecturer in Pharmacology, University of Bath; Honorary Immunologist, Royal National Hospital for Rheumatic Diseases, Upper Borough Walls, Bath, England.

F. D. Hart
MD, FRCP

Honorary Consulting Physician, Westminster Hospital, Chelsea Hospital for Women and the Hospital of St. John and St. Elizabeth, London, England.

D. W. G. Harron
PhD, MPS

Lecturer, Department of Therapeutics and Pharmacology, Queens University, Belfast, Northern Ireland.

I. Haslock
MD

Consultant Rheumatologist, South Tees Health District, Middlesbrough General Hospital, Middlesbrough, England.

B. L. Hazleman
MA, MB, FRCP

Consultant Rheumatologist, Director Rheumatology Research Unit, Addenbrooke's Hospital; Associate Lecturer, Cambridge University, Cambridge, England.

Carol Higham
MSc, MPS

Lecturer in Pharmacy, University of Manchester Rheumatic Diseases Centre, Hope Hospital, Salford, England.

P. J. L. Holt
MB, FRCP

Reader in Rheumatology and Physician in Charge, Rheumatism Research Centre, University of Manchester, The Royal Infirmary; Physician, Regional Paediatric Rheumatology Unit, Booth Hall Children's Hospital, Manchester, England.

S. P. Liyanage
MB, FRCP, DCH

Consultant Rheumatologist, Heatherwood Hospital, Ascot; King Edward VII Hospital, Windsor; and St Mark's Hospital, Maidenhead, England.

R. Madhok
MB, ChB, MRCP

Registrar, The Centre for Rheumatic Diseases, University Department of Medicine, The Royal Infirmary, Glasgow, Scotland.

J. M. H. Moll
BSc, DM, PhD,
FRCP

Consultant Physician in Rheumatology and Head, Sheffield Centre for Rheumatic Diseases, Nether Edge Hospital, Sheffield; Honorary Clinical Lecturer in Rheumatic Diseases, University of Sheffield, England.

**Vera C. M.
Neumann**
BA, MB, MRCP

Senior Registrar, Rheumatism Research Unit, University department of Medicine, General Infirmary at Leeds, England.

M. C. L'E. Orme
MA, MD, FRCP

Professor of Clinical Pharmacology, University of Liverpool; Consultant Physician, Liverpool AHA(T), Department of Pharmacology and Therapeutics, New Medical School, Ashton Street, Liverpool, England.

A. Rushton
MB, ChB, MRCP

Senior Medical Adviser and Deputy Manager, Clinical Research Department, Imperial Chemical Industries PLC, Pharmaceuticals Division, Alderley Park, Macclesfield, England.

A. J. Taggart
MD, MRCP

Consultant Physician and Senior Lecturer, Department of Therapeutics and Pharmacology, Queens University, Belfast, Northern Ireland.

V. Wright
MD, FRCP

Professor of Rheumatology, Rheumatism Research Unit, University department of Medicine, General Infirmary at Leeds, England.

Preface

This book is about the drugs used in the treatment and management of rheumatic disorders. The term 'therapeutics' used in the title is intended to mirror the relevance of drugs in the widest sense of the word. Thus, general principles underlying pharmaceutical and pharmacological study have been included together with more clinical matters concerned with applying specific rheumatic problems.

The *need* for another work on rheumatological drugs in itself, as opposed to the different approach intended, was prompted by the ever continuing and bewildering plethora of antirheumatic drugs flooding the market at present. We believe that such a burgeoning of new preparations is welcome in an era when in general there are still no 'cures' available. Moreover, we also feel that a continued update of this rapidly advancing field is essential, not only for its own sake, but also to place it in perspective with itself and with neighbouring fields.

When the volume was first envisaged it was felt that a realistic approach would be to divide the work into three main sections in order to highlight the general principles of therapeutics (Section I), the specifics of antirheumatic pharmacology (Section II), and the clinical application of these two disciplines (Section III). With this in mind, it was felt appropriate that editors with a special interest in each of these areas be responsible for sections covering these different therapeutic aspects. That this might engender some overlap between sections was considered justifiable if the general aim of providing a global view on rheumatological therapeutics be achieved.

Another point raised early in the planning stage was the question of including brief notes on 'para-therapeutic' details of rheumatic management in order to provide a perspective backcloth to the general theme of drug therapy. It is also hoped, therefore, that in providing brief comments on non-drug aspects, notably on remedial therapy and surgery, the readers will have placed before them a more general viewpoint on rheumatological therapeutics than might have resulted from a work totally confined to drugs.

A further aim was to present therapeutic material in a way that reasonably reflects what clinicians *actually do* in practice, as opposed to what they preach! To further this aim, contributors have been encouraged to include practical advice based on their day-to-day experiences, in addition to the more academic matters implied by their other term of reference – critical review of the past and present field.

It is hoped that the extensive glossary of international drug names at the end of the book will be of help to readers in other countries.

The book is aimed at clinicians in training and established posts mainly involved in the management of patients with rheumatic disorders. However, it is also hoped that it will be of value to those in related disciplines such as pharmaceutical and pharmacology researchers, orthopaedic surgeons, medical rehabilitationists, general practitioners, and remedial therapists.

J. M. H. Moll (Sheffield)
H. A. Bird (Harrogate)
A. Rushton (Macclesfield)

Acknowledgements

We wish to thank the following for secretarial assistance: Mrs P. Drake and Mrs P. Large (Sheffield), Mrs D. K. Smith and Mrs R. Schofield (Harrogate), and Mrs A. Withington (Macclesfield).

We also acknowledge the help of Mr J. Williamson in contributing towards the design of the cover.

Note on limited list
prescribing in the UK

The Secretary of State for Social Services has recently announced in parliament the government's intention to limit the range of drugs available for prescription on the NHS from 1 April 1985. The government feel committed to the principle of this scheme in order to contain the ever rising national drug bill.

The extent to which these proposals will affect rheumatological prescribing in the UK is not yet clear, and it is possible that the initial proposals will shortly be revised, perhaps with further revisions after this.

There has been much opposition to the government's proposals from various sectors of the medical profession, including the British Medical Association, but the outcome of present debate is not yet resolved.

Antirheumatic agents recently withdrawn (or restricted) in UK

Non-proprietary name	Proprietary name
zomepirac	Zomax (withdrawn)
alclofenac	Prinalgin (withdrawn)
fenclofenac	Flenac (withdrawn)
benoxaprofen	Opren (withdrawn)
indoprofen	Flosint (withdrawn)
indomethacin (as sodium trihydrate)	Osmosin (withdrawn)
flufenamic acid	Meralen (withdrawn)
feprazone	Methrazone (withdrawn)
oxyphenbutazone	Tanderil (withdrawn)
phenylbutazone	Butazolidin (restricted)

SECTION I

Pharmacological and therapeutic principles

INTRODUCTION

A. Rushton

The practice of therapeutics involves, above all else, complex decision making. The process has been sanctified by terms such as 'clinical judgement', which seems often to be regarded more as an art than a science. However, by analogy to the diagnostic aspects of medicine, therapeutics should be based upon objective assessment of factual knowledge.

The necessary factual knowledge can be divided into several components which include the pharmacological basis of therapy in a particular area of therapeutics, general principles of therapeutics (e.g. pharmacokinetics) and information on the efficacy and safety of individual drugs in specific conditions.

The underlying concept of this first section is to provide a broadly based springboard for the reader to dive into the more specific information on antirheumatic drugs and rheumatic diseases in the subsequent sections.

However, even in the more general subjects (e.g. pharmacokinetics) a rheumatological flavour has been included by appropriate exemplification.

The first chapter reviews the disappointing, yet tantalizing state of the pharmacological sciences in relation to rheumatic diseases. Clearly there are many options for therapeutic research, but the importance, to date, of 'empirical' therapeutics to the clinician is readily apparent.

The data base on pharmacokinetics is undoubtedly more mature, but the basic principles are as relevant to rheumatological therapeutics as they are to any branch of medicine. Moreover, the growing interest in chronokinetics and chronotherapeutics is particularly appropriate to rheumatology, in view of the diurnal variations in symptoms and immune status that occur in chronic inflammatory arthritis.

The study of drug interactions relies heavily upon pharmacokinetic principles and methodology. The clinical aspects of this area receive due attention and the fallibility of the test tube is emphasized, particularly in relation to protein-binding interactions.

Measurement of drug response is central to building the data base of knowledge. Separate chapters deal with efficacy and safety. The diversity of measurements used for the former in rheumatology probably reflects both disease complexity, as in rheumatoid arthritis, and inadequacy of current treatments. Chronic rheumatic disorders are, moreover, dynamic rather than static and often manifest a complex interplay of present disease activity and past tissue damage. This complicates the interpretation of efficacy data and, conversely, failure to appreciate disease dynamics may lead to false therapeutic expectations.

With regard to drug safety assessment, data collection methodology and guidelines for interpretation of results are applicable to therapeutics in general. However, many of the difficulties of this area have recently been highlighted in relation to antirheumatic drugs. In this, above all other aspects of therapeutics, there is a tendency for emotion to predominate over scientifically based judgement. It is hoped that the recent spate of drug withdrawals will serve as a stimulus for improvements in the processes of safety monitoring and data interpretation.

The balance of general therapeutics and specific rheumatological information in this section has not been easy to judge, but the efforts of the authors will be amply rewarded if the reader, on the one hand, finds useful practical information and, on the other, is stimulated to question the scientific basis of 'clinical traditions' that undoubtedly exist in rheumatological therapeutics.

CHAPTER 1

The pharmacological
basis of antirheumatic
drug therapy

N. D. Hall

1.1 INTRODUCTION

I am tempted to begin these introductory remarks by suggesting that antirheumatic therapy has in fact no pharmacological basis at all, or at least had none when the various compounds currently in use were first tested. Most chronic inflammatory joint diseases have in common a lack of understanding of aetiological factors and inadequate treatment by drugs with uncertain mechanisms of action and toxicity. In general, rheumatologists do not have available therapeutic agents designed to interact specifically with pathogenic processes, because these mechanisms have not been well characterized.

Thankfully, this is changing rapidly, with considerable advances now being made in our understanding of the major pathological feature associated with most rheumatic diseases – *inflammation*. Indeed, the development of research in this subject shares many features of the process itself – the literature has become vastly swollen, its generation causes considerable pain and may occasionally give rise to much heat and/or redness. We must all hope that a disease-modifying treatment emerges before the endstage, loss of function, develops. In the following sections, I will discuss current knowledge of the various factors associated with the inflammatory process, in particular, mediators, phagocytic cells, and the immune system. All of these are considered to be relevant to the pathogenesis of rheumatic disorders, although different aspects may play greater or lesser roles in the various diseases within this group.

The most common feature of the rheumatic diseases is pain in the joints, whether on moving or after rest. Pain is a cardinal sign of inflammation and is thought to result from sensitization of nerve fibres by inflammatory mediators (kinins, prostaglandins). As such, it is usually treated with non-steroidal anti-inflammatory drugs (NSAIDs) irrespective of the underlying disorder. A second major problem in many rheumatic diseases is joint swelling. This inflammatory response may result from various pathogenic mechanisms and may localize in different sites associated with particular conditions. Acute swelling is caused by vasodilatation and increased vascular permeability leading to the exudation of plasma proteins into the surrounding tissue. This process requires both mediators and polymorphonuclear (PMN) leucocytes (Section 1.2.1), and may therefore respond to NSAID therapy. However, certain diseases such as rheumatoid arthritis (RA) are also characterized by proliferation of the cells forming the synovial membrane of the joint. The cellularity of the proliferating synovium is further increased by large-scale infiltration of leucocytes, including lymphocytes, plasma cells, and monocyte/macrophages from the circulation (Zvaifler, 1973). These cells are active in the immune response and generate many factors (autoantibodies, immune complexes) which are thought to play a predominant role in the pathogenesis of RA.

Similar immunological activity is associated with other connective tissue diseases such as systemic lupus erythematosus (SLE). Joint symptoms are a major feature of this condition, although these are usually restricted to arthralgia or a non-erosive synovitis. More destructive lesions in SLE include damage to blood vessels and kidneys, and factors that may be responsible for this pattern of localization will be considered later in this section. The cellular component of inflammation, whether in RA or SLE, is more difficult to treat effectively, although immunomodulatory drugs (in RA) or cytotoxic regimes (RA, SLE) give good results in some patients.

Swelling is one of the causative factors in another symptom of rheumatic diseases – joint stiffness. Normal joint mobility requires smooth articulating cartilage surfaces lubricated with highly viscous synovial fluid. Plasma exudate will dilute the synovial fluid thereby reducing its effectiveness. However, stiffness is more generally a chronic problem caused by tissue changes (synovium, cartilage, bone) in and around the joint. In RA, the hypertrophied synovial tissue extends into the joint space and grows over the cartilage forming a pannus. This tissue is characterized by activated cells, especially macrophages, releasing lysosomal enzymes and other factors which degrade proteoglycan and collagen and destroy the normal smooth cartilage surface, thereby promoting stiffness and pain on movement. The erosions of cartilage and the underlying bone may be visualized radiologically and are a major pathological feature of RA. In other diseases, joint stiffness is associated with mechanisms quite distinct from the erosive, destructive lesions brought about by the mononuclear cells of the rheumatoid pannus. Osteoarthrosis (OA) is characterized by painful, stiff joints due to impaired biomechanical properties of the articular cartilage. There are only minimal changes in the synovium and little evidence of mononuclear cell involvement. The pathogenesis of OA probably involves biochemical activity in the cartilage leading to loss of the proteoglycan matrix. This may be as a result of some disturbance in chondrocyte metabolism.

Although very different from each other, both RA and OA involve what are essentially destructive changes to joint tissue. On the other hand, ankylosing spondylitis (AS) is characterized by excessive activity of the reconstructive arm of the inflammatory process – fibrosis and ankylosis. There is no clear indication of immunological abnormalities in AS, although histological studies show a mononuclear cell infiltrate around points of insertion of ligaments and capsules into bone, i. e. an enthesopathy (Ball, 1971). Major sites involved are the sacroiliac joints and intervertebral joints in the spine. As an 'inflammatory disease', AS may be treated with the same NSAIDs used in RA (with some exceptions, e. g. aspirin is relatively ineffective in spondylitis), although the inflammatory process in these two conditions appears quite different.

From the above it is clear that although rheumatic diseases share certain features in common, such as painful joints, they are rather dissimilar in their pathogenesis. Many questions relating the clinical signs and symptoms of rheumatic diseases to underlying pathogenic mechanisms remain to be answered. For example, it is not known why certain chronic inflammatory joint diseases are associated with erosive loss of cartilage and bone, whereas others are characterized by fibrosis and ankylosis. It is also uncertain why these diseases differ in the localization of inflammatory changes to different sites. It is reasonable to suppose that crystal-induced arthropathies are focused at points of crystal deposition, although little is known of the factors that control crystal formation. In diseases such as RA and SLE, with extensive immunological activity, immune complexes may act to induce an inflammatory response following fixation in a particular tissue. This could be the site at which the complexes are synthesized, for example IgG–IgG complexes in rheumatoid synovium (Munthe and Natvig, 1972). Alternatively, or in addition, complexes could be released from their point of synthesis into the circulation and thus interact with Fc receptors on endothelial cells or other tissues. A further possibility is that circulating antibodies may bind to antigens that have become trapped, thus forming immune complexes *in situ* (Jasin, 1975). The latter mechanism may be important in SLE, with circulating anti-DNA antibodies becoming fixed to DNA bound to exposed collagen in blood vessel walls or the kidneys (Izui *et al.*, 1976). Perhaps the major contributing factor to the initial localization of inflammatory disease *in joints* is the lack of a basement membrane between synovial blood vessels and the surrounding tissue. Increased vascular permeability induced by various mediators will therefore permit the rapid influx of large protein molecules, including immunoglobulins, immune complexes, and complement components, that are difficult to clear from the joint space and could interact with each other or with tissue components to trigger an inflammatory reaction (Kushner and Somerville, 1971).

Aetiological agents in the rheumatic diseases, such as infectious organisms, remain a subject for informed speculation (Hadler, 1976; Bennett, 1978). Whatever their identity, it is clear that several factors may modify the pattern of disease expression in individual patients or patient groups. An awareness of this importance of the host in determining the expression of disease manifestations has come about partly as a result of analysing genetic markers associated with specific diseases. In the field of rheumatology, such factors are well represented with associations of HLA-B27 with AS (Brewerton *et al.*, 1973) and some other spondarthritides, HLA-DR4 with RA (Stastny, 1978; Panayi *et al.*, 1978) and certain complement deficiencies with SLE (Glass *et al.*, 1976). The precise links between these genetic markers and the pathogenic mechanisms underlying each disease are still unclear, but further studies are sure to underscore the importance of these initial observations. It has recently been suggested (Jones *et al.*, 1983) that HLA-DR4 is a marker of likely disease severity in RA rather than of susceptibility to arthritis. This is in agreement with the observation that patients with extra-articular manifestations of severe RA (e. g. Felty's syndrome) are almost all HLA-DR4 positive (Dinant *et al.*, 1980).

1.2   INFLAMMATORY MEDIATORS

The release of several vasoactive substances is widely thought to mediate the major features of acute inflammation: vasodilatation, increased vascular permeability, and pain. As with all long-running plays, however, although the overall script remains the same, the individual members of the cast change as time passes. Thus, initial interest in histamine, 5-hydroxytryptamine (serotonin), and bradykinin has waned as, although these substances together with prostaglandins contribute to the carrageenan-induced oedema observed in rat paws (DiRosa *et al.*, 1971), evidence for a significant role in human inflammatory disease is poor (Zeitlin and Grennan, 1976). Centre-stage is currently held by other families of mediators, many derived from cell membrane phospholipids.

A simplified flow diagram of the major pathways involved in the production of inflammatory mediators from phospholipid is given in Fig. 1.1. The key event is the activation of phospholipase A_2 in the plasma membrane of various cell types. This activation, at least in neutrophils, can be triggered by numerous stimuli (see Section 1.3) and results in the release of fatty acids, particularly arachidonic (eicosatetraenoic) acid, from the C-2 position of the glycerol backbone of the phospholipid. Arachidonic acid may be converted into several important mediators of inflammation (Trang, 1980; Zeitlin, 1981) after

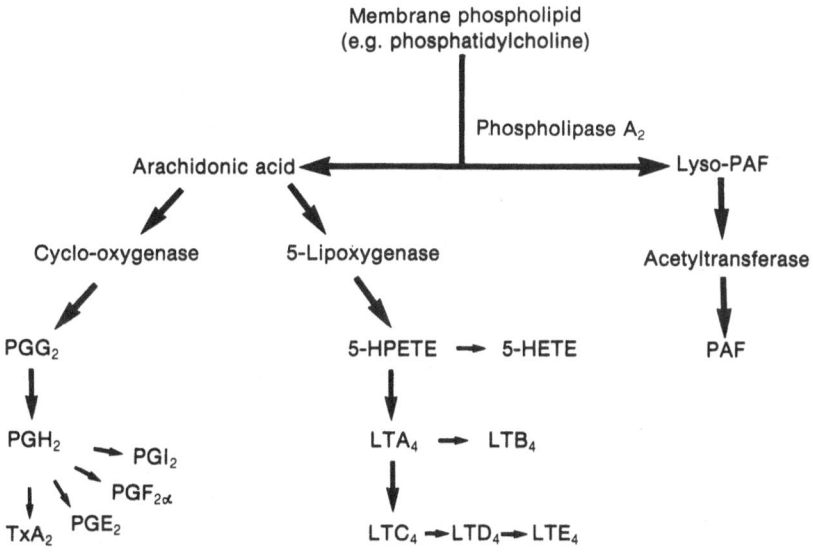

Figure 1.1 Flow diagram of major pathways generating inflammatory mediators from membrane phospholipid.

metabolism by either cyclo-oxygenase or lipoxygenase enzymes (Section 2.2.1). In addition to arachidonic acid, phospholipase A_2 may also generate a substance now recognized as lyso-PAF. This can be acetylated at the C-2 position to produce platelet activating factor, PAF (1-0-alkyl-2-acetyl-sn-glycero-3-phosphocholine). This substance is able to activate cell types other than platelets (e.g. neutrophils) and may therefore play an important role in inflammation (Section 1.2.2).

1.2.1 Metabolites of arachidonic acid

Cyclo-oxygenase catalyses the conversion of arachidonic acid into a cyclic endoperoxide, PGG_2. This is itself rapidly converted into PGH_2 which can give rise to several more stable products, including the prostaglandins E_2, $F_{2\alpha}$ and D_2 (reviewed by Trang, 1980; Zeitlin, 1981). Certain tissues contain enzymes that metabolize PGH_2 in different ways, leading to the generation of thromboxane A_2 (TxA_2) by platelets and prostacyclin (PGI_2) by vascular endothelium.

Further interest in the products of arachidonic acid metabolism has come from the discovery of a large number of hydroxy-fatty acids generated from this substrate by a family of lipoxygenase enzymes. These enzymes form hydroperoxide derivatives at different carbon atoms on the arachidonic acid (e.g. 5-, 8-, 9-, 11-, 12-, 15-lipoxygenases) and also differ in their tissue distribution. At present, the most widely studied lipoxygenase products are those in the 5-series synthesized by neutrophils (Fig. 1.1). Arachidonic acid is first converted into 5-hydroperoxyeicosatetraenoic acid (5-HPETE), which may either break down to form the corresponding hydroxyacid 5-HETE, or be metabolized to a 5,6-epoxide, leucotriene A_4 (LTA$_4$). This may be converted into a dihydroxyacid 5,12-diHETE (LTB$_4$) or, after reaction with glutathione, to LTC$_4$, LTD$_4$ and LTE$_4$ which together constitute slow reacting substance of anaphylaxis, SRS-A (Hammarström, 1983).

Several of the metabolites mentioned above have biological properties that are thought to be relevant to the inflammatory process. These effects may be brought about either by a direct action of the compounds themselves or, more often, by synergistic interactions between different mediators. Thus, prostaglandins of the E (PGE) series (Solomon et al., 1968) and prostacyclin (Szczeklik et al., 1978) are potent vasodilators in man, a direct action that probably explains the increased blood flow and skin redness associated with acute inflammation. However, these mediators do not by themselves cause pain but greatly potentiate the pain induced by low doses of histamine and bradykinin (Ferreira, 1972; Ferreira et al., 1978). A similar synergism between PGE and histamine or bradykinin has been noted in the induction of increased vascular permeability by the latter compounds (Crunkhorn and Willis, 1971). Potent vasodilators such as PGE$_2$ and PGI$_2$ may also synergize with another arachidonic acid metabolite, LTB$_4$, in increasing vascular permeability (Bray et al., 1981; Wedmore and Williams, 1981). In contrast to the effects of histamine and bradykinin, this reaction does not occur in the absence of neutrophils (Wedmore and Williams, 1981). Since LTB$_4$ is a potent chemotactic factor for PMN cells (Goetzl and Pickett, 1980; Ford-Hutchinson et al., 1980), this suggests that other chemotaxins might also be capable of mediating changes in vascular permeability. This is indeed so, and Wedmore and Williams (1981) have reported PMN-dependent oedema formation induced by complement fragment C5a (Fernandez et al., 1978) and synthetic peptide F-Met-Leu-Phe (Showell et al., 1976) in the presence of PGE$_2$. These data are summarized in Fig. 1.2. The precise role of the neutrophils in promoting plasma exudation is still unclear.

Much evidence has accumulated in recent years to show that the above mediators are produced in inflammatory sites in rheumatoid arthritis. Synovial fluid samples from such patients contain raised levels of PGE$_2$ (Morley, 1974), LTB$_4$ (Klickstein et al., 1980; Rae et al., 1982) and C5a (Ward and Zvaifler, 1971). Rheumatoid synovial fluid thus contains all the factors necessary to promote plasma exudation and oedema formation as proposed by Wedmore and Williams (1981). One other effect of PGE$_2$ should be mentioned in the context of rheumatic diseases, namely its promotion of bone resorption (Robinson et al., 1975). The relevance of this to erosive changes in rheumatoid joints is unclear, since NSAIDs, which effectively inhibit prostaglandin synthesis, (Section 1.4) do not appear to affect bone destruction in this disease.

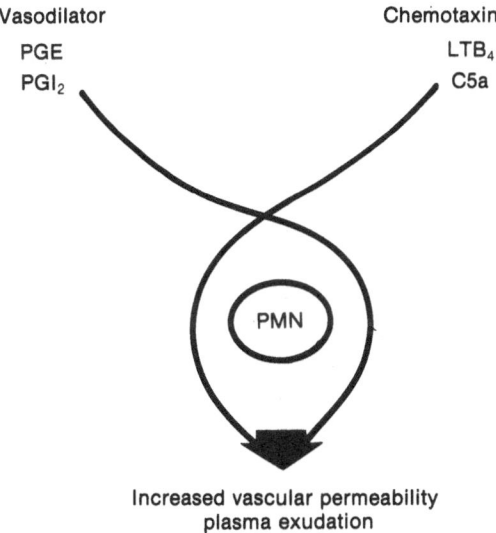

Vasodilator

PGE

PGI$_2$

Chemotaxin

LTB$_4$

C5a

PMN

Increased vascular permeability
plasma exudation

Figure 1.2 Interaction of mediators and PMN cells in the control of vascular permeability.

So far, the emphasis has been placed on the pro-inflammatory effects of the mediators. However, these are most apparent during acute inflammatory episodes, and different anti-inflammatory actions may emerge in chronic immune-mediated disease states (Kunkel *et al.*, 1981). The ability of arachidonic acid metabolites to modulate lymphocyte function is particularly intriguing (Bray, 1980). Inhibitory effects of prostaglandins on T cell proliferation have been observed (Goodwin *et al.*, 1977), and may be relevant to the depressed cellular responses to mitogens observed in Hodgkin's disease (Fisher and Bostick-Bruton, 1982) and progressive systemic sclerosis (Lockshin *et al.*, 1983). Prostaglandins may also induce suppressor T lymphocyte activity (Fischer *et al.*, 1981), thereby providing further evidence that inhibition of prostaglandin synthesis by NSAIDs could lead to increased immunological activity. More recently, these mediators have been shown to enhance immunoglobulin production by human cells stimulated with pokeweed mitogen (Staite and Panayi, 1982; Lydyard *et al.*, 1982). However, it has been suggested that, *in vitro*, rheumatoid lymphocytes are less sensitive to prostaglandins than healthy cells (Staite *et al.*, 1983). Decreased sensitivity to PGE$_1$ has also been observed in patients with progressive systemic sclerosis (Martin *et al.*, 1982). The possible contribution of mechanisms such as these and the recently described inhibition of T lymphocyte function by LTB$_4$ (Payan and Goetzl, 1983) to the pathogenesis of RA and other chronic inflammatory diseases clearly needs further study.

1.2.2 Phospholipid mediators

The identification of PAF as a phospholipid derivative (Demopoulos *et al.*, 1979) has stimulated many studies of the actions of this compound on cell types other than platelets. In man, a major source of PAF is the neutrophil (Lotner *et al.*, 1980). These cells are activated by PAF and undergo aggregation and degranulation (O'Flaherty *et al.*, 1981). Many of these effects of PAF may be secondary to its inducing the release of arachidonic acid from PMNs with subsequent generation of LTB_4 (Chilton *et al.*, 1982). This mechanism might also explain the increase in vascular permeability caused by intradermal administration of PAF. The ability of this compound to promote vascular changes and to activate neutrophils supports its inclusion as a potentially important mediator of inflammation. However, its precise role, especially as a putative stimulus for the generation of other active substances such as PGE_2 and LTB_4 awaits further elucidation.

1.3 PHAGOCYTIC CELLS

Phagocytic cells have been recognized as key elements in the inflammatory process since Metchnikoff's observations almost a century ago. Since then, many studies have led to the general hypothesis that such cells, both neutrophils and macrophages, are attracted to sites of inflammation by chemotactic factors and promote tissue damage by releasing lysosomal enzymes during phagocytosis of immune complexes or other particles (Hollander *et al.*, 1965). Of course, in the standard view (Fig. 1.3), this should not occur. Phagocytes

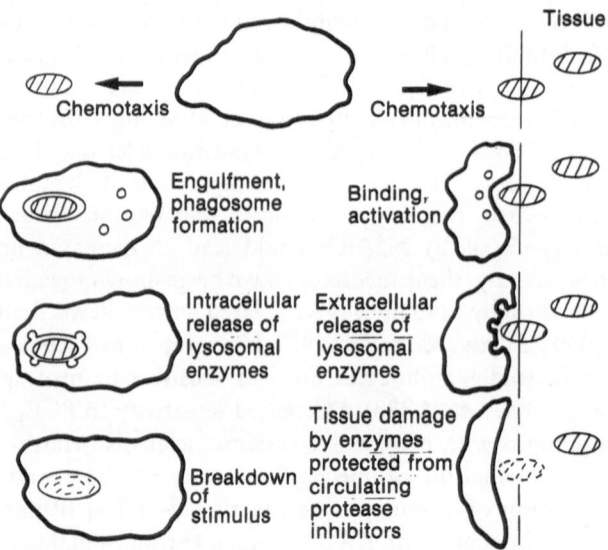

Figure 1.3 Phagocytic cell stimulation by soluble (left) or tissue-fixed (right) material, e.g. immune complexes.

move into the inflammatory site, and there bind and engulf the stimulus within an enclosed phagocytic vacuole. Lysosomes then fuse with the vacuole membrane and liberate their various enzymes to break down the phagocytosed material. Unfortunately, this clean picture of events is spoilt by some of the unsavoury eating habits of these cells when confronted by a stimulus that is either bound to a tissue surface or trapped within a tissue matrix (Jasin, 1975) (see also Fig. 1.3). Cell activation occurs before the phagocytic vacuole has fully closed, and so lysosomes secrete their digestive enzymes into the extracellular space, close to the tissue surface (Henson, 1971). Substantial damage may thereby ensue, as the enzymes are in an environment protected from protease inhibitors by the adhered phagocyte. This scheme, proposed as it was nearly 20 years ago, does not include other potential mediators of tissue damage released by activated phagocytes, nor does it give any information on the mechanisms that govern their secretion. Much work has been carried out in both these areas recently, and possible targets for future therapeutic intervention in inflammatory disease are being identified. When considering mechanisms of chronic disease, emphasis must be placed on the activity of macrophages as phagocytic cells capable of continuous enzyme production and release over several days (Baggiolini, 1982). However, most of the studies using human cells have concentrated on neutrophil activity, largely because of the relative availability of these cells.

In recent years, attention has been focused on the active oxygen species derived from stimulated phagocytic cells as potential mediators of tissue damage (Babior, 1978; Badwey and Karnovsky, 1980). These products of oxidative metabolism include the free radicals superoxide anion ($O_2^{\cdot-}$) and hydroxyl ($OH^{\cdot}$), and hydrogen peroxide (H_2O_2). They are secreted by neutrophils in considerable quantities following activation by a number of stimuli (see below). *In vitro*, at least, monocytes generate smaller amounts of these species than neutrophils (Reiss and Roos, 1978). Superoxide anion is produced by an NADPH-dependent reduction of molecular oxygen that occurs in the neutrophil membrane (Babior *et al.*, 1981), catalysed by 'NADPH oxidase', an unusual cytochrome b (Gabig *et al.*, 1982). It rapidly dismutates under physiological conditions to form hydrogen peroxide (Root and Metcalf, 1977). The primary function of this 'respiratory burst' is to generate mechanisms, such as H_2O_2-myeloperoxidase-Cl^- with the capacity to kill ingested bacteria (Rosen and Klebanoff, 1979a). The importance of oxidative metabolism by these cells is underlined by the recurrent infections suffered by patients with chronic granulomatous disease who lack the cytochrome b_{245} (NADPH) oxidase (Segal *et al.*, 1983).

In pathological states, active oxygen species may contribute significantly to the inflammatory process, with large quantities being released extracellularly by stimulated neutrophils (Babior *et al.*, 1973; Root *et al.*, 1975; Rosen and Klebanoff, 1979b). Superoxide anion has been implicated in the generation of chemotactic factors in plasma (Petrone *et al.*, 1980). Hydrogen peroxide is directly toxic to various cell types, including endothelial cells (Weiss *et al.*, 1981), in addition to its involvement in more potent cytotoxic systems such as H_2O_2-myeloperoxidase-$C1^-$ (Rosen and Klebanoff, 1979a) and hydroxyl radical formation. Hydroxyl radicals may be generated from super-oxide anion and hydrogen peroxide in an iron-catalysed reaction (Halliwell, 1978). They are amongst the most reactive chemical species known, interacting directly with many biological polymers including DNA (Brawn and Fridovich, 1981) and membrane lipids (Mead, 1976). Reaction with the latter brings about lipid peroxidation with subsequent breakdown of the fatty acids, disruption of the membrane structure and tissue damage.

The activation of neutrophils to secrete oxidative products may be brought about by numerous stimuli (Cheson *et al.*, 1977). These include soluble as well as particulate factors, supporting the independence of the respiratory burst from phagocytosis (Goldstein *et al.*, 1975). In inflamed tissue, possible stimuli include immune complexes (Weiss and Ward, 1982), crystals (Schumacher, 1977), bacterial products (Bennett, 1978), chemotactic peptides (Goldstein *et al.*, 1975), and LTB_4 (Goetzl and Pickett, 1980). The biochemical steps involved in this activation are now under intensive investigation. Early events include changes in membrane potential (Korchak and Weissmann, 1978) and phospholipid metabolism (Hirata and Axelrod, 1980; Lapetina, 1982). The latter may generate calcium ionophore activity (Lapetina *et al.*, 1981) which could contribute to changes in the mobilization of calcium ions both across the cell membrane (Naccache *et al.*, 1977) and intracellularly (Takeshige *et al.*, 1980; Smolen *et al.*, 1981). These Ca^{2+} fluxes appear to be crucial for subsequent neutrophil activation (Smolen *et al.*, 1982). The effects of Ca^{2+} on neutrophil function are mediated by the regulatory protein calmodulin (Smolen *et al.*, 1981). Ca^{2+}–calmodulin complexes have been shown to enhance directly the activity of NADPH oxidase (Jones *et al.*, 1982). Other calcium ionophores, such as A23187 (Romeo *et al.*, 1975; Zabucchi *et al.*, 1975) and LTB_4 (Goetzl and Pickett, 1980) also trigger neutrophil activation. Thus, Ca^{2+} mobilization is currently thought to play a pivotal role in stimulus–secretion coupling in neutrophils.

The important role of lysosomal enzyme secretion from phagocytic cells, both polymorphonuclear and mononuclear, in the pathogenesis of inflammatory joint diseases such as RA, is well established (Hollander *et al.*, 1965). Evidence of oxidative damage to synovial tissue, however, is more difficult to obtain. Lunec *et al.* (1981) have measured increased levels of free radical-induced lipid breakdown products in rheumatoid synovial fluid compared with samples from osteoarthrotic patients. Free radical-mediated alterations in IgG structure have also been reported (Jasin, 1983; Wickens *et al.*, 1983), and similar changes have been observed in rheumatoid samples (Wickens and Dormandy, 1982). These may lead to the formation of IgG aggregates which could mimic immune complexes in triggering phagocytic cells. At present however, most of the evidence concerning oxidative damage in RA remains circumstantial, such as the depolymerization of hyaluronic acid by hydroxyl radicals *in vitro* (McCord, 1974). Enzymes that protect against active oxygen species (superoxide dismutase, catalase) are absent from rheumatoid synovial fluid (Blake *et al.*, 1981), and other extracellular scavengers of these molecules such as serum sulphydryl groups (Hall *et al.*, 1984) may be depressed. The joint tissues may therefore be highly susceptible to oxidative damage, although more direct evidence of this is urgently required.

Many studies have been carried out on neutrophil and monocyte function in RA. Generally, monocytes from these patients show normal phagocytic activity (Temple and Loewi, 1977; Bar–Eli *et al.*, 1980), but depressed function has been shown in patients with vasculitis (Hurst and Nuki, 1981). Rheumatoid neutrophils may also show depressed function *in vitro*, especially following incubation in synovial fluid (Mowat and Baum, 1971; Turner *et al.*, 1973). The latter effect appears to be related to ingestion of immune complexes. Oxidative metabolism of rheumatoid PMN as measured by superoxide anion production is normal (Minty *et al.*, 1983). It appears, therefore, that the excessive tissue damage associated with phagocytic cell activity in RA is not due to an aberrant function of these cells, but rather reflects the massive local generation of stimulating factors, presumed to be immune complexes and products of complement activation and arachidonic acid metabolism.

1.4 ANTI-INFLAMMATORY DRUGS

It seems appropriate at this stage, before venturing into the role of the immune system in chronic rheumatic diseases, to discuss the interactions of drugs with the inflammatory mechanisms outlined in the preceding sections. The anti-inflammatory agents in current use may be conveniently divided into non-steroidal anti-inflammatory drugs (NSAIDs) and steroids, and these will be considered separately.

1.4.1 Non-steroidal anti-inflammatory drugs (NSAIDs)

This group of compounds has its origins in ancient history as illustrated by the varied and often curious uses of salicylates (reviewed by Gross and Greenberg, 1948). Aspirin has been followed by indomethacin, phenylbutazone and, more recently, by a galaxy of 'me-too' drugs based on different organic acids (propionic acid, phenylacetic acid, etc.). When considering the mode of action of these compounds as anti-inflammatory drugs, the starting point must be Vane's hypothesis (Vane, 1971) that these drugs act by inhibiting the synthesis of prostaglandins. It is clear that all NSAIDs are active inhibitors of cyclo-oxygenase *in vitro*, although their potencies in this assay cover a very wide range (Crook *et al.*, 1976). These drugs exhibit analgesic, antipyretic, and anti-inflammatory actions, as well as toxic effects on the gastrointestinal tract.

Prostaglandins promote pain (Ferreira, 1972), fever (Feldberg *et al.*, 1972) and swelling (Wedmore and Williams, 1981), and they may have a protective effect on the gastric mucosa (Rainsford, 1982). However, this neat association is probably not the whole story. In certain conditions, prostaglandins have also been shown to be anti-inflammatory and immunosuppressive (Section 1.2.1), thus questioning the wisdom of totally blocking their synthesis in patients with rheumatic diseases. Moreover, while clinical experience suggests that, broadly speaking, the NSAIDs are equally effective in patients, their potencies as cyclo-oxygenase inhibitors vary widely (Crook *et al.*, 1976). Salicylate, which has little effect on prostaglandin synthesis, is clinically indistinguishable from aspirin. Also, cyclo-oxygenase activity in rheumatoid synovial tissue may be abolished in patients taking low doses of aspirin (600 mg/day) which do not exert detectable anti-inflammatory effects. NSAIDs retain their anti-inflammatory activity in rats rendered deficient in prostaglandin precursors by dietary manipulation (Bonta *et al.*, 1977). Thus it seems that, although NSAIDs undoubtedly inhibit prostaglandin synthesis, this may be an insufficient explanation of their anti-inflammatory effects.

This conclusion begs the question – what else do they do? Unfortunately, a clear-cut answer is not available at present, although many other effects of these drugs, particularly on neutrophil function, have been observed. Various members of the NSAID group inhibit lysosomal enzyme secretion (Robinson, 1978; Smith and Iden, 1980) and superoxide anion production (Simchowitz *et al.*, 1979; Smolen and Weissmann, 1980; Edelson *et al.*, 1982) by human PMN cells and guinea-pig macrophages (Oyanagui, 1978). However, many of these studies employed drug concentrations well above physiological levels. More recently, NSAIDs have been shown to be sensitive inhibitors of chemiluminescence generated by H_2O_2-myeloperoxidase-Cl^- (Pekoe *et al.*, 1982), the major cytotoxic system of neutrophils. Thus, it seems possible that part of the anti-inflammatory activity of these drugs is due to interference with the oxidative metabolism of neutrophils. In this regard, it is interesting to note that a specific free radical scavenger, superoxide dismutase, has anti-inflammatory effects in man (Huber and Menander-Huber, 1980) and that other antioxidants also suppress inflammation in experimental systems (Bragt *et al.*, 1980).

1.4.2 Corticosteroids

There is no doubt that steroidal drugs are extremely potent anti-inflammatory agents, although their clinical use is severely restricted by toxic side effects. Chemical modification of the endogenous hormone hydrocortisone has allowed the separation of glucocorticoid from mineralocorticoid actions, but the former have not been uncoupled from anti-inflammatory activity.

Corticosteroids have many effects that probably contribute to their overall anti-inflammatory action. These drugs suppress the synthesis and release of prostaglandins (Lewis and Piper, 1975) by inhibiting phospholipase A_2 and thus preventing the generation of arachidonic acid from membrane phospholipid. Inhibition of phospholipase A_2 is mediated by a protein, lipocortin, the synthesis of which is induced by glucocorticoids (Hirata *et al.*, 1980). This is one example of a general mechanism whereby steroids modulate cell function by first binding to cytoplasmic receptors which then migrate as a steroid–receptor complex into the cell nucleus and interact with the genetic material. This results in the synthesis of new RNA and protein molecules (Peterkofsky and Tomkins, 1968). Lipocortin synthesis has a number of anti-inflammatory consequences in addition to inhibiting prostaglandin synthesis. Suppression of phospholipase A_2 activity also prevents the formation of lipoxygenase products such as LTB_4 and interferes with the generation of PAF (Fig. 1.1). This 'blanket' effect on the production of inflammatory mediators may help to explain the potency of steroids compared with NSAIDs. Other actions include effects on phagocytic cells, especially monocytes. Steroid administration depresses monocyte bactericidal activity (Rinehart *et al.*, 1975) and induces a profound monocytopenia (Fauci *et al.*, 1976). In contrast, steroid effects on neutrophil function occur only at high concentrations (Klempner and Gallin, 1978) and *in vivo* administration results in neutrophilia (Fauci *et al.*, 1976) due partly to release of PMN cells from the bone marrow (Bishop *et al.*, 1968).

The effects of glucocorticoids on the migration of various leucocyte populations may explain much of these drugs' anti-inflammatory and immunosuppressive actions (Parrillo and Fauci, 1979). In addition to the monocytopenia mentioned above, bolus administration of hydrocortisone causes a marked lymphopenia with a selective loss of T cells (Fauci *et al.*, 1976). This redistribution of mononuclear cells will prevent accumulation of these cells in inflamed tissues and will thus exert a suppressive effect on the chronic inflammatory process. The mechanisms underlying this effect are complex, but may include inhibition of vasodilatation and vascular permeability changes (secondary to effects on PGE and LTB_4 synthesis?), inhibition of chemotaxis (LTB_4-related?), and decreased adherence of inflammatory cells to vascular endothelium (McGregor, 1977).

1.5   IMMUNOLOGICAL MECHANISMS

It is likely that the enormous increase in research activity on aetiological and pathogenic factors in the rheumatic diseases has been closely linked with parallel advances in the science of immunology. In particular, the various mechanisms involved in regulating immunoglobulin synthesis have been scrutinized in view of the classical observations of autoantibodies in patients with RA, SLE, and other connective tissue diseases. This section will concentrate on those cellular interactions required for antibody production. These mechanisms will be examined in those diseases where autoantibody synthesis is most apparent, namely RA and SLE.

1.5.1 Cellular interactions required for antibody production

The immune response to most, if not all, antigens requires the presentation of antigen in an immunogenic form to the responding lymphocytes. Several cell types (antigen-presenting cells, APC) have been found to possess this antigen-presenting function *in vitro*, including monocyte/macrophages (Hersh and Harris, 1968; Rosenberg and Lipsky, 1981), dendritic (veiled) cells (Steinman and Nussenzweig, 1980), Langerhans cells (Braathen and Thorsby, 1983), and endothelial cells (Ashida *et al.*, 1981). In each case, antigen is presented to reactive T lymphocytes in association with protein determinants derived from genes within the major histocompatibility complex (MHC) encoded within the I region in mice and HLA-D in man (Möller, 1978). In man, antigens might be presented in association with determinants derived from three distinct loci, HLA-DR (Bergholtz and Thorsby, 1978), HLA-DS (DQ) (Gonwa *et al.*, 1983) and HLA-DP, but more studies are needed to establish this.

Antigen processing and presentation is followed by interaction and binding of specific T lymphocytes (Powell *et al.*, 1980). This formation of T cell-monocyte (APC) clusters is mutually stimulatory for both cell types. The monocyte secretes various molecules, including interleukin-1 (IL-1) (Oppenheim *et al.*, 1982) which augment T cell activity. IL-1 represents either a single entity or more probably a family of closely related proteins with many biological effects (see below), one of which is the induction of interleukin-2 (IL-2) production by a subpopulation of T cells (Smith *et al.*, 1980). IL-2 is a potent stimulator of T cell proliferation (Smith, 1980; Watson *et al.*, 1980) and the generation of cytotoxic T lymphocytes (Gillis *et al.*, 1981). Recently, natural killing by NK cells has also been shown to be dependent on IL-2 (Domzig *et al.*, 1983). In the context of antibody production, this lymphokine promotes proliferation of antigen-stimulated helper T cells via interaction with an IL-2 receptor (Tac) expressed on these cells (Miyawaki *et al.*, 1982; Leonard *et al.*, 1982). This clonal expansion of helper T cells amplifies the generation of helper factors that promote B cell activation and antibody synthesis. These helper factors are a heterogeneous group of proteins which need further characterization (Tada and Hayakawa, 1980) although one, T-cell replacing factor (TRF), has been shown to be important in the induction of B cell differentiation (Schimpl and Wecker, 1972; Leibson *et al.*, 1981). B cell triggering requires two signals – one antigen-specific causing activation (antigen and/or specific T helper factors), the other non-antigen-specific promoting differentiation (TRF). A summary of this necessarily simplified scheme is illustrated in Fig. 1.4.

As stated above, the monokine IL-1 has important actions on several cell types in addition to lymphocytes (Oppenheim and Gery, 1982). Thus, IL-1 appears to be similar if not identical to endogenous pyrogen and to leucocytic endogenous mediator (Sztein *et al.*, 1981). The latter factor acts on hepatocytes to switch on synthesis of the acute phase proteins (Kampschmidt, 1978).

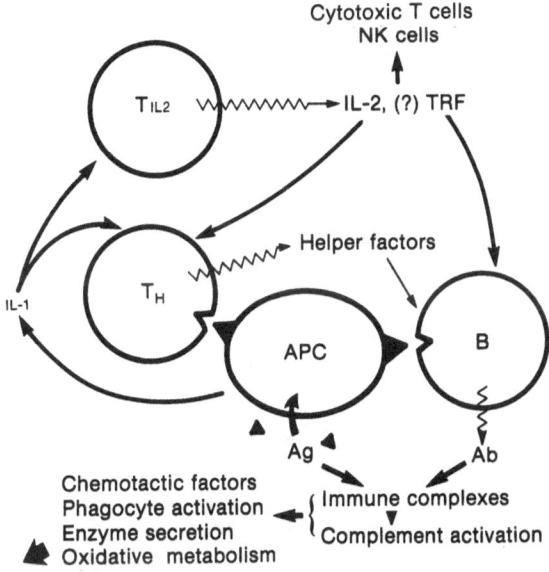

Cytotoxic T cells
NK cells

T_{IL2} ⟶ IL-2, (?) TRF

Helper factors

T_H

IL-1

APC

B

Ag   Ab

Chemotactic factors
Phagocyte activation
Enzyme secretion
Oxidative metabolism

Immune complexes
Complement activation

Tissue damage

Figure 1.4 Schematic illustration of cellular interactions involved in antibody production. The figure represents one possible sequence of events leading to antibody production. It is still uncertain whether the interaction of B cells with antigen requires antigen presenting cells or whether the B cells interact directly with helper T cells.

Several cell populations within connective tissue also respond to IL-1: synoviocytes are stimulated to secrete collagenase and prostaglandins (Mizel *et al.*, 1981), fibroblasts proliferate (Schmidt *et al.*, 1981), and chondrocytes are activated to degrade the cartilage matrix (Jasin and Dingle, 1981). Thus, IL-1 induces many cell functions that are relevant to the inflammatory process in general (fever, acute phase response) and to connective tissue in particular (synoviocyte, fibroblast, chondrocyte activation).

The cellular processes associated with antibody production are subject, in healthy individuals at least, to several control mechanisms which together limit the extent of immunoglobulin synthesis. These include suppressor T lymphocytes, immune complexes, the idiotypic network, and various mediators of inflammatory reactions. In man, suppressor T cells have been shown to inhibit both T cell proliferation (Shou *et al.*, 1976) and immunoglobulin synthesis by B cells (Moretta *et al.*, 1977; Gupta *et al.*, 1979). Specific antibody is able, after binding antigen, to switch off B cell activity via Fc-dependent mechanisms (Taylor, 1982). These may affect the B cell directly (Kölsch *et al.*, 1980) or interfere with T–B cell co-operation (Hoffman, 1980). The clonal expansion of antigen-specific T cells and the production of specific antibody will cause increases in the expression of certain idiotypes, and will therefore disturb the 'network' leading to suppression of the response (Roitt *et al.*, 1981). During inflammatory reactions, a number of mediators are generated which could influence the local immune response. Reference has already been made to the effects of arachidonic acid metabolites (PGE, LTB_4) on lymphocyte functions (Section 1.2.1). Other products of inflammatory cells, such as active oxygen species, can also modulate the immune response. These metabolites, especially hydrogen peroxide, can suppress lymphocyte activity (Hoffeld *et al.*, 1981; Nishida *et al.*, 1981) including suppressor cells (Zoschke *et al.*, 1982), but may, in other assay systems, be found necessary for lymphocyte activation (Novogrodsky *et al.*, 1982). Data like these serve to illustrate how very difficult it is to predict the overall effect of any particular putative modulator on the immune response in patients.

Before considering the involvement of the immune system in RA and SLE, it is appropriate to review briefly the surface markers that are often used to identify the functionally distinct lymphocytes described above. In particular, many studies have employed monoclonal antibodies (OKT, Leu) to detect specific subpopulations of T cells. The reagents OKT4/Leu 3a are reported to bind helper T cells, whereas OKT8/Leu 2a react with suppressor/cytotoxic cells (Reinherz and Schlossman, 1980). However, great care is required in the interpretation of data obtained with these reagents, especially when they are equated with specific cell functions. Recent results show that: (i) the OKT4[+] cell population includes suppressor cells in addition to helper cells (Thomas *et al.*, 1982), (ii) OKT4[+] cells also act as inducers of suppressor cells (Morimoto *et al.*, 1981, 1983), and (iii) functional T helper cells constitute only a minor subset within the OKT4[+] cell pool (Reinherz *et al.*, 1982). The OKT4[+] population of cells is clearly heterogeneous, and the expression of the marker cannot be equated with T helper cell function. A similar argument may be applied to the OKT8 marker, which is also detected on an apparently heterogeneous population of cells (Reinherz *et al.*, 1982).

T lymphocytes undergo distinct surface changes after activation, with the expression of HLA-DR antigens (Yu *et al.*, 1980) and receptors for IL-2 (Miyawaki *et al.*, 1982), transferrin (Haynes *et al.*, 1981; Goding and Burns, 1981), and hormones such as insulin (Helderman and Strom, 1978). Recently, it has been reported that HLA-DR and IL-2 receptor (Tac) show different kinetics of expression and are associated with different subpopulations of T cells after immunization with tetanus toxoid (Yachie *et al.*, 1983). Further work is needed to realise the full significance of these observations, but it suggests that the current association of HLA-DR antigen with general 'T cell activation' may be too simplistic.

1.5.2 Autoimmunity in the rheumatic diseases

Autoimmunity and autoimmune diseases may arise from a failure of the normal state of tolerance to self antigens. Self-tolerance is maintained by several mechanisms which vary for different antigens (Elson, 1980). Many self-reactive lymphocytes are deleted during development (clonal deletion), thus removing the possibility of autoantibody formation to certain antigens. However, low levels of autoantibodies and autoantigen-binding lymphocytes may be detected in the circulation of apparently normal individuals (Bankhurst and Williams, 1975; Elson *et al.*, 1979; Rodriguez *et al.*, 1982). It is generally thought that such self-reactive B cells do not generate significant levels of autoantibodies because suppressor T lymphocytes bring about a lack of T cell help.

The scheme shown in Fig. 1.5 suggests a number of ways whereby self-tolerance might be broken and autoimmunity might develop. The requirement for T helper cells could be met either by a failure of the suppressor system, or by helper factors generated in response to cross-reacting antigens (Cooke *et al.*, 1983). Alternatively, the B cells could be activated directly by a polyclonal stimulus such as Epstein–Barr virus (Depper and Zvaifler, 1981). These possibilities will be examined in relation to the known immunological disturbances in patients with RA and SLE.

Many studies (reviewed by Hall and Bacon, 1981) have shown a mild impairment of T cell functions in patients with RA. However, evidence is accumulating to indicate more dramatic disturbances of immunoregulation in the synovial tissue. Rheumatoid synovium has been referred to as an ectopic lymphoid organ with large numbers of lymphocytes and plasma cells (Zvaifler, 1973) generating immunoglobulin (Smiley *et al.*, 1968), including rheumatoid

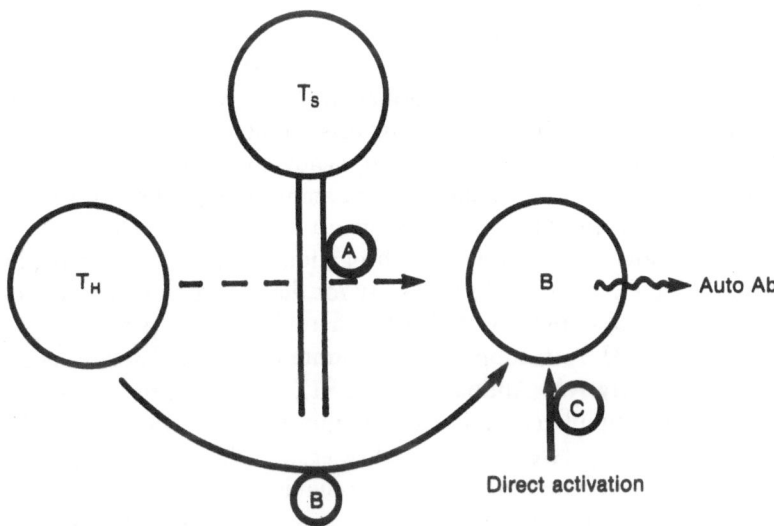

Figure 1.5 Possible mechanisms associated with autoantibody production. A – Failure of suppressor T cell function, leading to helper T cells triggering B lymphocytes. B – Circumvention of suppressor T cells – the provision of T cell help by, for example, a cross-reacting antigen. C – Direct activation of B lymphocytes by a polyclonal stimulus, for example, EB virus.

factors (Munthe and Natvig, 1972). The importance of lymphoid cells in the pathogenesis of RA is underlined by the rapid clinical improvement that results from removal of circulating lymphocytes by thoracic duct drainage (Paulus *et al.*, 1977). This technique also emphasizes the fact that the inflammatory reaction in the synovium is not self-perpetuating, but requires constant replenishment by circulating cells. Substantial evidence points to the activated state of lymphocytes in rheumatoid joints. Synovial fluid samples from these patients contain lymphokine (Stastny *et al.*, 1975) and IL-2-like activity (Wilkins *et al.*, 1983). Activated T lymphocytes have been identified both in synovial fluid (Galili *et al.*, 1981) and tissue (Burmester *et al.*, 1981), where they may arise after binding with HLA-DR positive macrophage-like (dendritic) cells (Poulter *et al.*, 1982). Surface marker studies of lymphocytes clustered around such cells in rheumatoid synovium show a preponderance of 'helper' phenotype cells and a lack of 'suppressor' cells (Duke *et al.*, 1982; Klareskog *et al.*, 1982). This has led to a hypothesis of RA as a disease of T lymphocyte/macrophage immunoregulation (Janossy *et al.*, 1981).

More important than the surface marker analysis of synovial lymphocytes is the finding of a lack of functional suppressor cells in this population (Chattopadhyay *et al.*, 1979a,b). Similar observations have been made in the peripheral blood of early RA patients (Abdou *et al.*, 1981), but normal suppressor cell activity has been assayed in patients with established disease (Dobloug *et al.*, 1981; Patel *et al.*, 1982). Rheumatoid blood mononuclear cells do, however, show some altered functions, notably depressed immunoglobulin production in response to pokeweed mitogen (Poikonen *et al.*, 1982). This may reflect abnormal T helper cell activity (Bellamy *et al.*, 1983) or defective monocyte accessory cell function (Plater-Zyberk *et al.*, 1983; McKeown *et al.*, 1984).

The general conclusion from these reports is that there is a localized defect in immunoregulation in the rheumatoid synovium. The reason for this is unknown, but a number of different mechanisms have been postulated: (i) lymphocytotoxic antibodies directed against regulatory T cells might be synthesized in synovial tissue and cause abrogation of suppressor activity. Such an antibody, reacting with T cells necessary for the induction of suppressor cells, has been identified in JRA (Juvenile Rheumatoid Arthritis) patients (Morimoto *et al.*, 1981, 1983). Anti-suppressor cell antibodies have also been detected in patients with early RA (Abdou *et al.*, 1981), (ii) some product of oxidative metabolism by stimulated phagocytes within the joint could cause the local inactivation of suppressor cells (Zoschke *et al.*, 1982). One might speculate that any, or a combination, of these mechanisms could allow B cell hyperactivity in the synovium and the subsequent production of autoantibodies, especially rheumatoid factors (Johnson, 1981). The self-association of IgG rheumatoid factors to form immune complexes (Pope *et al.*, 1974) could provide a major inflammatory stimulus within rheumatoid joints (Male and Roitt, 1981).

An alternative view of the mechanisms involved in autoantibody production in RA involves a role for the Epstein–Barr virus (EBV). This virus infects B lymphocytes, leading to the induction of immunoglobulin synthesis and the generation of immortalized cell lines (reviewed by Depper and Zvaifler, 1981). EBV stimulates rheumatoid factor production by both RA and healthy lymphocytes (Slaughter *et al.*, 1978). It has been shown that lymphoblastoid cell lines may be established more readily from rheumatoid than from healthy cells after EBV infection (Slaughter *et al.*, 1978; Bardwick *et al.*, 1980). The reason for this appears to be a defect in the suppressor T cells regulating EBV infection in RA (Depper *et al.*, 1981). This defect may explain the raised titres of EBV-associated antibodies in rheumatoid sera (Ferrell *et al.*, 1981), but may not be specific for RA, as similar findings have been reported in active multiple sclerosis (Fraser *et al.*, 1979). Any involvement of EBV in the pathogenesis of RA must remain speculative (Depper and Zvaifler, 1981), particularly when the polyclonal nature of this stimulus is compared with the restricted spectrum of autoantibodies, largely antiglobulins, detected in RA patients.

SLE is an autoimmune disease with evidence of a more generalized failure in immunoregulation. Many reports reveal a suppressor cell defect associated with disease activity (Sakane *et al.*, 1979, 1980). This loss of functional suppressor cells may be related to the actions of lymphocytotoxic antibodies. These antibodies show some selectivity for T cells bearing Fc_γ receptors (T_γ cells) (Okudaira *et al.*, 1979), a lymphocyte population associated with suppressor cell activity (Moretta *et al.*, 1977). Indeed, abrogation of suppressor cell activity has been shown after incubation of lymphocytes with sera from SLE patients plus complement (Koike *et al.*, 1979; Okudaira *et al.*, 1981). However, other autoantibodies may also contribute to the altered immunoregulation observed in SLE, notably by interfering with the recognition of Ia (HLA-DR) determinants (Okudaira *et al.*, 1982). In view of the important role of these determinants in antigen presentation (Section 1.5.1), such autoantibodies are likely to have dramatic effects on the immune response. This is reflected in the defective function of SLE lymphocytes in an autologous mixed lymphocyte reaction (Okudaira *et al.*, 1982; Smith and De Horatius, 1982).

Autoantibodies have also been implicated in the disordered immunoregulation observed in patients with other rheumatic diseases, notably mixed connective tissue disease. These patients display various autoantibodies against soluble nuclear antigens (Alarcon-Segovia, 1983). It has been suggested that one such antibody, anti-nRNP, can penetrate T_γ lymphocytes and abolish their suppressor cell function (Alarcon-Segovia and Ruiz-Arguelles, 1980). This property of the antibody depends on its Fc portion and might have pathogenic implications in other disease states (Alarcon-Segovia, 1981), although further studies are needed to verify this.

1.6 SECOND-LINE ANTIRHEUMATIC AGENTS

This group of drugs suffers a multitude of names such as slow-acting, long-acting, remission-inducing, disease-modifying, and penicillamine-like – in addition to that used in the section heading. The first two are safe enough, referring only to the kinetics of the clinical response in RA, but the next two alternatives are much more contentious, relying heavily on clinical interpretation rather than hard data. Perhaps the least satisfactory adjective is 'penicillamine-like' since we are unable to give a clear description of what penicillamine itself is like. In view of this, I have chosen the term 'second-line antirheumatic' to indicate the use of these compounds to supplement the first-line NSAID in active RA. The term also emphasizes that their beneficial effects are largely restricted to rheumatic disease (notably RA), as opposed to third-line drugs (to be discussed later) which are widely used in cancer chemotherapy. Most of the drugs in this category do not have anti-inflammatory activity as detected in the standard screening tests. Current thoughts on their modes of action revolve around modulation of the immune response, but it is highly likely that each compound in this group has a different mechanism whereby it exerts its antirheumatic effect. The agents to be considered under this heading include gold compounds (sodium aurothiomalate and auranofin), penicillamine, chloroquine (and hydroxychloroquine), levamisole, and sulphasalazine. Other groups of drugs with immunomodulating properties such as steroids and cytotoxic agents have been or are discussed in other sections.

1.6.1   Gold compounds

Gold compounds have been shown to possess several properties that might contribute to their overall effect on the rheumatoid disease process. However, many studies have been carried out *in vitro* using raised drug concentrations and may merely reflect heavy metal toxicity. Aurothiomalate has been shown to inhibit several lysosomal enzymes, including acid hydrolases released from macrophages (Persellin and Ziff, 1966) and the neutral protease elastase from PMN cells (Janoff, 1970). These enzymes may be inhibited intracellularly *in vivo*, as elemental gold is concentrated in the reticuloendothelial system (Gottlieb *et al.*, 1972) and may be readily detected within phagocytic cells in rheumatoid synovial tissue (Vernon-Roberts *et al.*, 1976; Nakamura and Igarashi, 1977). These observations on the distribution of gold *in vivo* may be responsible for several effects of these agents on phagocyte function. Both PMN cells (Mowat, 1978) and monocytes (Ho *et al.*, 1978) respond less well to chemotactic stimuli after treatment with aurothiomalate. This compound also suppresses phagocytic activity in rheumatoid patients (Jessop *et al.*, 1973). Auranofin inhibits chemotactic responses (Scheinberg *et al.*, 1981) and phagocytosis and oxidative metabolism by PMN (Davis *et al.*, 1982). Monocyte cytotoxicity is also inhibited by this drug (Russell *et al.*, 1982).

Effects of gold compounds on the immune system have been investigated in several assay systems. Aurothiomalate has been shown to inhibit complement activation *in vitro*, both by blocking C1 activity (Schultz *et al.*, 1974) and by preventing the formation of C3 convertase by the alternative pathway (Burge *et al.*, 1978). Both these effects are mediated by the gold component of the drug. The actions of gold compounds on mononuclear cell function are more complex. *In vitro*, it is clear that gold suppresses lymphocyte proliferation to antigens and mitogens (Lipsky and Ziff, 1977; Lies *et al.*, 1977). This effect is apparently caused by inhibiting monocyte accessory function in the culture system (Lipsky and Ziff, 1977, 1982). These observations *in vitro* contrast with studies carried out *ex vivo*, where a good clinical response to aurothiomalate is accompanied by a change in lymphocyte responsiveness from a depressed state to normal (Davis *et al.*, 1979; Highton *et al.*, 1981). This discrepancy may be due to cell traffic effects *in vivo*, where the inhibited monocytes may be localized in the synovium. Subsequent suppression of disease activity would permit the appearance of unaffected bone marrow-derived monocytes in the peripheral blood and hence a normalization of (blood) mononuclear cell function.

1.6.2 Penicillamine

Penicillamine was first used in the treatment of RA after the observation that it dissociated IgM-rheumatoid factor by reducing the disulphide bonds holding the molecule together (Ritzmann *et al.*, 1960). Although not now considered relevant to effects of penicillamine *in vivo*, this effect illustrates one important aspect of this drug's interactions with body tissues, namely sulphydryl–disulphide exchange. Another feature of penicillamine is its ability to chelate metal ions, including copper (Lyle, 1979). These observations explain the use of this drug in treating cystinuria and Wilson's disease, but their significance for the actions of penicillamine in RA remains obscure.

Interactions of the drug with sulphydryl groups and with copper have been shown to occur in rheumatoid patients. Penicillamine enhances serum sulphydryl–disulphide interchange reactions (Hall and Gillan, 1979) and dissociates IgA–alpha$_1$ antitrypsin complexes *in vivo* (Wollheim *et al.*, 1979). *In vitro*, the drug inhibits the sulphydryl-dependent heat denaturation of IgG (Gerber, 1978) and might therefore prevent the formation of autoantigenic IgG aggregates *in vivo*. A similar effect could also be achieved by a different mechanism, i. e. the scavenging of free radicals associated with the formation of aggregated IgG (Wickens *et al.*, 1983). Copper–penicillamine complexes have been shown to express superoxide dismutase-like activity, although at relatively high concentrations (Greenwald, 1981), and penicillamine and other thiols have recently been found to be potent inhibitors of myeloperoxidase activity (Matheson, 1982). This latter property could contribute to protecting tissue from oxidative damage (Rosen and Klebanoff, 1979a).

Studies of penicillamine effects on cell function have sometimes given conflicting results, usually because of drug concentration effects. Thus, penicillamine has been shown to inhibit chemotaxis by PMN cells *in vitro*, but only at non-physiological levels (Chwalinska-Sadowska and Baum, 1976). Phago-cytosis and lysosomal enzyme release by these cells were not affected, and other authors (Mowat, 1978) have failed to show an effect even on neutrophil chemotaxis. Lymphocyte responses to mitogens may be enhanced by 'low' doses of penicillamine and suppressed by higher doses (Room *et al.*, 1979). However, even this 'low' dose *in vitro* (10 ug ml^{-1}) is relatively high when compared with plasma levels observed in RA patients, especially when protein-binding is taken into account (unpublished observations). A clear-cut action of penicillamine at lower concentrations *in vitro* is the copper-catalysed inhibi-tion of T helper cell activity (Lipsky and Ziff, 1980). This could lead to diminished antibody and autoantibody (rheumatoid factor) levels in RA patients after penicillamine treatment. Such changes have been observed (Zuckner *et al.*, 1970; Pritchard and Nuki, 1978), and some patients become IgA-deficient (Stanworth and Hunneyball, 1979). However, the fall in serum rheumatoid factor levels may be slow or even non-existent (Bacon *et al.*, 1981) and convincing inhibition of T helper cell activity by penicillamine *in vivo* is still awaited. Evidence of sulphydryl group involvement in mononuclear cell function has recently been obtained in my own laboratory. It has been shown that monocyte accessory function is dependent on cell surface sulphydryl groups (McKeown *et al.*, 1984). Rheumatoid monocytes are defective in this assay, but normal cell function is regained either by treating the cells *in vitro* with 2-mercaptoethanol or by treating the patients with penicillamine. Similar effects of penicillamine on macrophage function have been observed in rats by Arrigoni-Martelli and co-workers (Binderup *et al.*, 1980a,b). These studies emphasize the importance of the sulphydryl moiety of the drug for its immuno-modulating effects, actions that may be shared by other sulphydryl-reactive compounds (Jaffe, 1980).

1.6.3 Chloroquine

Chloroquine and hydroxychloroquine are now being rehabilitated as second-line antirheumatic agents as it is generally conceded that with regular and careful ophthalmological examinations the risks of retinopathy are not as great as were previously thought. The established view on the mode of action of these compounds in RA has rested largely on their lysosomotropic properties (de Duve *et al.*, 1974). This effect probably provides adequate localized drug concentrations to inhibit some of the lysosomal enzymes *in situ*, and therefore contribute to an anti-inflammatory action. Inhibition of neutral protease by chloroquine has been reported (Perper and Oronsky, 1974), although release of the enzyme from stimulated neutrophils was not impaired. Generally, the effects of chloroquine *in vitro* have not, until recently, provided even a half-adequate explanation for its antirheumatic action. This gloomy picture may have changed, however, with the observation that low concentrations of chloroquine (10^{-6}M) cause a dramatic inhibition of interleukin-1 production by human monocytes (Scala and Oppenheim, 1983). In view of the important functions attributed to IL-1, both as an immunomodulator and as a mediator of cell activation in inflammatory responses (Oppenheim and Gery, 1982), this property of chloroquine could provide a full explanation of its effects in RA. Studies of IL-1 secretion in patients treated with the drug are now essential to confirm the initial *in vitro* observations.

1.6.4   Levamisole

Levamisole, an antihelminthic compound, has been shown to possess second-line antirheumatic actions in double-blind studies (Multicentre Study Group, 1978; Symoens and Schuermans, 1979) but its clinical use has waned in view of its unpredictable serious toxicity (Symoens *et al.*, 1979). The drug has a number of *in vitro* and *in vivo* effects on mononuclear cell function that have led to its being called 'immunorestorative' and 'thymomimetic' (Symoens and Rosenthal, 1977). *In vitro*, brief exposure of cells to high concentrations of levamisole stimulates monocyte functions (Schmidt and Douglas, 1976; Pike *et al.*, 1977), while lower concentrations increase the number of detectable E rosette-forming (T) lymphocytes (Verhaegen *et al.*, 1977a). Levamisole also enhances lymphocyte proliferation, an effect mediated by changes in cyclic GMP levels within the cells (Hadden *et al.*, 1975). Similar effects were obtained *in vitro* using imidazole, and one would speculate therefore that this action of levamisole involves the imidazole ring of its structure. Imidazole, however, unlike levamisole, failed to elicit these responses *in vivo* (Renoux, 1978). Levamisole is extensively metabolized *in vivo*, a major product being OMPI, a sulphydryl-containing derivative (De Brabander *et al.*, 1978). It is tempting to suggest, therefore, that this metabolite might have similar effects on mononuclear cells to those of penicillamine (Section 1.6.2). Effects of levamisole administration *in vivo* include increasing E rosette-forming cells in patients with various diseases (Verhaegen *et al.*, 1977b), generation of suppressor T cell activity (Moriya *et al.*, 1979), and enhancing neutrophil motility (Anderson *et al.*, 1979). The last two reports document effects of giving a single dose of levamisole (150 mg) to healthy volunteers. The possibility that levamisole might induce suppressor cell activity is intriguing, as it could explain both the stimulation of T cell proliferation (Scheinberg *et al.*, 1978) and the fall in serum immunoglobulins and rheumatoid factor levels associated with levamisole treatment (Multicentre Study Group, 1978). In summary, levamisole treatment is associated with enhancement of T cell, monocyte, and neutrophil functions. These effects are only apparent in individuals in whom initial cell function is depressed. The drug may be active *in vivo* after metabolism to the thiol, OMPI, and may therefore share certain actions with penicillamine.

1.6.5 Sulphasalazine

Sulphasalazine is another antirheumatic agent, once discarded, that is enjoying a revival. This has come about as the result of recent clinical studies comparing the drug with penicillamine (Neumann *et al.*, 1983) and with placebo and sodium aurothiomalate (Pullar *et al.*, 1983). Sulphasalazine therapy is associated with a fall in serum levels of acute phase proteins (Neumann *et al.*, 1983). As these are synthesized in the liver in response to a factor closely related or identical to IL-1 (Section 1.5.1), this may reflect an action of the drug on macrophages, the source of IL-1. However, it is equally possible that the drug is suppressing the chronic inflammatory process by some other mechanism, with the fall in acute phase proteins being a secondary phenomenon. There is plenty of scope for future studies with this compound!

1.7   THIRD-LINE (CYTOTOXIC) AGENTS

A small number of drugs, widely used in cancer chemotherapy, have been employed as 'last ditch' treatments for intractable rheumatoid disease. These compounds include the alkylating agents cyclophosphamide and chlorambucil, the purine analogue azathioprine, and the folate antagonist methotrexate. All these drugs have some degree of selective toxicity against dividing cells (Bertino, 1973). This is the basis for their use in RA (Hurd, 1973), in that they are intended to act on activated lymphocytes thereby suppressing immune responsiveness and associated disease activity. Unfortunately, activated lymphocytes are not the only rapidly dividing cells in rheumatoid patients, and use of cytotoxic drugs may lead to severe toxic effects on the gastrointestinal tract, gonads, and bone marrow cells.

Both cyclophosphamide and chlorambucil are activated in the liver, generating a highly reactive ethyleneimonium ion which binds avidly to guanine bases in DNA. This can lead to mismatching of base-pairs during DNA synthesis, loss of the guanine from the sugar-phosphate backbone, and covalent cross-linking between the DNA strands of the double helix – thus preventing their separation during DNA synthesis (Calabresi and Parks, 1970). Drug-treated cells are therefore unable to replicate their genetic material, and so die.

Azathioprine also acts as a pro-drug, being converted first into 6-mercaptopurine and later into the nucleotide 6-thioinosinic acid (Bertino, 1973). The latter metabolite mediates the cytotoxic effects of azathioprine by exerting pseudo-feedback inhibition of *de novo* purine synthesis and by blocking production of both adenine and guanine nucleotides. The dividing cell is thus starved of DNA precursors, and so replication ceases. Methotrexate is also an 'antimetabolite' drug, but acts on folate metabolism rather than directly on purine or pyrimidine bases. The drug is a potent inhibitor of dihydrofolate reductase, and so prevents formation of tetrahydrofolic acid (Bertino, 1973).

This co-factor is essential for several one-carbon transfer reactions involved in the synthesis of both thymidylate and purines; so the overall effect of the drug is again to deplete the dividing cells of DNA precursors.

As stated earlier, these drugs are used to treat severe RA because of their immunosuppressive properties. Cyclophosphamide appears to act preferentially on B lymphocytes (Poulter and Turk, 1972), causing marked loss of antibody-producing cells (Uyeki, 1967). However, this drug also affects T cell responses, being able to suppress delayed hypersensitivity responses when given after sensitization, but enhancing the response if administered beforehand (Mitsuoka *et al.*, 1976). The latter effect represents a toxic action on suppressor T cells or their precursors (Mitsuoka *et al.*, 1976; Sy *et al.*, 1977), a reaction that may also be demonstrated *in vitro* (Kaufmann *et al.*, 1980). In contrast to cyclophosphamide, azathioprine has little effect on antibody production, but causes dramatic suppression of T cell responses (Bach, 1976). Rheumatoid patients treated with cyclophosphamide show falls in serum immunoglobulin and rheumatoid factor levels and depressed delayed hypersensitivity to dinitrochlorobenzene (Townes *et al.*, 1976). However, primary antibody responses to *E. coli* Vi antigen were not affected by the drug. Similar results have been obtained by other workers (Alepa *et al.*, 1970). Taken together, these data indicate that the antirheumatic action of cyclophosphamide is not due to direct suppression of B lymphocyte function, but that the observed fall in circulating rheumatoid factor titres is probably a secondary phenomenon.

Thus, it is difficult to prove that immunosuppression explains the value of cyclophosphamide and azathioprine in the treatment of RA. However, this still seems to be the likeliest explanation in view of the known antirheumatic effects of physical means of suppressing lymphocyte function such as thoracic duct drainage (Paulus *et al.*, 1977), lymphapheresis (Wallace *et al.*, 1979) and total lymphoid irradiation (Kotzin *et al.*, 1981).

1.8 HETERODOX TREATMENTS

When considered in the light of the preceding section, heterodox treatments for inflammatory joint diseases may well take on a certain wholesome charm. However, evidence from properly conducted trials to support claims of clinical efficacy is often minimal or absent, and therefore it should not be too surprising to discover that studies of the pharmacology of such treatments are extremely rare. In view of this, this section will refer only to a small selection of the numerous regimens available.

Acupuncture has been used in China for several thousand years to induce relief from pain. The efficacy of such treatment has been confirmed in the West (Gaw *et al.*, 1975; Godfrey and Morgan, 1978), although no difference was found in these studies between needling along appropriate meridians or at random 'placebo' sites. There is growing interest in the mechanisms underlying the analgesic effects of acupuncture (Anon, 1981) particularly with the recent discovery of endogenous peptides, the enkephalins and endorphins, with analgesic properties. Naloxone, a drug that blocks the binding of morphine and opioid peptides to specific receptors, antagonizes the analgesic effects of acupuncture (Mayer et al., 1977). In addition, levels of β-endorphin and met-enkephalin rise in cerebrospinal fluid following low and high frequency electropuncture respectively (Clement-Jones et al., 1979, 1980). It is therefore interesting to speculate that acupuncture works by stimulating the release of endogenous opioid peptides which bind to specific receptors within the brain and thus induce pain relief. β-endorphin may be released in response to stress, thereby perhaps explaining the lack of site specificity in the response to needling mentioned above. Clearly, acupuncture has genuine effects which deserve further study.

A number of chemical and biological preparations are also available for treating arthritic patients, often at considerable cost. This latter observation may be relevant to the subjective assessment of the efficacy of these agents since most people would want to believe that spending their own money was doing them good. In one area at least – homoeopathy, the cost of raw materials should not be a problem as any possible active principle in the original extract is diluted beyond detectable limits before administration. This practice does not lend itself to scientific study, especially by pharmacologists, and no reports of laboratory-based research on homoeopathy have been published.

Copper bracelets are worn by many rheumatoid patients and probably cause some small absorption of copper through the skin. Copper salts may have anti-inflammatory actions, particularly in association with NSAIDs (Sorensen, 1976) or with D-penicillamine (Lipsky and Ziff, 1980). Copper is also essential for the oxidase activity of caeruloplasmin and may therefore contribute to antioxidant mechanisms in inflammatory conditions (Al-Timimi and Dormandy, 1977). However, the relevance of material absorbed from copper bracelets to these reactions is unknown, but probably minimal.

Bee venom extracts have been shown to possess anti-inflammatory activity in the rat model of adjuvant arthritis (Billingham et al., 1973; Zurier et al., 1973; Eiseman et al., 1982). The mechanism underlying this effect may be no more than counter-irritation, but has been shown in one study to involve release of corticosteroids (Zurier et al., 1973). In contrast, the activity of bee venom in an acute model of inflammation (carrageenan-induced rat paw oedema) was retained in adrenalectomized animals and could be purified as a small basic peptide (Billingham et al., 1973). More recently, administration of bee venom to rats has been shown to be accompanied by changes in hepatic microsomal enzymes that are often associated with immunomodulatory therapy (Eiseman et al., 1982), thus providing another possible explanation for its activity. Despite these interesting results, however, problems of dosage and route of administration ensure that the world bee population is in no immediate danger of extinction. The same may also be said of the New Zealand green-lipped mussel, extracts of which have attracted some attention in the press as a miracle drug for the treatment of arthritis. Sceptics might say that the most riveting aspect of this preparation is its odour of rotting fish. The mussel extract had no effect on adjuvant arthritis in rats (Cullen *et al.*, 1975) unless given intraperitoneally (Miller and Ormrod, 1980). Further studies suggest that the active principle is proteinaceous (Couch *et al.*, 1982). If the latter results are correct, it is very difficult to understand how this extract can exert anti-arthritic effects following oral administration. Such effects have been claimed in several anecdotal cases and in one larger group (Gibson *et al.*, 1980) although another study has failed to show improvement over placebo (Huskisson *et al.*, 1981).

1.9 PRESENT PROBLEMS AND FUTURE POSSIBILITIES

The time required for any new drug to progress from chemical synthesis to the general clinic is at least ten years. The beginning of this journey requires the existence of a relevant screening programme in the pharmacology laboratory to identify active compounds. Ideally, relevant screening assays are set up as a result of understanding some of the pathogenic mechanisms at work in the patient. Virtually all our present knowledge of the pathogenesis of inflammatory joint diseases has been accumulated in the last 25 years, with much being concentrated in the past decade. It follows from this, therefore, that the currently available anti-inflammatory drugs were developed before this information was available, using rather crude screening procedures such as carrageenan-induced oedema in rat paws (DiRosa *et al.*, 1971). The second-line antirheumatic drugs were not identified by screening at all, but rather were introduced into clinical studies as a result of serendipity, or at best incorrect reasoning. The development of suitable test systems to evaluate novel compounds is clearly vital since the screening assay is the major factor in defining the type of drug to be identified. Thus, carrageenan oedema is virtually guaranteed to detect cyclo-oxygenase inhibitors as anti-inflammatory drugs because of the important role of prostaglandins in this model. The major problem facing the pharmaceutical industry in this area is the lack of a suitable animal model that accurately mimics the pathogenesis of RA. Such a system would greatly facilitate the search for new antirheumatic agents, particularly of the second-line, immunomodulatory class. Current animal models of arthritis are inadequate in this regard, being unable to differentiate these drugs from anti-inflammatory compounds. The most extensively used test system is adjuvant arthritis induced in rats by intradermal injection of Freund's complete adjuvant (Pearson, 1956). This model is exacerbated (Arrigoni-Martelli, 1979) or unaffected by penicillamine (Liyanage and Currey, 1972), is exacerbated by levamisole (Dieppe *et al.*, 1976) and is unaffected by chloroquine (Newbould,

1963). Sodium aurothiomalate has been shown to suppress adjuvant arthritis when given prophylactically, but to be much less effective when used therapeutically (Sofia and Douglas, 1973). In contrast to the above, NSAIDs and steroids are able to suppress both primary and secondary lesions of adjuvant arthritis (Newbould, 1963). These drug effects are clearly the 'wrong way round' from the clinical rheumatologist's point of view and reflect the inadequacy of adjuvant arthritis as a model of RA. A broadly similar pattern of drug responses has also been noted in the antigen-induced model of synovitis in rabbits (Dumonde and Glynn, 1962). In a major study using 339 animals, Blackham and Radziwonik (1977) showed that steroids, most NSAIDs, cyclophosphamide and chloroquine suppressed the disease, whereas levamisole and penicillamine were inactive. The last drug has, however, been shown to exert an antiarthritic action in this model when administered for very long periods of time (Hunneyball et al., 1979). Recently, a different model of arthritis associated with autoimmunity to type II collagen has been described in rats (Trentham et al., 1977). A recent review by Trentham (1982) examines the similarities and differences between this model and rheumatoid arthritis. As with the other experimental arthritides, steroids, NSAIDs and cyclophosphamide suppress disease activity (Sloboda et al., 1981; Stuart et al., 1981). However, penicillamine also shows activity in this model (Sloboda et al., 1981) but gold (McCune et al., 1980; Sloboda et al., 1981) and levamisole (Stuart et al., 1981) do not. One further experimental model of RA is worthy of note. This is the spontaneously arising arthritis of the inbred mouse strain MRL/l. These mice exhibit erosions of articular cartilage, synovial proliferation, pannus formation and the generation of IgM and IgG antiglobulins (Dixon et al., 1980). Studies of antirheumatic drugs in this test system will be most interesting and might help to validate it as a model of RA.

In the light of current knowledge of inflammatory and immunological processes, several avenues suggest themselves for investigation of novel antirheumatic compounds. Production of inflammatory mediators such as LTB_4 and PAF is one possible target for pharmacological intervention. Indeed a NSAID, benoxaprofen, has been reported to inhibit human lipoxygenase activity (Harvey et al., 1983) but the drug was withdrawn from clinical use before long-term studies could be completed. A more general approach to anti-inflammatory therapy might be to inhibit phospholipase A_2 thereby blocking the synthesis of all cyclo-oxygenase and lipoxygenase products and also PAF. Steroids are known to have this effect, but an NSAID with similar action on the enzyme but without steroid-type toxicity would surely be a valuable compound. New drugs aimed at phagocytic cells in the inflammatory response could prevent activation of these cells or might interfere with tissue-damaging mechanisms generated by them. The former might be effected by blocking calcium fluxes across the cell membrane using specific channel-blocking drugs (Braunwald, 1982). Derivatives of the compounds presently available might show selectivity for inflammatory cell membranes. Lymphocytes also require calcium influx for activation (Whitney and Sutherland, 1973) and calcium channel antagonists might therefore be immunosuppressive. Recent thoughts on mechanisms of tissue damage in chronic inflammatory diseases have implicated active oxygen species in this process. The most toxic radical secreted by phagocytes is OH·, which is formed from superoxide anion and hydrogen peroxide in an iron-catalysed reaction. Removal of the catalytic iron should prevent OH· formation and so protect surrounding tissue. This hypothesis has led to the investigation of a specific iron-chelating drug, desferrioxamine in various animal models of inflammation (Blake *et al.*, 1983). This drug exhibited anti-inflammatory activity both in rats and in guinea pigs thus supporting the concept that oxidative metabolism of neutrophils and monocytes is an appropriate target for anti-inflammatory drugs.

The possible development of immunomodulatory compounds for the treatment of RA is particularly speculative. The major problem is in deciding first, whether the immune system *is* defective in this disease and secondly, how. Present evidence suggests a local (synovial) loss of immunoregulation that leads to excessive helper T cell–monocyte interaction. Drugs might therefore be sought either to enhance suppressor mechanisms or to inhibit T cell–monocyte clustering. Other possible sites of antirheumatic action include suppression of interleukin-1 and interleukin-2 production, or antagonism of the effects of these mediators on their respective target cells. Some evidence for the latter has been obtained with cyclosporin A, a potent immunosuppressive agent (Klaus, 1981), which may prevent the acquisition of receptors for IL-2 on lymphocytes following mitogenic stimulation (Larsson, 1980). Clinical and immunological studies of cyclosporin A in the treatment of RA are currently in progress. The difficulty with all putative immunomodulatory compounds, both present and future, is the limiting of their effects to the aberrant immune response in the synovial membrane. A more general suppression of immunity might render the patients susceptible to opportunistic infections and possibly malignancies, as illustrated by the Acquired Immune Deficiency Syndrome (AIDS). In view of this, biological manipulation of specific immune reactions, e. g. by idiotypic reagents, might represent a potentially less hazardous future for immunoregulatory therapy.

1.10 REFERENCES

Abdou, N. I., Lindsley, H. B., Racela, L. S., Pascual, E. and Hassanein, K. M. (1981) Suppressor T cell dysfunction and anti-suppressor cell antibody in active early RA. *J. Rheumatol.* 8, 9–18.

Alarcon-Segovia, D. (1981) Penetration of antinuclear antibodies into immunoregulatory T cells: pathogenetic role in the connective tissue diseases. *Clinics in Immunology and Allergy*, 1, 117–26.

Alarcon-Segovia, D. (1983) Antibodies to nuclear and other intracellular antigens in the connective tissue diseases. *Clinics in Rheumatic Diseases*, 9, 161–75.

Alarcon-Segovia, D. and Ruiz-Arguelles, A. (1980) Suppressor cell loss and dysfunction in mixed connective tissue disease. *Arthr. Rheum.*, **23**, 314–18.

Alepa, F. P., Zvaifler, N. J. and Sliwinski, A. J. (1970) Immunologic effects of cyclophosphamide treatment in rheumatoid arthritis. *Arthr. Rheum.* **13**, 754–60.

Al-Timimi, D. J. and Dormandy, T. L. (1977) The inhibition of lipid autoxidation by human caeruloplasmin. *Biochem. J.*, **168**, 283–8.

Anderson, R., Oosthuizen, R., Theron, A. and Van Rensburg, A. J. (1979) The *in vitro* evaluation of certain neutrophil and lymphocyte functions following the ingestion of 150 mg oral dose of levamisole: assessment of the extent and duration of stimulation of neutrophil chemotaxis, protein iodination and lymphocyte transformation. *Clin. Exp. Immunol.* **35**, 478–83.

Anon (1981) How does acupuncture work? *Br. Med. J.*, **283**, 746–8.

Arrigoni-Martelli, E. (1979) Penicillamine in experimental models of immunologically mediated inflammation. *Agents and Actions (Suppl.)*, **5**, 73–83.

Ashida, E. R., Johnson, A. R. and Lipsky, P. E. (1981) Human endothelial cell-lymphocyte interaction. Endothelial cells function as accessory cells necessary for mitogen-induced human T lymphocyte activation *in vitro. J. Clin. Invest.*, **67**, 1490–9.

Babior, B. M. (1978) Oxygen-dependent microbial killing by phagocytes. *N. Engl. J. Med.*, **298**, 659–68.

Babior, B. M., Kipnes, R. S. and Curnutte, J. T. (1973) Biological defence mechanisms: the production by leucocytes of superoxide, a potential bactericidal agent. *J. Clin. Invest.*, **52**, 741–4.

Babior, G. L., Rosin, R. E., McMurrich, B. J., Peters, W. A. and Babior, B. M. (1981) Arrangement of the respiratory burst oxidase in the plasma membrane of the neutrophil. *J. Clin. Invest.*, **67**, 1724–8.

Bach, J. F. (1976) The pharmacological and immunological basis for the use of immunosuppressive drugs. *Drugs*, **11**, 1–13.

Bacon, P. A., Blake, D. R., Alexander, G. J. M. and Hall, N. D. (1981) Alterations in immunological parameters associated with D-penicillamine therapy. In *Modulation of Autoimmunity and Disease: the Penicillamine Experience* (eds R. N. Maini and H. Berry), Praeger, Eastbourne, pp.10–15.

Badwey, J. A. and Karnovsky, M. L. (1980) Active oxygen species and the functions of phagocytic leucocytes. *Ann. Rev. Biochem.*, **49**, 695–726.

Baggiolini, M. (1982) Proteinases and acid hydrolases of neutrophils and macrophages and the mechanisms of their release. *Adv. Inflammation Res.*, **3**, 313–27.

Ball, J. (1971) Enthesopathy of rheumatoid and ankylosing spondylitis. *Ann. Rheum. Dis.*, **30**, 213–23.

Bankhurst, A. D. and Williams, R. C.Jr. (1975) Identification of DNA-binding lymphocytes in patients with systemic lupus erythematosus. *J. Clin. Invest.*, **56**, 1378–85.

Bardwick, P. A., Bluestein, H. G., Zvaifler, N. J., Depper, J. M. and Seegmiller, J. E. (1980) Altered regulation of Epstein–Barr virus-induced lymphocyte proliferation in rheumatoid arthritis lymphoid cells. *Arthr. Rheum.*, **23**, 626–32.

Bar-Eli, M., Ehrenfeld, M., Litvin, Y. and Gallily, R. (1980) Monocyte function in rheumatoid arthritis. *Scand. J. Rheumatol.*, **9**, 17–23.

Bellamy, N., Cairns, E. and Bell, D. A. (1983) Immunoregulation in rheumatoid arthritis: evaluation of T lymphocyte function in the control of polyclonal immunoglobulin synthesis *in vitro. J. Rheumatol.*, **10**, 19–27.

Bennett, J. C. (1978) The infectious etiology of rheumatoid arthritis. *Arthr. Rheum.*, **21**, 531–8.

Bergholtz, B. O. and Thorsby, E. (1978) HLA-D restriction of the macrophage-dependent response of immune human T lymphocytes to PPD *in vitro*: inhibition by anti-HLA-Dr antisera. *Scand. J. Immunol.*, **8**, 63–73.

Bertino, J. R. (1973) Chemical action and pharmacology of methotrexate, azathioprine and cyclophosphamide in man. *Arthr. Rheum.*, 16, 79–83.

Billingham, M. E. J., Morley, J., Hanson, J. M., Shipolini, R. A. and Vernon, C. A. (1973) An anti-inflammatory peptide from bee venom. *Nature*, 245, 163–4.

Binderup, L., Bramm, E. and Arrigoni-Martelli, E. (1980a) D-Penicillamine *in vivo* enhances lymphocyte DNA synthesis: role of macrophages. *Scand. J. Immunol.*, 11, 23–8.

Binderup, L., Bramm, E. and Arrigoni-Martelli, E. (1980b) Immunological effects of D-penicillamine during experimentally induced inflammation in rats. *Scand. J. Immunol.*, 12, 239–47.

Bishop, C. R., Athens, J. W., Boggs, D. R., Warner, H. R., Cartwright, G. E. and Wintrobe, M. M. (1968) Leucokinetic studies XIII A non-steady-state kinetic evaluation of the mechanism of cortisone-induced granulocytosis. *J. Clin. Invest.*, 47, 249–60.

Blackham, A. and Radziwonik, H. (1977) The effect of drugs in established rabbit monoarticular arthritis. *Agents and Actions*, 7, 473–80.

Blake, D. R., Hall, N. D., Bacon P. A., Dieppe, P. A., Halliwell, B. and Gutteridge, J. M. C. (1983) Effect of a specific iron chelating agent on animal models of inflammation. *Ann. Rheum. Dis.*, 42, 89–93.

Blake, D. R., Hall, N. D., Treby, D. A., Halliwell, B. and Gutteridge, J. M. C. (1981) Protection against superoxide and hydrogen peroxide in synovial fluid from rheumatoid patients. *Clin. Sci. Mol. Med.*, 61, 483–6.

Bonta, I. L., Bult, H., Vincent, J. E. and Zijlstra, F. J. (1977) Acute anti-inflammatory effects of aspirin and dexamethasone in rats deprived of endogenous prostaglandin precursors. *J. Pharm. Pharmacol.*, 29, 1–7.

Braathen, L. R. and Thorsby, E. (1983) Human epidermal Langerhans cells are more potent than blood monocytes in inducing some antigen-specific T-cell responses. *Br. J. Dermatol.*, 108, 139–46.

Bragt, P. C., Bansberg, J. I. and Bonta, I. L. (1980) Anti-inflammatory effects of free radical scavengers and antioxidants: further support for pro-inflammatory roles of endogenous hydrogen peroxide and lipid peroxides. *Inflammation*, 4, 289–99.

Braunwald, E. (1982) Mechanism of action of calcium-channel-blocking agents. *N. Engl. J. Med.*, 307, 1618–27.

Brawn, K. and Fridovich, I. (1981) DNA strand scission by enzymically generated oxygen radicals. *Arch. Biochem. Biophys.*, 206, 414–19.

Bray, M. A. (1980) Prostaglandins: fine tuning of the immune system? *Immunol. Today*, 1, 65–9.

Bray, M. A., Ford-Hutchinson, A. W. and Smith M. J. H. (1981) Leucotriene B$_4$: an inflammatory mediator *in vivo*. *Prostaglandins*, 22, 213–22.

Brewerton, D. A., Caffrey, M., Hart, F. D., James, D. C. O., Nicholls, A. and Sturrock, R. D. (1973) Ankylosing spondylitis and HLA 27. *Lancet*, i, 904–7.

Burge, J. J., Fearon, D. T. and Austen, K. F. (1978) Inhibition of the alternative pathway of complement by gold sodium thiomalate *in vitro*. *J. Immunol.*, 120, 1625–30.

Burmester, G. R., Yu, D. T. Y., Irani, A-M., Kunkel, H. G. and Winchester, R. J. (1981) Ia$^+$ T cells in synovial fluid and tissues of patients with rheumatoid arthritis. *Arthr. Rheum.*, 24, 1370–6.

Calabresi, P. and Parks, R. E.Jr. (1970) Alkylating agents, antimetabolites, hormones and other antiproliferative agents. in *The Pharmacological Basis of Therapeutics*, (eds. L. S. Goodman and A. Gilman), 4th edn., MacMillan, London, pp. 1348–95.

Chattopadhyay, C., Chattopadhyay, H., Natvig, J. B. and Mellbye, O. J. (1979a) Lack of suppressor cell activity in rheumatoid synovial lymphocytes. *Scand. J. Immunol.*, 10, 479–86.

Chattopadhyay, C., Chattopadhyay, H., Natvig, J. B., Michaelsen, T. E. and Mellbye, O. J. (1979b) Rheumatoid synovial lymphocytes lack concanavalin-A-activated suppressor cell activity. *Scand. J. Immunol.*, 10, 309–16.

Cheson, B. D., Curnutte, J. T. and Babior, B. M. (1977) The oxidative killing mechanisms of the neutrophil. *Prog. Clin. Immunol.*, 3, 1–65.

Chilton, F. H., O'Flaherty, J. T., Walsh, C. E., Thomas, M. J., Wykle, R. L., DeChatelet, L. R. and Waite, B. M. (1982) Platelet activating factor (PAF): stimulation of the lipoxygenase pathway in polymorphonuclear leucocytes (PMNL) by 1-0-alkyl-2-0-acetyl-sn-glycero-3-phosphocholine (AAGPC). *Fed. Proc.*, 41 667 (abs 2322).

Chwalinska-Sadowska, H. and Baum, J. (1976) The effect of D-penicillamine on polymorphonuclear leucocyte function. *J. Clin. Invest.*, 58, 871–9.

Clement-Jones, V., Lowry, P. J., McLoughlin, L., Besser, G. M., Rees, L. H. and Wen, H. L. (1979) Acupuncture in heroin addicts: changes in met-enkephalin and β-endorphin in blood and cerebrospinal fluid. *Lancet*, ii, 380–3.

Clement-Jones, V., Tomlin, S., Rees, L. H., McLoughlin, L., Besser, G. M. and Wen, H. L. (1980) Increased β-endorphin but not met-enkephalin levels in human cerebrospinal fluid after acupuncture for recurrent pain. *Lancet*, ii, 946–9.

Cooke, A., Lydyard, P. M. and Roitt, I. M. (1983) Mechanisms of autoimmunity: a role for cross-reactive idiotypes. *Immunol. Today*, 4, 170–5.

Couch, R. A. F., Ormrod, D. J., Miller, T. E. and Watkins, W. B. (1982) Anti-inflammatory activity in fractionated extracts of the green-lipped mussel. *N. Z. Med. J.*, 95, 803–6.

Crook, D., Collins, A. J., Bacon, P. A. and Chan, R. (1976) Prostaglandin synthetase activity from human rheumatoid synovial microsomes. *Ann. Rheum. Dis.*, 35, 327–32.

Crunkhorn, P. and Willis, A. L. (1971) Cutaneous reactions to intradermal prostaglandins. *Br. J. Pharmacol.*, 41, 49–56.

Cullen, J. C., Flint, M. H. and Leider, J. (1975) The effect of dried mussel extract on an induced polyarthritis in rats. *N. Z. Med. J.*, 81, 260–1.

Davis, P., Miller, C. L. and Russell, A. S. (1982) Effects of gold compounds on the function of phagocytic cells. I. Suppression of phagocytosis and the generation of chemiluminescence by polymorphonuclear leucocytes. *J. Rheumatol.* (Suppl. 8), 9, 18–24.

Davis, P., Percy, J. S. and Russell, A. S. (1979) *In vivo* and *in vitro* effects of gold salts on lymphocyte transformation responses and antibody-dependent cell-mediated cytotoxicity. *J. Rheumatol.*, 6, 527–33.

De Brabander, M., Aerts, F., Geuens, G., Van Ginchel, R., Van de Veire, R. and Van Belle, H. (1978) Levamisole, sulphydryls and microtubules: possible clues to the mechanism of its immunomodulatory activity. *Chem. Biol. Interactions*, 23, 45–63.

De Duve, C., de Garsy, T., Poole, B., Trouet, A., Tulkens, P. and van Hoof, F. (1974) Lysosomotropic agents. *Biochem. Pharmacol.*, 23, 2495–531.

Demopoulos, C. A., Pinckard, R. N. and Hanahan, D. J. (1979) Platelet-activating factor: evidence for 1-0-alkyl-2-acetyl-sn-glyceryl-3-phosphorylcholine as the active component (a new class of lipid chemical mediators). *J. Biol. Chem.*, 254, 9355–8.

Depper, J. M., Bluestein, H. G. and Zvaifler, N. J. (1981) Impaired regulation of Epstein–Barr virus-induced lymphocyte proliferation in rheumatoid arthritis is due to a T cell defect. *J. Immunol.*, 127, 1899–902.

Depper, J. M. and Zvaifler, N. J. (1981) Epstein–Barr virus: its relationship to the pathogenesis of rheumatoid arthritis. *Arthr. Rheum.*, 24, 755–61.

Dieppe, P. A., Willoughby, D. A., Stevens, C., Kirby, J. D. and Huskisson, E. C. (1976) 'Specific therapy' in new and conventional animal models. *Rheumatol. Rehabil.*, 15, 201–6.

Dinant, H. J., Hissink Muller, W., Van den Berg-Loonen, E. M., Nijenhuis, L. E. and Englefriet, C. P. (1980) HLA-DRw4 in Felty's syndrome. *Arthr. Rheum.*, 23, 1336.

DiRosa, M., Giroud, J. P. and Willoughby, D. A. (1971) Studies on the mediators of the acute inflammatory response induced in rats in different sites by carrageenan and turpentine. *J. Pathol. Bacteriol.*, 104, 15–29.

Dixon, F. J., Theofilopoulos, A. N., Izui, S. and McConahey, P. J. (1980) Murine SLE – aetiology and pathogenesis. in *Immunology 80: Progress in Immunology IV* (eds M. Fougereau and J. Dausset), Academic Press, London, pp. 959–95.

Dobloug, J. H., Chattopadhyay, C., Førre, Ø., Høyeraal, H. M. and Natvig, J. B. (1981) Con-A induced suppressor cell activity and T-lymphocyte subpopulations in peripheral blood lymphocytes of patients with rheumatoid arthritis and juvenile rheumatoid arthritis. *Scand. J. Immunol.*, 13, 367–73.

Domzig, W., Stadler, B. M. and Herberman, R. B. (1983) Interleukin 2 dependence of human natural killer (NK) cell activity. *J. Immunol.*, 130, 1970–3.

Duke, O., Panayi, G. S., Janossy, G. and Poulter, L. W. (1982) An immunohistological analysis of lymphocyte subpopulations and their microenvironment in the synovial membranes of patients with rheumatoid arthritis using monoclonal antibodies. *Clin. Exp. Immunol.*, 49, 22–30.

Dumonde, D. C. and Glynn, L. E. (1962) The production of arthritis in rabbits by an immunological reaction to fibrin. *Br. J. Exp. Pathol.*, 43, 373–83.

Edelson, H. S., Kaplan, H. B., Korchak, H. M., Smolen, J. E. and Weissmann, G. (1982) Dissociation by piroxicam of degranulation and superoxide anion generation from decrements in chlortetracycline fluorescence of activated human neutrophils. *Bioch. Biophys. Res. Commun.*, 104, 247–53.

Eiseman, J. L., Von Bredow, J. and Alvares, A. P. (1982) Effect of honeybee (*Apis mellifera*) venom on the course of adjuvant-induced arthritis and depression of drug metabolism in the rat. *Biochem. Pharmacol.*, 31, 1139–46.

Elson, C. J. (1980) Autoimmunity and the diverse pathways to B-cell unresponsiveness. *Immunol. Today*, 1, 42–5.

Elson, C. J., Naysmith, J. D. and Taylor, R. B. (1979) B cell tolerance and autoimmunity. *Int. Rev. Exp. Pathol.*, 19, 137–203.

Fauci, A. S., Dale, D. C. and Balow, J. E. (1976) Glucocorticosteroid therapy: mechanisms of action and clinical considerations. *Ann. Intern. Med.*, 84, 304–15.

Feldberg, W., Gupta, K. P., Milton, A. S. and Wendtland, S. (1972) Effect of bacterial pyrogen and antipyretics on prostaglandin activity in cerebrospinal fluid of unanaesthetised cats. *Br. J. Pharmacol.*, 46, 550P–1P.

Fernandez, H. N., Henson, P. M., Otani, A. and Hugli, T. E. (1978) Chemotactic response to human C3a and C5a anaphylatoxins. I. Evaluation of C3a and C5a leucotaxis *in vitro* and under simulated *in vivo* conditions. *J. Immunol.*, 120, 109–15.

Ferreira, S. H. (1972) Prostaglandins, aspirin-like drugs and analgesia. *Nature (New Biol.)*, 240, 200–3.

Ferreira, S. H., Nakamura, M. and Abreu Castro, M. S. (1978) The hyperalgesic effects of prostacyclin and PGE_2. *Prostaglandins*, 16, 31–37.

Ferrell, P. B., Aitcheson, C. T., Pearson, G. R. and Tan, E. M. (1981) Seroepidemiological study of relationships between Epstein–Barr virus and rheumatoid arthritis. *J. Clin. Invest.*, 67, 681–7.

Fischer, A., Durandy, A. and Griscelli, C. (1981) Role of prostaglandin E_2 in the induction of nonspecific T lymphocyte suppressor activity. *J. Immunol.*, **126**, 1452–5.

Fisher, R. I. and Bostick-Bruton, F. (1982) Depressed T cell proliferative responses in Hodgkin's disease: role of monocyte-mediated suppression via prostaglandins and hydrogen peroxide. *J. Immunol.*, **129**, 1770–4.

Ford-Hutchinson, A. W., Bray, M. A., Doig, M. V., Shipley, M. E. and Smith, M. J. H. (1980) Leucotriene B, a powerful chemokinetic and aggregating substance released from polymorphonuclear leucocytes. *Nature (London)*, **286**, 264–5.

Fraser, K. B., Millar, J. H. D., Haire, N. and McCrea, S. (1979) Increased tendency to spontaneous *in vitro* lymphocyte transformation in clinically active multiple sclerosis. *Lancet*, ii, 715–17.

Gabig, T. G., Schervish, E. W. and Santinga, J. T. (1982) Functional relationship of the cytochrome b to the superoxide-generating oxidase of human neutrophils. *J. Biol. Chem.*, **257**, 4114–19.

Galili, U., Rosenthal, L. and Klein, E. (1981) Activated T cells in the synovial fluid of arthritic patients. II *In vitro* activation of the autologous blood lymphocytes. *J. Immunol.*, **127**, 430–2.

Gaw, A. C., Chang, L. W. and Shaw, L-C. (1975) Efficacy of acupuncture on osteoarthritic pain. A controlled, double-blind study. *N. Engl. J. Med.*, **293**, 375–8.

Gerber, D. A. (1978) Inhibition of the denaturation of human gamma globulin by a mixture of D-penicillamine disulphide and copper. *Biochem. Pharmacol.*, **27**, 469–72.

Gibson, R. G., Gibson, S. L. M., Conway, V. and Chappell, D. (1980) *Perna canaliculus* in the treatment of arthritis. *Practitioner*, **224**, 955–60.

Gillis, S., Gillis, A. E. and Henney, C. S. (1981) Monoclonal antibody directed against interleukin 2. I Inhibition of T lymphocyte mitogenesis and the *in vitro* differentiation of alloreactive cytolytic T cells. *J. Exp. Med.*, **154**, 983–8.

Glass, D., Raum, D., Gibson, D., Stillman, J. S. and Schur, P. (1976) Inherited deficiency of the second component of complement. Rheumatic disease associations. *J. Clin. Invest.*, **58**, 853–61.

Godfrey, C. M. and Morgan, P. (1978) A controlled trial of the theory of acupuncture in musculoskeletal pain. *J. Rheumatol.*, **5**, 121–4.

Goding, J. W. and Burns, G. F. (1981) Monoclonal antibody OKT-9 recognises the receptor for transferrin on human acute lymphocytic leukemia cells. *J. Immunol.*, **127**, 1256–8.

Goetzl, E. J. and Pickett, W. C. (1980) The human PMN leucocyte chemotactic activity of complex hydroxy-eicosatetraenoic acids (HETEs). *J. Immunol.*, **125**, 1789–91.

Goldstein, I. M., Roos, D., Kaplan, H. B. and Weissmann, G. (1975) Complement and immunoglobulins stimulate superoxide production by human leucocytes independently of phagocytosis. *J. Clin. Invest.*, **56**, 1155–63.

Gonwa, T. A., Picker, L. J., Raff, H. V., Goyert, S. M., Silver, J. and Stobo, J. D. (1983) Antigen-presenting capabilities of human monocytes correlates with their expression of HLA-DS, an Ia determinant distinct from HLA-DR. *J. Immunol.*, **130**, 706–11.

Goodwin, J. S., Bankhurst, A. D. and Messner, R. P. (1977) Suppression of human T cell mitogenesis by prostaglandin. *J. Exp. Med.*, **146**, 1719–34.

Gottlieb, N. L., Smith, P. M. and Smith, E. M. (1972) Tissue gold concentration in a rheumatoid arthritic receiving chrysotherapy. *Arthr. Rheum.*, **15**, 16–22.

Greenwald, R. A. (1981) Effects of oxygen-derived free radicals on connective tissue macromolecules: inhibition by copper–penicillamine complex. *J. Rheumatol.* (suppl. 7), **8**, 9–13.

Gross, M. and Greenberg, L. A. (1948) *The Salicylates: A Critical Bibliographic Review*, Hillhouse Press, New Haven.

Gupta, S., Schwartz, S. A. and Good, R. A. (1979) Subpopulations of human T lymphocytes. VII Cellular basis of concanavalin A-induced T cell-mediated suppression of immunoglobulin production by B lymphocytes from normal humans. *Cell. Immunol.*, 44, 242–51.

Hadden, J. W., Coffey, R. G., Hadden, E. M., Lopez-Corrales, E. and Sunshine, G. H. (1975) Effects of levamisole and imidazole on lymphocyte proliferation and cyclic nucleotide levels. *Cell. Immunol.*, 20, 98–103.

Hadler, N. M. (1976) A pathogenetic model for erosive synovitis – lessons from animal arthritides. *Arthr. Rheum.*, 19, 256–66.

Hall, N. D. and Bacon, P. A. (1981) Lymphocyte subpopulations and their role in the rheumatic diseases. In *Immunological Aspects of Rheumatology* (ed. W. C. Dick), MTP Press, Lancaster, pp. 1–27.

Hall, N. D. and Gillan, A. H. (1979) Effects of antirheumatic drugs on protein sulphydryl reactivity of human serum. *J. Pharm. Pharmacol.*, 31, 676–80.

Hall, N. D., Maslen, C. L. and Blake, D. R. (1984) The oxidation of serum sulphydryl groups by hydrogen peroxide secreted by stimulated phagocytic cells in rheumatoid arthritis. *Rheumatol. Int.*, 4(1), 35–8.

Halliwell, B. (1978) Superoxide-dependent formation of hydroxyl radicals in the presence of iron chelates. *Fed. Eur. Biochem. Soc. Lett.*, 92, 321–6.

Hammarström, S. (1983) Leucotrienes. *Ann. Rev. Biochem.*, 52, 355–77.

Harvey, J., Parish, H., Ho, P. P. K., Boot, J. R. and Dawson, W. (1983) The preferential inhibition of 5-lipoxygenase product formation by benoxaprofen. *J. Pharm. Pharmacol.*, 35, 44–5.

Haynes, B. F., Hemler, M., Cotner, T., Mann, D. L., Eisenbarth, G. S., Strominger, J. L. and Fauci, A. S. (1981) Characterisation of a monoclonal antibody (5E 9) that defines a human cell surface antigen of cell activation. *J. Immunol.*, 127, 347–51.

Helderman, J. H. and Strom, T. B. (1978) Specific insulin binding site on T and B lymphocytes as a marker of cell activation. *Nature (London)*, 274, 62–3.

Henson, P. M. (1971) The immunologic release of constituents from neutrophil leucocytes. I. The role of antibody and complement on nonphagocytosable surfaces or phagocytosable particles. *J. Immunol.*, 107, 1535–46.

Hersh, E. M. and Harris, J. E. (1968) Macrophage–lymphocyte interaction in the antigen-induced blastogenic response of human peripheral blood leucocytes. *J. Immunol.*, 100, 1184–94.

Highton, J., Panayi, G. S., Shepherd, P., Griffin, J. and Gibson, T. (1981) Changes in immune function in patients with rheumatoid arthritis following treatment with sodium aurothiomalate. *Ann. Rheum. Dis.*, 40, 254–62.

Hirata, F. and Axelrod, J. (1980) Phospholipid methylation and biological signal transmission. *Science*, 209, 1082–90.

Hirata, F., Schiffmann, E., Venkatasubramanian, K., Salomon, D. and Axelrod, J. (1980) A phospholipase A_2 inhibitory protein in rabbit neutrophils induced by glucocorticoids. *Proc. Nat. Acad. Sci., USA*, 77, 2533–6.

Ho, P. P. K., Young, A. L. and Southard, G. L. (1978) Methyl ester of N-formylmethionyl-leucyl-phenylalanine: chemotactic responses of human blood monocytes and inhibition of gold compounds. *Arthr. Rheum.*, 21, 133–6.

Hoffeld, J. T., Metzger, Z. and Oppenheim, J. J. (1981) Oxygen-derived metabolites as suppressors of immune responses *in vitro*. *Lymphokines*, 2, 63–86.

Hoffman, M. K. (1980) Antibody regulates the co-operation of B cells with helper cells. *Immunol. Rev.*, 49, 79–91.

Hollander, J. L., McCarty, D. J.Jr, Astorga, G. and Castro-Murillo, E. (1965) Studies on the pathogenesis of rheumatoid joint inflammation. I The 'RA cell' and a working hypothesis. *Ann. Intern. Med.*, **62**, 271–80.

Huber, W. and Menander-Huber, K. B. (1980) Orgotein. *Clinics Rheum. Dis.*, **6**, 465–98.

Hunneyball, I. M., Stewart, G. A. and Stanworth, D. R. (1979) Effect of oral D-penicillamine treatment on experimental arthritis and associated immune responses in rabbits. III. Reduction of the monoarticular arthritis. *Ann. Rheum. Dis.*, **38**, 271–8.

Hurd, E. R. (1973) Immunosuppressive and anti-inflammatory properties of cyclophosphamide, azathioprine and methotrexate. *Arthr. Rheum.*, **16**, 84–8.

Hurst, N. P. and Nuki, G. (1981) Evidence for defect of complement-mediated phagocytosis by monocytes from patients with rheumatoid arthritis and cutaneous vasculitis. *Br. Med. J.*, **282**, 2081–3.

Huskisson, E. C., Scott, J. and Bryans, R. (1981) Seatone is ineffective in rheumatoid arthritis. *Br. Med. J.*, **282**, 1358–9.

Izui, S., Lambert, P-H. and Miescher, P. A. (1976) *In vitro* demonstration of a particular affinity of glomerular basement membrane and collagen for DNA. *J. Exp. Med.*, **144**, 428–43.

Jaffe, I. A. (1980) Thiol compounds with penicillamine-like activity and possible mode of action in rheumatoid arthritis. *Clinics Rheum. Dis.*, **6**, 633–45.

Janoff, A. (1970) Inhibition of human granulocyte elastase by gold sodium thiomalate. *Biochem. Pharmacol.*, **19**, 626–8.

Janossy, G., Panayi, G., Duke, O., Bofill, M., Poulter, L. W. and Goldstein, G. (1981) Rheumatoid arthritis: a disease of T lymphocyte/macrophage immunoregulation. *Lancet*, **ii**, 839–42.

Jasin, H. E. (1975) Mechanism of trapping of immune complexes in joint collagenous tissues. *Clin. Exp. Immunol.*, **22**, 473–85.

Jasin, H. E. (1983) Generation of IgG aggregates by the myeloperoxidase-hydrogen peroxide system. *J. Immunol.*, **130**, 1918–23.

Jasin, H. E. and Dingle, J. T. (1981) Human mononuclear cell factors mediate cartilage matrix degradation through chondrocyte activation. *J. Clin. Invest.*, **68**, 571–81.

Jessop, J. D., Vernon-Roberts, B. and Harris, J. (1973) Effects of gold salts and prednisolone on inflammatory cells. I Phagocytic activity of macrophages and polymorphs in inflammatory exudates studied by a 'skin-window' technique in rheumatoid and control patients. *Ann. Rheum. Dis.*, **32**, 294–300.

Johnson, P. M. (1981) Molecular nature and cross-reactions of rheumatoid factor. *Clinics Immunol. Allergy*, **1**, 103–15.

Jones, H. P., Ghai, G., Petrone, W. F. and McCord, J. M. (1982) Calmodulin-dependent stimulation of the NADPH oxidase of human neutrophils. *Biochim. Biophys. Acta*, **714**, 152–6.

Jones, V. E., Jacoby, R. K., Johnson, P. M., Phua, K. K. and Welsh, K. I. (1983) Association of HLA-DR4 with definite rheumatoid arthritis but not with susceptibility to arthritis. *Ann. Rheum. Dis.*, **42**, 223.

Kampschmidt, R. F. (1978) Leucocytic endogenous mediator. *J. Reticuloendothelial Soc.*, **23**, 287–97.

Kaufmann, S. H. E., Hahn, H. and Diamantstein, T. (1980) Relative susceptibilities of T cell subsets involved in delayed-type hypersensitivity to sheep red blood cells to the *in vitro* action of 4-hydroperoxycyclophosphamide. *J. Immunol.*, **125**, 1104–8.

Klareskog, L., Forsum, U., Scheynius, A., Kabelitz, D. and Wigzell, H. (1982) Evidence in support of a self-perpetuating HLA-DR-dependent delayed-type cell reaction in rheumatoid arthritis. *Proc. Nat. Acad. Sci., USA*, **79**, 3632–6.

Klaus, G. G. B. (1981) The effects of cyclosporin A on the immune system. *Immunol. Today*, **2**, 83–7.

Klempner, M. S. and Gallin, J. I. (1978) Inhibition of neutrophil Fc receptor function by corticosteroids. *Clin. Exp. Immunol.*, **34**, 137–42.

Klickstein, L. B., Shapleigh, C. and Goetzl, E. J. (1980) Lipoxygenation of arachidonic acid as a source of polymorphonuclear leucocyte chemotactic factors in synovial fluid and tissue in rheumatoid arthritis and spondyloarthritis. *J. Clin. Invest.*, **66**, 1166–70.

Koike, T., Kobayashi, S., Yoshiki, T., Itoh, T. and Shirai, T. (1979) Differential sensitivity of functional subsets of T cells to the cytotoxicity of natural T lymphocytotoxic auto-antibody of systemic lupus erythematosus. *Arthr. Rheum.*, **22**, 123–9.

Kölsch, E., Oberbarnscheidt, J., Bruner, K. and Heuer, J. (1980) The Fc receptor: its role in the transmission of differentiation signals. *Immunol. Rev.*, **49**, 61–78.

Korchak, H. M. and Weissmann, G. (1978) Changes in membrane potential of human granulocytes antecede the metabolic responses to surface stimulation. *Proc. Nat. Acad. Sci., USA*, **75**, 3818–22.

Kotzin, B. L., Strober, S., Engleman, E. G., Calin, A., Hoppe, R. T., Kansas, G. S., Terrell, C. P. and Kaplan, H. S. (1981) Treatment of intractable rheumatoid arthritis with total lymphoid irradiation. *N. Engl. J. Med.*, **305**, 969–76.

Kunkel, S. L., Ogawa, H., Conran, P. B., Ward, P. A. and Zurier, R. B. (1981) Suppression of acute and chronic inflammation by orally administered prostaglandins. *Arthr. Rheum.*, **24**, 1151–8.

Kushner, I. and Somerville, J. (1971) Permeability of human synovial membrane to plasma proteins. Relationship to molecular size and inflammation. *Arthr. Rheum.*, **14**, 560–70.

Lapetina, E. G. (1982) Regulation of arachidonic acid production: role of phospholipases C and A_2. *Trends Pharmacol. Sci.*, **3**, 115–18.

Lapetina, E. G., Billah, M. M. and Cuatrecasas, P. (1981) The phosphatidylinositol cycle and the regulation of arachidonic acid production. *Nature (London)*, **292**, 367–9.

Larsson, E-L. (1980) Cyclosporin A and dexamethasone suppress T cell responses by selectively acting at distinct sites of the triggering process. *J. Immunol.*, **124**, 2828–33.

Leibson, H. J., Marrack, P. and Kappler, J. W. (1981) B cell helper factors. I. Requirement for both interleukin 2 and another 40,000 mol wt factor. *J. Exp. Med.*, **154**, 1681–93.

Leonard, W. J., Depper, J. M., Uchiyama, T., Smith, K. A., Waldmann, T. A. and Greene, W. C. (1982) A monoclonal antibody that appears to recognise the receptor for human T cell growth factor; partial characterisation of the receptor. *Nature (London)*, **300**, 267–9.

Lewis, G. P. and Piper, P. J. (1975) Inhibition of release of prostaglandins as an explanation of some of the actions of anti-inflammatory corticosteroids. *Nature (London)*, **254**, 308–11.

Lies, R. B., Cardin, C. and Paulus, H. E. (1977) Inhibition by gold of human lymphocyte stimulation. An *in vitro* study. *Ann. Rheum. Dis.*, **36**, 216–8.

Lipsky, P. E. and Ziff, M. (1977) Inhibition of antigen- and mitogen-induced human lymphocyte proliferation by gold compounds. *J. Clin. Invest.*, **59**, 455–66.

Lipsky, P. E. and Ziff, M. (1980) Inhibition of human helper T cell function *in vitro* by D-penicillamine and $CuSO_4$. *J. Clin. Invest.*, **65**, 1069–76.

Lipsky, P. E. and Ziff, M. (1982) The mechanisms of action of gold and D-penicillamine in rheumatoid arthritis. *Adv. Inflammation Res.*, **3**, 219–35.

Liyanage, S. P. and Currey, H. L. F. (1972) Failure of oral D-penicillamine to modify adjuvant arthritis or immune response in the rat. *Ann. Rheum. Dis.*, 31, 521.

Lockshin, M. D., Markenson, J. A., Fuzesi, L., Kazanjian-Aram, S., Joachim, C. and Ordene, M. (1983) Monocyte-induced inhibition of lymphocyte response to phytohaemagglutinin in progressive systemic sclerosis. *Ann. Rheum. Dis.*, 42, 40–4.

Lotner, G. Z., Lynch, J. M., Betz, S. J. and Henson, P. M. (1980) Human neutrophil-derived platelet activating factor. *J. Immunol.*, 124, 676–84.

Lunec, J., Halloran, S. P., White, A. G. and Dormandy, T. L. (1981) Free-radical oxidation (peroxidation) products in serum and synovial fluid in rheumatoid arthritis. *J. Rheumatol.*, 8, 233–45.

Lydyard, P. M., Brostoff, J., Hudspith, B. N. and Parry, H. (1982) Prostaglandin E_2-mediated enhancement of human plasma cell differentiation. *Immunol. Lett.*, 4, 113–16.

Lyle, W. H. (1979) Penicillamine. *Clinics Rheum. Dis.*, 5, 569–601.

McCord, J. M. (1974) Free radicals and inflammation: protection of synovial fluid by superoxide dismutase. *Science*, 185, 529–31.

McCune, W. J., Trentham, D. E. and David, J. R. (1980) Gold does not alter the arthritic, humoral or cellular responses in rats with type II collagen-induced arthritis. *Arthr. Rheum.*, 23, 932–6.

McGregor, R. R. (1977) Granulocyte adherence changes induced by haemodialysis, endotoxin, epinephrine and glucocorticoids. *Ann. Intern. Med.*, 86, 35–9.

McKeown, M. J., Hall, N. D. and Corvalan, J. R. F. (1984) Defective monocyte accessory function due to surface sulphydryl (SH) oxidation in rheumatoid arthritis. *Clin. Exp. Immunol.*, 56, 607–13.

Male, D. K. and Roitt, I. M. (1981) Molecular analysis of complement-fixing rheumatoid synovial fluid immune complexes. *Clin. Exp. Immunol.*, 46, 521–9.

Martin, M. F. R., Dieppe, P. A., Whicher, J. and Bell, A. M. (1982) Defective acute phase responses in scleroderma. *Ann. Rheum. Dis.*, 41, 194.

Matheson, N. R. (1982) The effect of antiarthritic drugs and related compounds on the human neutrophil myeloperoxidase system. *Biochem. Biophys. Res. Commun.*, 108, 259–65.

Mayer, D. J., Price, D. D. and Rafii, A. (1977) Antagonism of acupuncture analgesia in man by the narcotic antagonist naloxone. *Brain Res.*, 121, 368–72.

Mead, J. F. (1976) Free radical mechanisms of lipid damage and consequences for cellular membranes. In *Free Radicals in Biology, Vol 1* (ed. W. A. Pryor), Academic Press, New York, pp. 51–68.

Miller, T. E. and Ormrod, D. (1980) The anti-inflammatory activity of *Perna canaliculus* (NZ green-lipped mussel). *N. Z. Med. J.*, 92, 187–93.

Minty, C. A., Hall, N. D. and Bacon, P. A. (1983) Depressed exocytosis by rheumatoid neutrophils *in vitro*. *Rheumatol. Int.*, 3, 139–42.

Mitsuoka, A., Baba, M. and Morikawa, S. (1976) Enhancement of delayed hypersensitivity by depletion of suppressor T cells with cyclophosphamide in mice. *Nature (London)*, 262, 77–8.

Miyawaki, T., Yachie, A., Uwadane, N., Ohzeki, S., Nagaoki, T. and Taniguchi, N. (1982) Functional significance of Tac antigen expressed on activated human T lymphocytes: Tac antigen interacts with T cell growth factor in cellular proliferation. *J. Immunol.*, 129, 2474–8.

Mizel, S. B., Dayer, J-M., Krane, S. M. and Mergenhagen, S. E. (1981) Stimulation of rheumatoid synovial cell collagenase and prostaglandin production by partially purified lymphocyte-activating factor (interleukin I). *Proc. Nat. Acad. Sci., USA*, 78, 2474–7.

Möller, G. (ed) (1978) Role of macrophages in the immune response. *Immunol. Rev.*, 40.

Moretta, L., Webb, S. R., Grossi, C. E., Lydyard, P. M. and Cooper, M. D. (1977) Functional analysis of two human T cell subpopulations: help and suppression of B cell responses by T cells bearing receptors for IgM or IgG. *J. Exp. Med.*, 146, 184–200.

Morimoto, C., Reinherz, E. L., Borel, Y., Mantzouranis, E., Steinberg, A. D. and Schlossman, S. F. (1981) Autoantibody to an immunoregulatory inducer population in patients with juvenile rheumatoid arthritis. *J. Clin. Invest.*, 67, 753–61.

Morimoto, C., Reinherz, E. L., Borel, Y. and Schlossman, S. F. (1983) Direct demonstration of the human suppressor inducer subset by anti-T cell antibodies. *J. Immunol.*, 130, 157–61.

Moriya, N., Miyawaki, T., Seki, H., Kubo, M., Nagaoki, T., Okuda, N. and Taniguchi, N. (1979) Induction of suppressor activity on B cell differentiation in human T cell subset with Fc (IgG) receptors by levamisole administration. *Scand. J. Immunol.*, 10, 535–41.

Morley, J. (1974) Prostaglandins and lymphokines in arthritis. *Prostaglandins*, 8, 315–25.

Mowat, A. G. (1978) Neutrophil chemotaxis in rheumatoid arthritis. Effect of D-penicillamine, gold salts and levamisole. *Ann. Rheum. Dis.*, 37, 1–8.

Mowat, A. G. and Baum, J. (1971) Chemotaxis of polymorphonuclear leucocytes from patients with rheumatoid arthritis. *J. Clin. Invest.*, 50, 2541–9.

Multicentre Study Group (1978) Levamisole in rheumatoid arthritis. *Lancet*, ii, 1007–12.

Munthe, E. and Natvig, J. B. (1972) Immunoglobulin classes, subclasses and complexes of IgG rheumatoid factor in rheumatoid plasma cells. *Clin. Exp. Immunol.*, 12, 55–70.

Naccache, P. H., Showell, H. J., Becker, E. L. and Sha'afi, R. I. (1977) Changes in ionic movements across rabbit polymorphonuclear leucocyte membranes during lysosomal enzyme release. *J. Cell Biol.*, 75, 635–49.

Nakamura, H. and Igarashi, M. (1977) Localisation of gold in synovial membrane of rheumatoid arthritis treated with sodium aurothiomalate. *Ann. Rheum. Dis.*, 36, 209–15.

Neumann, V. C., Grindulis, K. A., Hubball, S., McConkey, B. and Wright, V. (1983) Comparison between penicillamine and sulphasalazine in rheumatoid arthritis: Leeds–Birmingham trial. *Br. Med. J.*, 287, 1099–102.

Newbould, B. B. (1963) Chemotherapy of arthritis induced in rats by mycobacterial adjuvant. *Br. J. Pharmacol.*, 21, 127–36.

Nishida, Y., Tanimoto, K. and Akaoka, I. (1981) Effect of free radicals on lymphocyte response to mitogens and rosette formation. *Clin. Immunol. Immunopathol.*, 19, 319–24.

Novogrodsky, A., Ravid A., Rubin, A. L. and Stenzel, K. H. (1982) Hydroxyl radical scavengers inhibit lymphocyte mitogenesis. *Proc. Nat. Acad. Sci., USA*, 79, 1171–74.

O'Flaherty, J. T., Wykle, R. L., Miller, C. H., Lewis, J. C., Waite, M., Bass, D. A., McCall, C. E. and DeChatelet, L. R. (1981) 1-0-Alkyl-sn-glyceryl-3-phosphoryl-cholines: a novel class of neutrophil stimulants. *Am. J. Pathol.*, 103, 70–9.

Okudaira, K., Nakai, H., Hayakawa, T., Kastiwado, T., Tanimoto, K., Horiuchi, Y. and Juji, T. (1979) Detection of anti-lymphocyte antibody with two-color method in systemic lupus erythematosus and its heterogenous specificities against human T cell subsets. *J. Clin. Invest.*, 64, 1213–20.

Okudaira, K., Searles, R. P., Goodwin, J. S. and Williams, R. C.Jr (1982) Antibodies in the sera of patients with systemic lupus erythematosus that block the binding of monoclonal anti-Ia to Ia positive targets also inhibit the autologous mixed lymphocyte response. *J. Immunol.*, 129, 582–6.

Okudaira, K., Tanimoto, K. and Horiuchi, Y. (1981) Effect of antilymphocyte antibody in SLE on *in vitro* Ig synthesis. *Clin. Immunol. Immunopathol.*, 21, 162–70.

Oppenheim, J. J. and Gery, I. (1982) Interleukin 1 is more than an interleukin. *Immunol. Today*, 3, 113–19.

Oppenheim, J. J., Stadler, B. M., Siraganian, R. P., Mage, M. and Mathieson, B. (1982) Lymphokines: their role in lymphocyte responses. Properties of interleukin 1. *Fed. Proc.*, 41, 257–62.

Oyanagui, Y. (1978) Inhibition of superoxide anion production in non-stimulated guinea pig peritoneal exudate cells by anti-inflammatory drugs. *Biochem. Pharmacol.*, 27, 777–82.

Panayi, G. S., Wooley, P. and Batchelor, J. R. (1978) Genetic basis of rheumatoid disease: HLA antigens, disease manifestations and toxic reactions to drugs. *Br. Med. J.*, 2, 1326–8.

Parrillo, J. E. and Fauci, A. S. (1979) Mechanisms of glucocorticoid action on immune processes. *Ann. Rev. Pharmacol. Toxicol.*, 19, 179–201.

Patel, V., Panayi, G. S., Shepherd, P., Richter, M., Harkness, J. and Gibson, T. (1982) Lymphocyte studies in rheumatoid arthritis. V. Suppressor cell function in peripheral blood. *Scand. J. Rheumatol.*, 11, 133–7.

Paulus, H. E., Machleder, H. I., Levine, S., Yu, D. T. Y. and MacDonald, N. S. (1977) Lymphocyte involvement in rheumatoid arthritis. Studies during thoracic duct drainage. *Arthr. Rheum.*, 20, 1249–62.

Payan, D. G. and Goetzl, E. J. (1983) Specific suppression of human T lymphocyte function by leucotriene B_4. *J. Immunol.*, 131, 551–3.

Pearson, C. M. (1956) Development of arthritis, periarthritis and periostitis in rats given adjuvants. *Proc. Soc. Exp. Biol. Med.*, 91, 95–101.

Pekoe, G., Van Dyke, K., Mengoli, H., Peden, D. and English, D. (1982) Comparison of the effects of anti-oxidant non-steroidal anti-inflammatory drugs against myeloperoxidase and hypochlorous acid luminol-enhanced chemiluminescence. *Agents Actions*, 12, 232–8.

Perper, R. J. and Oronsky, A. L. (1974) Enzyme release from human leucocytes and degradation of cartilage matrix. Effects of antirheumatic drugs. *Arthr. Rheum.*, 17, 47–55.

Persellin, R. H. and Ziff, M. (1966) The effect of gold on lysosomal enzyme of the peritoneal macrophage. *Arthr. Rheum.*, 9, 57–65.

Peterkofsky, B. and Tomkins, G. M. (1968) Evidence for the steroid-induced accumulation of tyrosine-aminotransferase messenger RNA in the absence of protein synthesis. *Proc. Nat. Acad. Sci., USA*, 60, 222–8.

Petrone, W. F., English, D. K., Wong, K. and McCord, J. M. (1980) Free radicals and inflammation: superoxide-dependent activation of a neutrophil chemotactic factor in plasma. *Proc. Nat. Acad. Sci., USA*, 77, 1159–63.

Pike, M. C., Daniels, C. A. and Snyderman, R. (1977) Influenza-induced depression of monocyte chemotaxis: reversal by levamisole. *Cell. Immunol.*, 32, 234–8.

Plater-Zyberk, C., Clarke, M. F., Lam, K., Mumford, P. A., Room, G. R. W. and Maini, R. N. (1983) *In vitro* immunoglobulin synthesis by lymphocytes from patients with rheumatoid arthritis. I Effect of monocyte depletion and demonstration of an increased proportion of lymphocytes forming rosettes with mouse erythrocytes. *Clin. Exp. Immunol.*, 52, 505–11.

Poikonen, K., Oka, M., Möttönen, T., Jokinen, I. and Arvilommi, H. (1982) Synthesis of IgM, IgG and IgA in rheumatoid arthritis. *Ann. Rheum. Dis.*, 41, 607–11.

Pope, R. M., Teller, D. C. and Mannik, M. (1974) The molecular basis of self-association of antibodies to IgG (rheumatoid factors) in rheumatoid arthritis. *Proc. Nat. Acad. Sci., USA*, 71, 517–21.

Poulter, L. W., Duke, O., Hobbs, S., Janossy, G. and Panayi, G. (1982) Histochemical discrimination of HLA-DR positive cell populations in the normal and arthritic synovial lining. *Clin. Exp. Immunol.*, 48, 381–8.

Poulter, L. W. and Turk, J. L. (1972) Proportional increase in the θ-carrying lymphocytes in peripheral lymphoid tissue following treatment with cyclophosphamide. *Nature (New Biol.)*, 238, 17–18.

Powell, L. W., Hart, P., Neilsen, M. H. and Werdelin, O. (1980) Antigen-dependent physical interaction between human monocytes and T lymphocytes. *Scand. J. Immunol.*, 12, 467–73.

Pritchard, M. H. and Nuki, G. (1978) Gold and penicillamine: a proposed mode of action in rheumatoid arthritis, based on synovial fluid analysis. *Ann. Rheum. Dis.*, 37, 493–503.

Pullar, T., Hunter, J. A. and Capell, H. A. (1983) Sulphasalazine in rheumatoid arthritis: a double blind comparison of sulphasalazine with placebo and sodium aurothiomalate. *Br. Med. J.*, 287, 1102–4.

Rae, S. A., Davidson, E. M. and Smith, M. J. H. (1982) Leucotriene B₄, an inflammatory mediator in gout. *Lancet*, ii, 1122–4.

Rainsford, K. D. (1982) Analysis of the gastrointestinal side-effects of nonsteroidal anti-inflammatory drugs, with particular reference to comparative studies in man and laboratory species. *Rheumatol. Int.*, 2, 1–10.

Reinherz, E. L., Morimoto, C., Fitzgerald, K. A., Hussey, R. E., Daley, J. F. and Schlossman, S. F. (1982) Heterogeneity of human T4⁺ inducer T cells defined by a monoclonal antibody that delineates two functional subpopulations. *J. Immunol.*, 128, 463–8.

Reinherz, E. L. and Schlossman, S. F. (1980) Regulation of the immune response – inducer and suppressor T-lymphocyte subsets in human beings. *N. Engl. J. Med.*, 303, 370–3.

Reiss, M. and Roos, D. (1978) Differences in oxygen metabolism of phagocytosing monocytes and neutrophils. *J. Clin. Invest.*, 61, 480–8.

Renoux, G. (1978) Modulation of immunity by levamisole. *Pharmacol. Therap. A*, 2, 397–423.

Rinehart, J. J., Sagone, A. L., Balcerzak, S. P., Ackerman, G. A. and LoBuglio, A. F. (1975) Effects of corticosteroid therapy on human monocyte function. *N. Engl. J. Med.*, 292, 236–41.

Ritzmann, S. E., Coleman, S. L. and Levin, W. C. (1960) The effect of some mercaptanes upon a macrocryogelglobulin: modifications induced by cysteamine, penicillamine and penicillin. *J. Clin. Invest.*, 39, 1320–9.

Robinson, B. V. (1978) The pharmacology of phagocytosis. *Rheumatol. Rehabil.*, Suppl., 37–46.

Robinson, D. R., Tashjian, A. H.Jr. and Levine, L. (1975) Prostaglandin-stimulated bone resorption by rheumatoid synovia. *J. Clin. Invest.*, 56, 1181–8.

Rodriguez, M. A., Ceuppens, J. L. and Goodwin, J. S. (1982) Regulation of IgM rheumatoid factor production in lymphocyte cultures from young and old subjects. *J. Immunol.*, 128, 2422–8.

Roitt, I. M., Cooke, A., Male, D. K., Hay, F. C., Guarnotta, G., Lydyard, P. M., de Carvalho, L. P. and Thanavala, Y. (1981) Idiotypic networks and their possible exploitation for manipulation of the immune response. *Lancet*, i, 1041–5.

Romeo, D., Zabucchi, G., Miani, N., Rossi, F. (1975) Ion movement across leucocyte plasma membrane and excitation of their metabolism. *Nature (London)*, 253, 542–4.

Room, G., Roffe, L. and Maini, R. N. (1979) Inhibitory effect of D-penicillamine on human lymphocyte cultures stimulated by phytohaemagglutinin, the antagonistic action of L-cysteine and synergistic inhibition by copper sulphate. *Scand. J. Rheumatol.* (suppl. 28), 47–57.

Root, R. K. and Metcalf, J. A. (1977) H_2O_2 release from human granulocytes during phagocytosis: relationship to superoxide anion formation and cellular catabolism of H_2O_2: studies with normal and cytochalasin B treated cells. *J. Clin. Invest.*, **60**, 1266–79.

Root, R. K., Metcalf, J., Oshino, N. and Chance, B. (1975) H_2O_2 release from human granulocytes during phagocytosis: I Documentation, quantitation and some regulating factors. *J. Clin. Invest.*, **55**, 945–55.

Rosen, H. and Klebanoff, S. J. (1979a) Bactericidal activity of a superoxide anion-generating system. *J. Exp. Med.*, **149**, 27–39.

Rosen, H. and Klebanoff, S. J. (1979b) Hydroxyl radical generation by polymorphonuclear leucocytes measured by electron spin resonance spectroscopy. *J. Clin. Invest.*, **64**, 1725–9.

Rosenberg, S. A. and Lipsky, P. E. (1981) The role of monocytes in pokeweed mitogen-stimulated human B cell activation: separate requirements for intact monocytes and a soluble monocyte factor. *J. Immunol.*, **126**, 1341–5.

Russell, A. S., Davis, P. and Miller, C. (1982) The effect of a new antirheumatic drug, triethylphosphine gold (auranofin) on *in vitro* lymphocyte and monocyte cytotoxicity. *J. Rheumatol.*, **9**, 30–5.

Sakane, T., Steinberg, A. D. and Green, I. (1980) Studies of immune functions of patients with systemic lupus erythematosus. V. T cell suppressor function and autologous mixed lymphocyte reaction during active and inactive phases of disease. *Arthr. Rheum.*, **23**, 225–31.

Sakane, T., Steinberg, A. D., Reeves, J. P. and Green, I. (1979) Studies of immune functions of patients with systemic lupus erythematosus. T cell subsets and antibodies to T cell subsets. *J. Clin. Invest.*, **64**, 1260–9.

Scala, G. and Oppenheim, J. J. (1983) Antigen presentation by human monocytes: evidence for stimulant processing and requirement for interleukin I. *J. Immunol.*, **131**, 1160–6.

Scheinberg, M. A., Santos, L. and Finkelstein, A. (1981) Gold inhibition of human monocyte function. *Arthr. Rheum.*, **24**, S117.

Scheinberg, M. A., Santos, L., Mendes, N. F. and Musatti, C. (1978) Decreased lymphocyte response to PHA, Con-A, and calcium ionophore (A 23187) in patients with RA and SLE, and reversal with levamisole in rheumatoid arthritis. *Arthr. Rheum.*, **21**, 326–9.

Schimpl, A. and Wecker, E. (1972) Replacement of T cell function by a T cell product. *Nature (New Biol.)*, **237**, 15–17.

Schmidt, M. E. and Douglas, S. D. (1976) Effects of levamisole on human monocyte function and immunoprotein receptors. *Clin. Immunol. Immunopathol.*, **6**, 299–305.

Schmidt, J. A., Mizel, S. B. and Green, I. (1981) A fibroblast proliferation factor isolated from human MLR supernatants has physical and functional properties similar to human interleukin 1 (IL-1). *Fed. Proc.*, **40**, 1084.

Schultz, D. R., Volanakis, J. E., Arnold, P. J., Gottlieb, N. L., Sakai, K. and Stroud, R. M. (1974) Inactivation of C1 in rheumatoid synovial fluid, purified C1 and C1 esterase, by gold compounds. *Clin. Exp. Immunol.*, **17**, 395–406.

Schumacher, H. R.Jr (1977) Pathogenesis of crystal-induced synovitis. *Clinics Rheum. Dis.*, **3**, 105–31.

Segal, A. W., Cross, A. R., Garcia, R. C., Borregaard, N., Valerius, N. H., Soothill, J. F. and Jones, O. T. G. (1983) Absence of cytochrome b_{245} in chronic granulomatous disease. *N. Engl. J. Med.*, **308**, 245–51.

Shou, L., Schwartz, S. A. and Good, R. A. (1976) Suppressor cell activity after concanavalin A treatment of lymphocytes from normal donors. *J. Exp. Med.*, **143**, 1100–10.

Showell, H. J., Freer, R. J., Zigmond, S. H., Schiffmann, E., Aswanikumer, S., Corcoran, B. and Becker, E. L. (1976) The structure–activity relations of synthetic peptides as chemotactic factors and inducers of lysosomal enzyme secretion for neutrophils. Effect of metabolic inhibitors and anti-inflammatory drugs. *J. Exp. Med.*, **143**, 1154–69.

Simchowitz, L., Mehta, J. and Spilberg, I. (1979) Chemotactic factor-induced generation of superoxide radicals by human neutrophils. *Arthr. Rheum.*, **22**, 755–63.

Slaughter, L., Carson, D. A., Jensen, F. C., Holbrook, T. L. and Vaughan, J. H. (1978) *In vitro* effects of Epstein–Barr virus on peripheral blood mononuclear cells from patients with rheumatoid arthritis and normal subjects. *J. Exp. Med.*, **148**, 1429–34.

Sloboda, A. E., Birnbaum, J. E., Oronsky, A. L. and Kerwar, S. S. (1981) Studies on type II collagen-induced polyarthritis in rats: effect of anti-inflammatory and antirheumatic agents. *Arthr. Rheum.*, **24**, 616–24.

Smiley, J. D., Sachs, C. and Ziff, M. (1968) *In vitro* synthesis of immunoglobulin by rheumatoid synovial membrane. *J. Clin. Invest.*, **47**, 624–32.

Smith, J. B. and DeHoratius, R. J. (1982) Deficient autologous mixed lymphocyte reactions correlate with disease activity in systemic lupus erythematosus and rheumatoid arthritis. *Clin. Exp. Immunol.*, **48**, 155–62.

Smith, K. A. (1980) T cell growth factor. *Immunol. Rev.*, **51**, 337–57.

Smith, K. A., Lachman, L. B., Oppenheim, J. J. and Favata, M. F. (1980) The functional relationship of the interleukins. *J. Exp. Med.*, **151**, 1551–6.

Smith, R. J. and Iden, S. S. (1980) Pharmacological modulation of chemotactic factor-elicited release of granule-associated enzymes from human neutrophils. *Biochem. Pharmacol.*, **29**, 2389–95.

Smolen, J. E., Korchak, H. M. and Weissmann, G. (1981) The roles of extracellular and intracellular calcium in lysosomal enzyme release and superoxide anion generation by human neutrophils. *Biochim. Biophys. Acta*, **677**, 512–20.

Smolen, J. E., Korchak, H. M. and Weissmann, G. (1982) Stimulus–response coupling in neutrophils. *Trends Pharmacol. Sci.*, **3**, 483–5.

Smolen, J. E. and Weissmann, G. (1980) Effects of indomethacin 5,8,11,14-eicosatetraynoic acid, and *p*-bromophenacyl bromide on lysosomal enzyme release and superoxide anion generation by human polymorphonuclear leucocytes. *Biochem. Pharmacol.*, **29**, 533–8.

Sofia, R. D. and Douglas, J. F. (1973) The prophylactic and therapeutic effects of gold sodium thiomalate against adjuvant-induced polyarthritis in rats. *Agents Actions*, **3**, 335–43.

Solomon, L. M., Juklin, L. and Kirschbaum, M. B. (1968) Prostaglandin on cutaneous vasculature. *J. Invest. Dermatol.*, **51**, 280–2.

Sorenson, J. R. J. (1976) Copper chelates as possible active forms of the antiarthritic agents. *J. Med. Chem.*, **19**, 135–48.

Staite, N. D., Ganczakowski, M., Panayi, G. S. and Unger, A. (1983) Prostaglandin-mediated immunoregulation: reduced sensitivity of *in vitro* immunoglobulin production to indomethacin in rheumatoid arthritis. *Clin. Exp. Immunol.*, **52**, 535–42.

Staite, N. D. and Panayi, G. S. (1982) Regulation of human immunoglobulin production *in vitro* by prostaglandin E_2. *Clin. Exp. Immunol.*, **49**, 115–22.

Stanworth, D. R. and Hunneyball, I. M. (1979) The influence of D-penicillamine treatment on the humoral immune system. *Scand. J. Rheumatol.* (Suppl. 28), 37–46.

Stastny, P. (1978) Association of the B cell alloantigen DRw4 with rheumatoid arthritis. *N. Engl. J. Med.*, **298**, 869–71.

Stastny, P., Rosenthal, M., Andreis, M. and Ziff, M. (1975) Lymphokines in the rheumatoid joint. *Arthr. Rheum.*, **18**, 237–43.

Steinman, R. M. and Nussenzweig, M. C. (1980) Dendritic cells: features and functions. *Immunol. Rev.*, **53**, 127–47.

Stuart, J. M., Myers, L. K., Townes, A. S. and Kang, A. H. (1981) Effect of cyclophosphamide, hydrocortisone and levamisole on collagen-induced arthritis in rats. *Arthr. Rheum.*, **24**, 790–4.

Sy, M-S., Miller, S. D. and Claman, H. N. (1977) Immune suppression with supraoptimal doses of antigen in contact sensitivity. I Demonstration of suppressor cells and their sensitivity to cyclophosphamide. *J. Immunol.*, **119**, 240–4.

Symoens, J. and Rosenthal, M. (1977) Levamisole in the modulation of the immune response: the current experimental and clinical state. *J. Reticuloendothelial Soc.*, **21**, 175–221.

Symoens, J. and Schuermans, Y. (1979) Levamisole – a basic antirheumatic drug. *Clinics Rheum. Dis.*, **5**, 603–29.

Symoens, J., Veys, E., Mielants, H. and Pinals, R. (1979) Adverse reactions to levamisole. *Cancer Treat. Rep.*, **62**, 1721–30.

Szczeklik, A., Gryclewski, R. J., Nizenkowski, R., Musial, J., Pieton, R. and Mruk, J. (1978) Circulatory and anti-platelet effects of intravenous prostacyclin in healthy man. *Pharmacol. Res. Commun.*, **10**, 545–56.

Sztein, M. B., Vogel, S. N., Sipe, J. D., Murphy, P. A., Mizel, S. B., Oppenheim, J. J. and Rosenstreich, D. L. (1981) The role of macrophages in the acute-phase response: SAA inducer is closely related to lymphocyte activating factor and endogenous pyrogen. *Cell. Immunol.*, **63**, 164–76.

Tada, T. and Hayakawa, K. (1980) Antigen-specific helper and suppressor factors. in *Immunology 80: Progress in Immunology IV* (eds, M. Fougereau and J. Dausset), Academic Press, London, pp. 389–402.

Takeshige, K., Nabi, Z. F., Tatschek, B. and Minakami, S. (1980) Release of calcium from membranes and its relation to phagocytic metabolic changes: a fluorescence study on leucocytes loaded with chlortetracycline. *Biochem. Biophys. Res. Commun.*, **95**, 410–15.

Taylor, R. B. (1982) Regulation of antibody responses by antibody towards the immunogen. *Immunol. Today*, **3**, 47–51.

Temple, A. and Loewi, G. (1977) The effect of sera from patients with connective tissue diseases on red cell binding and phagocytosis by monocytes. *Immunology*, **33**, 109–14.

Thomas, Y., Rogozinski, L., Irigoyen, O. H., Shen, H. H., Talbe, M. A., Goldstein, G. and Chess, L. (1982) Functional analysis of human T cell subsets defined by monoclonal antibodies. V Suppressor cells within the activated OKT4[+] population belong to a distinct subset. *J. Immunol.*, **128**, 1386–90.

Townes, A. S., Sowa, J. M. and Shulman, L. E. (1976) Controlled trial of cyclophosphamide in rheumatoid arthritis. *Arthr. Rheum.*, **19**, 563–73.

Trang, L. E. (1980) Prostaglandins and inflammation. *Seminars Arthr. Rheum.*, **9**, 153–90.

Trentham, D. E. (1982) Collagen arthritis as a relevant model for rheumatoid arthritis. Evidence pro and con. *Arthr. Rheum.*, **25**, 911–16.

Trentham, D. E., Townes, A. S. and Kang, A. H. (1977) Autoimmunity to type II collagen: an experimental model of arthritis. *J. Exp. Med.*, **146**, 857–68.

Turner, R. A., Schumacher, H. R. and Myers, A. R. (1973) Phagocytic function of polymorphonuclear leucocytes in rheumatic diseases. *J. Clin. Invest.*, **52**, 1632–5.

Uyeki, E. M. (1967) Effects of several antitumour agents on spleen hemolysin plaque-forming cells. *Biochem. Pharmacol.*, 16, 53–8.

Vane, J. R. (1971) Inhibition of prostaglandin synthesis as a mechanism of action for aspirin-like drugs. *Nature (New Biol.)*, 231, 232–5.

Verhaegen, H., De Cock, W. and De Cree, J. (1977a) The effects of azathioprine and levamisole on rosette-forming cells of healthy subjects and cancer patients. *Clin. Exp. Immunol.*, 29, 311–15.

Verhaegen, H., De Cree, J., De Cock, W. and Verbruggen, F. (1977b) Restoration by levamisole of low E-rosette forming cells in patients suffering from various diseases. *Clin. Exp. Immunol.*, 27, 313–18.

Vernon-Roberts, B., Dore, J. L., Jessop, J. D. and Henderson, W. J. (1976) Selective concentration and localisation of gold in macrophages of synovial and other tissue during and after chrysotherapy in rheumatoid patients. *Ann. Rheum. Dis.*, 35, 477–86.

Wallace, D. J., Goldfinger, D., Gatti, R., Lowe, C., Fan, P., Bluestone, R. and Klinenberg, J. R. (1979) Plasmapheresis and lymphoplasmapheresis in the management of rheumatoid arthritis. *Arthr. Rheum.*, 22, 703–10.

Ward, P. A. and Zvaifler, N. J. (1971) Complement-derived leucotactic factors in inflammatory synovial fluids of humans. *J. Clin. Invest.*, 50, 606–16.

Watson, J., Mochizuki, D. and Gillis, S. (1980) T cell growth factors: interleukin 2. *Immunol. Today*, 1, 113–17.

Wedmore, C. V. and Williams, T. J. (1981) Control of vascular permeability by polymorphonuclear leucocytes in inflammation. *Nature (London)*, 289, 646–50.

Weiss, S. J. and Ward, P. A. (1982) Immune complex induced generation of oxygen metabolites by human neutrophils. *J. Immunol.*, 129, 309–13.

Weiss, S. J., Young, J., LoBuglio, A. F., Slivka, A. and Nimeh, N. F. (1981) Role of hydrogen peroxide in neutrophil-mediated destruction of cultured endothelial cells. *J. Clin. Invest.*, 68, 714–21.

Whitney, R. B. and Sutherland, R. M. (1973) Requirements for calcium ions in lymphocyte transformation stimulated by phytohaemagglutinin. *J. Cell. Physiol.*, 80, 329–38.

Wickens, D. G. and Dormandy, T. L. (1982) Further studies of fluorescent free-radical products in synovial fluid. *Clin. Rheumatol.*, 1, 151–2.

Wickens, D. G., Norden, A. G., Lunec, J. and Dormandy, T. L. (1983) Fluorescence changes in human gamma-globulin induced by free-radical activity. *Biochim. Biophys. Acta*, 742, 607–16.

Wilkins, J. A., Warrington, R. J., Sigurdson, S. L. and Rutherford, W. J. (1983) The demonstration of an interleukin 2-like activity in the synovial fluids of rheumatoid arthritis patients. *J. Rheumatol.*, 10, 109–13.

Wollheim, F. A., Jeppsson, J. O. and Laurell, C. B. (1979) D-penicillamine treatment in rheumatoid arthritis monitored by plasma alpha 1 antitrypsin-IgA complexes and plasma and urinary sulphur-containing amino acids. *Scand. J. Rheumatol.* (suppl. 28), 21–27.

Yachie, A., Miyawaki, T., Uwadana, N., Ohzeki, S. and Taniguchi, N. (1983) Sequential expression of T cell activation (Tac) antigen and Ia determinants on circulating human T cells after immunisation with tetanus toxoid. *J. Immunol.*, 131, 731–5.

Yu, D. T. Y., Winchester, R. J., Fu, S. M., Gibofsky, A., Ko, H. S. and Kunkel, H. G. (1980) Peripheral blood Ia-positive T cells. Increases in certain diseases and after immunisation. *J. Exp. Med.*, 151, 91–100.

Zabucchi, G., Soranzo, M. R., Rossi, F. and Romeo, D. (1975) Exocytosis in human polymorphonuclear leucocytes induced by A23187 and calcium. *Fed. Eur. Biochem. Soc. Lett.*, 54, 44–8.

Zeitlin, I. J. (1981) Arachidonate metabolites in inflammation. *Clinics Rheum. Dis.,* 7, 781–97.

Zeitlin, I. J. and Grennan, D. M. (1976) The role of the inflammatory mediators in joint inflammation, in *Recent Advances in Rheumatology* (eds W. W. Buchanan and W. C. Dick), Churchill Livingston, London, pp. 195–212.

Zoschke, D. C., Draime, S. and Messner, R. P. (1982) Phagocytic cell-derived hydrogen peroxide and T cell regulation. *Arthr. Rheum.,* 25, S27.

Zuckner, J., Ramsey, R. H., Dorner, R. W. and Gantner, G. E. (1970) D-Penicillamine in rheumatoid arthritis. *Arthr. Rheum.,* 13, 131–8.

Zurier, R. B., Mitnick, H., Bloomgarden, D. and Weissmann, G. (1973) Effect of bee venom on experimental arthritis. *Ann. Rheum. Dis.,* 32, 466–70.

Zvaifler, N. J. (1973) The immunopathology of joint inflammation in rheumatoid arthritis. *Adv. Immunol.,* 16, 265–336.

CHAPTER 2

Pharmacokinetics

Allister J. Taggart

and

Dean W. G. Harron

2.1 INTRODUCTION

Pharmacokinetics is a science that has emerged in the last thirty years with the development of laboratory techniques for measuring drug concentrations in body fluids. It is a quantitative means of analysing the way in which the body handles drugs, with particular regard to their absorption, distribution, metabolism and excretion. The variability in drug response between different patients and in the same patients at different times is a fundamental problem of all drug therapy and may lead to inadequate or excessive treatment – a therapeutic dose for one individual may be toxic for another. Pharmacokinetics attempts to quantify this variation in order to predict drug response more accurately and optimize therapy.

2.2 DRUG ABSORPTION

2.2.1 Routes of administration

Most drugs are administered by mouth for convenience, but in particular cases other routes may be more appropriate. Parenteral administration is required for drugs that are poorly absorbed from the gastrointestinal tract or rapidly metabolized before reaching the systemic circulation (see Section 2.5.2). The intravenous route may be used to achieve a more rapid effect and has the added advantage of 100% bioavailability. A drug's bioavailability is a measure of the extent of its absorption into the systemic circulation. Since complete absorption is assured with intravenous injection, this is the standard by which other routes of administration are compared. The rate of absorption may be expressed in terms of C_{max}, the peak plasma concentration, or t_{max}, the time taken to reach that peak, but neither is as important as the extent of drug absorption.

Although it is often assumed to be so, the intramuscular route is not a completely reliable way of administering drugs. Drugs must remain in solution at the site of injection if they are to be absorbed efficiently but compounds like diazepam and phenytoin are poorly soluble at physiological pH and tend to precipitate in muscle tissue. Digoxin should not be given intramuscularly because its absorption is erratic and it causes painful muscle necrosis (Steiness *et al.*, 1974). Absorption may also be affected by regional blood flow. The effect of insulin can vary according to the site of injection and factors such as age and cardiac function may also be important.

Despite these drawbacks, intramuscular injection is an important means of drug administration. One advantage that it shares with intravenous therapy is the guarantee of a patient's compliance with treatment. This is sometimes a reason for choosing intramuscular gold instead of an oral preparation as second-line therapy in rheumatoid arthritis. Long-acting parenteral phenothiazines have been used in psychiatry for many years to assure patient compliance (Johnson and Freeman, 1972). More recently, pharmacologists have developed formulations that are administered by the transdermal, vaginal and conjunctival routes (Heilmann, 1978). The first of these routes may improve systemic bioavailability of certain compounds over oral administration whereas the second and third are predominantly used to treat local conditions. Significant systemic absorption has however been reported following vaginal or ocular dosing of, for example, certain β-adrenoceptor antagonists (Patel *et al.*, 1983; Schoene *et al.*, 1984).

Similarly, in the case of intra-articular steroids, the doses that are commonly used for large joints produce significant adrenocortical suppression (Bird *et al.*,

TABLE 2.1
Factors affecting gastrointestinal drug absorption

Presence of food or other drugs in the gut
Rate of gastric emptying
Gut transfer time
Intestinal disease
Drug formulation
Gastric pH
Gut flora

1979; Reeback *et al.*, 1980). Although novel drug delivery systems (e. g. liposome encapsulation) may increase the utility of 'local' drug administration, the gastrointestinal tract remains the primary route of absorption for drug therapy, including the antirheumatic drugs. Absorption usually occurs by passive diffusion through the gut mucosa, although it is sometimes achieved by active transport or pinocytosis. The rate and extent of drug absorption depends on a number of variables (Table 2.1).

2.2.2 Factors affecting gut absorption

(a) *Gastric emptying and gut motility*

Pharmacokinetic studies are usually carried out on subjects who are fasting in order to standardize the rate of gastric emptying. The clinical setting is much more variable and patients often take their medication with meals. Food tends to delay gastric emptying which in turn affects the rate of drug delivery to the rest of the gut. The small intestine has a much greater absorptive capacity than the stomach, thus administration with food affects the speed rather than the extent of drug absorption. There are exceptions to this general rule. For example, the bioavailability of D-penicillamine is halved if it is taken with food (Bergstrom *et al.*, 1981; Schuna *et al.*, 1983). This may be a consequence of its strong chelating properties (Lyle *et al.*, 1977). In contrast, food may enhance the absorption of drugs which are subject to a substantial first-pass effect (Section 2.5.2). The reasons for this are not clear, but food may decrease the degree of first-pass metabolism. Other drug therapy and disease may also affect drug absorption. Anticholinergic agents and narcotic analgesics can delay drug absorption by causing gastric stasis and an acute attack of migraine can have a similar effect (Nimmo, 1976). These drugs also reduce intestinal motility and may therefore increase the absorption of drugs which are slow in dissolving (e. g. dicoumarol). This shows how variable such absorption inter-actions can be. In diarrhoeal states, gut transit may be too fast to permit full absorption of some drugs; if the intestinal mucosa is also diseased absorption may be impaired further (Heizer *et al.*, 1971). Motility is probably not so critical for the non-steroidal anti-inflammatory drugs (NSAIDs) because of their rapid absorption, but it can be important for controlled-release prep-arations which are less readily absorbed (Crosland-Taylor *et al.*, 1965). Drug absorption is sometimes affected by binding or chelation with other drugs within the gut lumen. If oral iron is taken with D-penicillamine, an insoluble complex is formed in the gut and the bioavailability of both medicaments is reduced (Lyle *et al.*, 1977).

(b) *Drug formulation*

The form in which a drug is constituted can have an important effect on its pharmacokinetic profile. Tablets and capsules contain a variety of constituents in addition to the active drug. These include diluents, binding agents, lubricants and dyes. The most important properties of a tablet are its disintegration characteristics, particle size and dissolution rate. The practical importance of these factors was illustrated by a problem with digoxin bioavailability which arose in 1969. Changes in the drug's manufacturing process affected the particle size and dissolution rate of digoxin tablets and led to a 50% drop in bioavailability (Binnion, 1974; Shaw and Carless, 1974). A second example is more relevant to rheumatology. A recent study has shown a significant difference in the bioavailability of two enteric-coated formulations of prednisolone (Lee *et al.*, 1979). When the formulation with the greater bioavailability was compared with plain prednisolone, their overall absorption was very similar, although the enteric formulation delayed the onset of steroid uptake.

In the field of rheumatology, much effort has been devoted to developing formulations which modify the undesirable characteristics of antirheumatic drugs. Aspirin has been manipulated in this way because of the high frequency of gastric upset associated with its use. As salicylate ions accumulate in the gastric mucosa, they cause an alteration in cell defence so that hydrogen ions are permitted to diffuse in from the gastric juice (Ivey and Clifton, 1974). The 'back diffusion' of ions causes mucosal damage which can be reduced by altering the formulation of aspirin to impair absorption in the stomach. This has been achieved by enteric coating, buffering with alkalis or combination with aluminium salts. Absorption of aspirin in the small intestine rather than the stomach reduces dyspepsia and gives a slower onset but longer duration of effect (Buchanan *et al.*, 1979).

More recently, sustained release formulations have been developed for aspirin and several other NSAIDs. Some of these use a plastic matrix to encapsulate the drug whilst others surround it in a semi-permeable membrane which permits the entry of water into the tablet with the gradual dissolution of its contents. Sustained-release formulations enable a drug with a short half-life to be administered only once or twice a day. In theory, this flattens the plasma concentration curve, and reduces side effects that are related to high drug levels. These aims, however, are not always fulfilled (Adams *et al.*, 1982). A reduced frequency of daily dosing may also improve patient compliance (Taggart *et al.*, 1981).

Another approach to the problem of dyspepsia is the use of suppository formulations. The rectal absorption of drugs occurs via the portal vein, and is usually as complete as absorption by the oral route. The surface area of the rectum is much smaller than that of the small intestine so the rate of absorption is not as rapid. This may explain why peak drug levels are often lower with suppository formulations and some side effects are reduced (Alvan *et al.*, 1975; Baber *et al.*, 1980). In individual patients, however, the disadvantages of suppositories may outweigh the advantages. Some patients develop rectal irritation and diarrhoea whilst others find them distasteful to use or difficult to insert because of their arthritic hand deformities.

(c)   *Gut pH and drug ionization*

The ionization of a drug is of theoretical rather than practical importance in determining the extent of absorption. Its main influence is on the site of absorption which has more effect on the side effects of a preparation. Compounds that exist in a polar or ionized form do not cross biological membranes easily. Weak acids tend to be ionized in an alkaline environment and the opposite is true for alkalis. The NSAIDs are mostly weak acids so they tend to be readily absorbed in the acid environment of the stomach. Despite this, most drug absorption takes place in the small intestine because of its large surface area and extensive blood perfusion. These factors usually outweigh the influence of drug ionization.

(d)   *Gut flora*

Some drugs are subject to metabolism by resident gut flora which can have a significant effect on their bioavailability and therapeutic effect. Sulphasalazine is a useful remittive agent in the management of ulcerative colitis and rheumatoid arthritis (Misiewicz *et al.*, 1965; Neumann *et al.*, 1983). Between 10 and 20% of the drug is absorbed unchanged in the small intestine but the remainder reaches the large bowel where it is split into 5-aminosalicylic acid and sulphapyridine by gut flora. The sulphapyridine moiety is mostly absorbed but 5-aminosalicylic acid is excreted in the faeces (Das and Dubin, 1976). The drug's beneficial effect in colitis is thought to be due to the local effect of salicylate in the colon (Dew *et al.*, 1982) so gut flora are vital to its efficacy in rheumatoid arthritis, sulphapyridine appears to be the active moiety (Neumann *et al* 1986) but it is not yet clear whether it achieves its 'second line' effect by a local or a systemic action.

2.2.3   Absorption and elimination kinetics

The absorption and elimination of drugs are subject to many different variables but the rate at which they occur obeys basic rules that may be expressed mathematically. The intestinal absorption and glomerular filtration of most drugs are passive processes that proceed at rates proportional to the amount of substrate remaining. These processes obey *first order* or *exponential* kinetics and may be expressed thus:

$$\frac{\mathrm{d}D}{\mathrm{d}t} = -kD \tag{2.1}$$

where D = the amount of drug still to be processed at time t

and k = the first-order constant (absorption or elimination).

In contrast, active processes such as drug metabolism, biliary excretion and renal tubular secretion are capable of being saturated if the drug concentration exceeds a certain level. When this happens, the process proceeds at a constant rate which is independent of the substrate concentration. The process then obeys *zero order* kinetics which may be expressed thus:

$$\frac{-\mathrm{d}D}{\mathrm{d}t} = K \tag{2.2}$$

where D = the amount of drug still to be processed at time t

and K = the rate of the process (absorption, metabolism, excretion, etc.).

Most drugs obey first order kinetics but some display dose-dependent characteristics with first order kinetics at lower doses and zero order at higher levels. This may be hazardous because the serum drug concentration can rise dramatically when saturation point is reached. The elimination of aspirin is dose-dependent. The half-life of a 300 mg tablet is only 3 hours but this rises to 20 hours for a 10 g dose (Levy, 1965).

2.3   DRUG DISTRIBUTION

2.3.1   Plasma protein binding

Drugs are transported throughout the body in both bound and unbound forms. Albumin is the major binding protein in plasma and serves as a means of drug storage as well as transport. Only the unbound fraction is pharmacologically active and available for metabolism or excretion. The degree to which a drug is protein bound depends on its binding characteristics and on the concentration of drug and albumin in the plasma. The albumin level is affected by several factors including age and disease. These are considered in Section 2.7.2.

A drug binds with a plasma protein in a reversible process which is governed by the law of mass action:

$$\text{drug + protein} \quad \underset{k_2}{\overset{k_1}{\rightleftharpoons}} \quad \text{drug–protein complex} \tag{2.3}$$

The rate constants k_1 and k_2 determine the affinity of the drug for the binding protein but in practice protein binding is not a hindrance to the removal of drug from the plasma. The dissociation of drug from its carrier protein occurs at a rapid rate but the diffusion of drug into the tissues is much slower.

In the slightly alkaline pH (7.4) of plasma acidic compounds are largely ionized and this tends to increase their degree of protein binding. The NSAIDs are highly protein bound but they are also poorly distributed throughout the body. This means that the drug bound to plasma proteins forms a major proportion of the total body stores. As a result, NSAIDs are prone to displacement interactions with other acidic compounds such as the oral anticoagulants and sulphonylureas. Albumin has two independent binding sites for acidic drugs (Sjoholm, 1978) so drug interactions only occur if two compounds are competing for the same binding site. Although both phenylbutazone and ibuprofen are highly protein bound and poorly distributed, only phenylbutazone competes for the same binding sites as warfarin and tolbutamide. This competitive displacement, however, plays little, if any, role in the well-recognized clinical interactions between phenylbutazone and these drugs (see Chapter 3).

2.3.2 Drug compartments

Drug compartments are a mathematical concept that is used to describe the distribution of a drug throughout the body. Each compartment is a theoretical rather than an anatomical space. In a one-compartmental model there is immediate equilibrium between the plasma and the peripheral tissues. Both are considered as a single homogeneous entity so that plasma drug levels are expected to correlate with clinical response. In practice, these conditions only apply to a few drugs (Riegelman *et al.*, 1968).

In contrast, the two-compartment model is appropriate for many drugs. In this system, the plasma and highly perfused organs like the heart, liver and kidneys are regarded as the central compartment. Less well perfused tissues (muscle, skin, fat) are the peripheral or deep compartment to which the drug is more slowly distributed. A drug enters and leaves the system via the central

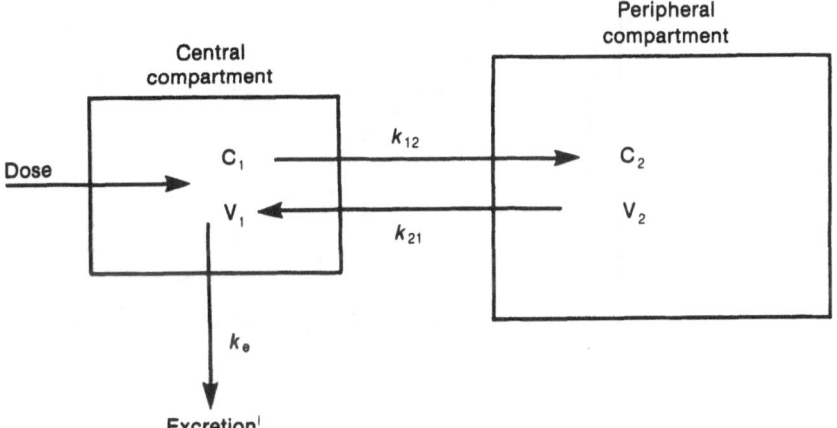

Figure 2.1 Schematic diagram of a two-compartment model. Drug is introduced and eliminated only from the central compartment. k_{12} and k_{21} represent the rate constants for the transfer of drug between the two compartments and k_e is the overall elimination rate constant. C_1, C_2, V_1 and V_2 are the drug concentrations and volumes of distribution in the central and peripheral compartments.

compartment and passes from one zone to the other at rates which are governed by first order kinetics (Fig. 2.1). This model is applicable to several antirheumatic drugs and has been well described for indomethacin (Kwan *et al.*, 1976), chloroquine (McChesney *et al.*, 1967) and gold (Gerber *et al.*, 1974). Extensive tissue binding in the deep compartment is thought to explain why 40% of a dose of gold remains unexcreted two months after injection (Gerber *et al.*, 1974). Some workers have devised more complex multi-compartmental models for certain drugs but these are not widely applicable.

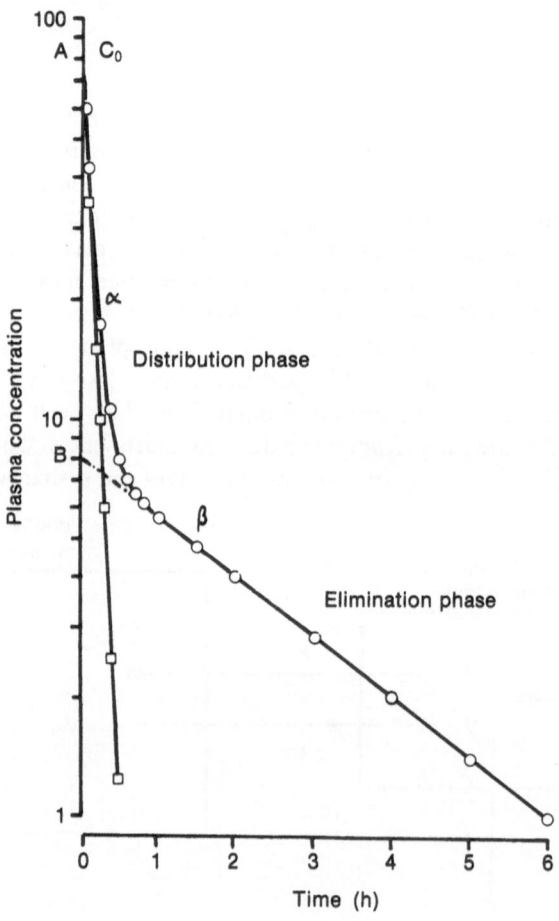

Figure 2.2 Schematic diagram of the semi-logarithmic plot of drug plasma concentration as a function of time following rapid I.V. injection (as predicted by a two-compartment model). B is the intercept at $t=0$ determined by extrapolation of the β or elimination phase. A is calculated using the method of residuals (Gibaldi and Perrier, 1975). C_0 is equal to $A+B$.

2.3.3 Plasma concentration curves

The plasma concentration curve is a useful tool from which several kinetic parameters are derived. The curve is obtained by measuring the plasma concentration of a drug several times during the distribution and elimination of a single dose. These values are then plotted on a logarithmic scale against unit time.

A single intravenous bolus is the simplest method of drug administration for pharmacokinetic analysis as it bypasses the process of drug absorption. In a one-compartment model, the plasma concentration graph is a straight line. The profile for a two-compartment model is more complex (Fig. 2.2). Following intravenous injection, there is a rapid fall in plasma concentration as the compound is distributed throughout the central and peripheral compartments. This is the alpha or distribution phase. As elimination starts to predominate over distribution, the graph enters a beta or elimination phase with a slower rate of decay. Both phases have their own half-lives which are derived from the slope of the graph. Whilst the distribution half-life is a parameter that is rarely used, the elimination half-life is often quoted.

2.3.4 Plasma elimination half-life $(t_{1/2})$

The plasma elimination half-life is defined as the time taken for the plasma concentration of a drug to fall by 50%. This remains constant provided that the drug continues to obey first-order kinetics. The half-life is derived thus:

$$t_{1/2}\beta = \frac{\log_n 2}{\beta} \tag{2.4}$$

$$t_{1/2}\beta = \frac{0.693}{\beta} \tag{2.5}$$

$$t_{1/2}\beta = \frac{0.693}{k_{el}} \tag{2.6}$$

where β = the slope of the elimination phase of the plasma concentration curve

and k_{el} = the first-order elimination rate constant.

The plasma elimination half-life is a useful indicator of the duration of action of a drug and hence the optimum frequency of administration. It also enables one to calculate the time required to reach a constant or 'steady state' plasma concentration with repeated dosing. This is the point at which drug absorption is balanced by drug elimination. If a compound is administered at a fixed dosage and interval, steady-state conditions will be reached after approximately five half-lives (van Rossum, 1968). Although there are still fluctuations in plasma drug levels after each dose, the average drug concentration remains

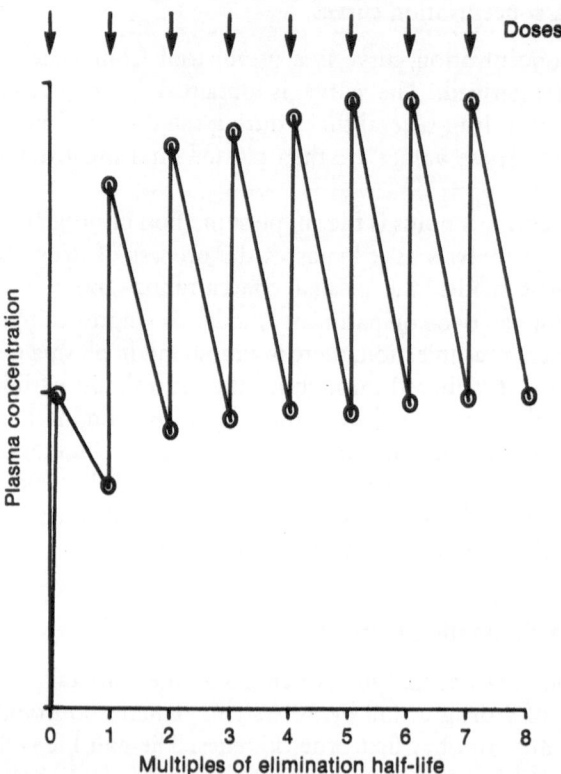

Figure 2.3 Theoretical accumulation of an intravenous drug bolus administered once every elimination half-life.

stable (Fig. 2.3). At this stage, the full therapeutic effect of a drug should be evident, provided that the dosage schedule is appropriate. Compounds with short half-lives reach steady-state conditions much quicker than those with long half-lives but their plasma drug levels fluctuate more between doses. In renal failure, the elimination half-life of many drugs is prolonged and accumulation can go on for days or even weeks. In this situation, dosage adjustments are often necessary in order to prevent the development of adverse effects. If treatment is discontinued, the same conditions apply as for drug accumulation. About five elimination half-lives must elapse before the drug will be totally eliminated from the body (Harrison *et al.*, 1977).

The plasma concentration of a drug at 'steady state' is determined by a number of factors including the elimination half-life or its counterpart, the elimination rate constant. Thus:

$$C_{ss} = \frac{FD}{V_d k_{el} T} \tag{2.7}$$

where

   C_{ss} = the steady-state drug concentration

   F = the fraction of the dose absorbed

   D = the drug dosage

   V_d = the apparent volume of distribution

   k_{el} = the first-order elimination rate constant

   T = the dosage interval

Of the five parameters that determine the drug concentration at steady state, two are controlled by the prescriber (D and T). F is the equivalent of the bioavailability and has been discussed earlier. V_d and k_{el} are the main causes of variation in the steady-state concentration.

2.3.5 Apparent volume of distribution (V_d)

The apparent volume of distribution is defined as the hypothetical volume into which a drug dose would have to be distributed in order to achieve the same concentration as that in plasma. Although it is purely a theoretical concept, V_d gives a useful indication of the extent to which a drug is distributed throughout the peripheral tissues. It may be derived from the plasma concentration curve if the drug obeys first-order kinetics:

$$V_d = \frac{D}{C_o} \qquad (2.8)$$

where V_d = the apparent volume of distribution

        D = the drug dosage

        C_o = the plasma drug concentration at zero time.

C_o is a theoretical value obtained by extrapolating the straight line of the elimination phase back to the vertical axis (Fig. 2.2). V_d can only be derived in this way if the drug is given intravenously or its systemic bioavailability is known accurately. An alternative way of calculating V_d is to measure the total area under the plasma concentration curve (AUC). Thus:

$$V_d = \frac{D}{\text{AUC}\, k_{el}} \qquad (2.9)$$

If steady state has been reached and there is no net transfer of drug from the central to peripheral compartments, then:

$$V_{d(ss)} = \frac{D}{C_{ss}} \qquad (2.10)$$

The apparent volume of distribution is an indicator of the extent of tissue binding as well as a measure of drug distribution. If a drug is avidly bound to the tissues, its clearance from the body is prolonged and the apparent volume of distribution is large.

Most of the NSAIDs are highly bound to plasma proteins and have limited volumes of distribution but this is not true for all antirheumatic agents. The antimalarial, chloroquine, is used in the treatment of connective tissue diseases and has a large volume of distribution (Mackenzie and Scherbel, 1980). It is extensively bound to tissues like the liver, lungs, kidney and heart (Di Maio and Henry, 1974). The drug also accumulates in the retina leading to retinal damage in a small proportion of patients (Bernstein *et al.*, 1963). The apparent volume of distribution is affected by factors such as age and disease. These are considered in Section 2.7.2.

2.3.6   Clearance

Creatinine clearance is a term familiar to physicians in relation to renal function. Drug clearance is a similar concept used to describe the elimination of a drug from a body system. It may be applied to plasma, blood or any body tissue from which a drug is cleared. The total body clearance is the sum of the individual clearance rates and is defined as the apparent volume from which a drug is cleared in a unit of time (ml per minute). The concept embraces drug metabolism as well as excretion but only refers to parent drug and not to metabolites.

Just as the apparent volume of distribution relates the plasma concentration of a drug to the total amount in the body, so clearance links the concentration to the rate at which the drug is eliminated from the body. In mathematical terms:

$$Cl_B = V_d \, K_{el} \tag{2.11}$$

$$= V_d \frac{0.693}{t_{1/2}} \tag{2.12}$$

where Cl_B = the total body clearance.

Clearance should not be confused with the elimination half-life although the two are related. The half-life is an indirect indicator of the rate of drug elimination and is influenced by changes in the apparent volume of distribution as well as clearance. The clearance rate is a much more reliable parameter and provides information about the factors likely to affect drug disposition. Hepatic and renal clearance are considered later in the chapter.

2.4   PLASMA DRUG LEVELS AND THERAPEUTIC EFFECT

The relevance of pharmacokinetics to antirheumatic therapy has been questioned because there is often a discrepancy between plasma drug levels and therapeutic effect. This is particularly true of the NSAIDs. Some of these drugs have half-lives which are not in harmony with the onset and duration of their therapeutic effect. Flurbiprofen has a half-life of four hours (Adams and Buckler, 1979) but only needs to be taken twice daily. Indeed, it has been suggested that twice daily dosing may be more effective than four times a day (Kowanko *et al.*, 1981). At the other end of the scale, piroxicam has an elimination half-life of 38 hours (Hobbs and Twomey, 1979) but its analgesic effects are evident within a few hours of dosing, long before the drug has accumulated in the body (Blum and Wagenhauser, 1980). Some studies have shown considerable variation in the individual response to NSAIDs, to an extent that is not compatible with known pharmacokinetic data (Huskisson *et al.*, 1976; Gall *et al.*, 1982; Scott *et al.*, 1982). Others have tried to relate plasma levels and dosage to the clinical effects of these drugs but with little success (Orme *et al.*, 1976, 1981; Grennan *et al.*, 1983).

Against this disappointing scenario must be set examples where kinetic parameters do show a relationship to clinical effects. The plasma concentration of aspirin has been correlated with both its toxic and therapeutic effects (Bardare *et al.*, 1978; Makela *et al.*, 1979) and, in a recent study in patients with rheumatoid arthritis, there was a correlation between serum naproxen levels and therapeutic effect (Day *et al.*, 1982).

How do we reconcile this conflicting evidence? There are a number of reasons why the concentration of drug in the blood may not correlate with its clinical effects. In the first place, there are serious weaknesses in the methods for assessing the activity of rheumatic disease. Pain, swelling and tenderness are the cardinal signs of joint inflammation but they are difficult to quantify. Observer errors and spontaneous variation in disease activity contribute to the difficulties of patient assessment (Lansbury *et al.*, 1962; Co-operating Clinics, 1965). In some cases a 75% shift from baseline may be necessary before a change can be ascribed to drug therapy (Lansbury *et al.*, 1962). The figure may be even greater if assessments are not carried out by the same observer and at the same time of day (Wright, 1959; Lansbury *et al.*, 1962). The selection of patients for study is also important. Predetermined entrance criteria are essential in any therapeutic trial in order to eliminate those patients who do not have active disease.

The measurement of plasma drug levels may also present problems. If a compound is converted into active metabolites then measurements of the parent compound will underestimate the amount of active drug present. Pharmacological assays usually measure the total drug concentration and fail to distinguish between bound and unbound drug. Since only the unbound fraction is 'active', the total drug concentration is unlikely to reflect the situation in the tissues. Even if unbound drug levels are measured, the correlation with therapeutic effect is not necessarily better (Day *et al.*, 1982; Grennan *et al.*, 1983). A compound may selectively concentrate at its site of action so that its effects persist long after it has disappeared from the plasma. This 'hit and run' effect is characteristic of many NSAIDs (Huskisson, 1978).

Even if we could measure tissue drug levels routinely, this would still not take account of the variation in end-organ sensitivity. In their study of the pharmacokinetics of ibuprofen, Grennan *et al.* (1983) concluded that kinetic factors were responsible for only a small proportion of the variability in the individual response to NSAIDs. This means that pharmacodynamic variables must be important. Variations in the sensitivity of tissue receptors are difficult to study directly, but the discovery of receptors on the surface of peripheral blood cells has made research into pharmacodynamics a realistic proposition. Much of this work has been done with adrenoceptors (Lees, 1981). This has revealed that receptor numbers can vary dramatically under the influence of many different factors including drug therapy. Since the changes that occur in peripheral blood receptors can be related to drug response (Ford *et al.*, 1979), it seems reasonable to assume that they reflect what is happening at the drug's site of action.

Unfortunately, this type of approach is not directly applicable to rheumatology. Antirheumatic drug receptors have not been isolated in peripheral blood cells and a major stumbling block is our uncertainty as to the precise mode of action of these drugs. Despite this, there has been some progress; most NSAIDs inhibit the action of prostaglandin synthetase and this enzyme is found in platelets as well as connective tissue. Orme *et al.* (1981) used the production of malonyldialdehyde in platelets as an index of prostaglandin synthetase activity. They found that plasma levels of indomethacin and flurbiprofen are correlated with the inhibition of malonyldialdehyde production in those who respond to treatment but not in non-responders. Whilst these findings are far from conclusive, they do suggest that differences in tissue metabolism may account for some of the variations in the response to these drugs.

2.5 METABOLISM

During the process of evolution, animal species have developed systems with the capability to dispose of harmful compounds that enter the body. These systems are sufficiently adaptable to be able to deal with most drugs and chemicals. Whilst some drugs are excreted unchanged by the kidneys, most are metabolized. Although metabolism occurs principally in the liver, it also occurs in the plasma, gut wall, lungs and kidneys.

Hepatic metabolism occurs mainly in the microsomes of the smooth endoplasmic reticulum. The major chemical reactions are hydrolysis, oxidation, reduction, and glucuronidation. Some drugs are subject to one metabolic process whereas others undergo several reactions.

Drugs are more readily absorbed in a lipid soluble rather than a polar form, but the opposite is true of their elimination. Compounds that are lipid soluble have a low renal clearance because they diffuse back through the renal tubular epithelium after glomerular filtration. Metabolizing enzymes convert nonpolar groups into polar, water-soluble metabolites which are easier to excrete. The preparation of drugs for excretion is the major function of metabolism, but there are several others.

Some drugs are converted from inactive pro-drugs into active metabolites. Most pro-drugs that are used in rheumatology were developed with the objective of reducing the incidence of dyspepsia. Benorylate is a paracetamol ester of aspirin which is absorbed intact and then broken down into two active moieties. Sulindac and fenbufen are both non-steroidal pro-drugs which are metabolized to their active constituents in the liver. Although these compounds may cause less dyspepsia, they do not abolish it because the active metabolites are able to reach the gastric mucosa via the systemic circulation.

In other cases, the metabolic process may convert an active drug into one or more active metabolites. The NSAID, phenylbutazone, is metabolized to oxyphenbutazone and γ-hydroxyphenbutazone. Oxyphenbutazone has potent anti-inflammatory properties but γ-hydroxyphenbutazone has only uricosuric effects. Some metabolites may have toxic effects; isoniazid and paracetamol produce toxic metabolites which cause liver damage if they accumulate in sufficient quantities (Mitchell *et al.*, 1974). The nephrotoxicity of salicylates and paracetamol is also due to toxic metabolites (Mitchell *et al.*, 1977).

2.5.1 Hepatic clearance

The activity of liver metabolizing enzymes may be expressed mathematically in terms of the hepatic blood clearance:

$$\text{hepatic blood clearance} = Cl_H E_H \qquad (2.13)$$

where Cl_H = the hepatic blood flow and E_H = the hepatic extraction ratio.

The hepatic blood clearance is defined as the volume of blood flowing through the liver which is cleared of drug per unit of time. It is a composite of the biliary clearance and the hepatic metabolic clearance. The extraction ratio is a measure of the efficiency with which a drug is extracted by an organ of elimination:

$$E = \frac{C_A - C_V}{C_V} \qquad (2.14)$$

where E = the extraction ratio, C_A = the concentration of drug in arterial blood entering the organ and C_V = the concentration of drug in venous blood leaving the organ.

Hepatic clearance involves several steps, any one of which may be the rate limiting factor. Drugs with a high extraction ratio (e. g. lignocaine, propranolol, tricyclic antidepressants) are efficiently removed by the hepatocyte so liver perfusion is the factor that limits their clearance. Such drugs are said to be flow dependent. For compounds with a low extraction ratio (e. g. salicylic acid, phenylbutazone), C_V is similar to C_A and changes in the hepatic blood flow have little effect on clearance. Factors that affect the rate of extraction are more important for these drugs. They include the degree of plasma protein binding, rate of hepatic metabolism and biliary clearance. A change in the rate of drug metabolism will be reflected in the half-life of compounds with a low extraction ratio but not in those that are flow dependent.

2.5.2 First-pass effect

When a drug is taken orally, it is absorbed by the gut and enters the portal venous system before passing through the liver to the systemic circulation. If a compound is extensively metabolized in the gut wall or has a high hepatic extraction ratio, very little enters the systemic circulation after its 'first pass' through the liver. The first-pass effect is of considerable importance for a drug like lignocaine whose systemic bioavailability is only 30% but of less significance in the case of propranolol which has an active metabolite, 4-hydroxy-propranolol. The oral bioavailability of a drug is related to its hepatic extraction ratio thus:

$$\text{oral bioavailability} = 1 - E_H \qquad (2.15)$$

In some cases, a significant first-pass effect can be overcome by increasing the oral dose so that the liver's extraction capacity is swamped. Another way is to administer the drug by an alternative route in order to bypass the gut. This is the reason for giving glyceryl trinitrate sublingually or transdermally.

2.5.3 Biliary excretion and enterohepatic recirculation

All drugs are excreted in the bile but some to a much greater extent than others. The rate of biliary excretion may be expressed as the biliary clearance which is comparable to the hepatic, renal or total body clearance:

$$\text{biliary drug clearance} = \frac{\text{bile flow} \times \text{concentration of drug in bile}}{\text{concentration of drug in plasma}} \qquad (2.16)$$

A drug is excreted in the bile in substantial quantities if it is polar and has a molecular weight greater than 250. Glucuronides fulfil both criteria and are the predominant metabolites in bile.

Some drugs are excreted in bile and reabsorbed in the intestine to complete an enterohepatic circulation. This applies to antirheumatic agents like sulphasalazine, indomethacin, and sulindac. Between 10 and 20% of sulphasalazine is absorbed unchanged, but most of this is re-excreted in the bile where it undergoes further enterohepatic recirculation (Das and Dubin, 1976). Indomethacin is excreted in the bile as the glucuronide which is hydrolysed by gut flora. This releases the parent compound which is then reabsorbed. The extent of this process is variable, but may account for the whole of an oral dose of indomethacin (Kwan *et al.*, 1976; Duggan and Kwan, 1979). The intermittent nature of bile flow can lead to wide fluctuations in the plasma levels of such a drug.

2.6 EXCRETION

Although some drugs are excreted in the saliva, breast milk and sweat, these routes are of little importance in comparison to biliary and renal excretion. Biliary excretion has been discussed in the previous section but, for most drugs, it is an insignificant means of clearance. The kidneys are by far the most important route for drug excretion.

If a drug is partially metabolized by the liver and partially excreted unchanged, the total clearance will be the sum of both processes:

$$\text{total drug clearance} = \text{renal clearance} + \text{hepatic clearance} \qquad (2.17)$$

Renal clearance does not take account of the excretion of metabolites, so a drug that is extensively metabolized by the liver will have a negligible renal clearance even though its metabolites may all be eliminated by the kidneys. If a drug is removed completely by glomerular filtration, its renal clearance will be equivalent to the creatinine clearance. Many compounds are secreted and absorbed by the renal tubules as well as being filtered at the glomerulus. Their overall clearance is the net result of all three processes.

2.6.1 Glomerular filtration

Only compounds with a molecular weight of less than $60\,000 - 70\,000$ can pass through the glomerular basement membrane. Plasma proteins are too large to be filtered, so only the unbound drug fraction enters the renal tubule. If the renal clearance of a drug exceeds the creatinine clearance then tubular secretion must be contributing to drug elimination.

2.6.2 Tubular secretion

Renal tubular secretion is an active process which occurs predominantly in the proximal convoluted tubule. Weak organic acids and bases are eliminated in this way by separate membrane 'pumps'. Each pump is a non-specific mechanism which can handle a number of drugs simultaneously. The simultaneous secretion of several drugs can lead to the competitive inhibition of one by another. This is the mechanism by which probenecid reduces the clearance of penicillin.

Whilst glomerular filtration is a passive process that does not remove drug bound to plasma proteins, tubular secretion is efficient enough to clear both bound and unbound fractions. Unbound drug can be removed from plasma at such a rate that there is time for dissociation of drug–protein complexes and additional drug excretion.

Changes in protein binding affect the renal clearance of a drug in much the same way as the hepatic clearance. If a drug has a high renal extraction ratio (e.g. penicillin) its clearance is dependent on renal blood flow. Drugs with a low extraction ratio (e.g. phenobarbitone) are more susceptible to factors such as a change in plasma protein binding.

2.6.3   Tubular reabsorption

Tubular reabsorption occurs throughout the length of the nephron and has an important influence on the renal clearance of water and electrolytes as well as some drugs. Molecules such as glucose, vitamins and amino acids are reabsorbed actively but the reabsorption of drugs is usually a passive process.

The ease with which a drug is reabsorbed depends on its molecular weight and degree of polarity. Polar drugs find it difficult to diffuse back across the renal tubular epithelium, just like the intestinal mucosa. A change in a drug's polarity can therefore have significant effects on its rate of excretion. Weakly acidic drugs, with a pK_a between 3.0 and 7.5, are predominantly ionized if the urinary pH is greater than 7.5. Alkalization of the urine enhances the elimination of such drugs and is the rationale of forced alkaline diuresis which is used in the treatment of aspirin poisoning (Lawson *et al.*, 1969). The same principle applies to the acidification of the urine. This enhances the elimination of drugs like amphetamine and pethidine which have a pK_a between 7.5 and 10.5.

Irrespective of pH, drug elimination may be promoted by increased urinary output. Drugs which are extensively reabsorbed by the renal tubules are flow dependent; in the presence of a diuresis, their reabsorption is reduced and drug elimination is enhanced. Weak acids and bases display flow-dependent as well as pH-dependent characteristics so that changes in both can influence the quantity of drug excreted. Forced diuresis is only of value where renal clearance accounts for a substantial proportion of drug excretion.

2.7   THE VARIABILITY OF THE HUMAN DRUG RESPONSE

Although all stages of drug handling are subject to variability, metabolism is the principal source of variation between individuals. The activity of metabolizing enzymes is subject to a number of different factors which may be broadly classified as genetic or environmental.

2.7.1   Genetic factors

Comparisons between identical and non-identical twins have shown that genetic factors have an important influence on the rate of drug metabolism. They may act via one gene (monogenic) or several (polygenic). Monogenic factors tend to have a major effect on metabolism as, for example, in the case of drug acetylation. Isoniazid, procainamide, hydrallazine and the sulphonamides are all metabolized by hepatic acetylation. A Caucasian population is

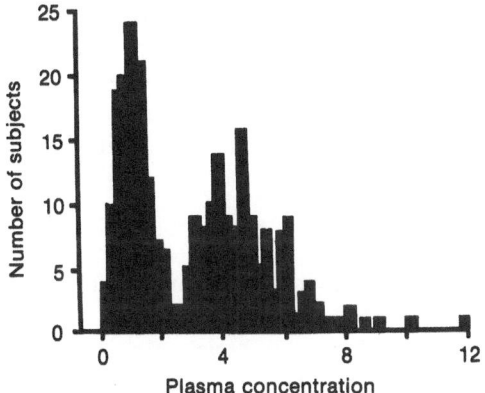

Figure 2.4 Monogenic drug metabolism. 6-hour plasma isoniazid concentrations in 483 subjects given a single oral drug dose of 9.8 mg/kg. The bimodal distribution represents slow and fast acetylation of the drug. (Adapted from Evans *et al.*, 1960.)

divided into about equal proportions of fast and slow acetylators (Karlsson and Molin, 1975). Slow acetylators have higher levels of these drugs in the plasma and are subject to a greater frequency of adverse effects (Perry *et al.*, 1967). If we plot the plasma levels of a population taking equivalent doses of a drug like isoniazid, the fast and slow acetylators are aggregated around two peaks in a bimodal distribution (Fig. 2.4). Most metabolic processes, however, are controlled by several genes. Each has a small effect which summates with others to influence the same metabolic process. Plasma levels from a population taking a drug that is subject to polygenic metabolic influences are distributed normally about a single peak (Fig. 2.5).

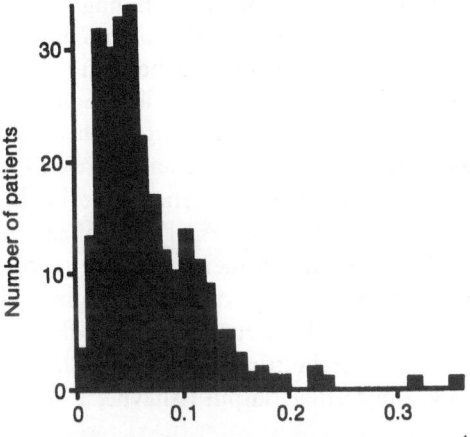

Figure 2.5 Polygenic drug metabolism. Unimodal distribution of steady-state plasma nortriptyline concentrations in 263 patients taking 25 mg of drug three times daily. (Reproduced with permission, F. Sjoqvist and Adis Press Ltd.)

Although genetic factors have an important influence on the activity of metabolizing enzymes, they have little effect on the rate of renal clearance. One exception is the tubular defect, renal tubular acidosis, which may be inherited as a dominant or recessive trait. The role of genetic factors in the control of drug absorption and distribution has yet to be clarified.

2.7.2   Environmental factors

Genetic factors combine with environmental influences to determine individual drug response. Other drug therapy, diet, habits, age, and disease can all affect the body's handling of a drug.

(a)   *Drug therapy*

The disposition of one drug may be affected by another in a number of different ways. The identification and mechanistic investigation of these 'drug interactions' represent a growth subject, which is reviewed in depth in Chapter 3.

(b)   *Diet*

Malnutrition can alter almost every pharmacokinetic process from drug absorption to excretion. Changes in tissue uptake and receptor sensitivity may also contribute to the variation in drug response (Krishnaswamy, 1978). Whilst there have been relatively few studies of drug kinetics in human malnutrition, some trends have emerged.

Patients who are markedly underweight generally have hypoalbuminaemia which leads to a reduction in plasma protein binding. Reduced protein binding increases the rate of drug delivery to the tissues but also enhances drug clearance (Levy, 1976). These changes have been shown for both tetracycline (Shastri and Krishnaswamy, 1976) and phenylbutazone (Krishnaswamy *et al.*, 1981), although the net outcome was different for these drugs when measured in terms of apparent volume of distribution; an increase for tetracycline and a reduction for phenylbutazone. This difference is probably due to changes in tissue binding and illustrates the dangers of generalizing about the effects of disease on different drugs. Although there are some reports of impaired drug metabolism in malnutrition, liver function seems to be well preserved until a late stage (Krishnaswamy, 1978). Drugs which are flow-dependent are most likely to be affected, since malnutrition can impair hepatic and renal blood flow by a reduction in the cardiac output (Alleyne, 1966).

(c)   *Habits*

Cigarette smoking, alcohol, and caffeine are all potent inducers of liver enzyme activity as measured by the rate of antipyrine metabolism (Vestal *et al.*, 1975). Nicotine can induce its own metabolism and that of drugs like theophylline (Jenne *et al.*, 1975) and pentazocine (Keeri-Szanto and Pomeroy, 1971). Alcohol may enhance or inhibit the metabolism of other drugs depending on the pattern of drinking. A 'binge' of alcohol will potentiate the effects of phenobarbitone by inhibiting metabolism (Rubin *et al.*, 1970) whilst chronic alcohol abuse tends to induce liver enzymes (Misra *et al.*, 1971). The development of hepatic cirrhosis will reduce or negate the latter effect.

(d) *Age*

(i) Absorption

From infancy to senescence, changes occur in the handling of drugs and these factors can have important implications for the treatment of disease. Neonates undergo a rapid period of maturation with changes in gastric pH, gut motility and biliary function. It is not surprising, therefore, that drug absorption in a newborn baby may differ considerably from that in an older child or adult. The absorption of some drugs is delayed in infancy (e. g. paracetamol – Levy *et al.*, 1975) and in others the overall absorption is reduced (e. g. phenobarbitone – Wallin *et al.*, 1974). Many drugs, like the sulphonamides, are unaffected (Sereni *et al.*, 1968), and some are even absorbed more efficiently (e.g. penicillin – Huang and High, 1953). The percutaneous absorption of lipid-soluble drugs is enhanced in neonates, and this has been the cause of several accidental deaths. Some of these have occurred because of the rapid absorption of boric acid from skin creams used for nappy rash.

Whilst neonates show erratic changes in absorption, older children absorb drugs just as quickly and completely as adults. In the elderly, there are several theoretical reasons why drug absorption might be reduced. Delayed gastric emptying, relative achlorhydria and poor intestinal motility all occur in old age, and each is capable of reducing drug absorption. Active transport mechanisms are also impaired, but this has little effect on bioavailability since most drugs are absorbed passively. In spite of these theoretical reasons, there is little evidence of a major change in drug absorption in old age. Antirheumatic drugs such as phenylbutazone and indomethacin are absorbed normally in the elderly (Traeger *et al.*, 1973; Triggs *et al.*, 1975).

(ii) Distribution

Age affects the distribution of drugs via changes in body composition and drug binding. The total body water makes up 85% of the body weight in a premature baby, 70% in a full-term infant, and only 60% in an adolescent or adult. Thus, babies require proportionately larger doses of water-soluble drugs (e.g. penicillins, cephalosporins, aminoglycosides) in order to achieve the same plasma drug levels as adults. Protein binding is reduced in infancy because of lower serum albumin levels and the reduced binding capacity of fetal albumin (Morselli, 1976). These changes raise the proportion of unbound drug in the plasma and increase the apparent volume of distribution. Where a drug is highly protein bound and has a small volume of distribution (e.g. salicylate) this can lead to significant potentiation of drug effects (Koch-Weser and Sellers, 1976). For a drug that is weakly protein bound and widely distributed (e.g. digoxin) the consequences are less certain. The binding of digoxin in peripheral tissues is much greater for neonates and children than for adults. This leads to a further increase in the drug's apparent volume of distribution and explains why children can tolerate proportionately larger doses than adults (Reuning *et al.*, 1973). At the other end of the scale, the elderly need less digoxin than younger adults because of a lower lean body weight, poorer renal function, and reduced tissue binding of the drug (Ewy *et al.*, 1969).

(iii)   Metabolism

In the neonatal and perinatal periods, hepatic metabolism is not fully developed and drug clearance may be impaired. This applies particularly to the processes of oxidation and glucuronidation, and affects drugs like paracetamol, salicylate, and phenylbutazone (Bochner *et al.*, 1978). The failure of conjugation of chloramphenicol can lead to cardiovascular collapse and the so-called 'grey baby syndrome'. Microsomal enzyme systems mature rapidly within the first month of life and by one year of age they are comparable to those of adulthood. Indeed, some drugs like diazoxide, theophylline, and carbamazepine are metabolized more rapidly in childhood.

Just as the efficiency of hepatic metabolism improves in childhood so it declines in old age. Hepatic blood flow falls in the elderly so the metabolism of flow dependent drugs also declines with age (Castleden *et al.*, 1975). The effects are less consistent for drugs with a low extraction ratio. Antipyrine metabolism is unaffected by hepatic blood flow (Branch *et al.*, 1974; Nies *et al.*, 1976) but its clearance is also impaired in the elderly (Vestal *et al.*, 1975). A number of groups have reported prolonged half-lives in old age (Jori *et al.*, 1972; Traeger *et al.*, 1973; Briant *et al.*, 1975), but these results are difficult to interpret because of failure to measure drug clearance. Although the two are closely related, one cannot assume that a change in half-life is equivalent to an alteration in drug clearance. This is well illustrated by a study by Klotz *et al.* (1975). They showed that the elimination half-life of diazepam was prolonged in the elderly, but since the apparent volume of distribution also rose, there was no change in drug clearance. This emphasizes the point that clearance is superior to half-life as an indicator of drug elimination.

(iv)   Excretion

Ageing affects renal function and the renal clearance of drugs. Indeed, the deterioration in renal function is the most important kinetic change of old age. The creatinine clearance is depressed in infancy but rises to a maximum at the age of about six months. It remains high during childhood but declines with age at an annual rate of about 1% (Crooks *et al.*, 1976). Whilst a healthy young adult may have a creatinine clearance of 80–120 ml.min^{-1}, the figure is only 20–40 ml.min^{-1}, in an elderly person with no renal disease. This decline in renal function may be concealed by a normal serum creatinine because the production of creatinine falls with age.

Dosage adjustments are necessary in old age for drugs with a low therapeutic ratio which either have active metabolites or are excreted unchanged. Recent experience with the NSAID benoxaprofen has emphasized the dangers of drug accumulation in the elderly. Kinetic studies revealed an elimination half-life of 30 – 35 hours in normal adults, but this was extended to 111 hours in subjects over 75 years (Hamdy *et al.*, 1982). In retrospect, it was not surprising that the drug produced significant adverse effects in such patients (Taggart and Alderdice, 1982).

(e) *Disease*

Despite the fact that drugs are primarily used to treat illness, surprisingly little is known about the effects of disease on drug handling. Most of the work in this area has been done in cardiac, liver, and renal disease.

(i) Heart

Cardiac failure can affect the metabolism of drugs with a high extraction ratio (e.g. lignocaine, propranolol) by effects on liver blood flow. In one study, the half-life of lignocaine was 10.2 hours for a group of patients with cardiac failure, but only 1.4 hours for matched controls (Prescott *et al.*, 1976). The effect on a drug with a low extraction ratio (antipyrine) was much less. Heart disease may also affect the response to cardioactive drugs like digoxin. It increases the sensitivity of the myocardium so that cardiotoxicity becomes more frequent and more severe (Beller *et al.*, 1971; Smith and Willerson, 1971).

(ii) Liver

Since the liver is the main organ of metabolism, one might expect that liver disease would affect drug metabolism. This is true for some drugs and diseases, but not all. Although cardiac failure is the main cause of a reduction in the metabolism of flow dependent drugs, liver cirrhosis can have a similar effect through the development of portal hypertension. Portal-systemic shunting can also lower drug clearance by reducing the extent of first-pass metabolism. Drugs with a low extraction ratio are influenced more by changes in hepatocellular function and protein binding.

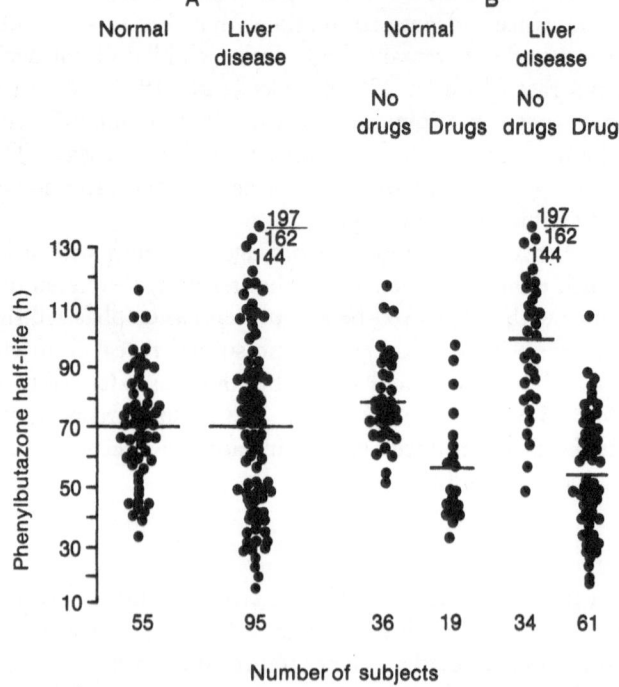

Figure 2.6 Plasma elimination half-life of phenylbutazone in patients with liver disease and in matched controls. The data were analysed as a whole (A) and separately according to other drug therapy (B). (Adapted from Levi *et al.*, 1968.)

Kinetic studies in liver disease have produced some confusing and contradictory results. One reason for these discrepancies is the failure to standardize drug therapy. Levi *et al.* (1968) found no difference in the half-life of phenylbutazone in patients with liver disease when compared with controls. However, when the figures were analysed according to other drug therapy, significant differences did emerge (Fig. 2.6). Patients who were taking other medication were no different from matched controls, but patients and controls who were taking phenylbutazone alone were quite distinct. Half-lives were prolonged in both of these groups, and particularly in those with liver disease. These findings suggest that enzyme induction by other drug therapy can compensate for the impairment of metabolism in liver disease.

The effect of liver disease on protein binding provides another source of confusion. Plasma protein binding is diminished in liver disease but the reduction in serum albumin accounts for only a proportion of this change (Koch-Weser and Sellers, 1976). Liver damage also appears to cause qualitative changes in serum albumin which affect its binding capacity. Together, these changes increase the proportion of unbound drug in the plasma which expands the apparent volume of distribution.

Some drugs which are metabolized in the liver cause hepatic damage if taken in excessive dosage. This leads to a vicious circle where further liver damage occurs as more drug accumulates. In paracetamol overdosage, changes in the drug's half-life have proved to be a useful prognostic indicator which can assist the physician in his choice of therapy (Prescott *et al.*, 1971).

(iii)   Kidney

Since the kidneys are the main organs of excretion, renal disease can have a major influence on drug handling, particularly in those compounds that are excreted unchanged. Uraemia affects drug disposition in a number of different ways. Drug absorption may be reduced if the diarrhoea which occurs in renal failure is severe. Plasma protein binding is reduced because of the impairment of the binding affinity of albumin and the reduction in its serum concentration secondary to proteinuria. A highly bound drug like phenytoin is significantly displaced from its binding sites in uraemia (Reidenberg *et al.*, 1971). The rise in the proportion of unbound drug causes a compensatory increase in drug clearance so that there is a fall in the total drug concentration, even though the amount of free drug remains the same. This may explain why uraemic epileptics may respond to lower plasma phenytoin (total) levels than usual (Odar-Cederlof *et al.*, 1970).

Whilst the volume of distribution of phenytoin is increased, the opposite is true for digoxin. Uraemia impairs the *tissue* binding of digoxin which overrides the effect of changes in *plasma* binding (Koup *et al.*, 1975). Some drug effects may be enhanced by an increase in tissue sensitivity (e.g. chlorpromazine, narcotic analgesics) but the most profound effects of renal disease are due to changes in drug excretion.

Although some drugs are secreted and/or absorbed by the renal tubules, the creatinine clearance remains a reliable guide to the renal clearance. Dosage reductions are only necessary if a drug has a low toxic:therapeutic ratio and either has active metabolites or is excreted unchanged. Such a reduction may be achieved by increasing the dosage interval or reducing each dose. Increasing the dosage interval lowers the trough plasma level but a reduction in dose reduces the peak. A combination of both maintains a smoother plasma concentration overall. An increase in the dosage interval is the normal adjustment with antibiotics like the aminoglycosides although a combination of measures will do equally well. With cardiotoxic drugs like digoxin or procainamide, dosage reduction is more appropriate to avoid peaks, which can cause cardiac arrhythmias. Dosage reductions of any form are rarely necessary unless the renal function falls below 50% of normal. Nomograms are available to calculate the dosage of drugs like digoxin and gentamicin in renal failure but these are of limited value (Johnston *et al.*, 1979). There is no substitute for the regular observation of the patient and estimation of plasma drug levels.

NSAIDs with a long half-life (e.g. phenylbutazone) should be avoided in patients with significant renal impairment unless they are extensively metabolized to inactive metabolites (piroxicam). Some NSAIDs may actually accentuate renal failure. Two groups have reported cases of acute renal shutdown after treatment with indomethacin in patients with underlying renal damage (Walshe and Venuto, 1979; Tan *et al.*, 1979). If this is a true drug effect, it could be due to the inhibition of renal prostaglandins which are important mediators of renin secretion and regulators of renal blood flow. Support for this idea has come from studies of creatinine clearance and renal blood flow in patients taking various NSAIDs (Kimberly and Plotz, 1977; Kimberly *et al.*, 1978). Chloroquine and penicillamine must be used in reduced dosage in uraemia because they are partially excreted by the kidney. Gold has a half-life of several days and is contraindicated in uraemia. Generally, it is wise to avoid all compounds that are excreted unchanged.

(iv)   Lungs

Respiratory disease may also affect drug disposition (du Souich *et al.*, 1978). Hypoxia can alter hepatic and renal clearance by effects on protein binding but the overall effect may be difficult to predict. Work with animals has shown that acute hypoxia decreases the hepatic clearance of some drugs (Cumming and Mannering, 1970) whilst chronic hypoxia increases it (Medina and Merritt, 1970). Studies in dogs have demonstrated changes in the myocardial concentration and distribution of digoxin under hypoxic conditions (Harron *et al.*, 1982). Pulmonary hypertension may also affect drug handling by effects on the cardiac output. In general, severe respiratory disease is most likely to affect flow-dependent drugs and those which are excreted unchanged.

(v)   Rheumatic disease

The effect of rheumatic inflammation on drug disposition is largely unknown. Studies with salicylate suggest that its apparent volume of distribution is reduced in rheumatoid disease (Koch-Weser *et al.*, 1980) whilst phenylbutazone kinetics seem unaffected by it (Aarbakke *et al.*, 1977). A study of steroid kinetics in children has reported a significant increase in the half-life of prednisolone in systemic lupus erythematosus when compared with non-inflammatory diseases (Green *et al.*, 1978).

The kinetics of propranolol have been investigated in patients with chronic inflammatory disease and significant increases, about fourfold, in peak plasma concentrations were observed in rheumatoid arthritics with an erythrocyte sedimentation rate exceeding 20 mm hr^{-1}(Schneider *et al.*, 1979). The clinical significance of this change is probably minor for a drug like propranolol with a wide therapeutic ratio (Schneider and Bishop, 1982) but the disposition of drugs with a narrow therapeutic ratio (e.g. lignocaine) merits investigation in patients with chronic rheumatic inflammation.

2.8 CHRONOPHARMACOLOGY AND CHRONOTHERAPEUTICS

In Section 2.7, we considered some of the factors which contribute to the variability in the human drug response. It is now clear that the time at which a drug is administered may also be important. Chronopharmacology is the study of the influence of biological rhythms on the pharmacokinetics and pharmacodynamics of a drug. It is a discipline which has emerged from the study of circadian rhythms and their effect on biological activity. Much of the early work was carried out in the field of endocrinology, but more recently this approach has been applied to other specialities, including rheumatology.

2.8.1 Chronopharmacokinetics

Time-related changes in pharmacokinetics have been documented for a number of drugs, some of which are listed in Table 2.2. Much of this work

TABLE 2.2
Some drugs in which chronopharmacokinetic changes have been documented

Groups	Drugs
Analgesics/NSAIDs	Aspirin Sodium salicylate Paracetamol Phenacetin Amidopyrine Indomethacin
Tranquillizers/Anti-depressants	Diazepam Clorazepate Hexobarbitone Nortriptyline
Cardioactive agents	β-Methyl digoxin Propranolol
Bronchodilators	Aminophylline Theophylline Theophylline sustained release
Antibiotics	Sulphanilamide Sulfamyazine Ampicillin Erythromycin
Miscellaneous	cisplatinum Ferrous sulpathe Lithium carbonate Phenytoin Hydrocortisone Prednisolone

consisted of single-dose studies in normal volunteers. In most instances the effects were substantial and of potential practical importance. Prednisolone and indomethacin are examples of relevance to rheumatology.

The diurnal variation in adrenal cortical activity has been appreciated for many years, so it is no surprise that corticosteroids were an early choice for chronokinetic study in man. In 1970, Morselli *et al.* reported a diurnal variation in the rate of disappearance of intravenous cortisol from the plasma of psychiatric patients. Plasma clearance was enhanced when the drug was given at 4 p. m. instead of 8 a. m., and this difference was reflected in the drug's elimination half-life. Recent work has shown that the kinetics of prednisolone are also subject to diurnal variation. English *et al.* (1983) have shown that bioavailability and unbound plasma concentrations are maximal if dosing is between 6 a. m. and noon. The drug's half-life is correspondingly shortened in response to the high concentrations of free drug. These findings are partly explained by the diurnal variation in concentrations of transcortin, the plasma protein that binds to corticosteroids (Angeli *et al.*, 1978). Circadian changes in liver metabolism and adrenal activity may also be relevant. The clinical significance of these findings is uncertain, but the implication is that steroids are likely to be more potent, as well as less toxic, when given in the morning.

Clench *et al.* (1981) have studied indomethacin kinetics after a single drug dose given at five different times of day (Fig. 2.7). Peak plasma concentra-

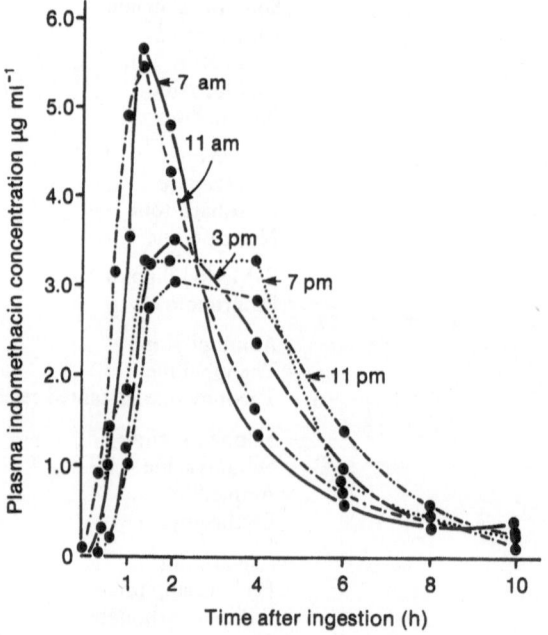

Figure 2.7 Plasma indomethacin concentrations in nine healthy subjects who received a single oral drug dose (100 mg) at five different times of day. (Reproduced with permission, Clench *et al.*, 1981 and Springer–Verlag.)

tions are higher when the drug is taken in the morning (7 a. m. or 11 a. m.). Absorption and elimination rates are also maximal but the bioavailability remains unchanged. Indomethacin peaks are often associated with adverse effects (Turakka and Airaksinen, 1974; Alvan *et al.*, 1975), so the time of administration may influence the frequency of drug toxicity. Large doses of indomethacin can be given at night with few adverse effects for treating early morning stiffness (Huskisson *et al.*, 1970). It has been suggested that sleep may mask the drug's toxic effects, but this study suggests that chronokinetic factors are also important. A recent study of the chronopharmacokinetics of indomethacin suppositories has failed to demonstrate such variation so the circadian rhythm may be dependent on the function of the upper gastro-intestinal tract (Taggart *et al.*, 1986).

Although the importance of chronokinetics is now recognized, little is known of the causative mechanisms. Drug absorption may be subject to circadian variation, particularly with acidic drugs like the NSAIDs. Plasma protein levels undergo rhythmic changes throughout a 24-hour period (Angeli *et al.*, 1978; Touitou *et al.*, 1979), with consequent variation in drug distribution and clearance. Animal studies have shown that the activity of liver enzymes has a diurnal rhythm, so this may affect drug metabolism (Radzia-lowski and Bousquet, 1968). Changes in renal enzyme activity can affect tubular function and secretion. With the cytotoxic drug, cisplatinum, maximal therapeutic effect appears to coincide with a minimal danger from nephrotoxicity (Hrushesky *et al.*, 1980). With drugs like salicylate, circadian changes in renal excretion are mediated by the rhythmic variation in urinary pH and maximal drug excretion follows night-time administration (Reinberg *et al.*, 1967, 1975).

2.8.2 Chronesthesy

Circadian rhythms may influence the pharmacodynamics as well as the pharmacokinetics of drug therapy. The effect of these rhythms on our sensitivity to drugs and other environmental factors is known as chronesthesy. In some instances, it can be ascribed to changes in tissue receptors (Hughes *et al.*, 1976; Wirz-Justice *et al.*, 1980), but various mechanisms are likely to be involved. There is evidence of a rhythmic variation in the reactivity of the bronchial mucosa to drugs and allergens (Reinberg *et al.*, 1971; Smolensky *et al.*, 1981). Similar changes have been shown in allergic skin reactions and in the duration of local anaesthesia (Pollmann, 1981; Reinberg and Reinberg, 1977).

Changes in pharmacokinetic and pharmacodynamic parameters can have an important influence on the outcome of drug therapy, but it is a mistake to assume that circadian rhythms always act in unison. Peak plasma levels may coincide with a drop in end-organ sensitivity, which is another reason why drug kinetics may not necessarily predict therapeutic effect (Smolensky *et al.*, 1981).

2.8.3 Chronotherapeutics

Chronopharmacology has contributed to our understanding of the variability in the human drug response, but it may also be of practical therapeutic value (Editorial, 1978). The L1210 mouse has provided a dramatic example of the potential benefits of chronotherapeutics. The mortality rate from leukaemia in this animal model can be reduced by up to 80% with the use of a chemo-therapy regime that varies sinusoidally with time (Scheving et al., 1977). Tumour rhythms have also been described in human neoplasms (Gautherie and Gros, 1977), but it remains to be seen whether practical benefits will accrue from the approach.

Promising results have already been achieved using chronoradiotherapy in human oro-facial tumours. Gupta and Deka (1975) have timed the administration of radiotherapy according to the circadian variation in tumour temperature. Seventy per cent regression rates were achieved when treatment was given at the peak of tumour temperature, but only 30% when it was given eight hours earlier (Deka, 1975).

If chronoradiotherapy is in its infancy, then chronocorticotherapy has entered a healthy childhood. Some of the early work in chronotherapeutics concerned the use of corticosteroids in the treatment of inflammatory diseases like asthma and rheumatoid arthritis. Physicians are generally aware that adrenal suppression may be minimized if corticosteroids are given as a single dose in the morning (Nichols et al., 1965). It is perhaps less well known that the drug's therapeutic effect may also be influenced by its time of administration.

Several studies have shown that bronchodilatation is maximal when steroids are given as a once daily, morning dose (Reinberg et al., 1974, 1977). Rheumatologists have been reluctant to adopt the same approach because morning stiffness is a common problem in inflammatory arthritis, and bedtime dosing is regarded as the most effective way of managing it (De Andrade et al., 1964). Theoretically, a morning dose of prednisolone should be just as effective as a night time dose for the treatment of early morning stiffness (Kowanko et al., 1982), but this does not appear to be borne out by a recent controlled trial (De Silva et al., 1984).

Steroids are widely used for their immunosuppressive as well as for their anti-inflammatory properties. Cellular immune responses display circadian rhythms with a peak of activity at 7 a. m. (Cove-Smith et al., 1978). This may explain why the commonest time for the rejection of a renal transplant is in the early morning (Knapp et al., 1979). It may also explain why recipients who take their immunosuppressive therapy in divided doses seem to do better than those who take their medication at night (Knapp et al., 1980). If this is the explanation, then it may be best to give all immunosuppressives as a single dose in the morning. This has been the practice of the Renal Unit in Belfast which has the highest rate of graft survival in the UK (McGeown et al., 1977).

Whilst there may be other explanations for these results, they have been striking enough to prompt further study into the chronotherapy of immunosuppression (Salaman, 1983).

Immune responses are pertinent to rheumatology as well as to nephrology. Harkness *et al.* (1982) have shown circadian rhythmicity in several aspects of cellular immunity in patients with rheumatoid arthritis. They have also found corresponding changes in clinical disease activity. Signs and symptoms such as joint stiffness, grip strength, and joint tenderness are at their worst in the early morning (Wright, 1959; Scott, 1960; Kowanko *et al.*, 1981). Traditionally this has been blamed on the period of overnight inactivity, but it may, in fact, be due to increased activity in the immune system. As interest grows in the subject of chronoimmunology, more evidence is accumulating for circadian rhythmicity in various aspects of the immune response (Ritchie *et al.*, 1983). These findings are likely to have important implications for the speciality of rheumatology.

2.9 REFERENCES

Aarbakke, J., Bakke, O. M., Milde, E. J. and Davies, D. S. (1977) Disposition and oxidative metabolism of phenylbutazone in man. *Eur. J. Clin. Pharmacol.*, 11, 359–66.

Adams, K. R. H., Halliday, L. D. C., Sibeon, R. G., Baber, N., Littler, T. and Orme, M. L'E. (1982) A clinical and pharmacokinetic study of indomethacin in standard and slow release formulations. *Br. J. Clin. Pharmacol.*, 14, 286–9.

Adams, S. S. and Buckler, J. W. (1979) Ibuprofen and flurbiprofen. *Clin. Rheum. Dis.*, 5, 359–80.

Alleyne, G. A. O. (1966) Cardiac function in severely malnourished Jamaican children. *Clin. Sci.*, 30, 553–62.

Alvan, G., Orme, M., Bertilsson, L., Ekstrand, R. and Palmer, L. (1975) Pharmacokinetics of indomethacin in man. *Clin. Pharmacol. Ther.*, 18, 364–73.

Angeli, A., Frajria, R., De Paoli, R., Fonzo, D. and Ceresa, F. (1978) Diurnal variation of prednisolone binding to serum corticosteroid-binding globulin in man. *Clin. Pharmacol. Ther.*, 23, 47–53.

Baber, N., Sibeon, R., Laws, E., Halliday, L., Orme, M. and Littler, T. (1980) Indomethacin in rheumatoid arthritis: comparison of oral and rectal dosing. *Br. J. Clin. Pharmacol.*, 10, 387–92.

Bachmann, F. (1980) Synovial fluid concentrations of piroxicam. *Rheumatology in the Eighties: an advance in therapy – piroxicam* (ed. J. A. Boyle), Excerpta Medica, Princeton.

Bardare, M., Cislaghi, G. U., Mandelli, M. and Sereni, F. (1978) Value of monitoring plasma salicylate levels in treating juvenile rheumatoid arthritis. *Arch. Dis. Child.*, 53, 381–5.

Beller, G. A., Smith, T. W., Abelmann, W. H., Haber, E. and Hood, W. B. (1971) Digitalis intoxication. A prospective study with serum level correlations. *N. Engl. J. Med.*, 284, 989–97.

Bergstrom, R. F., Kay, D. R., Harkcom, T. M. and Wagner, J. G. (1981) Penicillamine kinetics in normal subjects. *Clin. Pharmacol. Ther.*, 30, 404–13.

Bernstein, H., Zvaifler, N., Rubin, M. and Mansour, A. M. (1963) The ocular deposition of chloroquine. *Invest. Opthalmol.*, 2, 384–92.

Binnion, P. F. (1974) The absorption of digoxin tablets. *Clin. Pharmacol. Ther.*, **16**, 807–12.

Bird, H. A., Ring, E. F. J. and Bacon, P. A. (1979) A thermographic and clinical comparison of three intra-articular steroid preparations in rheumatoid arthritis. *Ann. Rheum. Dis.*, **38**, 36–9.

Blum, W. and Wagenhauser, F. (1980) The speed of onset of action of piroxicam in patients with osteoarthritis: a placebo controlled study. *Rheumatology in the Eighties: an advance in therapy – piroxicam* (ed. J. A. Boyle), Excerpta Medica, Princeton.

Bochner, F., Carruthers, G., Kampmann, J. and Steiner, J. (1978) *Handbook of Clinical Pharmacology*, Little Brown, Boston.

Branch, R. A., Shand, D. G., Wilkinson, G. R. and Nies, A. S. (1974) Increased clearance of antipyrine and D-propranolol after phenobarbital treatment in the monkey. *J. Clin. Invest.*, **53**, 1101–7.

Briant, R. H., Liddle, D. E., Dorrington, R. and Williams, F. M. (1975) Plasma half-life of two analgesic drugs in young and elderly adults. *N. Z. Med. J.*, **82**, 136–7.

Buchanan, W. W., Rooney, P. J. and Rennie, J. A.N. (1979) Aspirin and the salicylates. *Clin. Rheum. Dis.*, **5**, 499–540.

Castleden, C. M., Kaye, C. M. and Parsons, R. L. (1975) The effect of age on plasma levels of propranolol and practolol in man. *Br. J. Clin. Pharmacol.*, **2**, 303–6.

Clench, J., Reinberg, A., Dziewanowska, Z., Ghata, J. and Smolensky, M. (1981) Circadian changes in the bioavailability and effects of indomethacin. *Eur. J. Clin. Pharmacol.*, **20**, 359–69.

Co-operating Clinics Committee of the American Rheumatism Association (1965) A seven day variability study of 499 patients with peripheral rheumatoid arthritis. *Arthr. Rheum.*, **8**, 302–35.

Cove-Smith, J. R., Kabler, P., Pownall, R. and Knapp, M. S. (1978) Circadian variation in an immune response in man. *Br. Med. J.*, **ii**, 253–4.

Crooks, J., O'Malley, K. and Stevenson, I. H. (1976) Pharmacokinetics in the elderly. *Clin. Pharmacokinet.*, **1**, 280–96.

Crosland-Taylor, P., Keeling, D. H. and Cromie, B. W. (1965) A trial of slow-release tablets of ferrous sulphate. *Curr. Ther. Res.*, **7**, 244–8.

Cumming, J. F. and Mannering, G. T. (1970) Effect of phenobarbital administration on the oxygen requirement for hexobarbital metabolism in the isolated, perfused rat liver and in the intact rat. *Biochem. Pharmacol.*, **19**, 973–8.

Das, K. M. and Dubin, R. (1976) Clinical pharmacokinetics of sulphasalazine. *Clin. Pharmacokinet.*, **1**, 406–25.

Day, R. O., Furst, D. E., Dromgoole, S. H., Kamm, B., Roe, R. and Paulus, H. E. (1982) Relationship of serum naproxen concentration to efficacy in rheumatoid arthritis. *Clin. Pharmacol. Ther.*, **31**, 733–40.

DeAndrade, J. R., McCormick, J. N. and Hill, A. G. S. (1964) Small doses of prednisolone in the management of rheumatoid arthritis. *Ann. Rheum. Dis.*, **23**, 158–62.

Deka, A. C. (1975) Application of chronobiology to radiotherapy of tumours of the oral cavity. Thesis, *Postgrad. Inst. Med. Educ. Res.*, Chandigarh, India.

De Silva, M., Binder, A. and Hazleman, B. (1984) The timing of prednisolone dosage and its effect on morning stiffness in rheumatoid arthritis. *Ann. Rheum. Dis.*, **43**, 790–3.

Dew, M. J., Hughes, P., Harries, A. D., Williams, G., Evans, B. K. and Rhodes, J. (1982) Maintenance of remission in ulcerative colitis with oral preparation of 5-amino salicylic acid. *Br. Med. J.*, **285**, 1012.

DiMaio, V. J.M. and Henry, L. D. (1974) Chloroquine poisoning. *South. Med. J.*, **67**, 1031–5.

Duggan, D. E. and Kwan, K. C. (1979) Enterohepatic recirculation of drugs as a determinant of therapeutic ratio. *Drug. Metab. Rev.*, 9, 21–4.

Editorial (1978) Chronotherapeutics, a new clinical science. *Br. Med. J.*, i, 1376.

English, J., Dunne, M. and Marks, V. (1983) Diurnal variation in prednisolone kinetics. *Clin. Pharmacol. Ther.*, 33, 381–5.

Evans, D. A. P., Manley, K. A. and McKusick, V. A. (1960) Genetic control of isoniazid metabolism in man. *Br. Med. J.*, ii, 485–91.

Ewy, G. A., Chapman, C. and Hayter, C. J. (1969) Digoxin metabolism in the elderly. *Circulation*, 44, 810–4.

Ford, A. R., Aronson, J. K., Grahame-Smith, D. G. and Carver, J. G. (1979) Changes in cardiac glycoside receptor sites, rubidium uptake and intracellular sodium concentrations in the erythrocytes of patients receiving digoxin during the early phases of treatment of cardiac failure in regular rhythm and of atrial fibrillation. *Br. J. Clin. Pharmacol.*, 8, 125–34.

Gall, E. P., Caperton, E. M., McComb, J. E. *et al.* (1982) Clinical comparison of ibuprofen, fenoprofen calcium, naproxen and tolmetin sodium in rheumatoid arthritis. *J. Rheumatol.*, 9, 402–7.

Gautherie, M. and Gros, C. (1977) Circadian rhythm alteration of skin temperature in breast cancer. *Chronobiologia*, 4, 1–17.

Gerber, R. C., Paulus, H. E., Jennrich, R. I. *et al.* (1974) Gold kinetics following aurothiomalate therapy: use of a whole-body radiation counter. *J. Lab. Clin. Med.*, 83, 778–89.

Gibaldi, M. and Perrier, D. (1975) Drugs and the pharmaceutical sciences. *Pharmacokinetics*, Vol. 1, Marcel Dekker, New York.

Green, O. C., Winter, R. J., Kawahara, F. S. *et al.* (1978) Pharmacokinetic studies of prednisolone in children. *J. Pediatr.*, 93, 299–303.

Grennan, D. M., Aarons, L., Siddiqui, M., Richards, M., Thompson, R. and Higham, C. (1983) Dose–response study with ibuprofen in rheumatoid arthritis: clinical and pharmacokinetic findings. *Br. J. Clin. Pharmacol.*, 15, 311–16.

Gupta, B. D. and Deka, A. C. (1975) Application of chronobiology to radiotherapy of tumor of oral cavity. *Chronobiologia*, 2 (Suppl. 1), 125.

Hamdy, R. C., Murnane, B., Perera, N., Woodcock, K. and Koch, I. M. (1982) The pharmacokinetics of benoxaprofen in elderly subjects. *Eur. J. Rheum. Inflamm.*, 5, 69–75.

Harkness, J. A. L., Richter, M. B., Panayi, G. S. *et al.* (1982) Circadian variation in disease activity in rheumatoid arthritis. *Br. Med. J.*, 284, 551–4.

Harrison, D. C., Meffin, P. J. and Winkle, R. A. (1977) Clinical pharmacokinetics of antiarrhythmic drugs. *Prog. Cardiovasc. Dis.*, 20, 217–42.

Harron, D. W. G., Swanton, J. G., Collier, P. S. and Cullen, A. B. (1982) Digoxin distribution between plasma and myocardium in hypoxic and non-hypoxic dogs. *Experentia*, 38, 839–40.

Heilmann, K. (1978) *Therapeutic Systems – Pattern-specific Drug Delivery: Concept and Development*, Georg Theime, Stuttgart.

Heizer, W. D., Smith, T. W. and Goldfinger, S. E. (1971) Absorption of digoxin in patients with malabsorption syndromes. *N. Engl. J. Med.*, 285, 257–9.

Hobbs, D. C. and Twomey, T. M. (1979) Piroxicam pharmacokinetics in man: aspirin and antacid interaction studies. *J. Clin. Pharmacol.*, 19, 270–81.

Hrushesky, W., Levi, F. and Kennedy, B. J. (1980) Cis-diammine-dichloroplatinum (DPP) toxicity to the human kidney reduced by circadian timing. *Proc. Am. Soc. Clin. Oncol.*, 21, C45.

Huang, N. N. and High, R. H. (1953) Comparison of serum levels following the administration of oral and parenteral preparations of penicillin to infants and children of various age groups. *J. Pediatr.*, 42, 657–68.

Hughes, A., Jacabon, H. J., Wagner, R. K. and Jungblut, P. W. (1976) Ovarian independent fluctuations of estradiol receptor levels in mammalian tissues. *Mol. Cell. Endocrinol.*, 5, 379–88.

Huskisson, E. C., Woolf, D. L., Balme, H. W., Scott, J. and Franklyn, S. (1976) Four new anti-inflammatory drugs: responses and variations. *Br. Med. J.*, i, 1048–9.

Huskisson, E. C. (1978) Non-steroidal anti-inflammatory analgesics: basic clinical pharmacology and therapeutic use. *Drugs*, 15, 387–92.

Ivey, K. J. and Clifton, J. A. (1974) Back diffusion of hydrogen ions across gastric mucosa of patients with gastric ulcer and rheumatoid arthritis. *Br. Med. J.*, i, 16–19.

Jenne, J. W., Nagasawa, H. T., McHugh, R. *et al.* (1975) Decreased theophylline half-life in cigarette smokers. *Life Sci.*, 17, 195–8.

Johnson, D. A. W. and Freeman, H. (1972) Long-acting tranquillisers. *Practitioner*, 208, 395–400.

Johnston, G. D., Harron, D. W. G. and McDevitt, D. G. (1979) Can digoxin prescribing be improved? A comparison between intuitive and assisted dose selection. *Eur. J. Clin. Pharmacol.*, 16, 229–35.

Jori, A., Di Salle, E. and Quadri, A. (1972) Rate of aminopyrine disappearance from plasma in young and aged humans. *Pharmacology*, 8, 273–9.

Karlsson, E. and Molin, L. (1975) Polymorphic acetylation of procainamide in healthy subjects. *Acta Med. Scand.*, 197, 299–302.

Keeri-Szanto, M. and Pomeroy, J. R. (1971) Atmospheric pollution and pentazocine metabolism. *Lancet*, i, 947–9.

Kimberly, R. P., Bowden, R. E., Keiser, H. R. and Plotz, P. H. (1978) Reduction of renal function by newer nonsteroidal anti-inflammatory drugs. *Am. J. Med.*, 64, 804–7.

Kimberly, R. P. and Plotz, P. H. (1977) Aspirin-induced depression of renal function. *N. Engl. J. Med.*, 296, 418–24.

Klotz, U., Avant, G. R., Hoyumpa, A., Schenker, S. and Wilkinson, G. R. (1975) The effects of age and liver disease on the disposition and elimination of diazepam in adult man. *J. Clin. Invest.*, 55, 347–59.

Knapp, M. S., Byrom, N. P., Pownall, R. and Mayor, P. (1980) Time of day of taking immunosuppressive agents after renal transplantation: a possible influence on graft survival. *Br. Med. J.*, 281, 1382–5.

Knapp, M. S., Cove-Smith, J. R., Dugdale, R., Mackenzie, N. and Pownall, R. (1979) Possible effect of time on renal allograft rejection. *Br. Med. J.*, i, 75–7.

Koch-Weser, J. and Sellers, E. M. (1976) Drug therapy. Binding of drugs to serum albumin (second of two parts). *N. Engl. J. Med.*, 294, 526–31.

Koch-Weser, J., Simon, L. S. and Mills, J. A. (1980) Drug therapy: non-steroidal anti-inflammatory drugs (first of two parts). *N. Engl. J. Med.*, 302, 1179–85.

Koup, J. R., Jusko, W. J., Elwood, C. M. and Kohli, R. K. (1975) Digoxin pharmacokinetics: role of renal failure in dosage regimen design. *Clin. Pharmacol. Ther.*, 18, 9–21.

Kowanko, I. C., Knapp, M. S., Pownall, R. and Swannell, A. J. (1982) Domiciliary self-measurement in rheumatoid arthritis and the demonstration of circadian rhythmicity. *Ann. Rheum. Dis.*, 41, 453–5.

Kowanko, I. C., Pownall, R., Knapp, M. S., Swannell, A. J. and Mahoney, P. G. C. (1981) Circadian variations in the signs and symptoms of rheumatoid arthritis and in the therapeutic effectiveness of flurbiprofen at different times of day. *Br. J. Clin. Pharmacol.*, 11, 477–84.

Krishnaswamy, K. (1978) Drug metabolism and pharmacokinetics in malnutrition. *Clin. Pharmacokinet.*, 3, 216–40.

Krishnaswamy, K., Ushasri, V. and Nadamuni Naidu, A. (1981) The effect of malnutrition on the pharmacokinetics of phenylbutazone. *Clin. Pharmacokinet.*, 6, 152–9.

Kwan, K. C., Breault, G. O., Umbenhauer, E. R., McMahon, F. G. and Duggan, D. E. (1976) Kinetics of indomethacin absorption, elimination and enterohepatic circulation in man. *J. Pharmacokinet. Biopharm.*, 4, 255–80.

Lansbury, J., Baier, H. N. and McCraken, S. (1962) Statistical study of variation in systemic and articular indexes. *Arthr. Rheum.*, 5, 445–56.

Lawson, A. A. H., Proudfoot, A. T., Brown, S. S. *et al.* (1969) Forced diuresis in the treatment of acute salicylate poisoning in adults. *Quart. J. Med.*, 38, 31–48.

Lee, D. A.H., Taylor, G. M., Walker, J. G. and James, V. H.T. (1979) The effect of food and tablet formulation on plasma prednisolone levels following administration of enteric-coated tablets. *Br. J. Clin. Pharmacol.*, 7, 523–8.

Lees, G. M. (1981) A hitch-hiker's guide to the galaxy of adrenoceptors. *Br. Med. J.*, 283, 173–8.

Levi, A. J., Sherlock, S. and Walker, D. (1968) Phenylbutazone and isoniazid metabolism in patients with liver disease in relation to previous drug therapy. *Lancet*, i, 1275–9.

Levy, G. (1965) Pharmacokinetics of salicylate elimination in man. *J. Pharm. Sci.*, 54, 959–67.

Levy, G. (1976) Effect of plasma protein binding of drugs on duration and intensity of pharmacological activity. *J. Pharm. Sci.*, 65, 1264–5.

Levy, G., Khanna, N. N., Soda, D. M., Tsuzuki, O. and Stern, L. (1975) Pharmacokinetics of acetaminophen in the human neonate: formation of acetaminophen glucuronide and sulfate in relation to plasma bilirubin concentration and D-glucaric acid excretion. *Pediatrics*, 55, 818–25.

Lyle, W. H., Pearcey, D. F. and Hui, M. (1977) Inhibition of penicillamine-induced cupriuresis by oral iron. *Proc. Roy. Soc. Med.*, 70 (Suppl: 3), 48–9.

McChesney, E. W., Fasco, M. J. and Banks, W. F. (1967) The metabolism of chloroquine in man during and after repeated oral dosage. *J. Pharmacol. Exp. Ther.*, 10, 366–71.

McGeown, M. G., Kennedy, J. A., Loughbridge, W. G. G. *et al.* (1977) One hundred kidney transplants in the Belfast City Hospital. *Lancet*, ii, 648–51.

Mackenzie, A. H. and Scherbel, A. L. (1980) Chloroquine and hydroxychloroquine in rheumatological therapy. *Clin. Rheum. Dis.*, 6, 545–66.

Makela, A. L., Yrjana, T. and Mattila, M. (1979) Dosage of salicylate for children with juvenile rheumatoid arthritis. *Acta Paediatr. Scand.*, 68, 423–30.

Medina, M. A. and Merritt, J. H. (1970) Drug metabolism and pharmacologic action in mice exposed to reduced barometric pressure. *Biochem. Pharmacol.*, 19, 2812–16.

Misiewicz, J. J., Lennard-Lones, J. E., Connell, A. M., Baron, J. H. and Jones, F. A. (1965) Controlled trial of sulphasalazine in maintenance therapy for ulcerative colitis. *Lancet*, i, 185–8.

Misra, P. S., Lefevre, A., Ishii, H., Rubin, E. and Lieber, C. S. (1971) Increase of ethanol, meprobamate and pentobarbital metabolism after chronic ethanol administration in man and in rats. *Am. J. Med.*, 51, 346–51.

Mitchell, J. R., Thorgeirsson, S. S., Potter, W. Z., Jollow, D. J. and Keiser, H. (1974) Acetaminophen-induced hepatic injury: protective role of glutathione in man and rationale for therapy. *Clin. Pharmacol. Ther.*, 16, 676–84.

Mitchell, J. R., McMurtry, R. J., Statham, C. N. and Nelson, S. D. (1977) Molecular basis for several drug-induced nephropathies. *Am. J. Med.*, 62, 518–26.

Morselli, P. L. (1976) Clinical pharmacokinetics in neonates. *Clin. Pharmacokinet.*, 1, 81–98.

Morselli, P. L., Marc, V., Garattini, S. and Zaccala, M. (1970) Metabolism of exogenous cortisol in humans – I. Diurnal variation in plasma disappearance rate. *Biochem. Pharmacol.*, 19, 1643–7.

Neumann, V. C., Grindulis, K. A., Hubball, S., McConkey, B. and Wright, V. (1983) Comparison between penicillamine and sulphasalazine in rheumatoid arthritis: Leeds–Birmingham Trial. *Br. Med. J.*, 287, 1099–1102.

Neumann, V. C., Taggart, A. J., LeGallez, P., Astbury, C., Hill, J. and Bird, H. A. (1986) A study to determine the active moiety of sulphasalazine in rheumatoid arthritis. *J. Rheumatol.*, 13, in press.

Nichols, T., Nugent, C. A. and Tyler, F. H. (1965) Diurnal variation in suppression of adrenal function by glucocorticoids. *J. Clin. Endocrinol.*, 25, 343–9.

Nies, A. S., Shand, D. G. and Wilkinson, G. R. (1976) Altered hepatic blood flow and drug disposition. *Clin. Pharmacokinet.*, 1, 135–55.

Nimmo, W. S. (1976) Drugs, diseases and gastric emptying. *Clin. Pharmacokinet.*, 1, 189–203.

Odar-Cederlof, I., Lunde, P. K. M. and Sjoqvist, F. (1970) Abnormal pharmacokinetics of diphenylhydantoin in a patient with uraemia. *Lancet*, ii, 831–2.

Orme, M., Baber, N., Keenan, J., Halliday, L., Sibeon, R. and Littler, T. (1981) Pharmacokinetics and biochemical effects in responders and non-responders to non-steroidal anti-inflammatory drugs. *Scand. J. Rheum. (Suppl.)*, 39, 19–27.

Orme, M., Holt, P. J. L., Hughes, G. R. V. et al. (1976) Plasma concentration of phenylbutazone and its therapeutic effect – studies in patients with rheumatoid arthritis. *Br. J. Clin. Pharmacol.*, 3, 185–91.

Patel, L. G., Warrington, S. J. and Pearson, R. M. (1983) Propranolol concentrations in plasma after insertion into the vagina. *Br. Med. J.*, 287, 1247–8

Perry, H. M., Sakamoto, A. and Tan, E. M. (1967) Relationship of acetylating enzyme to hydrallazine toxicity. *J. Lab. Clin. Med.*, 70, 1020–1.

Pollmann, L. (1981) Etude de la chronobiologie des dents. *Rev. Stomatol. Chir. Maxillofac.*, 82, 201–3.

Prescott, L. F., Adjepon-Yamoah, K. K. and Talbot, R. G. (1976) Impaired lignocaine metabolism in patients with myocardial infarction and cardiac failure. *Br. Med. J.*, i, 939–41.

Prescott, L. F., Wright, N., Roscoe, P. and Brown, S. S. (1971) Plasma-paracetamol half-life and hepatic necrosis in patients with paracetamol overdosage. *Lancet*, i, 519–22.

Radzialowski, F. M. and Bousquet, W. F. (1968) Daily rhythmic variation in hepatic drug metabolism in the rat and mouse. *J. Pharmacol. Exp. Ther.*, 163, 229–38.

Reeback, J. S., Chakraborty, J., English, J., Gibson, T. and Marks, V. (1980) Plasma steroid levels after intra-articular injection of prednisolone acetate in patients with rheumatoid arthritis. *Ann. Rheum. Dis.*, 39, 22–4.

Reidenberg, M. M., Odar-Cederlof, I., von Bahr, C. et al., (1971) Protein binding of diphenylhydantoin and desmethylimipramine in plasma from patients with poor renal function. *N. Engl. J. Med.*, 285, 264–7.

Reinberg, A., Clench, J., Ghata, J., Halberg, T. et al. (1975) Rythmes circadiens des parametres de l'excretion urinaire du salicylate (chronopharmacokinetique) chez l'homme adulte sain. *C. R. Acad. Sci. (Paris)*, 280, 1697–700.

Reinberg, A., Gervais, P., Morin, M. and Abulker, C. (1971) Rythme circadien humain du seuil de la reponse bronchique a l'acetylcholine. *C. R. Acad. Sci. (Paris)*, 272, 1879–81.

Reinberg, A., Guillet, P., Gervais, P., Ghata, J., Vignaud, D. and Abulker, C. (1977) One month chronocorticotherapy (Dutimelan 8–15 mite). Control of the asthmatic condition without adrenal suppression and circadian rhythm alteration. *Chronobiologia*, 4, 295–312.

Reinberg, A., Halberg, F. and Falliers, C. (1974) Circadian timing of methylpredniso-lone effects in asthmatic boys. *Chronobiologia*, 1, 333–47.

Reinberg, A. and Reinberg, M. (1977) Circadian changes of the duration of action of local anaesthetic agents. *Naunyn Schmiedebergs Arch. Pharmacol.*, 297, 149–59.

Reinberg, A., Zagula-Mally, Z., Ghata, J. and Halberg, F. (1967) Circadian rhythms in duration of salicylate excretion referred to phase of excretory rhythms and routine. *Proc. Soc. Exp. Biol.*, 124, 826–32.

Reuning, R. H., Sams, R. A. and Notari, R. E. (1973) Role of pharmacokinetics in drug dosage adjustment. I. Pharmacologic effect kinetics and apparent volume of distribution of digoxin. *J. Clin. Pharm.*, 13, 127–41.

Riegelman, S., Loo, J. C. K. and Rowland, M. (1968) Shortcomings in pharmacokinetic analysis by conceiving the body to exhibit properties of a single compartment. *J. Pharm. Sci.*, 57, 117–23.

Ritchie, A. W.S., Oswald, I., Spedding Micklem, H. *et al.* (1983) Circadian variation of lymphocyte subpopulations: a study with monoclonal antibodies. *Br. Med. J.*,286, 1773–5.

van Rossum, J. (1968) Pharmacokinetics of accumulation. *J. Pharm. Sci.*, 57, 2162–4.

Rubin, E., Gang, H., Misra, P. and Lieber, C. S. (1970) Inhibition of drug metabolism by acute intoxication: a hepatic microsomal mechanism. *Am. J. Med.*, 49, 801–6.

Salaman, J. R. (1983) Steroids and immunosuppression. *Br. Med. J.*, 286, 1373–5.

Scheving, L. E., Burns, E. R., Pauly, J. E., Halberg, F. and Haus, E. (1977) Survival and cure of leukemic mice after circadian optimization of treatment with cyclophos-phamide and arabinosyl cytosine. *Cancer Res.*, 37, 3648–55.

Schneider, R. E. and Bishop, H. (1982) β-blocker plasma concentrations and inflamma-tory disease: clinical implications. *Clin. Pharmacokinet.*, 7, 281–4.

Schneider, R. E., Bishop, H. and Hawkins, C. F. (1979) Plasma propranolol concentra-tions and the erythrocyte sedimentation rate. *Br. J. Clin. Pharmacol.*, 8, 43–7.

Schoene, R. B., Abuan, T., Ward, B. S. and Beasley, C. H. (1984) Effects of topical betaxolol, timolol and placebo on pulmonary function in asthmatic bronchitis. *Am. J. Ophthalmol.*, 97, 86–92.

Schuna, A., Osman, M. A., Patel, R. B., Welling, P. G. and Sundstrom, W. R. (1983) Influence of food on the bioavailability of penicillamine. *J. Rheumatol.*, 10, 95–7.

Scott, D. L., Roden, S., Marshall, T. and Kendall, M. J. (1982) Variations in responses to non-steroidal anti-inflammatory drugs. *Br. J. Clin. Pharmacol.*, 14, 691–4.

Scott, J. T. (1960) Morning stiffness in rheumatoid arthritis. *Ann. Rheum. Dis.*, 19, 361.

Sereni, F., Perletti, L., Marubini, E. and Mars, G. (1968) Pharmacokinetic studies with a long-acting sulfonamide in subjects of different ages. *Pediatr. Res.*, 2 29–37.

Shastri, A. K. and Krishnaswamy, K. (1976) Undernutrition and tetracycline half-life. *Clin. Chim. Acta*, 66, 157–64.

Shaw, T. R. D. and Carless, J. E. (1974) The effect of particle size on the absorption of digoxin. *Eur. J. Clin. Pharmacol.*, 7, 269–73.

Sjoholm, I. (1978) Binding of drugs to human serum albumin. *Proceedings of the XIth FEBS Meeting*, Copenhagen 1977, 50, 71.

Sjoqvist, F., Borga, O. and Orme, M.L'E. (1980) Fundamentals of clinical pharma-cology in *Drug Treatment* (ed. G. S. Avery), Churchill Livingstone, London, Vol.1, p. 61.

Smith, T. W. and Willerson, J. T. (1971) Suicidal and accidental digoxin ingestion: report of five cases with serum digoxin level correlations. *Circulation*, 44, 29–36.

Smolensky, M. H., Reinberg, A. and Queng, J. T. (1981) The chronobiology and chronopharmacology of allergy. *Ann. Allergy*, 47, 234–52.

du Souich, P., McClean, A. J., Lalka, D., Erill, S. and Gibaldi, M. (1978) Pulmonary disease and drug kinetics. *Clin. Pharmacokinet.*, 3, 257–66.

Steiness, E., Svendsen, O. and Rasmussen, F. (1974) Plasma digoxin after parenteral administration. Local reaction after intramuscular injection. *Clin. Pharmacol. Ther.*, 16, 430–4.

Taggart, A. J., Johnston, G. D. and McDevitt, D. G. (1981) Does the frequency of daily dosage influence compliance with digoxin therapy? *Br. J. Clin. Pharmacol.*, 1, 31–4.

Taggart, A. J., McElnay, J. C., Kerr, B. and Passmore, P. (1986) Chronopharmacokinetics of indomethacin suppositories in healthy volunteers. *Br. J. Clin. Pharmacol.*, 21, in press.

Taggart, H. McA. and Alderdice, J. M. (1982) Fatal cholestatic jaundice in elderly patients taking benoxaprofen. *Br. Med. J.*, 284, 1372.

Tan, S. Y., Shapiro, R. and Kish, M. A. (1979) Reversible acute renal failure induced by indomethacin. *J. Am. Med. Assoc.*, 241, 2732–3.

Touitou, Y., Touitou, C., Bogdan, A., Beck, H. and Reinberg, A. (1979) Circadian rhythms in serum total proteins: observed differences according to age and mental health. *Chronobiologia*, 6, 164.

Traeger, A., Kunze, M. and Ankermann, H. (1973) Zur pharmakokinetik von indomethazin bei alten menschen. *Z. Alternsforsch*, 27, 151–5.

Triggs, E. J., Nation, R. L., Long, A. and Ashley, J. J. (1975) Pharmacokinetics in the elderly. *Eur. J. Clin. Pharmacol.*, 8, 55–62.

Turakka, H. and Airaksinen, M. M. (1974) Biopharmaceutical assessment of phenylbutazone and indomethacin preparations. *Ann. Clin. Res.*, Suppl. 11, 34–41.

Vestal, R. E., Norris, A. H., Tobin, J. D., Cohen, B. H., Shock, N. W. and Andres, R. (1975) Antipyrine metabolism in man: influence of age, alcohol, caffeine and smoking. *Clin. Pharmacol. Ther.*, 18, 425–32.

Wallin, A., Jalling, B. and Boreus, L. O. (1974) Plasma concentrations of phenobarbital in the neonate during prophylaxis for neonatal hyperbilirubinemia. *J. Pediatr.*, 85, 392–8.

Walshe, J. J. and Venuto, R. C. (1979) Acute oliguric renal failure induced by indomethacin: possible mechanism. *Ann. Intern. Med.*, 91, 47–9.

Whitlam, J. B., Brown, K. F., Crooks, M. J. and Room, G. F.W. (1981) Transsynovial distribution of ibuprofen in arthritic patients. *Clin. Pharmacol. Ther.*, 29, 487–92.

Wirz-Justice, A., Kafka, M. S., Naber, D. and Wehr, T. A. (1980) Circadian rhythms in rat brain: α- and β- adrenergic receptors are modified by chronic imipramine. *Life Sci.*, 27, 341–7.

Wright, V. (1959) Some observations on diurnal variation of grip. *Clin. Sci.*, 18, 17–23.

CHAPTER 3

Drug interactions

M. C. L'E. Orme

3.1 INTRODUCTION

The physician of the 1980s has a vast therapeutic armamentarium at his disposal with which to treat his patient. While in some countries, e. g. Germany, the number of preparations may exceed 10 000, in the UK some 3000 preparations are listed in the monthly index of medical supplies (MIMS). There are perhaps 1000 pharmacologically active drugs available for prescription and the potential pairs of drugs that might interact is therefore about 500 000. Patients admitted to hospital on average receive 4 or 5 drugs during the course of a hospital admission, and one in every five patients receives at least ten drugs (Crooks and Moir, 1974). There is little doubt that in the last ten years the exposure of patients to drugs has increased and this applies to both hospital and general practice.

Clearly the potential for drug interaction is very large and many physicians are frightened at the mention of drug interactions because of the size of the subject. The problem is largely of our own making since most of the drug interactions described are not clinically relevant. There are three main reasons for this. First, many interactions are initially described from studies in animals, and when the studies are eventually carried out in patients no such interaction may be seen. As an example, Conney (1967) lists over 200 compounds that are inducers of hepatic microsomal drug metabolizing enzymes in animals, and yet the number of drugs that induce these enzymes in man is very small, probably in single figures (Park and Breckenridge, 1981). Secondly, many studies are performed *in vitro*, and this is particularly true of protein binding studies.

TABLE 3.1
Mechanisms of drug interaction

(1)	Outside the patient (e.g. in infusion bottle).
(2)	In the gastrointestinal tract.
(3)	During distribution of drug to its site of action (e.g. protein binding displacement).
(4)	During metabolism (e.g. enzyme induction and inhibition).
(5)	At the receptor.
(6)	During excretion from the body.

What occurs in the test tube may not be relevant *in vivo*. Indomethacin was initially reported to displace warfarin from its protein binding sites in plasma (Solomon *et al.*, 1968), and it was predicted that indomethacin would potentiate warfarin in the clinical setting. In practice no such interaction occurs (Vesell *et al.*, 1975; Pullar and Capell, 1982) and many patients on warfarin have no doubt been denied a valuable treatment for their gout because of this problem. Thirdly, drug interactions are often described as a result of a single case report. While this is without doubt a valuable method to pass on information it does lead to fallacious results at times. It may take a detailed study in many patients to disprove the single case report, and even then editors are less interested in negative information than in positive data.

It has been conventional in the past to discuss drug interactions under their sites or mechanisms of interaction, as listed in Table 3.1. This is often a valuable method, particularly since if the mechanism of an interaction is understood, then in the future it may be possible to predict interactions. Drug interactions with antirheumatic drugs have only recently come to the forefront, and thus information on their mechanism of interaction is lacking. Model studies have been performed with some of the NSAIDs, looking at the effect on antipyrine clearance and metabolism. Chalmers *et al.* (1973) showed that flurbiprofen prolonged the half-life of antipyrine, while ibuprofen had no such effect (Greenblatt and Abernethy, 1983). Prolongation of the antipyrine half-life is usually attributed to inhibition of drug metabolism, as has been shown for phenylbutazone (see Section 3.3.1) and azapropazone (Williamson *et al.*, 1984). Indeed, in the process of researching this chapter, I was surprised to find that a literature search provided over 2000 references, most of them from the last six years. The title of 'Drug interactions with antirheumatic drugs' in most peoples' minds equates with 'drug interactions with NSAIDs' since there is very little information concerning interactions with gold, penicillamine or corticosteroids. This chapter will therefore concentrate on the NSAIDs, with particular emphasis on the clinical areas where problems have been reported. The reader is referred to a number of recent reviews for additional information

(Brooks *et al.*, 1977; Reinicke and Vesel, 1979; Hayes, 1981; Miller, 1981; Day *et al.*, 1982; Heuer, 1983; Verbeek *et al.*, 1983).

3.2   ANTACIDS

Antacids and NSAIDs are often taken together, not infrequently without the knowledge of the doctor since over the counter preparations of both types of drugs are readily available. Many so-called non-systemic antacids, such as aluminium and magnesium hydroxide, can increase urinary pH as well as increasing the pH of the stomach contents. As a result, both absorption and elimination of NSAIDs – predominantly weak organic acids – may be affected. It is however difficult to generalize on the effect that is likely to be produced but in most cases the clinical importance of this interaction is not very great. Although magnesium and aluminium hydroxide increase the rate of absorption of aspirin, there is no overall effect on the amount of aspirin absorbed (Nayak *et al.*, 1977). However in children, Levy *et al.* (1975) reported lower serum concentrations of salicylate when antacids were given with the aspirin. Since the clearance of salicylate is increased if the pH of the urine is increased it is possible that the therapeutic effect of aspirin would be diminished in patients taking regular antacid therapy. However, in practice, this does not seem to be a clinical problem.

In some cases NSAIDs and antacid are formulated in the same tablet (e. g. aspirin, phenylbutazone), because of the known tendency of NSAIDs to cause gastrointestinal irritation. In the case of oxyphenbutazone, both the rate and extent of absorption are increased by combination of the drug with aluminium hydroxide and magnesium trisilicate (Dugal *et al.*, 1980). With moderate and high doses of aspirin, gastrointestinal damage is almost invariable and the administration of large amounts of sodium bicarbonate almost abolishes gastrointestinal blood loss (Leonards and Levy, 1969). However, since systemic alkalosis is likely to result, this regime is not recommended. The administration of buffered tablets of aspirin, containing small amounts of antacid, does decrease the epigastric discomfort caused by aspirin, but does not greatly reduce the gastrointestinal damage (Leonards and Levy, 1969; Lanza *et al.*, 1980).

Coadministration of aluminium hydroxide and diflunisal reduced the plasma concentration versus time curve (AUC) of diflunisal by 40% in four healthy volunteers (from 1008.4 $\mu g/ml^{-1} \times h$ to 607.7 $\mu g/ml^{-1} \times h$, Verbeeck *et al.*, 1979). A smaller effect was seen when diflunisal was given with a mixture of aluminium and magnesium hydroxide (Holmes *et al.*, 1979). The studies of Tobert *et al.* (1981) show that aluminium hydroxide reduces the absorption of diflunisal (as found by Verbeeck *et al.*, 1979), but magnesium hydroxide increases the absorption of diflunisal. In the presence of food however these antacids have no effect on the absorption of diflunisal (Tobert *et al.*, 1981).

The absorption of indomethacin is decreased by both aluminium hydroxide (Garnham *et al.*, 1977) and aluminium–magnesium antacid mixtures (Galeazzi, 1977). Emori *et al.* (1976) reported that a magnesium–aluminium gel only delayed the absorption of indomethacin without significantly affecting the overall absorption. Aluminium hydroxide antacids reduce the absorption of naproxen but a combined aluminium–magnesium antacid mixture has no overall effect on naproxen absorption (Segre *et al.*, 1974a; Segre, 1979). However, sodium bicarbonate seems to increase the rate of absorption of both naproxen (Segre, 1979) and indomethacin (Garnham *et al.*, 1977). The rate and extent of absorption of ketoprofen (Brazier *et al.*, 1981), tolmetin (Ayres *et al.*, 1977), fenoprofen (Chernish *et al.*, 1972), azapropazone (Faust-Tinnefeldt *et al.*, 1977) and piroxicam (Hobbs and Twomey, 1979) are not affected by concurrent use of magnesium–aluminium hydroxide mixtures.

In general it would be wise to use aluminium–magnesium mixtures in preference to aluminium hydroxide, if an antacid is required in patients taking NSAIDs.

3.3   ORAL ANTICOAGULANTS

3.3.1   Phenylbutazone and anticoagulants

Interactions between oral anticoagulants and NSAIDs have been recognized for some years, and most clinical problems have occurred with phenylbutazone. Nordoy in 1959 was the first to recognize the interaction; bleeding occurred when phenylbutazone was given to patients on warfarin. Further reports of this interaction followed (Eisen, 1964; Hoffbrand and Kininmonth, 1967; Aggeler *et al.*, 1967) and have also included oxyphenbutazone with phenindione (Hobbs *et al.*, 1965) and with dicoumarol (Weiner *et al.*, 1965). Solomon *et al.* (1968) and O'Reilly (1973) showed that phenylbutazone displaced warfarin from its protein binding sites, and the studies by Aggeler *et al.* (1967) and O'Reilly and Aggeler (1968) were compatible with this mechanism. Since indomethacin (Solomon *et al.*, 1968) and other NSAIDs compete for protein binding sites with warfarin (Wanwimolruk *et al.*, 1982) it has been assumed that all NSAIDs will prolong the action of warfarin, even though Hoffbrand and Kininmonth (1967) had found no clinical effect of indomethacin on warfarin. The interaction of phenylbutazone with warfarin affects all patients exposed to it (Udall, 1969) and involves other anticoagulants such as marcoumar (Seiler and Duckert, 1968) and phenprocoumon (O'Reilly, 1982a).

It is now clear that the interaction has very little to do with protein binding displacement but is due to a stereoselective interaction. Racemic warfarin

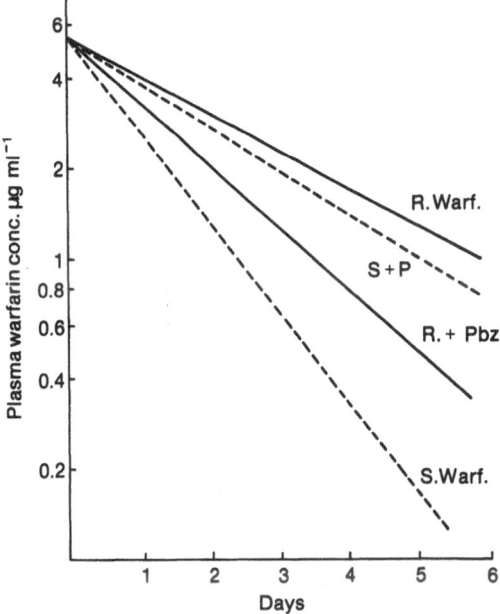

Figure 3.1 Plasma warfarin concentration decay over a six-day period after the oral administration of R(+) warfarin and S(−) warfarin to human volunteers before and after phenylbutazone (PBZ) (100 mg t.i.d. for 10 days). (Reproduced by kind permission of the editor and authors of the *J. Clin. Invest.* 53, 1607, (1974).)

consists of two enantiomers, S- and R-warfarin, and S-warfarin is 5 times more potent than R-warfarin as an anticoagulant. Phenylbutazone inhibits the metabolism of S-warfarin but induces the metabolism of R-warfarin as shown in Fig. 3.1. There is no net change in the total warfarin concentration in plasma, but a greater proportion of the warfarin is present as S-warfarin, the more potent enantiomer (Lewis *et al.*, 1974; O'Reilly *et al.*, 1980). A similar interaction is seen between warfarin and sulphinpyrazone (O'Reilly, 1982b). Azapropazone, which is structurally related to phenylbutazone, also displaces warfarin from plasma protein binding (McElnay and D'Arcy, 1977) and prolongs the prothrombin time in patients on warfarin (Green *et al.*, 1977; Powell-Jackson, 1977). The mechanism is probably inhibition of drug metabolism rather than displacement from protein binding.

3.3.2   Aspirin and anticoagulants

Large doses of salicylate may depress the vitamin K-dependent synthesis of coagulation factors VII, IX and X with a resultant increase in the prothrombin time (Fausa, 1970; O'Reilly *et al.*, 1971). In general, doses of at least 4 g of aspirin daily are required to produce this effect. Salicylate displaces warfarin from its plasma protein binding sites *in vitro* (Schary *et al.*, 1978; Donaldson *et al.*, 1982), but this mechanism is of little relevance in clinical practice. Studies in patients taking warfarin and salicylate together (up to 3 g aspirin daily) have not shown any alteration in prothrombin time (Udall, 1969). There is, however, a clear risk of bleeding if patients taking warfarin are given aspirin because of the effects of salicylate on platelet aggregation and cutaneous bleeding time (O'Brien, 1968; O'Reilly *et al.*, 1971). Diflunisal, a recent aspirin derivative, did not prolong the prothrombin time of patients taking warfarin (Serlin *et al.*, 1980) but, once diflunisal therapy was stopped, there was a fall in the prothrombin time for about two weeks, and this was associated with a decrease in the concentration of free warfarin in plasma (i. e. non-protein bound). The explanation of this effect is probably related to the recovery from protein binding displacement. In contrast, diflunisal prolonged the prothrombin time in three patients taking acenocoumarin (Tempero *et al.*, 1977).

3.3.3   Other NSAIDs and anticoagulants

It is clear now that most of the other NSAIDs, in spite of displacing warfarin from protein binding sites, do not produce any significant effect on the degree of hypoprothrombinaemia induced by warfarin (see Table 3.2). Nevertheless they should be used with care in patients taking warfarin because of their effects on gastric mucosa and platelet aggregation. The following NSAIDs have been shown to have no significant interaction with oral anticoagulants: indomethacin with warfarin (Vesell *et al.*, 1975; Pullar and Capell, 1982); sulindac with phenprocoumon (Schenk *et al.*, 1980); sulindac with warfarin (Loftin and Vesell, 1979), although these authors and Carter (1979) both report one patient in whom warfarin was potentiated by sulindac; ibuprofen with phenprocoumon (Boekhout-Mussert and Loeliger, 1974) and ibuprofen with warfarin (Penner and Abbrecht, 1975); flurbiprofen with phenprocoumon (Marbet *et al.*, 1977), but in two patients on acenocoumarin, flurbiprofen enhanced the hypoprothrombinaemic effect (Stricker and Delhez, 1982); naproxen with warfarin (Jain *et al.*, 1979; Slattery *et al.*, 1979) and naproxen with phenprocoumon (Angelkort, 1978); indoprofen with warfarin (Jacono *et al.*, 1981); tolmetin with warfarin (Whitsett *et al.*, 1975) and with phenprocoumon (Rust *et al.*, 1975); diclofenac with phenprocoumon (Krzywanek and Breddin, 1977) or with acenocoumarin (Michot *et al.*, 1975); alclofenac with phenprocoumon or acenocoumarin (Kaufmann, 1977); zomepirac with warfarin (Minn and Zinny, 1980) and benoxaprofen with warfarin (Chatfield *et al.*, 1978).

In contrast, oxametacin, a near relative to indomethacin, significantly decreased the thrombotest in 12 patients on warfarin (Baele *et al.*, 1983) and piroxicam also potentiated the effect of acenocoumarin in some patients (Brogden *et al.*, 1981). Fenbufen has been reported to lower plasma warfarin concentrations in volunteers but the change in prothrombin time was small

TABLE 3.2
Interaction between oral anticoagulants and NSAIDs

NSAID	Anticoagulant	Effect on prothrombin time	Effect on warfarin kinetics in vivo
Phenylbutazone	Warfarin	Prolonged	Inhibition of S warfarin metabolism
	Dicoumarol	Prolonged	
	Marcoumar	Prolonged	
	Phenprocoumon	Prolonged	
Oxyphenbutazone	Warfarin	Prolonged	Inhibition of S warfarin metabolism
Azapropazone	Warfarin	Prolonged	?
Aspirin	Warfarin	Prolonged with high dose aspirin	None
Diflunisal	Warfarin	None	See text
Indomethacin	Warfarin	None	None
Sulindac	Warfarin, Phenprocoumon	None	None
Fenbufen	Warfarin	Sl. shortening	Fall in plasma warfarin concn.
Ibuprofen	Warfarin	None	—
	Phenprocoumon	None	—
Flurbiprofen	Phenprocoumon	None	—
	Acenocoumarol	Prolonged (2 patients)	—
Naproxen	Warfarin	None	None
Naproxen	Phenprocoumon	Temporary prolongation	?
Mefenamic acid	Warfarin	Slight prolongation	?
Indoprofen	Warfarin	None	—
Tolmetin	Warfarin	None	—
Piroxicam	Acenocoumarin	Prolongation	—
Diclofenac	Phenprocoumon	None	—
Alclofenac	Acenocoumarin	None	—
Zomepirac	Warfarin	None	—

(1.9 seconds), and it is doubtful if this is of clinical significance (Savitsky et al., 1980). Glafenine, a popular NSAID in Holland, significantly enhanced the activity of phenprocoumon in 20 patients (Boejinga and Van der Vijgh, 1977). Finally mefenamic acid has been reported to cause a large increase in the free warfarin concentrations in plasma (Sellers and Koch-Weser, 1970) and to potentiate significantly the effects of warfarin in vivo (Holmes, 1967; Baragar and Smith, 1978).

In summary, phenylbutazone, oxyphenbutazone, and azapropazone should not be given to patients taking oral anticoagulants, and it is perhaps wise to avoid mefenamic acid. However, drugs like indomethacin, naproxen, ibuprofen, and flurbiprofen can be given to patients being treated with warfarin, provided care is taken.

3.4 ANTICONVULSANTS

3.4.1 Phenytoin

Phenylbutazone was reported in 1973 by Andreasen *et al.* to prolong the plasma half-life of phenytoin. In a group of 14 pairs of twins a daily dose of 500mg phenylbutazone lengthened the half-life of phenytoin from 13.7 ± 4.8 (mean $\pm$ SD) to 22.0 ± 5.5 hours. The prolongation appeared to be due more to environmental than to genetic factors and is in keeping with the known ability of phenylbutazone to inhibit drug metabolizing enzymes (Lewis *et al.*, 1974). It is surprising that no other interactions have been reported between these two drugs whereas azapropazone, a drug that is chemically related to phenylbutazone, has featured in this context. Roberts *et al.* (1981) reported one patient who developed ataxia and nystagmus when azapropazone was given, and this was associated with high plasma concentrations of phenytoin. Geaney *et al.* (1982) showed that azapropazone increased the plasma concentration of phenytoin from 20µmol 1^{-1} to 41µmol 1^{-1} in five volunteers – this finding is also in keeping with inhibition of drug metabolism by azapropazone. Phenytoin, with its capacity limited metabolism, is very easily affected by such inhibitors of drug metabolism. Sandyk (1982) reported a patient who had been taking phenytoin 500 mg/day for 5 years with no untoward effects, and who developed nystagmus due to high concentrations of phenytoin after being given ibuprofen 400 mg q. i. d.

An interaction between phenytoin and aspirin has been widely reported and here there is a reasonable consistency of opinion. Aspirin displaces phenytoin from its binding sites on plasma albumin and *in vivo* this leads to a fall in the total plasma phenytoin concentration of about 20–25% (Olanow *et al.*, 1979; Paxton, 1980; Fraser *et al.*, 1980). There is, however, no increase in the free (i.e. unbound) phenytoin concentration in plasma, which is the therapeutically active part (Olanow *et al.*, 1979; Paxton, 1980), although the free fraction may increase (Fraser *et al.*, 1980). In this situation the displaced phenytoin is available for metabolic clearance. Leonard *et al.* (1981) found a small increase in the free phenytoin concentration in plasma during high dose aspirin therapy (975 mg q. i. d.) but not during low dose therapy (325 mg q. i. d.). The rise in free concentration was small, from 0.97 µg ml^{-1} to 1.13 µg ml^{-1}, and probably not of significance in the long term. Inoue and Walsh (1983) found that the fall in total plasma phenytoin concentrations in one patient given aspirin was associated with the development of a low serum folate concentration. Interactions between NSAIDs and phenytoin do not seem to be of major clinical significance, but nevertheless any patient who is taking phenytoin and who is given a NSAID should be considered from the drug interaction point of view. The metabolism of phenytoin is so easily inhibited that it is often worth checking a plasma phenytoin concentration a week or so after starting the new drug.

3.4.2   Valproic acid

Aspirin also displaces valproic acid from its protein binding sites, as does phenylbutazone (Fleitman *et al.*, 1980). However, the former interaction seems more complicated than this, since the half-life of valproic acid is increased (Orr *et al.*, 1982) and the free concentration of valproate is increased by 60% (Farrell *et al.*, 1982). These observations suggest that, in addition to the protein binding displacement, the clearance of valproate, probably through the kidney, is impaired by aspirin. In contrast to these findings, Schobben *et al.* (1978) reported that salicylate increased the excretion of valproate in the urine by enhancing the clearance of the glucuronide metabolite of valproic acid. Comparative studies in rhesus monkeys (Viswanathan and Levy, 1981) confirmed that the predominant effect of aspirin is to displace valproic acid from protein binding sites with no increase in the free concentration of the drug. In general the interaction between aspirin and valproic acid is not of clinical significance.

3.5   ANTIDIABETIC DRUGS

NSAIDs have been known to interact with antidiabetic drugs for at least 20 years, and the subject has been reviewed elsewhere (Hansen and Christensen, 1977; Diwan and Kulkarni, 1983). Wishinski *et al.* (1962) reported that salicylate displaced tolbutamide and chlorpropamide from protein binding sites *in vitro* and this could lead *in vivo* to increased free concentrations of the antidiabetic drugs, and hence an increased hypoglycaemic effect. However, it is now recognized that such protein binding interactions are very unusual, and any increased free drug concentration will be rapidly cleared by metabolism. Cherner *et al.* (1963) described prolonged hypoglycaemia in a patient receiving tolbutamide who had also been given aspirin, but the amount of aspirin consumed was very small. Stowers *et al.* (1959) reported that large doses of aspirin may potentiate the effects of hypoglycaemic drugs, perhaps by interfering with the renal tubular secretion of drugs like chlorpropamide. However, it may also be that any such interaction is partly caused by the hypoglycaemic effect of salicylates (Giugliano and D'Onofrio, 1980). It seems unlikely that aspirin will cause a significant interaction with oral hypoglycaemic agents, except when large doses of aspirin are used.

Enhancement of the effect of oral hypoglycaemic drugs is well recognized for phenylbutazone and oxyphenbutazone. Initial reports described potentiation by phenylbutazone of the action of tolbutamide (Christensen et al., 1963; Gulbrandsen, 1959; Slade and Iosefa, 1967; Tannenbaum et al., 1974), and this was confirmed in animal studies (Mahfouz et al., 1970). Phenylbutazone was also shown to enhance the effect of chlorpropamide (Thomsen et al., 1970), glibenclamide (Hirns and Königstein, 1969), and acetohexamide (Field et al., 1967). The mechanism of this interaction is almost certainly inhibition of the metabolism of the hypoglycaemic drug by phenylbutazone or oxyphenbutazone. Although Field et al. (1967) suggested that the interaction with acetohexamide was due to the inhibition of the renal excretion of hydroxyhexamide, the active metabolite of acetohexamide, this mechanism is not appropriate to most hypoglycaemic drugs. Kristensen and Christensen (1969) showed that phenylbutazone and oxyphenbutazone prolong the plasma half-life of tolbutamide from 4.5 to 10.5 hours, and similar prolongation of tolbutamide half-life in plasma was reported by Pond et al. (1977) and by Szita et al. (1980). Ober (1974) reported that pheylbutazone reduced the renal excretion of carboxytolbutamide, the main metabolite of tolbutamide, while at the same time increasing plasma tolbutamide concentrations. Azapropazone, which is structurally related to phenylbutazone, also prolongs the plasma half-life of tolbutamide (from 7.7 ± 1.6 hours to 25.2 ± 6.1 hours in three volunteers, Andreasen et al., 1981). There is little doubt that phenylbutazone, oxyphenbutazone, and azapropazone should not be used in patients receiving oral hypoglycaemic drugs. Fortunately there are other effective NSAIDs that do not interact with oral hypoglycaemic agents. Pedrazzi et al. (1981) showed no clinical interaction between indoprofen and glipizide, although blood glipizide concentrations were not measured. In a similar study, Melander and Wählin-Bohl (1981) showed that indoprofen did increase plasma glipizide concentrations; but, like Pedrazzi et al. (1981), they found no change in blood glucose levels on indoprofen. Naproxen had no effect on the pharmacodynamic effect of tolbutamide and no effect on tolbutamide plasma concentrations (Sachse et al., 1979; Whiting et al., 1979). Similarly, no significant interaction has been shown between flurbiprofen and tolbutamide (Cremoncini et al., 1980), tolmetin and glibenclamide (Chlud and Kaik, 1977), ketoprofen and tolbutamide, chlorpropamide, or glibenclamide (Voigt and Klassen, 1982), and sulindac and tolbutamide (Ryan et al., 1977). Diclofenac (Chlud, 1976; Fowler, 1979) and diflunisal (Tempero et al., 1977; Steelman et al., 1978) also do not interact with oral antidiabetic drugs.

3.6 ANTIHYPERTENSIVE AGENTS

3.6.1 Indomethacin and hypotensive drugs

Attenuation of the hypotensive effects of beta-adrenoceptor blocking drugs by NSAIDs has recently been reported, and is now recognized as an important clinical problem. Most of the reported interactions have involved indomethacin, but it is clear that other NSAIDs can be involved and that the effect is also seen with other antihypertensive drugs. Durao *et al.* (1977) noted that in seven patients the use of indomethacin prevented the full antihypertensive effect of both propranolol and pindolol. This observation has been confirmed in double-blind studies by Watkins *et al.* (1980) and Wing *et al.* (1981). Watkins *et al.* (1980) also found that indomethacin impaired the antihypertensive effect of both propranolol and thiazide diuretics. Wing *et al.* (1981) showed that in 12 patients the addition of indomethacin 25 mg t. i. d. to various antihypertensive regimens caused the mean blood pressure to increase from 136/83 to 152/89. There is no general agreement in the literature as to the effects of indomethacin alone on the blood pressure. Patak *et al.* (1975), Mills *et al.* (1982), Steiness and Waldorff (1982), and Thadani *et al.* (1983) all found an increase in blood pressure in control subjects when indomethacin was given. However, Lopez–Ovejero *et al.* (1978), Salvetti *et al.* (1982), and Silberbauer *et al.* (1982) found no such alteration in blood pressure. It has been suggested that indomethacin may act as a vasoconstrictor, especially in the splanchnic circulation, and this effect has been shown in both rabbits (Hierton, 1981) and dogs (Gerkens *et al.*, 1977; Humphrey and Zins, 1983). In animal studies, other NSAIDs such as naproxen (Hierton, 1981) have no such effect, and there is some evidence that this disparity is also true in man (Wennmalm *et al.*, 1983). Whether this mechanism underlies the clinical interaction is certainly not clear. Watkins *et al.* (1980) showed that indomethacin reduced the urinary excretion of the main metabolite of prostaglandin $F_{2\alpha}$ by about 50%. It has been suggested that indomethacin inhibits the propranolol-induced formation of vasodilatory prostaglandins (Romero and Strong, 1977). Indomethacin also inhibits the antihypertensive effect of beta-adrenoceptor blockers other than propranolol (Lopez-Ovejero *et al.*, 1978) such as oxprenolol (Salvetti *et al.*, 1982) and atenolol (Pitkäjärvi *et al.*, 1983). However, indomethacin does not interfere with the beta-adrenoceptor blockade produced by these drugs (Rolf-Smith *et al.*, 1983) nor does it worsen angina in patients receiving beta-adrenoceptor blocking drugs (Thadani *et al.*, 1983). The interaction with atenolol is difficult to evaluate since the absorption of atenolol is reduced in some patients with inflammatory diseases (Kirch *et al.*, 1983).

Indomethacin also attenuates the hypotensive response to other antihypertensive drugs such as captopril (Abe *et al.*, 1980; Fujita *et al.*, 1981; Silberbauer *et al.*, 1982). This interaction seems to be more noticeable in patients with low renin hypertension, who would be expected to respond less well to captopril, than in patients with a high renin type of hypertension (Fujita *et al.*, 1981). It is interesting in this context to note that indomethacin has been shown to potentiate the hypertensive effect of infused angiotensin II (Vierhopper *et al.*, 1981; Fujita *et al.*, 1982). Prostaglandins do not appear to mediate the effects of captopril (De Forrest *et al.*, 1982).

Indomethacin also inhibits the antihypertensive effect of prazosin, but only in about half the patients studied (Rubin *et al.*, 1980). There also appears to be variation in the effect on hydrallazine, but, in normal volunteers, Jackson and Pickles (1983) showed no such inhibitory effect on the blood pressure response. It may be that the effect of indomethacin is different in patients with hypertension compared to normal volunteers.

3.6.2   Other NSAIDs

There is relatively little information available on other NSAIDs and their potential interaction with antihypertensive drugs. Aspirin has either no effect on blood pressure (Mills *et al.*, 1982) or causes only a very slight increase in blood pressure (Sziegoleit *et al.*, 1982) in control hypertensive patients. However, aspirin has been shown to prevent the hypotensive effect of pindolol and propranolol (Sziegoleit *et al.*, 1982) and verapamil (Das, 1982). Schäfer-Korting *et al.* (1983) found no pharmacokinetic interaction between aspirin and atenolol. It is interesting that the platelet anti-aggregation effects of aspirin were enhanced by propranolol rather than attenuated, but it is not clear if this effect is clinically significant (Keber *et al.*, 1979).

Flurbiprofen, when given in a dose of 300 mg daily to 10 hypertensive patients, was shown to inhibit the hypotensive effect of propranolol but not that of atenolol (Webster *et al.*, 1983). Sulindac may also be a NSAID that is free of this interaction. Steiness and Waldorff (1982) showed that sulindac did not impair the hypotensive effect of thiazide diuretics, while indomethacin did impair it. They attributed this disparity to lack of effect of sulindac on renal prostaglandins.

It is clear that much more information is required in this area. However, it would be unwise to give indomethacin to a hypertensive patient, whatever therapy they were receiving for their hypertension. The answer to the question 'What other NSAID can I give such patients?' is at the moment unresolved.

3.7   DIGITALIS GLYCOSIDES

The possibility that NSAIDs might interact with digitalis glycosides was first raised by Solomon *et al.* (1971). They described a patient in whom the plasma concentration of digitoxin was markedly decreased when phenylbutazone was given. Although phenylbutazone displaced digitoxin from protein binding sites in plasma, the extent of the change in plasma digitoxin made a protein binding interaction unlikely, and the authors suggested that phenylbutazone might have induced the metabolism of digitoxin. Solomon and Abrams (1972) showed that phenylbutazone shortened the plasma half-life of digitoxin, in keeping with this hypothesis. However, phenylbutazone is not normally considered to be an enzyme inducer in man, although it does induce the metabolism of R-warfarin (Lewis *et al.*, 1974). A chemically related drug, azapropazone, has been shown not to interact significantly with digitoxin (Faust-Tinnefeldt *et al.*, 1979) and in a separate study the same group showed that azapropazone did not alter the plasma half-life of digitoxin (Faust-Tinnefeldt and Gilfrich, 1977).

In a study in dogs, Wilkerson and Glenn (1977) found that aspirin, indomethacin, and ibuprofen all reduced the dose of ouabain required to cause premature ventricular beats or ventricular tachycardia. They also reported that guanethidine prevented this interaction and postulated that adrenergic mechanisms were involved. In a further study, Wilkerson *et al.* (1980) showed that the toxicity of digoxin was also increased in dogs given aspirin, ibuprofen or indomethacin. The cause of this interaction appeared to be pharmacokinetic since all three NSAIDs caused a significant increase in the plasma concentration of digoxin. Aspirin 650 mg q. i. d. increased the plasma digoxin concentration from 1.12 ± 0.15 to 2.58 ± 0.24 ng ml^{-1}, while the increase with ibuprofen was from 0.9 ± 0.16 to 3.5 ± 0.65 ng ml^{-1}. Clearly, if these NSAIDs were to cause similar changes in digoxin plasma concentrations in patients then a major drug interaction would have been identified. In general, this seems not to be so, although the literature is confusing. In six volunteers, Finch *et al.* (1983) showed that indomethacin (50 mg t. i. d.) had no effect on the pharmacokinetics of digoxin; but in preterm infants Koren *et al.* (1983) found that indomethacin (0.3 mg kg^{-1}) increased the plasma concentration of digoxin from 2.2 ± 0.7 ng ml^{-1} to 3.2 ± 0.7 ng ml^{-1}. This was associated with a prolonged digoxin plasma half-life, apparently due to an indomethacin-induced reduction in glomerular filtration rate.

Fenster *et al.* (1982) showed that aspirin did not affect the kinetics of digoxin in eight adult men, while both flurbiprofen (Gross *et al.*, 1980) and fenbufen (Dunky *et al.*, 1979) produced either no or minimal changes in the steady-state plasma digoxin concentration. Similarly, piroxicam did not show any pharmacokinetic interaction with digoxin (Brodgen *et al.*, 1981). In a study with ibuprofen however, Quattrochi *et al.* (1983) found an average 59% increase in the plasma digoxin concentration when ibuprofen in doses up to 1000 mg day^{-1} was given to a group of 12 patients. In general, it seems that there is no systematic interaction between NSAIDs and digoxin. However, in view of the known ability of many NSAIDs to reduce the glomerular filtration rate in some patients, if unexpected toxicity is seen in a patient taking digoxin and who is given a NSAID, then this interaction should be suspected.

3.8 DIURETICS

3.8.1 Indomethacin and diuretics

It is now recognized that prostaglandins may function as natriuretic factors (Dunn and Hood, 1977), and they have been postulated as mediating the effects of certain diuretics (Attalah, 1979). It would not be too surprising therefore to find that NSAIDs interfere with the clinical efficacy of certain diuretics, perhaps by inhibiting prostaglandin synthetase activity. Elliott (1962) was the first to note an interaction between NSAIDs and diuretics when he showed that aspirin antagonized the diuretic effect of propranolol. Since that time there has been a lot of research activity, mostly involving indomethacin, but there are still many unanswered questions.

There is little doubt that indomethacin antagonizes the diuretic effect of loop diuretics such as frusemide and bumetanide. In some patients the interaction of indomethacin with frusemide also results in a loss of hypotensive control (Patak *et al.*, 1975; Pedrinelli *et al.*, 1982). It would appear that renal blood flow plays a major mechanistic role in this interaction. It is known that loop diuretics increase renal blood flow, concomitant with an increase in renal prostaglandins, particularly prostaglandin E_2 (Weber *et al.*, 1977). In dogs indomethacin inhibits the frusemide-induced increase in renal blood flow (Williamson *et al.*, 1975; Nies *et al.*, 1983), and comparable studies in the rat (Spät *et al.*, 1977) and rabbit (Oliw *et al.*, 1976) have shown a similar interaction between indomethacin and frusemide.

Tiggeler *et al.* (1977) described four patients in whom indomethacin inhibited the diuretic effect of large doses of frusemide, but the diuretic effect was restored by spironolactone. Indomethacin in standard clinical dosage decreases the natriuretic and diuretic effects of frusemide (Brater, 1979; Smith *et al.*, 1979; Chennavasin *et al.*, 1980). Plasma concentrations of frusemide are increased by indomethacin (Smith *et al.*, 1979) and this might seem unexpected, but the diuretic effect of frusemide is related to the tubular concentration of the drug and this is reduced by indomethacin, due to an impairment of the renal clearance of frusemide (Smith *et al.*, 1979). Studies in dogs show a similar mechanism and the ability of the loop of Henle to respond to frusemide is apparently not affected (Data *et al.*, 1978). However, it would appear that the interaction cannot be fully explained on this basis (Chennavasin *et al.*, 1980). It is of interest here to note that plasma concentrations of indomethacin are not significantly affected by frusemide (Brooks *et al.*, 1974a). Indomethacin is known to suppress plasma renin activity, and this may lead to hyperkalaemia (MacCarthy *et al.*, 1979; Mor *et al.*, 1983) but indomethacin does not significantly suppress the rise in plasma renin activity induced by frusemide (Dessaulles and Schwartz, 1979). Studies in dogs (Anderson *et al.*, 1983), however, suggest that the effect of indomethacin on plasma renin activity may be of importance in the interaction of indomethacin with frusemide. A low dose of indomethacin showed an effect of the drug on frusemide-induced diuresis without a concomitant reduction in renal prostaglandins (Kondo *et al.*, 1983). Indomethacin also blocks the audiological effects of frusemide (Arenberg and Goodfriend, 1980).

The diuretic effect of other loop diuretics is also inhibited by indomethacin. Thus the effects of bumetanide (Pedrinelli *et al.*, 1980; Brater *et al.*, 1981) are inhibited by indomethacin and studies in dogs link this action to changes in renal blood flow (Olsen, 1975). The effects of ethacrinic acid are also impaired by indomethacin (Williamson *et al.*, 1974). There is no clear picture as to the effect of indomethacin on other diuretics. The diuretic effects of theophylline seem to be impaired by indomethacin (Oliw *et al.*, 1977). Indomethacin did not impair the diuretic effect of hydrochlorthiazide in man (Williams *et al.*, 1982; Favre *et al.*, 1983) or in the chimpanzee (Fanelli *et al.*, 1980) but the effect of bemetizide, a thiazide diuretic acting on the loop of Henle, was impaired by indomethacin (Düsing *et al.*, 1983). The diuretic effect of triamterene was not altered by indomethacin (Favre *et al.*, 1983) but the combination of these two drugs has been reported to cause renal failure (Favre *et al.*, 1982).

3.8.2 Other NSAIDs

Following the initial report of Elliott (1962) concerning aspirin and spironolactone, Tweedale and Ogilvie (1973) confirmed the blunting effect of aspirin on the diuretic effect of spironolactone. In animal studies, aspirin inhibited the increase in renal blood flow caused by arachidonic acid (Anderson *et al.*, 1983) and in the clinical situation aspirin has been shown to inhibit the diuretic effect of two loop diuretics, frusemide (Valette and Apoil, 1979; Bartoli *et al.*, 1980) and piretanide (Valette and Apoil, 1979). In two women taking aspirin, the addition of a carbonic anhydrase inhibitor caused salicylate intoxication, probably due to the acidaemia arising from the use of carbonic anhydrase inhibitors (Anderson *et al.*, 1978). Diflunisal caused a 25% increase in plasma concentrations of hydrochlorthiazide but the clinical significance of this effect is probably not very great (Tempero *et al.*, 1977). However, Favre *et al.* (1983) showed that diflunisal inhibited the diuretic effect of frusemide, spironolactone and hydrochlorthiazide.

There is relatively little information on the other NSAIDs. Allan *et al.* (1981) reported one patient in whom indomethacin inhibited the diuretic effect of frusemide, but diuresis was restored when flurbiprofen was substituted for the indomethacin. In contrast, Rawles (1982) showed that flurbiprofen inhibited the diuretic effect of frusemide and Symmons *et al.* (1983) also showed that flurbiprofen inhibited the effects of frusemide but to a larger extent than indomethacin. In another clinical report ibuprofen and naproxen apparently inhibited the diuretic effect of frusemide and diuresis was only restored when these NSAIDs were stopped (Yeung Laiwah and Mactier, 1981). Both indoprofen and sulindac have been reported not to interact with frusemide. In 12 patients on frusemide, indoprofen had no significant effect on the frusemide-induced diuresis (Passeri *et al.*, 1981). Calin (1981) suggested that sulindac may not inhibit the frusemide-induced diuresis, because of the lack of effect of sulindac on renal prostaglandin, but no data to this effect are available. In three patients who developed renal impairment on ibuprofen and naproxen, the symptoms and signs resolved when sulindac was given (Bunning and Barth, 1982). Finally, although azapropazone caused some fluid retention in patients, it did not affect the frusemide-induced diuresis (Williamson *et al.*, 1983).

This area of drug interaction is still very confused, partly because a clear picture of the mechanism has not yet emerged. It does not appear that inhibition of prostaglandin synthesis in the kidney is the main cause of this interaction. It is clear that indomethacin can inhibit the diuresis of loop diuretics, but probably not of thiazide diuretics (although the hypotensive effect will be impaired). If a patient taking a NSAID develops a failure of diuresis while receiving a diuretic this interaction should be considered. Until more information is available the choice of an alternative diuretic will be by trial and error.

3.9   INTERACTIONS BETWEEN NSAIDs

3.9.1   Aspirin and indomethacin

Treatment with combinations of NSAIDs is quite common although the value of such combination therapy is doubtful. Aspirin is widely used with other NSAIDs (Grennan *et al.*, 1977) and there is a sizeable literature on these interactions. The most widely studied combination is that of aspirin and indomethacin but the work in this area is contradictory (see Table 3.3). Jeremy and Towson (1970), using radiolabelled compounds, found that aspirin reduced the plasma concentration of indomethacin and they explained the lack of additive clinical effect on this interaction. Champion *et al.* (1972), however, could find no evidence that 3.6 g aspirin daily had any effect on the plasma concentration of indomethacin in patients or in volunteers. The scene was thus set for continuing controversy which is also seen in the animal models for this interaction. Van Arman *et al.* (1973) reported that aspirin antagonized the effect of indomethacin and phenylbutazone in the rat, whereas Garrett *et al.* (1983) using a different rat model could find no evidence that aspirin interacted with a number of NSAIDs. Yesair *et al.* (1970) found that salicylate reduced the plasma concentration of indomethacin in rats.

In general, it appears that aspirin will produce a significant reduction in the plasma concentration of indomethacin given concurrently (Rubin *et al.*, 1973, 1974; Helleberg *et al.*, 1977; Kwan *et al.*, 1978; Correll and Jensen, 1979). Even here there are disparities, for Kaldestadt *et al.* (1975) showed that aspirin reduced the peak concentration in plasma of orally administered indomethacin

TABLE 3.3

Pharmacokinetic and pharmacodynamic interactions in man between indomethacin and aspirin (see text)

Reference	Effect on indomethacin plasma concn.	Effect of indomethacin on plasma concn. of aspirin	Clinical effect compared to indomethacin alone
Jeremy and Towson (1970)	Reduced	—	—
Champion et al. (1972)	None	—	—
Rubin et al. (1973)	Reduced	None	—
Lindquist et al. (1974)	None	None	—
Kaldestadt et al. (1975)	Reduced (Indomethacin orally)	None	—
	None (Indomethacin rectally)	None	—
Brooks et al. (1975)	None	—	None
Farnham et al. (1975)	Increased (rate of absorption)	—	—
Helleberg et al. (1977)	Reduced (high dose aspirin)	—	—
	None (low dose aspirin)	—	
Pawlotsky et al. (1977)	None	—	Reduced
Kwan et al. (1978)	Reduced	—	—
Pawlotsky et al. (1978)	—	—	Reduced
Correll and Jensen (1979)	Reduced	None	
Torgyan et al. (1979)	—	—	None (sodium salicylate used)
Helleberg (1981)	—	—	None
Alvan et al. (1981)	—	—	Indomethacin enhanced effect of aspirin

but not of rectally administered indomethacin. This finding suggests a mechanism for the interaction and it is likely that the absorption of indomethacin from the upper gastrointestinal tract is reduced by aspirin (Kwan et al., 1978).

The clearance of indomethacin from the plasma may also be enhanced by aspirin (by some 20–25%), perhaps because of displacement of indomethacin from its protein binding sites in plasma (Helleberg et al., 1977) or because of increased biliary clearance (Kwan et al., 1978). Several studies, like those of Champion et al. (1972), have failed to show any significant effect of aspirin on plasma concentrations of indomethacin (Lindquist et al., 1974; Brooks et al., 1975; Pawlotsky et al., 1977, 1978) but, in general, these studies have tended to use the less accurate and specific spectrofluorometric assay. Thus the studies of Kwan et al. (1978) using sensitive and more specific analytical methods for indomethacin are to be preferred in this regard. Some studies have even suggested that the plasma concentration of indomethacin is increased by aspirin (Garnham et al., 1975; Helleberg, 1981). However Garnham et al. (1975) used a buffered aspirin preparation and found only an increased rate of absorption of indomethacin.

In spite of these controversies there is general agreement that the plasma concentration of aspirin is not altered by indomethacin (Rubin et al., 1973, 1974; Lindquist et al., 1974; Kaldestadt et al., 1975; Corell and Jensen, 1979).

The clinical significance of this interaction is probably not very great and no change in overall anti-inflammatory activity is to be expected (Brooks et al., 1975; Torgyan et al., 1979; Helleberg, 1981). Pawlotsky et al. (1977, 1978) however, using the sigma ESR and articular index as a measure of the clinical effect reported that aspirin reduced the therapeutic effect of indomethacin. In contrast, there are reports that indomethacin increased the therapeutic effect of aspirin, particularly low dosage aspirin (2 g daily) (Alvan and Ekstrand, 1981; Ekstrand et al., 1981). Brooks et al. (1975) reported that side effects were more common with the combination therapy of indomethacin plus aspirin, than with indomethacin alone, but Torgyan et al. (1979) suggested that the blood loss from the gastrointestinal tract may be less with the combination therapy, than with indomethacin alone. In a further twist to this interaction story, Livio et al. (1982) reported that indomethacin prevented the inhibitory effects of aspirin on platelet cyclo-oxygenase activity.

3.9.2 Aspirin and other NSAIDs

The protein binding of phenylbutazone may be altered by aspirin (Chignell and Stark Weather, 1971) and phenylbutazone appeared to inhibit the uricosuric effect of aspirin (Oyer et al., 1966). It would appear, however, that there is no significant interaction between aspirin and phenylbutazone either in man or in animals (Mielens et al., 1968). Table 3.4 summarizes the interactions in man between aspirin and the other NSAIDSs. In general, aspirin lowers the plasma concentration of the various NSAIDs but usually without any effect on the overall clinical response. Plasma concentrations of naproxen (Segre et al., 1974b; Boost, 1975), flurbiprofen (Brooks and Khong, 1977), ibuprofen (Grennan et al., 1979; Day et al., 1982), ketoprofen (Williams et al., 1981), fenoprofen (Rubin et al., 1973, 1974), fenbufen (Chiccarelli et al., 1980), tolmetin (Cressman et al., 1976), meclofenamate (Baragar and Smith, 1978), diclofenac (Müller et al., 1977; Fowler, 1979; Willis et al., 1980), and difluni-

TABLE 3.4
Pharmacokinetic interactions in man between NSAIDs and aspirin

Drug	Drug levels reduced by aspirin	Clinical effect	Salicylate levels reduced by drug	References
Naproxen	Yes (a,b)	Enhanced (c)	No (b)	(a) Boost (1975), (b) Segre et al. (1974b) Willkens and Segal (1975)
Flurbiprofen	Yes	—	—	Brooks and Khong (1977)
Buprofen	Yes	Enhanced	—	Grennan et al. (1979); Day et al. (1982)
Ketoprofen	Yes	—		Williams et al. (1981)
Fenoprofen	Yes	—	No	Rubin et al. (1974)
Fenbufen	Yes	—	—	Chicarelli et al. (1980)
Tolmetin	Yes	—	—	Cressman et al. (1976)
Piroxicam	No	—	—	Hobbs and Twomey (1979)
Sudoxicam	No	—	—	Wiseman et al. (1975)
Sulindac	—	None		Pawlotsky (1978)
Meclofenamate	Yes	—	—	Baragar and Smith (1978) (c) Willkins and Segre (1975)
Diclofenac	Yes (a,b,c)	—	Yes (a)	(a) Müller et al. (1977), (b) Fowler (1979), (c) Willis et al. (1980)
Zomepirac	No (Reduced)			Desiraju et al. (1983)
Diflunisal	Yes (a,b)		No (b)	(a) Steelman et al. (1978), (b) Schulz et al. (1979)
Dextropro-poxyphene paracetamol			No	Hemming et al. (1981)

sal (Steelman et al., 1978; Schultz et al., 1979) are all reduced by concomitant aspirin therapy. In general, the average reduction in plasma concentration was between 25 and 30%. The mechanism of the interaction is not clear; some workers have suggested a reduced absorption of the NSAID (Brooks and Khong, 1977; Chiccarelli et al., 1980) while others have proposed a reduction in the protein binding of the NSAID (Rubin et al., 1974; Segre et al., 1974b; Cressman et al., 1976; Williams et al., 1981). Willis et al. (1980) also suggested that the biliary clearance of diclofenac was enhanced by aspirin. Williams et al. (1981) also showed that salicylate reduced the metabolic conversion of ketoprofen into its conjugated metabolites, while the metabolism to non-conjugated derivatives was enhanced.

A number of studies have shown no effect of aspirin on plasma NSAID concentrations. Thus aspirin did not reduce the plasma concentration of sudoxicam (Wiseman et al., 1975), piroxicam (Hobbs and Twomey, 1979) or zomepirac (Desiraju et al., 1983). Indeed, aspirin caused an increase in the plasma zomepirac concentrations from 2.0 ± 0.8 to 3.5 ± 1.8 µg ml^{-1}. There was very little evidence of any effect of the NSAIDs on salicylate concentrations, although salicylate concentrations were reduced by diclofenac (Müller et al., 1977). Naproxen (Segre et al., 1974b), fenoprofen (Rubin et al., 1974), diflunisal (Schulz et al., 1979) and dextropropoxyphene plus paracetamol (Hemming et al., 1981) did not have any effect on plasma salicylate concentrations.

There is very little evidence that these interactions are of much clinical significance. Willkens and Segre (1975) showed that the addition of naproxen to patients taking aspirin caused a modest but noticeable improvement in the clinical assessments. The combination of aspirin and ibuprofen is slightly more effective than either drug alone (Grennan et al., 1979; Day et al., 1982). In both instances aspirin was given in high doses (3.6–5.2 g daily).

3.9.3 Other NSAIDs

Few studies have examined the interaction between other NSAIDs. Diflunisal had no effect on the kinetics of naproxen (Dresse et al., 1978) but increased the plasma concentration of indomethacin by a factor of 2 or 3, apparently due to a reduced conjugation and biliary clearance of indomethacin (Tjandramaga et al., 1983). Finally flurbiprofen had no effect on the plasma concentrations of indomethacin (Rudge et al., 1982).

It would seem from these studies that although small falls in the plasma concentrations of NSAIDs are seen when aspirin is given, there is little or no clinical significance to these observations. The additional anti-inflammatory effect of aspirin compensates for any potential loss in therapeutic activity.

3.10 LITHIUM

Leftwich et al. (1977) originally reported that indomethacin was antidiuretic in a patient with lithium-induced diabetes insipidus. They reported that indomethacin increased the plasma concentration of lithium. A similar observation was reported by Singer et al. (1978) with phenylbutazone increasing lithium concentrations from 0.7 to 1.44 nmol l^{-1}. Indomethacin seems to increase the plasma lithium concentration by between 30 and 50% on average, probably by decreasing the renal clearance of lithium (Frolich et al., 1979). There is, however, no clear pattern as to which NSAIDs will affect lithium and which will not. Reimann et al. (1983) reported that whereas indomethacin increased plasma lithium concentrations, aspirin had no such effect. Clometacin, a drug chemically related to indomethacin, increased lithium plasma concentrations in three patients, and in six other women reduced the lithium clearance from 18.5 to 11.0 ml min^{-1} (Edou *et al.*, 1983). Diclofenac increased plasma lithium concentrations by 26% in five female volunteers due to a fall in the renal clearance of lithium (Reimann and Frölich, 1981), and recently three cases of lithium toxicity have been associated with piroxicam administration (Kerry *et al.*, 1983). In a study comparing indomethacin and ibuprofen in six patients taking lithium, indomethacin caused the expected increase in plasma lithium concentrations but ibuprofen had no such effect. This interaction is clearly of considerable clinical significance. Since there is no clear picture of which NSAID to use with safety, it would be wise to check plasma lithium concentrations in all patients receiving a NSAID with their lithium and to reduce the dose of lithium if any increase in the plasma lithium concentration is seen.

3.11 METHOTREXATE

There is a potentially dangerous interaction if salicylates are given to patients taking methotrexate. Salicylate inhibits the renal clearance of methotrexate by about 30–40% (Liegler *et al.*, 1969) and in addition there is some displacement of methotrexate from its plasma protein binding sites (Shen and Azarnoff, 1978). The resulting interaction has caused death because of pancytopenia (Mandel, 1976). There is some evidence that phenylbutazone may produce similar problems with methotrexate (Adams and Hunter, 1976) and, in animal studies, a number of other NSAIDs inhibit the renal clearance of methotrexate, for example indomethacin, naproxen and ibuprofen (Nierenberg, 1983). Clearly NSAIDs should be used with great care in patients taking methotrexate, and the dose of methotrexate should probably be reduced by one third. Phenylbutazone is also reported to potentiate the effect of chlorambucil (Schiffman *et al.*, 1978).

3.12 PROBENECID

In 1968 Skeith *et al.* reported that the renal excretion of indomethacin was reduced by concurrent administration of probenecid, although the observation was based on total radioactivity profiles after the administration of ^{14}C-indomethacin. The interaction was investigated in further detail by Brooks *et al.* (1974b) and Baber *et al.* (1978) since the use of probenecid might prolong the plasma half-life of indomethacin and thus enhance its beneficial effects. This might be preferable to increasing the dose of indomethacin with its accompanying side effects due to high peak concentrations in plasma. In practice both studies showed an enhanced clinical effect of probenecid plus indomethacin compared to indomethacin alone and this was associated with an increased plasma indomethacin concentration. There was no increase in side effects. The effect appeared to be due to a reduced biliary excretion of indomethacin with little effect on the renal excretion of indomethacin.

Studies with other NSAIDs have shown similar interactions between probenecid and naproxen (Runkel et al., 1978), carprofen (Yü and Perel, 1980), diflunisal (Meffin et al., 1981), and ketoprofen (Upton et al., 1982). All these drugs are metabolized by conjugation with glucuronic acid and then excreted in part in the bile. Probenecid appears to inhibit the glucuronidation of both naproxen (Runkel et al., 1978) and ketoprofen (Upton et al., 1982) with a decreased excretion in the urine of glucuronide conjugates of these drugs. It seems likely that drugs which do not undergo glucuronidation will not be affected by probenecid (Day et al., 1982).

The clinical value of this beneficial interaction is probably limited but the occasional use of probenecid can enhance the therapeutic effect of NSAIDs such as indomethacin.

3.13   GOLD AND PENICILLAMINE

There are various reports of interactions with these drugs, but in view of the potential toxicity of these drugs, any other drug therapy should be kept to a minimum. The absorption of penicillamine has been reported to be inhibited by iron salts, probably because of chelation in the gut lumen (Lyle et al., 1977).

3.14   CORTICOSTEROIDS

Patients may be taking NSAIDs as well as corticosteroids for their rheumatic disease and there are occasional reports of interactions in this area. Plasma concentrations of salicylate appear to decrease during long-term costicosteroid therapy (Klinenberg and Miller, 1965; Graham et al., 1977). The clearance of salicylate in these patients is increased largely through the kidney. In contrast, azapropazone concentrations in plasma are not affected by prednisolone therapy (Faust-Tinnefeldt and Geissler, 1978).

Several drugs that are used for non-rheumatic disorders are known to induce the metabolism of glucurocorticoids, such as phenytoin (Petereit and Meikle, 1977), phenobarbitone and rifampicin (Jubiz and Meikle, 1979). In such cases the dose of prednisolone may have to be increased considerably to regain control of the disease. Unfortunately a marked interindividual variation in the response to such enzyme inducing agents makes it very difficult to predict the dosage requirements. In contrast a recent study has shown that indomethacin and naproxen increase the free concentrations of prednisolone in plasma, without an increase in the total prednisolone concentrations (Rae et al., 1982). If confirmed, this may explain the steroid-sparing effects of such drugs.

3.15 ALLOPURINOL

Although allopurinol is not strictly an antirheumatic drug, it is widely used in patients with gout and there are a number of relevant interactions with this drug. Allopurinol, being an inhibitor of xanthine oxidase, will inhibit the metabolism of drugs that are metabolized by this enzyme. Thus azathioprine and 6-mercaptopurine are potentiated by allopurinol (Elion, 1978). It is recommended that the dose of azathioprine and mercaptopurine should be reduced *to approximately 25%* of previous levels if allopurinol is used concurrently (Calabresi and Parks, 1980).

It has been suggested that allopurinol is an inhibitor of drug microsomal oxidation (Vesell *et al.*, 1970) but this has not been fully confirmed. Allopurinol does not inhibit the metabolism of phenylbutazone (Horwitz *et al.*, 1977) and only in high doses (600 mg day^{-1}) has it been shown to inhibit the metabolism of theophylline (Manfredi and Vesell, 1981). In a more standard dosage of 300 mg day^{-1} no such interaction is seen (Grygiel *et al.*, 1979).

3.16 SULPHINPYRAZONE

Sulphinpyrazone is chemically related to the pyrazolones, phenylbutazone and azapropazone, so it is not too surprising to find that it is an inhibitor of drug metabolism. It has been reported to inhibit the metabolism of warfarin (O'Reilly, 1982b) and tolbutamide (Miners *et al.*, 1982), while inducing the metabolism of theophylline (Birkett *et al.*, 1983) and antipyrine (Walter *et al.*, 1981). The interaction is of considerable interest since in the case of warfarin, like phenylbutazone, sulphinpyrazone only inhibits the S-enantiomer (the more potent one) of warfarin (O'Reilly, 1982b). It is suggested that sulphinpyrazone may have a dual effect on two different forms of cytochrome P450. It may inhibit the form of P450 involved in the metabolism of tolbutamide and S-warfarin (like phenylbutazone – Lewis *et al.*, 1974) while enhancing the form of cytochrome P450 mediating the metabolism of theophylline, antipyrine and R-warfarin. In the case of warfarin, the effect of the two interactions is to enhance the hypoprothrombinaemic effect because the metabolism of the more potent enantiomer, S-warfarin, is inhibited.

Salicylate inhibits the uricosuric effects of sulphinpyrazone and probenecid (Yü *et al.*, 1963) and thus only occasional doses of aspirin should be given to patients taking these drugs for their uricosuric activities.

3.17 OTHER DRUGS

The oral contraceptive steroids are taken by a large number of women but do not appear to cause significant interaction problems. Although salicylate concentrations may be reduced in users of oral contraceptive steroids (Gupta *et al.*, 1982), there is no effect on phenylbutazone metabolism (O'Malley *et al.*, 1972; Gupta *et al.*, 1982).

Cimetidine, although it is known to inhibit the metabolism of other drugs, has no significant effect on the pharmacokinetics of indomethacin (Howes *et al.*, 1983) or ibuprofen (Conrad and Mayersohn, 1983). Consolo *et al.* (1970) reported that desmethylimipramine delayed the absorption of phenylbutazone, perhaps due to the delay in gastric emptying produced by the anticholinergic effect of desmethylimipramine. No significant interaction was reported between naproxen and diazepam (Stitt *et al.*, 1977) but Hobkirk *et al.* (1977) found the combination of diazepam and indomethacin helped night time rheumatic pain more than indomethacin alone. In a follow up to this observation, Bird *et al.* (1983) tried the combination of indomethacin and haloperidol in a double-blind study. However, the study had to be discontinued at the half-way stage because of profound drowsiness and confusion in the patients receiving indomethacin and haloperidol. Phenobarbitone, which is a well-known enzyme inducing agent, has been shown to lower fenoprofen concentrations by enhancing the metabolic clearance of fenoprofen (Helleberg *et al.*, 1974). Aspirin has been reported to impair the absorption of vitamin C (Basu, 1982) and to prolong the plasma half-life of penicillin from 44.5 to 72.4 minutes (Kampmann *et al.*, 1972). The latter interaction was also seen with indomethacin as well as aspirin and was thought to be due to competition for the tubular excretion of penicillin.

Lee *et al.* (1979) reported an episode of severe hypertension in a patient who was taking indomethacin and who received an appetite suppressant containing phenylpropanolamine. They wondered if indomethacin had increased the sensitivity to indirect amines but there is no direct evidence for this. Indeed, Brink *et al.* (1980) reported that indomethacin reduced the responsiveness of airway muscle to histamine. Aspirin (0.5–1.0 g) has been reported to enhance the therapeutic effect of nitroglycerin probably by increasing the plasma concentration of nitroglycerin (Weber *et al.*, 1983). Finally in this miscellaneous section, levamisole (50 mg t. i. d.) has no effect on the pharmacokinetics of salicylate in volunteers given 3.9 g of aspirin daily (Rumble *et al.*, 1979) and dimethylsulphoxide has been reported to inhibit the bioactivation of sulindac (Swanson *et al.*, 1983).

3.18   CONCLUSIONS

It is clear that the spotlight is being turned on to the subject of drug interactions with antirheumatic drugs and many articles are being published at present. In some cases the interactions discussed are of little clinical importance, but this must not be allowed to camouflage the clinically important interactions. There is no doubt that phenylbutazone (plus oxyphenbutazone and other pyrazolones) should not be given to patients taking oral anticoagulants, but that is no reason to deprive such patients of other NSAIDs where such drugs are clinically indicated. The interactions with aspirin and antacids are largely of academic interest but there are real problems in the combined use of NSAIDs with diuretics (especially loop diuretics) and with antihypertensive drugs. Clarification is required in this latter area and it is hoped that further studies will resolve these issues.

3.19 REFERENCES

Abe, K., Itoh, T., Imai, Y., Sato, M., Haruyama T., Sakurai Y., Goto, T., Otsuka Y. and Yoshinaga, K. (1980) Implication of endogenous prostaglandin system in the antihypertensive effect of captopril SQ 14225 in low renin hypertension. *Jap. Circ. J.*, 44, 422–5.

Adams, J. D. and Hunter, G. A. (1976) Drug interactions in psoriasis. *Aust. J. Dermatol.*, 17, 39–40.

Aggeler, P. M., O'Reilly, R. A., Leong, L. and Kowitz, P. E. (1967) Potentiation of anticoagulant effect of warfarin by phenylbutazone. *N. Engl. J. Med.*, 276, 496–501.

Allan, S. G., Knox, J. and Kerr, F. (1981) Interaction between diuretics and indomethacin. *Br. Med. J.*, 283, 1611.

Alvan, G. and Ekstrand, R. (1981) Clinical effects of indomethacin and additive clinical effect of indomethacin during salicylate maintenance therapy. *Scand. J. Rheumatol.*, 39, (Suppl.), 29–32.

Anderson, C. J., Kaufman, P. L. and Sturm, R. J. (1978) Toxicity of combined therapy with carbonic anhydrase inhibitors and aspirin. *Am. J. Ophthalmol.*, 86, 516–19.

Anderson, W. P., Bartley, P. J., Casley, D. J. and Selig, S. E. (1983) Comparison of aspirin and indomethacin pre-treatment on the responses to reduced renal artery pressure in conscious dogs. *J. Physiol.*, 336, 101–12.

Andreasen, P. B., Froland, A., Skovsted, L., Anderson, S. A. and Hauge, M. (1973) Diphenylhydantoin half life in man and its inhibition by phenylbutazone: the role of genetic factors. *Acta Med. Scand.*, 193, 561–4.

Andreasen, P. B., Simonsen, K., Brocks, K., Dimo, B. and Bouchelouche, P. (1981) Hypoglycaemia induced by azapropazone – tolbutamide interaction. *Br. J. Clin. Pharmacol.*, 12, 581–3.

Angelkort, B. (1978) Zum Einfluss von naproxen auf die thrombozytare Blutstillung und die Antikoagulantien – Behandlung mit phenprocoumon. *Fortschr. Med.*, 15, 1249–52.

Arenberg, I. K. and Goodfriend, T. L. (1980) Indomethacin blocks the acute audiologic effects of furoside in Ménière's disease. *Arch. Otolarynyol.*, 106, 383–6.

Attallah, A. A. (1979) Interaction of prostaglandins with diuretics. *Prostaglandins*, 18, 369–75.

Ayres, J. W., Wiedler, D. J., Mackichen, J., Sakmar, E., Hallmark, M. R., Lemanowicz, E. F. and Wagner, J. G. (1977) Pharmacokinetics of tolmetin with and without concomitant administration of antacid in man. *Eur. J. Clin. Pharmacol.*, 12, 421–8.

Baber, N., Halliday, L., Sibeon, R., Littler, T. and Orme, M. (1978) The interaction between indomethacin and probenecid. A clinical and pharmacokinetic study. *Clin. Pharmacol. Ther.*, 24, 298–307.

Baele, G., Rasquin, K. and Barbier, F. (1983) Effects of oxametacin on coumarin anticoagulation and on platelet function in humans. *Arzneim. Forsch.*, 33, 149–52.

Baragar, F. D. and Smith, T. C. (1978) Drug interaction studies with sodium meclofenamate (Meclomen). *Curr. Ther. Res.*, 23, S51–S59.

Bartoli, E., Arras, S., Faedda, R., Soggia, G., Satta, A. and Olmeo, N. A. (1980) Blunting of furosemide diuresis by aspirin in man. *J. Clin. Pharmacol.*, 20, 452–8.

Basu, T. K. (1982) Vitamin C – aspirin interactions. *Int. J. Vit. Nutr. Res.*, 23, 83–90.

Bird, H. A., le Gallez, P. and Wright, V. (1983) Drowsiness due to haloperidol/indomethacin in combination. *Lancet*, i, 830–1.

Birkett, D. J., Miners, J. O. and Attwood, J. (1983) Evidence for a dual action of sulphinpyrazone on drug metabolism in man: theophylline – sulphinpyrazone interaction. *Br. J. Clin. Pharmacol.*, 15, 567–9.

Boejinga, J. K. and Van der Vijgh, W. J. (1977) Double blind study of the effect of glafenine (Glifanan) on oral anticoagulant therapy with phenprocoumon (Marcumar). *Eur. J. Clin. Pharmacol.*, 12, 291–6.

Boekhout-Mussert, M. J. and Loeliger, E. A. (1974) Influence of ibuprofen on oral anticoagulation with phenprocoumon. *J. Int. Med. Res.*, 2, 297–83.

Boost, G. (1975) Klinisch-pharmakologische und Pharmakokinetische Studien mit Naproxen. *Arzneim. Forsch.*, 25, 281–7.

Brater, D. C. (1979) Analysis of the effect of indomethacin on the response to furosemide in man: effect of dose of furosemide. *J. Pharmacol. Exp. Ther.*, 210, 386–390.

Brater, D. C., Fox, W. R. and Chennavasin, P. (1981) Interaction studies with bumetanide and furosemide. Effects of probenecid and of indomethacin on response to bumetanide in man. *J. Clin. Pharmacol.*, 21, 647–53.

Brazier, J. L., Tamisier, J. N., Ambert, D. and Bannier, A. (1981) Bioavailability of ketoprofen in man with and without concomitant administration of aluminium phosphate. *Eur. J. Clin. Pharmacol.*, 19, 305–7.

Brink, C., Grimauld, C., Guillot, C. and Orehek, J. (1980) The interaction between indomethacin and contractile agents on human isolated airway muscle. *Br. J. Pharmacol.*, 69, 383–8.

Brogden, R. N., Heel, R. C., Speight, T. M. and Avery, G. S. (1981) Piroxicam: a review of its pharmacological properties and therapeutic efficacy. *Drugs*, 22, 165–87.

Brooks, P. M., Bell, M. A., Lee, P., Rooney, P. J. and Dick, W. C. (1974a) The effect of frusemide on indomethacin plasma levels. *J. Clin. Pharmacol.*, 1, 485–9.

Brooks, P. M., Bell, M. A., Mason, D. I. and Buchanan, W. W. (1977) Interactions of anti-rheumatic drugs. *Agents Actions* (Suppl. 1), 85–95.

Brooks, P. M., Bell, M. A., Sturrock, R. D., Famoey, J. P. and Dick, W. C. (1974b) The clinical significance of the indomethacin–probenecid interaction. *Br. J. Clin. Pharmacol.*, 1, 287–90.

Brooks, P. M. and Khong, T. K. (1977) Flurbiprofen–aspirin interaction: a double-blind crossover study. *Curr. Med. Res. Opinion*, 5, 53–7.

Brooks, P. M., Walker, J. J., Bell, M. A., Buchanan, W. W. and Rhymer, A. R. (1975) Indomethacin–aspirin interaction: a clinical appraisal. *Br. Med. J.*, 3, 69–71.

Bunning, R. D. and Barth, W. F. (1982) Sulindac – a potentially renal sparing non-steroidal anti-inflammatory drug. *J. Am. Med. Assoc.*, 248, 2864–7.

Calabresi, P. and Parks, R. E. (1980) Chemotherapy of neoplastic diseases. in *The Pharmacological Basis of Therapeutics* (eds A. G. Gilman, L. S. Goodman and A. Gilman), MacMillans, New York, pp. 1249–313.

Calin, A. (1981) Non-steroidal anti inflammatory drugs and frusemide-induced diuresis. *Br. Med. J.*, 283, 1399–400.

Carter, S. A. (1979) Potential effect of sulindac on response of prothrombin time to oral anticoagulants. *Lancet*, ii, 698–9.

Chalmers, I. M., Bell, M. A. and Buchanan, W. W. (1973) Effect of flurbiprofen on the metabolism of antipyrine in man. *Ann. Rheum. Dis.*, 32, 58–61.

Champion, G. D., Paulus, H. E., Mongan, E., Okun, R., Pearson, C. M. and Sarkissian, E. (1972) The effect of aspirin on serum indomethacin. *Clin. Pharmacol. Ther.*, 13, 239–44.

Chatfield, D. H., Green, J. N., Kao, J. C., Tarrant, M. E. and Woodage, T. J. (1978) Plasma protein binding and interaction studies with benoxaprofen. *Biochem. Pharmacol.*, 27, 887–90.

Chennavasin, P., Seiwell, R. and Brater, D. C. (1980) Pharmacokinetic-dynamic analysis of the indomethacin–frusemide interaction in man. *J. Pharmacol. Exp. Ther.*, 215, 77–81.

Cherner, R., Groppe, C. W. and Rupp, J. J. (1963) Prolonged tolbutamide-induced hypoglycaemia. *J. Am. Med. Assoc.*, 185, 883–4.

Chernish, S. M., Rubin, A., Rodda, B. E. and Ridolfo, A. S. (1972) The physiological disposition of fenoprofen IV. The effects of position of subject, food ingestion, antacid ingestion on the plasma levels of orally administered fenoprofen. *J. Med.*, 3, 249–57.

Chiccarelli, F. S., Eisner, H. J. and Van Lear, G. E. (1980) Metabolic and pharmacokinetic studies with fenbufen in man. *Arzneim. Forsch.*, 30, 728–35.

Chignell, C. F. and Stark Weather, D. K. (1971) Optical studies of drug protein complexes V. The interaction of phenylbutazone, flufenamic acid, and dicoumarol with acetyl salicylic acid treated human serum albumin. *Mol. Pharmacol.*, 7, 229–37.

Chlud, K. (1976) Investigations with possible interactions between diclofenac and glibenclamide. *Z. Rheumaforsch.*, 35, 377–82.

Chlud, K. and Kaik, B. (1977) Clinical studies of the interaction between tolmetin and glibenclamide. *Int. J. Clin. Pharmacol.*, 15, 409–10.

Christensen, L. K., Hansen, J. M. and Kristenson, M. (1963) Sulphaphenazole induced hypoglycaemic attacks in tolbutamide-treated diabetics. *Lancet*, ii, 1298–301.

Conney, A. H. (1967) Pharmacological implications of enzyme induction. *Pharmacol. Rev.*, 19, 317–66.

Conrad, K. A. and Mayersohn, M. (1983) Cimetidine does not affect single dose ibuprofen kinetics in volunteers. *Proc. 2nd World Conf. Clin. Pharmacol. Ther.*, Abstract No. 668.

Consolo, S., Morselli, P. L., Zaccala, M. and Garattini, S. (1970) Delayed absorption of phenylbutazone caused by desmethylimipramine in humans. *Eur. J. Pharmacol.*, 10, 239–42.

Corell, T. and Jensen, K. M. (1979) Interaction of salicylates and other non-steroidal anti-inflammatory agents in rats as shown by gastro-ulcerogenic and anti-inflammatory activities, and plasma concentrations. *Acta Pharmacol. Toxicol.*, 45, 225–31.

Cremoncini, C., Vignati, E., Cremoncini, M., Libroia, A. and Valente, M. C. (1980) Study on interaction between oral antidiabetic drugs and flurbiprofen. *Br. J. Clin. Pract.*, Suppl. 9, 27–9.

Cressman, W. A., Wortham, F. and Plostnieks, J. (1976) Absorption and excretion of tolmetin in man. *Clin. Pharmacol. Ther.*, 19, 224–33.

Crooks, J. and Moir, D. C. (1974) The detection of drug interaction in a hospital environment, in *Clinical Effects of Interaction between Drugs* (eds L. E. Cluff and J. C. Petrie) Excerpta Medica, Amsterdam, pp. 255–62.

Das, U. N. (1982) Modification of anti-hypertensive action of verapamil by inhibition of endogenous prostaglandin synthesis. *Prostaglandins Leukotrienes Med.*, 9, 167–9.

Data, J. L., Rane, A., Gerkens, J., Wilkinson, G. R., Nies, A. S. and Branch, R. A. (1978) The influence of indomethacin on the pharmacokinetics, diuretic response and hemodynamics of frusemide in the dog. *J. Pharmacol. Exp. Ther.*, 206, 431–8.

Day, R. O., Graham, G. G., Champion, G. D. and Lee, E. (1982) Clinically significant drug interactions with anti-rheumatic drugs, in *Anti-Rheumatic Drugs* (ed. E. Huskisson), Praeger, Basle, pp. 37–54.

De Forrest, J. M., Waldron, T. L. and Antonaccio, M. J. (1982) Renal response to captopril in conscious dogs pretreated with indomethacin. *Am. J. Physiol.*, 243, F543–F548.

Desiraju, R. K., Nayak, R. K., Pritchard, J. F. (1983) Zomepirac–aspirin interactions in man. *Clin. Pharmacol. Ther.*, 33, 250.

Dessaulles, E. and Schwartz, J. (1979) A comparative study of the action of frusemide and methylchlorthiazide on renin release by rat kidney slices and the interaction with indomethacin. *Br. J. Pharmacol.*, 65, 193–6.

Diwan, P. V. and Kulkarni D. R. (1983) Influence of non-steroidal anti-inflammatory agents on tolbutamide hypoglycaemia. *Ind. J. Med. Res.*, 78, 147–50.

Donaldson, D. R., Sreeharan, N., Crow, M. J. and Rajad, S. M. (1982) Assessment of the interaction of warfarin with aspirin and dipyridamole. *Thrombosis Haemostasis*, 47, 77.

Dresse, A., Gerard, M. A., Quinaux, N., Fischer, P. and Gerardy, J. (1978) Effect of diflunisal on the human plasma levels and on the urinary excretion of naproxen. *Arch. Int. Pharmacodynam. Ther.*, 236, 276–84.

Dugal, R., Dupuis, C., Bertrand, M. and Gagnon, M. A. (1980) The effect of buffering on oxyphenbutazone absorption kinetics and systemic availability. *Biopharm. Drug Disposition*, 1, 307–21.

Dunky, A., Ogris, E., Eberl, R. and Sailer, V. (1979) Interaction study with digoxin and fenbufen. *IXth Eur. Rheumatol. Congr.*, Wiesbaden, Abstract No. 315.

Dunn, M. J. and Hood, V. L. (1977) Prostaglandins and the kidney. *Am. J. Physiol.*, 233, F169–F184.

Durao, V., Prata, M. M. and Goncalves, L. M. P. (1977) Modification of antihypertensive effect of β-adrenoceptor-blocking agents by inhibition of endogenous prostaglandin synthesis. *Lancet*, ii, 1005–7.

Düsing, R., Nicholas, V., Glatte, B., Glänzer, K., Kipnowski, J. and Kramer, H. J. (1983) Interaction of bemetizide and indomethacin in the kidney. *Br. J. Clin. Pharmacol.*, 16, 377–84.

Edou, D., Godin, M., Colonna, L., Petit, M. and Fillastre, J. P. (1983) Interaction médicamenteuse: clométacine-lithium. *Presse Méd.*, 12, 1551.

Eisen, M. J. (1964) Combined effect of sodium warfarin and phenylbutazone. *J. Am. Med. Assoc.*, 189, 64–5.

Ekstrand, R., Alvan, G., Magnusson, A., Oliw, E., Palmer, L. and Rane, A. (1981) Additive clinical effect of indomethacin suppositories during salicylate therapy in rheumatoid patients. *Scand. J. Rheumatol.*, 10, 69–75.

Elion, G. B. (1978) Allopurinol and other inhibitors of urate synthesis, in *Handbook of Experimental Pharmacology* (eds W. N. Kelley and I. M. Weiner), Vol. 51, Springer-Verlag, Berlin, pp. 485–514.

Elliot, H. C. (1962) Reduced adrenocortical steroid excretion rates in man following aspirin administration. *Metabolism*, 11, 1015–18.

Emori, H. W., Paulus, H. E., Bluestone, R., Champion, G. D. and Pearson, C. (1976) Indomethacin serum concentrations in man. Effects of dosage, food and antacids. *Ann. Rheum. Dis.*, 35, 333–8.

Fanelli, G. M., Bohm, D. L., Camp, A. E. and Shum, W. K. (1980) Inability of indomethacin to modify hydrochlorthiazide diuresis and natriuresis by the chimpanzee kidney. *J. Pharmacol. Exp. Ther.*, 213, 596–9.

Farrell, K., Orr, J. M., Abbott, F. S., Ferguson, S., Sheppard, I., Godolphin, W. and Bruni, J. (1982) The effect of acetylsalicylic acid on serum free valproate concentrations and valproate clearance in children. *J. Paediatr.*, 101, 142–4.

Fausa, O. (1970) Salicylate-induced hypoprothrombinaemia. A report of four cases. *Acta Med. Scand.*, 188, 403–8.

Faust-Tinnefeldt Von, G. and Geissler, H. E. (1978) Azapropazone and rheumatic combination therapy considering drug interactions: azapropazone, aurothioglucose and azapropazone prednisolone. *Arzneim. Forsch.*, 28, 337–41.

Faust-Tinnefeldt Von, G., Geissler, H. E. and Gilfrich, H. J. (1979) Azapropazone – Plasmaspiogel während kombinierten Anwendung mit Digitoxin. *Medizin. Welt*, 30, 181–2.

Faust-Tinnefeldt Von, G., Geissler, H. E. and Mutschler, E. (1977) Azapropazone Plasmaspiegel unter Begleitmedikation mit einen Antacidun oder Laxans. *Arzneim. Forsch.*, 27, 2411–14.

Faust-Tinnefeldt Von, G. and Gilfrich, H. J. (1977) Kinetics of digitoxin during antirheumatic therapy with azapropazone. *Arzneim. Forsch.*, 27, 2009–11.

Favre, L., Glasson, Ph., Riondel, A. and Valloton, M. B. (1983) Interaction of diuretics and non-steroidal anti-inflammatory drugs in man. *Clin. Sci.*, 64, 407–15.

Favre, L., Glasson, P. and Vallotton, M. B. (1982) Reversible acute renal failure from combined triamterene and indomethacin: a study in healthy subjects. *Ann. Intern. Med.*, 96, 317–20.

Fenster, P. E., Comess, K. A., Hanson, C. D. and Finley, P. R. (1982) Kinetics of the digoxin–aspirin combination. *Clin. Pharmacol. Ther.*, 32, 428–30.

Field, J. B., Ohta, M., Boyle, C. and Remer, A. (1967) Potentiation of acetohexamide hypoglycaemia by phenylbutazone. *N. Engl. J. Med.*, 277, 889–94.

Finch, M. B., Kelly, J. G., Johnston, G. D. and McDevitt, D. G. (1983) Evidence against a digoxin–indomethacin interaction. *Br. J. Clin. Pharmacol.*, 16, 212–13P.

Fleitman, J. S., Bruni, J., Perrin, J. H. and Wilder, B. J. (1980) Albumin binding interactions of sodium valproate. *J. Clin. Pharmacol.*, 20, 514–17.

Fowler, P. D. (1979) Diclofenac sodium (voltarol). Drug interactions and special studies. *Rheumatol. Rehabil.*, Suppl. 2, 60–8.

Fraser, D. G., Ludden, T. M., Evens, R. P. and Sutherland, E. W. (1980) Displacement of phenytoin from plasma binding sites by salicylate. *Clin. Pharmacol. Ther.*, 27, 165–9.

Frölich, J. C., Leftwich, R., Ragheb, M., Oates, J. A., Reimann, I. and Buchanan, D. (1979) Indomethacin increases plasma lithium. *Br. Med. J.*, 1, 1115–16.

Fujita, T., Yamashita, W. and Yamashita, K. (1981) Effect of indomethacin on antihypertensive action of captopril in hypertensive patients. *Clin. Exp. Hypertension*, 3, 939–52.

Fujita, T., Ando, K., Sato, Y. and Yamashita, K. (1982) Effect of indomethacin on responses to [Sar-ileu]-angiotensin II. *Clin. Pharmacol. Ther.*, 32, 366–70.

Galeazzi, R. L. (1977) The effect of an antacid on the bioavailability of indomethacin. *Eur. J. Clin. Pharmacol.*, 12, 65–8.

Garnham, J. C., Raymond, K., Shotton, E. and Turner, P. (1975) The effect of buffered aspirin on plasma indomethacin. *Eur. J. Clin. Pharmacol.*, 8, 107–13.

Garnham, J. C., Kaspi, T., Kaye, C. M. and Oh, V. M. S. (1977) The different effects of sodium bicarbonate and aluminium hydroxide on the absorption of indomethacin in man. *Postgrad. Med. J.*, 53, 126–9.

Garrett, R., Manthey, B., Vernon-Roberts, B. and Brooks, P. M. (1983) Assessment of non-steroidal anti-inflammatory drug combinations by the polyurethane sponge implantation model in the rat. *Ann. Rheum. Dis.*, 42, 439–42.

Geaney, D. P., Carver, J. G., Aronson, J. K. and Warlow, C. P. (1982) Interaction of azapropazone with phenytoin. *Br. Med. J.*, 284, 1373.

Gerkens, J. F., Shand, D. G., Flexner, C., Nies, A. S., Oates, J. A. and Data, J. L. (1977) Effect of indomethacin and aspirin on gastric blood flow and acid secretion. *J. Pharmacol. Exp. Ther.*, 203, 646–52.

Giugliano, D. and D'Onofrio, F. (1980) Acetylsalicylic acid in human diabetes, in *Guidelines to Metabolic Therapy*, Vol. 9, Upjohn Company, Kalamazoo, Michigan, USA, pp. 3–4.

Graham, G. G., Champion, G. D., Day, R. O. and Paul, P. D. (1977) Patterns of plasma concentrations and urinary excretion of salicylate in rheumatoid arthritis. *Clin. Pharmacol. Ther.*, 22, 410–20.

Green, A. E., Hort, J. F., Korn, H. E. T. and Leach H. (1977) Potentiation of warfarin by azapropazone. *Br. Med. J.*, 1, 1532.

Greenblatt, D. J. and Abernethy, D. R. (1983) Ibuprofen does not impair antipyrine clearance. *Clin. Pharmacol. Ther.*, 33, 267.

Grennan, D. M., Ferry, D. G., Ashworth, M. E., Kenny, R. E. and MacKinnon, M. (1979) The aspirin–ibuprofen interaction in rheumatoid arthritis. *Br. J. Clin. Pharmacol.*, 8, 497–503.

Grennan, D. M., Karetai, M. and Palmer, D. G. (1977) Drug prescribing in rheumatoid arthritis in Otago. *N. Z. Med. J.*, 86, 130–2.

Gross, D., Rau, R. and Hind, I. D. (1980) Effect of flurbiprofen on steady-state levels and excretion of digoxin. *Br. J. Clin. Pract.*, Suppl. 9, 20–6.

Grygiel, J. J., Wing, L. M. H., Farkas, J. and Birkett, D. J. (1979) Effects of allopurinol on theophylline metabolism and clearance. *Clin. Pharmacol. Ther.*, 26, 660–7.

Gulbrandsen, R. (1959) Okt tolbutamid-effect. ted hjelp au fenylbutazon. *Tiddsskrift for den Norska Laegeforening*, 79, 1127–8.

Gupta, K. C., Joshi, J. V., Hazari, K., Pohujani, S. M. and Satoskar, R. S. (1982) Effect of low estrogen combination oral contraceptive on metabolism of aspirin and phenylbutazone. *Int. J. Clin. Pharmacol. Ther. Toxicol.*, 20, 511–3.

Hansen, J. M. and Christensen, L. K. (1977) Drug interactions with oral sulphonylurea drugs. *Drugs*, 13, 24–34.

Hayes, A. H. (1981) Therapeutic implications of drug interactions with acetaminophen and aspirin. *Arch. Intern. Med.*, 141, 301–4.

Helleberg, L. (1981) Clinical pharmacokinetics of indomethacin. *Clin. Pharmacokinet.*, 6, 245–58.

Helleberg, L., Rubin, A., Wolen, R. L., Rodda, B. E., Ridolfo, A. S. and Gruber, C. M. J. (1974) A pharmacokinetic interaction in man between phenobarbitone and fenoprofen, a new anti-inflammatory agent. *Br. J. Clin. Pharmacol.*, 1, 371–4.

Helleberg, L., Gylding-Sabroe, J. and Sylvest, J. (1977) The effect of aspirin upon the physiological disposition of indomethacin in man. *Scand. J. Rheumatol.*, 6, 71.

Hemming, J. D., Bird, H. A., Pickup, M. E., Saunders, A., Lowe, J. R. and Dixon, J. S. (1981) Bioavailability of aspirin in the presence of dextropropoxyphene/paracetamol combination. *Pharmacotherapeutica*, 2, 543–6.

Heuer, L. J. (1983) Interaktion zwischen Antihypertensiva und Antirheumatika. *Deutsch Medizin. Wochenschr.*, 108, 268–71.

Hierton, C. (1981) Effects of indomethacin, naproxen and paracetamol on regional blood flow in rabbits. *Acta Pharmacol. Toxicol.*, 49, 327–33.

Hirns, S. and Königstein, R. P. (1969) HB419 Ein neues orales Antidiabetikum und sein Anwendung im hohen Alter. *Wiener Medizin. Wochenschr.*, 119, 632–3.

Hobbs, C. B., Miller, A. L., Thornley, J. H. (1965) Potentiation of anticoagulant therapy by oxyphenbutaxone. *Postgrad. Med. J.*, 41, 563–65.

Hobbs, D. C. and Twomey, T. M. (1979) Piroxicam pharmacokinetics in man: aspirin and antacid interaction studies. *J. Clin. Pharmacol.*, 19, 270–81.

Hobkirk, D., Rhodes, M. and Haslock, I. (1977) Night medication in rheumatoid arthritis. II Combined therapy with indomethacin and diazepam. *Rheumatol. Rehabil.*, 16, 125–7.

Hoffbrand, B. I. and Kininmonth, D. A. (1967) Potentiation of anticoagulants. *Br. Med. J.*, 2, 838–9.

Holmes, E. L. (1967) Pharmacology of the fenamates. IV Toleration by normal human subjects. *Ann. Phys. Med.*, 9 (Suppl.), 36–49.

Holmes, G. I., Irvin, J. D., Schrogie, J. J., Davies, R. O., Breault, G. O., Rogers, J. D., Huber, P. B. and Zinny, M. A. (1979) Effects of Maalox on the bioavailability of diflunisal. *Clin. Pharmacol. Ther.*, 25, 229.

Horwitz, D., Thorgeirsson, S. S. and Mitchell, J. R. (1977) The influence of allopurinol and size of dose on the metabolism of phenylbutazone in patients with gout. *Eur. J. Clin. Pharmacol.*, 12, 133–6.

Howes, C. A., Pullar, T., Sourindhrin, I., Mistra, P. C., Capell, H., Lawson, D. H. and Tilstone, W. J. (1983) Reduced steady-state plasma concentrations of chlorpromazine and indomethacin in patients receiving cimetidine. *Eur. J. Clin. Pharmacol.*, 24, 99–102.

Humphrey, S. J. and Zins, G. R. (1983) The effects of indomethacin on systemic hemodynamics and blood flow in the conscious dog. *Res. Commun. Chem. Pathol. Pharmacol.*, 39, 229–40.

Inoue, F. and Walsh, R. J. (1983) Folate supplements and phenytoin–salicylate interaction. *Neurology*, 33, 115–16.

Jackson, S. H. D. and Pickles, H. (1983) Indomethacin does not attenuate the effects of hydralazine in normal subjects. *Eur. J. Clin. Pharmacol.*, 25, 303–6.

Jacono, A., Caso, P., Gualtieri, S., Raucci, D., Bianchi, A., Vigorito, C., Bergamini, N. and Iadeviaa, V. (1981) Clinical study of possible interactions between indoprofen and oral anticoagulants. *Eur. J. Rheumatol. Inflammation*, 4, 32–5.

Jain, A., McMahon, F. G., Slattery, J. T. and Levy, G. (1979) Effect of naproxen on steady-state serum concentration and anticoagulant activity of warfarin. *Clin. Pharmacol. Ther.*, 25, 61–6.

Jeremy, R. and Towson, J. (1970) Interaction of aspirin and indomethacin in the treatment of rheumatoid arthritis. *Med. J. Aust.*, 2, 127–9.

Jubiz, W. and Meikle, A. W. (1979) Alterations of glucocorticoid actions by other drugs and disease states. *Drugs*, 18, 113–21.

Kaldestadt, E., Hansel, T. and Brath, H. K. (1975) Interaction of indomethacin and acetylsalicylic acid as shown by the serum concentrations of indomethacin and salicylate. *Eur. J. Clin. Pharmacol.*, 9, 199–207.

Kampmann, J., Hansen, J. M., Siersback-Nielsen, K. and Laursen, H. (1972) Effect of some drugs on penicillin half-life in blood. *Clin. Pharmacol. Ther.*, 13, 516–19.

Kaufmann, E. (1977) Effect of alclofenac on the prothrombin level in patients under treatment with anticoagulants. *Schweizische Medizin. Wochenschr.*, 107, 882–7.

Keber, I., Jerse, M., Keber, D. and Stegnar, M. (1979) The influence of combined treatment with propranolol and acetylsalicylic acid on platelet aggregation in coronary heart disease. *Br. J. Clin. Pharmacol.*, 7, 287–91.

Kerry, R. J., Owen, G. and Michaelson, S. (1983) Possible toxic interaction between lithium and piroxicam. *Lancet*, i, 418–19.

Kirch, W., Spahn, H., Ohnhaus, E., Köhler, H., Heinz, U. and Mutschler, E. (1983) Influence of inflammatory disease on the clinical pharmacokinetics of atenolol and metoprolol. *Biopharm. Drug Dis.*, 4, 73–81.

Klinenberg, J. R. and Miller, F. (1965) Effect of corticosteroids on salicylate concentration. *J. Am. Med. Assoc.*, **194**, 601–4.

Kondo, K., Oka, T., Ohashi, K., Touru, M. and Ebihara, A. (1983) Drug interaction between furosemide and indomethacin: effect of small dose of indomethacin on furosemide-induced natriuresis. *Proc. 2nd World Congr. Clin. Pharmacol.*, Abstract No. 251.

Koren, G., Zarfin, Y., Perlman, M. and MacLeod, S. M. (1983) Influence of indomethacin on digoxin pharmacokinetics in pre-term infants. *Proc. 2nd World Conf. Clin. Pharmacol. Ther.*, Abstract No. 32.

Kristensen, M. and Christensen, L. K. (1969) Drug-induced changes of the blood glucose lowering effect of oral hypoglycaemic agents. *Acta diabetica latina*, **6** (Suppl. 1), 116–36.

Krzywanek, H. J. and Breddin, K. (1977) Beeinflusst Diclofenac die orale Antikoagulantienstherapie und die Plaettchenaggregation. *Medizin. Welt*, **28**, 1843–5.

Kwan, K. C., Breault, G. O., Davis, R. L., Lei, B. W., Czerwinski, A. W., Besselaar, G. H. and Duggan, D. E. (1978) Effects of concomitant aspirin administration on the pharmacokinetics of indomethacin in man. *J. Pharmacokin. Biopharm.*, **6**, 451–76.

Lanza, F. L., Royger, G. L. and Nelson, R. S. (1980) Endoscopic evaluation of the effects of aspirin, buffered aspirin, and enteric-coated aspirin on gastric and duodenal mucosa. *N. Engl. J. Med.*, **303**, 136–8.

Lee, K. Y., Beilin, L. J. and Vandongen, R. (1979) Severe hypertension after ingestion of an appetite suppressant (phenylpropanolamine) with indomethacin. *Lancet*, i, 1110–11.

Leftwich, R., Walker, L. and Smigel, M. (1977) Indomethacin is antidiuretic in lithium-induced diabetes insipidus. *Clin. Res.*, **25**, 272A.

Leonard, R. F., Knott, P. J., Rankin, G. O., Robinson, D. S. and Melnick, D. E. (1981) Phenytoin–salicylate interaction. *Clin. Pharmacol. Ther.*, **29**, 56–60.

Leonards, R. F. and Levy, G. (1969) Reduction or prevention of aspirin-induced occult gastrointestinal blood loss in man. *Clin. Pharmacol. Ther.*, **10**, 571–4.

Levy, G., Lampman, T., Kamath, B. L. and Garettson, L. K. (1975) Decreased serum salicylate concentrations in children with rheumatic fever treated with antacid. *N. Engl. J. Med.*, **293**, 323–5.

Lewis, R. J., Trager, W. F., Chan, K. K., Breckenridge, A., Orme, M., Rowland, M. and Schary, W. (1974) Warfarin. Stereochemical aspects of its metabolism and the interaction with phenylbutazone. *J. Clin. Invest.*, **53**, 1607–17.

Liegler, D. G., Henderson, E. S., Hahn, M. A. and Oliverio, V. T. (1969) The effect of organic acids on renal clearance of methotrexate in man. *Clin. Pharmacol. Ther.*, **10**, 849–57.

Lindquist, B., Jensen, K. M., Johansson, H. and Hansen, T. (1974) Effect of concurrent administration of aspirin and indomethacin on serum concentrations. *Clin. Pharmacol. Ther.*, **15**, 247–52.

Livio, M., Del Maschio, A., Cerletti, C. and de Gaetano, G. (1982) Indomethacin prevents the long-lasting inhibitory effect of aspirin on human platelet cyclooxygenase activity. *Prostaglandins*, **23**, 787–96.

Loftin, J. P. and Vesell, E. S. (1979) Interaction between sulindac and warfarin: different results in normal subjects and in an unusual patient with a potassium-losing renal tubular defect. *J. Clin. Pharmacol.*, **19**, 733–42.

Lopez-Ovejero, J. A., Weber, M. A., Drayer, J. M., Sealey, J. E. and Laragh, J. H. (1978) Effects of indomethacin alone and during diuretic or β-adrenoceptor blocking therapy on blood pressure and the renin system in essential hypertension. *Clin. Sci. Mol. Med.*, **55**, 203S–205S.

Lyle, W. H., Pearcey, D. F. and Hui, M. (1977) Inhibition of penicillamine-induced cupresis by oral iron. *Proc. R. Soc. Med.*, 70 (Suppl. 3), 48–9.

MacCarthy, E. P., Frost, G. W. and Stokes, G. S. (1979) Indomethacin-induced hyperkalaemia. *Med. J. Aust.*, 1, 550.

McElnay, J. C. and D'Arcy, P. F. (1977) Interaction between azapropazone and warfarin. *Br. Med. J.*, 2, 773–4.

Mahfouz, M., Abdel-Maguid, R. and El-Dakhakny, M. (1970) Potentiation of the hypoglycaemic action of tolbutamide by different drugs. *Arzneim. Forsch.*, 20, 120–2.

Mandel, M. A. (1976) The synergistic effect of salicylates on methotrexate toxicity. *Plastic Reconstruct. Surg.*, 57, 733–7.

Manfredi, R. and Vesell, E. S. (1981) Inhibition of theophylline metabolism by long-term allopurinol administration. *Clin. Pharmacol. Ther.*, 29, 224–9.

Marbet, G. A., Duckert, F., Walter, M., Six, P. and Airenne, H. (1977) Interaction study between phenprocoumon and flurbiprofen. *Curr. Med. Res. Opinion*, 5, 26–31.

Meffin, P. J., Veenendaal, J. R. and Brooks, P. M. (1981) Diflunisal–probenecid co-disposition: Michaelis–Menten kinetics with competitive inhibition. *Clin. Exp. Pharmacol. Physiol.*, 9, 605–11.

Melander, A. and Wåhlin-Bohl, E. (1981) Interaction of glipizide and indoprofen. *Eur. J. Rheumatol. Inflammation*, 4, 22–5.

Michot, F., Ajdacic, K. and Glaus, L. (1975) A double blind clinical trial to determine if an interaction exists between diclofenac sodium and the oral anticoagulant acenocoumarol (nicoumalone). *J. Int. Med. Res.*, 3, 153–7.

Mielens, Z. E., Drobeck, H. P., Rozitis, J. and Sansone, V. J. (1968) Interaction of aspirin with non-steroidal anti-inflammatory drugs in rats. *J. Pharm. Pharmacol.*, 20, 567–9.

Miller, D. R. (1981) Combination use of non-steroidal anti-inflammatory drugs. *Drug Intell. Clin. Pharm.*, 15, 3–7.

Mills, E. H., Whitworth, J. A., Andrews, J. and Kincaird-Smith, P. (1982) Non-steroidal anti-inflammatory drugs and blood pressure. *Aust. N. Z. J. Med.*, 12, 478–82.

Miners, J. O., Foenander, T., Wanwimolruk, S., Gallus, S. and Birkett, D. J. (1982) The effect of sulphinpyrazone on oxidative drug metabolism in man: inhibition of tolbutamide elimination. *Eur. J. Clin. Pharmacol.*, 22, 321–6.

Minn, F. L. and Zinny, M. A. (1980) Zomepirac and warfarin: a clinical study to determine if interaction exists. *J. Clin. Pharmacol.*, 20, 418–21.

Mor, R., Pitlik, S. and Rosenfeld, J. B. (1983) Indomethacin- and moduretic-induced hyperkalaemia. *Israeli J. Med. Sci.*, 19, 535–7.

Müller, F. O., Hundt, H. K. and Müller, D. G. (1977) Pharmacokinetic and pharmaco-dynamic implications of long-term administration of non steroidal anti-inflammatory agents. *Int. J. Clin. Pharmacol. Biopharm.*, 15, 397–402.

Nayak, R. K., Smyth, R. D., Polk, A., Herczeg, T., Carter, V., Visalli, A. J. and Reavey-Cantwell, M. H. (1977) Effect of antacids on aspirin dissolution and bioavailability. *J. Pharmacokin. Biopharm.*, 5, 597–613.

Nierenberg, D. W. (1983) Competitive inhibition of methotrexate accumulation in rabbit kidney slices by non-steroidal anti-inflammatory drugs. *J. Pharmacol. Exp. Ther.*, 226, 1–6.

Nies, A. S., Gal, J., Fadul, S. and Gerber, J. G. (1983) Indomethacin–furosemide interaction: the importance of renal blood flow. *J. Pharmacol. Exp. Ther.*, 226, 27–32.

Nordoy, S. (1959) Combined treatment with phenylbutazone and anticoagulants. *Tidssksift for den Norske Laegeforening*, 79, 143.

O'Brien, J. R. (1968) The effect of salicylates on human platelets. *Lancet*, i, 779–83.

O'Malley, K., Stevenson, I. H. and Crooks, J. (1972) Impairment of human drug metabolism by oral contraceptive steroids. *Clin. Pharmacol. Ther.*, 13, 552–7.

O'Reilly, R. A. (1973) The binding of sodium warfarin to plasma albumin and its displacement by phenylbutazone. *Ann. N. Y. Acad. Sci.*, 226, 293–308.

O'Reilly, R. A. (1982a) Phenylbutazone and sulfinpyrazone interaction with oral anticoagulant phenprocoumon. *Arch. Intern. Med.*, 142, 1634–7.

O'Reilly, R. A. (1982b) Stereoselective interaction of sulphinpyrazone with racemic warfarin and its separated enantiomers in man. *Circulation*, 65, 202–7.

O'Reilly, R. A. and Aggeler, P. M. (1968) Phenylbutazone potentiation of anticoagulant effect: fluorometric assay of warfarin. *Proc. Soc. Exp. Biol. Med.*, 128, 1080–1.

O'Reilly, R. A., Sahud, M. A. and Aggeler, P. M. (1971) Impact of aspirin and chlorthalidone on the pharmacodynamics of oral anticoagulants in man. *Ann. N. Y. Acad. Sci.*, 179, 173–86.

O'Reilly, R. A., Trager, W. F., Motley, C. H. and Howald, W. (1980) Stereoselective interaction of phenylbutazone with [^{12}C/^{13}C] warfarin pseudoracemates in man. *J. Clin. Invest.*, 65, 746–53.

Ober, K. F. (1974) Mechanism of interaction of tolbutamide and phenylbutazone in diabetic patients. *Eur. J. Clin. Pharmacol.*, 7, 291–4.

Olanow, C. W., Finn, A. and Prussak, C. (1979) The effect of salicylate on phenytoin pharmacokinetics. *Trans. Am. Neurol. Assoc.*, 104, 109–10.

Oliw, E., Ängaard, E. and Fredholm, B. (1977) Effect of indomethacin on the renal actions of theophylline. *Eur. J. Pharmacol.*, 43, 9–16.

Oliw, E., Kover, G., Larsson, C. and Ängaard, E. (1976) Reduction by indomethacin of furosemide effects in the rabbit. *Eur. J. Pharmacol.*, 38, 95–100.

Olsen, U. B. (1975) Indomethacin inhibition of bumetanide diuresis in dogs. *Acta Pharmacol. Toxicol.*, 37, 65–78.

Orr, J. M., Abbott, F. S., Farrell, K., Ferguson, S., Sheppard, I. and Godolphin, W. (1982) Interaction between valproic acid and aspirin in epileptic children: serum protein binding and metabolic effects. *Clin. Pharmacol. Ther.*, 31, 642–9.

Oyer, J. H., Wagner, S. L. and Schmid, F. R. (1966) Suppression of salicylate-induced uricosuria by phenylbutazone. *Am. J. Med. Sci.*, 251, 1–7.

Park, B. K. and Breckenridge, A. M. (1981) Clinical implications of enzyme induction and enzyme inhibition. *Clin. Pharm.*, 6, 1–24.

Passeri, M., Ferretti, G., Monica, C., Fanfani, A. and Bergamini, N. (1981) Study of the possible interactions of indoprofen on the diuretic effect of furosemide. *Eur. J. Rheumatol. Inflammation*, 4, 36–40.

Patak, R. V., Mookerjee, B. K., Bentzel, C. J., Hysert, P. E., Babe, M. and Lee, J. B. (1975) Antagonism of the effects of furosemide by indomethacin in normal and hypertensive man. *Prostaglandins*, 10, 649–59.

Pawlotsky, Y., Durand, B., Delbary, A., Le Treut, A., Catheline, M. and Bourel, M. (1977) Reduction de l'activité de l'indométhacine par l'aspirine. Intéret des mesures de l'indice articulaire et de la sigma V. S. *Nouvelle Presse Méd.*, 6, 255–58.

Pawlotsky, Y., Chales, G., Grosbois, B., Miane, B. and Bourel, M. (1978) Comparative interaction of aspirin with indomethacin and sulindac in chronic rheumatic diseases. *Eur. J. Rheumatol. Inflammation*, 1, 18–20.

Paxton, J. W. (1980) Effects of aspirin on salivary and serum phenytoin kinetics in healthy subjects. *Clin. Pharmacol. Ther.*, 27, 170–8.

Pedrazzi, F., Bommartini, F., Freddo, J. and Emanueli, A. (1981) A study of the possible interactions of indoprofen with hypoglycaemic sulphonylureas in diabetic patients. *Eur. J. Rheumatol. Inflammation*, 4, 26–31.

Pedrinelli, R., Magagna, A., Arzilli, F., Sassano, P. and Salvetti, A. (1980) Influence of indomethacin on the natriuretic and renin-stimulating effect of bumetanide in essential hypertension. *Clin. Pharmacol. Ther.*, 28, 722–31.

Pedrinelli, R., Magagna A. and Salvetti, A. (1982) The effect of oxprenolol and indomethacin on renin and aldosterone of normal subjects during low sodium diet. *Eur. J. Clin. Invest.*, 12, 107–11.

Penner, J. A. and Abbrecht, P. H. (1975) Lack of interaction between ibuprofen and warfarin. *Curr. Ther. Res.*, 18, 862–71.

Petereit, M. S. and Meikle, A. W. (1977) Effectiveness of prednisolone during phenytoin therapy. *Clin. Pharmacol. Ther.*, 22, 912–16.

Pitkäjärvi, T., Pyykönen, M. L., Ylitalo, P., Nurmi, A-K., Seppälä, E. and Vapaatalo, H. (1983) Interaction of indomethacin and atenolol in essential hypertension. *Proc. 2nd World Conf. Clin. Pharmacol. Ther.*, Abstract No. 5.

Pond, S. M., Birkett, D. J. and Wade, D. N. (1977) Mechanisms of inhibition of tolbutamide metabolism: phenylbutazone, oxyphenbutazone, sulphaphenazole. *Clin. Pharmacol. Ther.*, 22, 573–9.

Powell-Jackson, P. R. (1977) Interaction between azapropazone and warfarin. *Br. Med. J.*, 1, 1193–4.

Pullar, T. and Capell, H. A. (1982) Interaction of indomethacin and warfarin. *Br. Med. J.*, 284, 198.

Quattrochi, F. P., Robinson, J. D., Curry, R. W., Grieco, M. L. and Schulman S. G. (1983) The effect of ibuprofen on serum digoxin concentrations. *Drug Intell. Clin. Pharm.*, 17, 286–8.

Rae, S. A., Williams, I. A., English, J. and Baylis, E. M. (1982) Alteration of plasma prednisolone levels by indomethacin and naproxen. *Br. J. Clin. Pharm.*, 14, 459–61.

Ragheb, M., Ban, T. A., Buchanan, D. and Frolich, J. C. (1980) Interaction of indomethacin and ibuprofen with lithium in manic patients under a steady-state lithium level. *J. Clin. Psychiatr.*, 41, 397–8.

Rawles, J. M. (1982) Antagonism between non-steroidal anti-inflammatory drugs and diuretics. *Scott. Med. J.*, 27, 37–40.

Reimann, I. W. and Frölich, J. C. (1981) Effects of diclofenac on lithium kinetics. *Clin. Pharmacol. Ther.*, 30, 348–53.

Reimann, I. W., Diener, U. and Frölich, J. C. (1983) Indomethacin but not aspirin increases plasma lithium ion levels. *Arch. Gen. Psychiatr.*, 40, 283–6.

Reinicke, C. and Vesel, G. (1979) Pharmacokinetic interactions between non-steroidal antirheumatism agents. *Vutreshni Bolesti*, 18, 76–82.

Roberts, C. J. C., Daneshmend, T. K., Macfarlane, D. and Dieppe, P. A. (1981) Anticonvulsant intoxication precipitated by azapropazone. *Postgrad. Med. J.*, 57, 191–2.

Rolf-Smith, S., Gibson, R., Bradley, D. and Kendall, M. J. (1983) Failure of indomethacin to modify β-adrenoceptor blockade. *Br. J. Clin. Pharmacol.*, 15, 267–8.

Romero, J. C. and Strong, C. G. (1977) The effect of indomethacin blockade of prostaglandin synthesis on blood pressure of normal rabbits and rabbits with renovascular hypertension. *Circ. Res.*, 40, 35–41.

Rubin, A., Chernish, S. M., Crabtree, R., Gruber, C. M., Helleberg, L., Rodda, B. E., Warrick, P., Wolen, R. L. and Ridolfo, A. S. (1974) A profile of the physiological disposition and gastrointestinal effects of fenoprofen in man. *Curr. Med. Res. Opinion*, 2, 529–43.

Rubin, A., Rodda, B. E., Warrick, P., Gruber, C. M. and Ridolfo, A. S. (1973) Interaction of aspirin with non-steroidal anti-inflammatory drugs in man. *Arthr. Rheum.*, 16, 635–45.

Rubin, P. C., Jackson, G. and Blaschke, T. F. (1980) Studies on the clinical pharmacology of prazosin II: the influence of indomethacin and of propranolol on the action and disposition of prazosin. *Br. J. Clin. Pharmacol.*, 10, 33–40.

Rudge, S. R., Lloyd-Jones, J. K. and Hind, I. D. (1982) Interaction between flurbiprofen and indomethacin in rheumatoid arthritis. *Br. J. Clin. Pharmacol.*, 13, 448–51.

Rumble, R. H., Brooks, P. M. and Roberts, M. S. (1979) Interaction between levamisole and aspirin in man. *Br. J. Clin. Pharmacol.*, 7, 631–3.

Runkel, R., Mroszczak, E., Chaplin, M., Sevelius, H. and Segre, E. (1978) Naproxen–probenecid interaction. *Clin. Pharmacol. Ther.*, 24, 706–13.

Rust, O., Biland, L., Thilo, D., Nyman, D. and Duckert, F. (1975) Testing of the antirheumatic drug tolmetin for interaction with oral anticoagulants. *Schweizische medizin. Wochenschr.*, 105, 752–3.

Ryan, J. R., Jain, A. K., McMahon, F. G. and Vargas, R. (1977) On the question of an interaction between sulindac and tolbutamide in the control in diabetes. *Clin. Pharmacol. Ther.*, 21, 231–3.

Sachse Von, G., Willms, B. and Becker, R. (1979) Interaction between naproxen and tolbutamide on metabolism in diabetes. *Arzneim. Forsch.*, 29, 835–6.

Salvetti, A., Arzilli, F., Pedrinelli, R., Beggi, P. and Motolese, M. (1982) Interaction between oxprenolol in essential hypertensive patients. *Eur. J. Clin. Pharmacol.*, 22, 197–201.

Sandyk, R. (1982) Phenytoin toxicity induced by interaction with ibuprofen. *S. Afr. Med. J.*, 62, 592.

Savitsky, J. P., Terzakis, T., Bina, P., Chicarelli, F. and Haynes, J. (1980) Fenbufen–warfarin interaction in healthy volunteers. *Clin. Pharmacol. Ther.*, 27, 284.

Schäfer-Korting, M., Kirch, W., Axthelm, T., Köhler, H. and Mutschler, E. (1983) Atenolol interaction with aspirin, allopurinol and ampicillin. *Clin. Pharmacol. Ther.*, 33, 283–8.

Schary, W. L., Aarons, L. J. and Rowland, M. (1978) Representation and interpretation of drug displacement interactions. *Biochem. Pharmacol.*, 27, 139–46.

Schenk, H., Klein, G., Haralambus, I. and Goebel, R. (1980) Coumarintherapie unter dem Antirheumaticum Sulindac. *Z. Rheumatol.*, 39, 102–8.

Schiffman, F. J., Uehara, Y., Fisher, J. M. and Rabinovitz, M. (1978) Potentiation of chlorambucil activity by phenylbutazone. *Cancer Lett.*, 4, 211–16.

Schobben, F., Vree, T. B. and van der Kleijn, E. (1978) Pharmacokinetics, metabolism and distribution of 2-N-Propyl pentanoate (sodium valproate) and the influence of salicylate co-medication, in *Advances in Epileptology – 1977* (eds M. Meinardi and T. Rowan), Swets and Zeitlinger, Amsterdam, pp. 271–7.

Schulz P., Perrier, C. V., Ferber-Perret, F., Vandenheuval, W. J. and Steelman, S. L. (1979) Diflunisal, a new-acting analgesic and prostaglandin inhibitor: effect of concomitant acetylsalicylic acid therapy on ototoxicity and on disposition of both drugs. *J. Int. Med. Res.*, 7, 61–8.

Segre, E. (1979) Drug interactions with naproxen. *Eur. J. Rheumatol. Inflammation*, 2, 12–18.

Segre, E. J., Chaplin, M., Forchielli, E., Runkel, R. and Sevelius, H. (1974b) Naproxen–aspirin interactions in man. *Clin. Pharmacol. Ther.*, 15, 374–9.

Segre, E. J., Sevelius, H. and Varady, J. (1974a) Effect of antacids on naproxen absorption. *N. Engl. J. Med.*, 291, 582–3.

Seiler, K. and Duckert, F. (1968) Properties of 3-(1-phenyl-propyl)-4-oxycoumarin (Marcoumar) in the plasma when tested in normal cases and under the influence of drugs. *Thromb. Diathes. Haemorrhag.*, 19, 89–96.

Sellers, E. M. and Koch-Weser, J. (1970) Displacement of warfarin from human albumin by diazoxide, and ethacrynic, mefenamic and nalidixic acids. *Clin. Pharmacol. Ther.*, 11, 524–9.

Serlin, M. J., Mossman, S., Sibeon, R. G., Tempero, K. F. and Breckenridge, A. M. (1980) Interaction between diflunisal and warfarin. *Clin. Pharmacol. Ther.*, 28, 493–8.

Shen, D. D. and Azarnoff, D. L. (1978) Clinical pharmacokinetics of methotrexate. *Clin. Pharmacokinet.*, 3, 1–13.

Silberbauer, K., Stanek, B. and Templ, H. (1982) Acute hypotensive effect of captopril in man modified by prostaglandin synthesis inhibition. *Br. J. Clin. Pharmacol.*, 14 (Suppl. 2), 87S–93S.

Singer, L., Imbs, J. L., Schmidt, M., Mack, G., Sebban, M. and Danion, J. M. (1978) Baisse de la clairance rénale du lithium sous l'effet de la phénylbutazone. *Encéphale*, 4, 33–40.

Skeith, M. D., Simkin, P. A. and Healey, L. A. (1968) The renal excretion of indomethacin and its inhibition by probenecid. *Clin. Pharmacol. Ther.*, 9, 89–93.

Slack, B. L., Warner, M. E. and Keiser, H. R. (1978) The effect of prostaglandin synthetase inhibition on the action of hydralazine. *Circulation*, 58, 21.

Slade, I. H. and Iosefa, R. N. (1967) Fatal hypoglycemic coma from the use of tolbutamide in elderly patients: Report of two cases. *J. Am. Geriatr. Soc.*, 15, 948–50.

Slattery, J. T., Levy, G., Jain, A. and McMahon, F. G. (1979) Effect of naproxen on the kinetics of elimination and anticoagulant activity of a single dose of warfarin. *Clin. Pharmacol. Ther.*, 25, 51–60.

Smith, D. E., Brater, D. C., Lin, E. T. and Benet, L. Z. (1979) Attenuation of furosemide's diuretic effect by indomethacin: pharmacokinetic evaluation. *J. Pharmacokinet. Biopharm.*, 7, 265–74.

Solomon, H. M. and Abrams, W. B. (1972) Interactions between digitoxin and other drugs in man. *Am. Heart J.*, 83, 277–80.

Solomon, H. M., Reich, S., Spirt, N. and Abrams, W. B. (1971) Interactions between digitoxin and other drugs *in vitro* and *in vivo*. *Ann. N. Y. Acad. Sci.*, 179, 362–8.

Solomon, H. M., Schrogie, J. J. and Williams, D. (1968) The displacement of phenylbutazone ^{14}C and warfarin ^{14}C from human albumin by various drugs and fatty acids. *Biochem. Pharmacol.*, 17, 143–51.

Spät, A., Józan, S., Gaál, K. and Mózes, T. (1977) Effect of indomethacin on the adrenal response to furosemide in the rat. *J. Endocrinol.*, 73, 401–2.

Steelman, S. L., Cirillo, V. J. and Tempero, K. F. (1978) The chemistry, pharmacology and clinical pharmacology of diflunisal. *Curr. Med. Res. Opinion*, 5, 506–14.

Steiness, E. and Waldorff, S. (1982) Different interactions of indomethacin and sulindac with thiazides in hypertension. *Br. Med. J.*, 285, 1702–3.

Stitt, F. W., Latour, R. and Frane, J. W. (1977) A clinical study of naproxen-diazepam drug interaction on tests of mood and attention. *Curr. Ther. Res.*, 21, 149–56.

Stowers, J. M., Constable, L. W. and Hunter, R. B. (1959) A clinical and pharmacological comparison of chlorpropamide and other sulphonylureas. *Ann. N. Y. Acad. Sci.*, 74, 689–95.

Stricker, B. H. and Delhez, J. L. (1982) Interactions between flurbiprofen and coumarins. *Br. Med. J.*, 285, 812–13.

Swanson, B. N., Boppana, V. K., Vlasses, P. H., Rotmensch, H. H. and Ferguson, R. K. (1983) Dimethylsulphoxide inhibits bioactivation of sulindac. *J. Lab. Clin. Med.*, 102, 95–101.

Symmons, D. P. M., Kendall, M. J., Rees, J. A. and Hind, I. D. (1983) The effect of flurbiprofen on the response to frusemide in healthy volunteers. *Int. J. Clin. Pharmacol. Ther. Toxicol.*, 21, 350–4.

Sziegoleit, W., Rausch, J., Polák Gy., Gyorgy, M., Dekov, E. and Békés, M. (1982) Influence of acetylsalicylic acid on acute circulatory effects of the beta-blocking agents pindolol and propranolol in humans. *Int. J. Clin. Pharmacol. Ther. Toxicol.*, 20, 423–30.

Szita, M., Gachalyi, B., Tornyossy, M. and Kaldor, A. (1980) Interaction of phenylbutazone and tolbutamide in man. *Int. J. Clin. Pharmacol. Ther. Toxicol.*, 18, 378–80.

Tannenbaum, H., Anderson, L. G. and Saeldner, J. S. (1974) Phenylbutazone–tolbutamide drug interaction. *N. Engl. J. Med.*, 290, 344.

Tempero, K. F., Cirillo, V. J. and Steelman, S. L. (1977) Diflunisal: a review of pharmacokinetic and pharmacodynamic properties, drug interactions, and special tolerability studies in humans. *Br. J. Clin. Pharmacol.*, 4 (Suppl. 1), 31S–36S.

Thadani, U., Kellerman, D., Martin, T. and Glenn, T. (1983) Effects of indomethacin on haemodynamics and exercise tolerance in angina pectoris. *Clin. Pharmacol. Ther.*, 33, 211.

Thomsen, P. E. B., Ostenfeld, H. O. L. and Kristensen, M. (1970) Chlorpropamide-phenylbutazone as the cause of hypoglycaemia. A case of an unfortunate drug combination. *Ugeskrift for Laeger*, 137, 1722–4.

Tiggeler, R. E. W., Koena, R. A. P. and Wijdeveld, P. G. A. B. (1977) Inhibition of furosemide-induced natriuresis by indomethacin in patients with the nephrotic syndrome. *Clin. Sci. Mol. Med.*, 52, 149–51.

Tjandramaga, T. B., Verbesselt, R., Van Hecken, A., de Schepper, P. J. (1983) Diflunisal–indomethacin interaction: evidence for impaired indomethacin-glucuronide formation. *Proc. 2nd World Conf. Clin. Pharmacol. Ther.*, Abstract No. 28.

Tobert, J. A., De Schepper, P., Tjandramaga, T. B., Mullie, A., Buntinx, A. P., Meisinger, M. A. P., Huber, P. B., Hall, T. L. P. and Yeh, K. C. (1981) Effects of antacids on the bioavailability of diflunisal in the fasting and postprandial states. *Clin. Pharmacol. Ther.*, 30, 385–9.

Torgyan, S., Wagner, L., Neumann, T., Pakuts, B. and Csanyi, M. (1979) A comparative study with indomethacin and combined indomethacin–sodium salicylate in rheumatoid arthritis. *Int. J. Clin. Pharmacol. Biopharm.*, 17, 439–41.

Tweedale, M. G. and Ogilvie, R. I. (1973) Antagonism of Spironolactone-induced natriuresis by aspirin in man. *N. Engl. J. Med.*, 289, 198–200.

Udall, J. A. (1969) Drug interference with warfarin. *Am. J. Cardiol.* 23, 143.

Upton, R. A., Williams, R. L., Buskin, J. N. and Jones, R. M. (1982) Effects of probenecid on ketoprofen kinetics. *Clin. Pharmacol. Ther.*, 31, 705–12.

Valette, H. and Apoil, E. (1979) Interaction between salicylate and two loop diuretics. *Br. J. Clin. Pharmacol.*, 8, 592–4.

Van Arman, C. G., Nuss, G. W. and Risley, E. A. (1973) Interactions of aspirin, indomethacin and other drugs in adjuvant induced arthritis in the rat. *J. Pharmacol. Exp. Ther.*, 187, 400–14.

Verbeeck, R., Tjandramaga, T. B., Mullie, A., Verbesselt, R. and De Schepper, P. J. (1979) Effect of aluminium hydroxide on diflunisal absorption. *Br. J. Clin. Pharmacol.*, 7, 519–22.

Verbeek, R. K., Blackburn, J. L. and Loewen, G. R. (1983) Clinical pharmacokinetics of non-steroidal anti-inflammatory drugs. *Clin. Pharmacokinet.*, 8, 297–331.

Vesell, E. S., Passananti, G. T. and Green, F. E. (1970) Impairment of drug metabolism in man by allopurinol and nortryptiline. *N. Engl. J. Med.*, 283, 1484–8.

Vesell, E. S., Passananti, G. T. and Johnson, A. O. (1975) Failure of indomethacin and warfarin to interact in normal human volunteers. *J. Clin. Pharmacol.*, 15, 486–95.

Vierhopper, H., Waldhausl, W. and Nowotny, P. (1981) Effect of indomethacin upon angiotensin-induced changes in blood pressure and plasma aldosterone in normal man. *Eur. J. Clin. Invest.*, 11, 85–9.

Viswanathan, C. T. and Levy, R. H. (1981) Plasma protein binding interaction between valproic and salicylic acids in rhesus monkeys. *J. Pharm. Sci.*, 70, 1279–81.

Voigt, U. and Klassen, E. (1982) Zur Prüfung von Ketoprofen auf Interaktionon mit oraler Antidiabetika. *Medizin. Welt*, 33, 1592–3.

Walter, E., Staiger, Ch., De Vries, J., Zimmerman, R. and Weber, E. (1981) Induction of drug metabolising enzymes by sulphinpyrazone. *Eur. J. Clin. Pharmacol.*, 19, 353–8.

Wanwimolruk, S., Birkett, D. J. and Brooks, P. M. (1982) Protein binding of some non-steroidal anti-inflammatory drugs in rheumatoid arthritis. *Clin. Pharmacokinet.*, 7, 85–92.

Watkins, J., Abbott, E. C., Hensby, C. N., Webster, J. and Dollery, C. T. (1980) Attenuation of hypotensive effect of propranolol and thiazide diuretics by indomethacin. *Br. Med. J.*, 281, 702–5.

Weber, P. C., Scherer, B. and Larsson, C. (1977) Increase of free arachidonic acid by furosemide in man as the cause of prostaglandin and renin release. *Eur. J. Pharmacol.*, 41, 329–32.

Weber, S., Daoud, H., Richard, M. O., Rey, E., Olive, G., Guerin, F. and Degeorges, M. (1983) Influence of aspirin on the haemodynamic effects of nitroglycerin. *Proc. 2nd World Conf. Clin. Pharmacol. Ther.*, Abstract No. 138.

Webster, J., Hawksworth, G. M., McLean, I. and Petrie, J. C. (1983) Attenuation of the antihypertensive effect of single doses of propranolol and atenolol by flurbiprofen. *Proc. 2nd World Conf. Clin. Pharmacol. Ther.*, Abstract No. 2.

Weiner, M., Siddiqui, A. A., Bostanci, N. and Dayton, P. G. (1965) Drug interaction – the effect of combined administration on the halflife of coumarin and pyrazolone drugs in man. *Fed. Proc.*, 24, 153.

Wennmalm, A., Eriksson, S., Hagerfeldt, L., Law, D., Patrono, C. and Pinca, E. (1983) Effect of prostaglandin synthesis inhibitors on basal and carbon dioxide stimulated cerebral blood flow in man, in *Advances in Prostaglandin, Thromboxane and Leukotriene Research* (eds B. Samuelsson, R. Paoletti and P. W. Ramwell), Vol. 12, Raven Press, New York.

Whiting, B., Lorenzi, M., Robins, D. S. and Williams, R. (1979) The influence of naproxen on glucose metabolism and tolbutamide pharmacologic effect. *Clin. Pharmacol. Ther.*, 25, 253.

Whitsett, T. L., Barry, J. P., Czerwinski, A. W., Hall, W. H. and Hampton, J. W. (1975) Interaction of tolmetin and warfarin: A clinical investigation, in *Tolmetin a New Non-steroidal Anti-inflammatory Agent* (ed. J. Ward), Excerpta Medica, Princeton.

Wilkerson, R. D. and Glenn, T. M. (1977) Influence of non-steroidal anti-inflammatory drugs on ouabain toxicity. *Am. Heart J.*, 94, 454–9.

Wilkerson, R. D., Mockridge, P. B. and Massing, G. K. (1980) Effect of selected drugs on serum digoxin concentration in dogs. *Am. J. Cardiol.* 45, 1201–10.

Williams, R. L., Davies, R. O., Berman, R. S., Holmes, G. I., Huber, P., Gee, W. L., Lin, E. T. and Benet, L. Z. (1982) Hydrochlorthiazide pharmacokinetics and pharmacologic effect: the influence of indomethacin. *J. Clin. Pharmacol.* 22, 32–41.

Williams, R. L., Upton, R. A., Buskin, J. N. and Jones, R. M. (1981) Ketoprofen–aspirin interactions. *Clin. Pharmacol. Ther.*, 30, 226–31.

Williamson, H. E., Bourland, W. A. and Marchand, G. R. (1974) Inhibition of ethacrinic acid-induced increase in renal blood flow by indomethacin. *Prostaglandins*, 8, 297–301.

Williamson, H. E., Bourland, W. A. and Marchand, G. R. (1975) Inhibition of furosemide induced increase in renal blood flow by indomethacin. *Proc. Soc. Exp. Biol. Med.*, 148, 164–7.

Williamson, P., Ene, D. and Roberts, C. (1983) Effects of azapropazone and frusemide on renal sodium and urate excretion. *Proc. 2nd World Conf. Clin. Pharmacol. Ther.*, Abstract No. 249.

Williamson, P. J., Daneshmend, T. K., Ene, M. D. and Roberts, C. J. C. (1984) Antipyrine kinetics during administration of azapropazone and frusemide. *Br. J. Clin. Pharmacol.*, 17, 627P.

Willis, J. V., Kendall, M. J. and Jack, D. B. (1980) A study of the effect of aspirin on the pharmacokinetics of oral and intravenous diclofenac sodium. *Eur. J. Clin. Pharmacol.*, 18, 415–18.

Willkens, R. F. and Segre, E. J. (1975) Combination therapy with naproxen and aspirin in rheumatoid arthritis. *Arthr. Rheum.*, 19, 677–82.

Wing, L. M. H., Bune, A. J. C., Chalmers, J. P., Graham, J. R. and West, M. J. (1981) The effects of indomethacin in treated hypertensive patients. *Clin. Exp. Pharmacol. Physiol.*, 8, 537–41.

Wiseman, E. H., Chang, Y-H. and Hobbs, D. C. (1975) Interaction of sudoxicam and aspirin in animals and man. *Clin. Pharmacol. Ther.*, 18, 441–8.

Wishinsky, H., Glasser, E. J. and Perkal, S. (1962) Protein interactions of sulphonylurea compounds. *Diabetes*, 2 (Suppl), 18–25.

Witzgall, H., Hirsch, F., Scherer, B. and Weber, P. C. (1982) Acute haemodynamic and hormonal effects of captopril are diminished by indomethacin. *Clin. Sci.*, 62, 611–15.

Yesair, D. W., Remington, L., Callahan, M. and Kensler, C. J. (1970) Comparative effects of salicylic acid, phenylbutazone, probenecid and other anions on the metabolism, distribution and excretion of indomethacin by rats. *Biochem. Pharmacol.*, 19, 1591–600.

Yeung Laiwah, A. C. and Mactier, R. A. (1981) Antagonistic effect of non-steroidal anti-inflammatory drugs on frusemide induced cardiac failure. *Br. Med. J.*, 283, 714.

Yü, T. F. and Perel J. (1980) Pharmacokinetic and clinical studies of carprofen in gout. *J. Clin. Pharmacol.*, 20, 347–51.

Yü, T. F., Dayton, P. G. and Gutman, A. B. (1963) Mutual suppression of the uricosuric effects of sulfinpyrazone and salicylate: a study in interactions between drug. *J. Clin. Invest.*, 42, 1330–9.

CHAPTER 4

Adverse reactions

A. Rushton

4.1 INTRODUCTION

The rheumatological literature abounds with adverse reaction information and, relatively recently, several examples have been dramatically brought to public awareness in relation to product withdrawal. Political interest has also burgeoned and parliamentary questions concerning adverse reaction reporting, product liability and regulatory authority responsivity are now commonplace. The present situation is not, of course, unique to rheumatological therapeutics but continuing close attention will undoubtedly be the safety of antirheumatic drugs.

In this chapter, I do not intend to provide a detailed listing of adverse reactions attributed to antirheumatic drugs. For such comprehensive information the reader is referred to appropriate sources (Del Favero, 1983; Rainsford and Velo, 1984). However, illustrative examples of general principles are included and more information will be given in subsequent chapters that cover individual drugs or therapeutic classes.

Adverse drug reactions (ADRs) have been classified in different ways. One of the simplest classifications separates ADRs into Type A and Type B (Rawlins and Thompson, 1981). According to this classification Type A reactions result from the recognized pharmacological action of a drug, and are usually predictable, assuming that the pharmacology has been adequately investigated and documented. Type B reactions are aberrant effects which do not result from a drug's 'normal' pharmacology. The frequency of such effects, which usually cannot be predicted from toxicological screening programmes, is generally low but morbidity and mortality may be high. Although a few ADRs may not readily fall into either of these two categories, more complex classifications, e.g. overdosage, intolerance, side effects, secondary effects, idiosyncrasy, and hypersensitivity (Rosenheim and Moulton, 1958), do not offer any real advantage in relation to diagnosis or management of individual cases.

Rheumatological examples of Type A reactions include the gastrointestinal microbleeding associated with cyclo-oxygenase inhibitors (Chernish et al., 1979; Yeung Laiwah et al., 1981) and the CNS effects of indomethacin. In the former the pharmacological mechanism has been suggested by studies that demonstrated prevention of the microbleeding by orally administered prostaglandin E_2 (Johansson et al., 1980; Cohen et al., 1980). The relationship of gastrointestinal microbleeding to induction of peptic ulceration is not clearly established but it is likely that inhibition of prostaglandin synthesis also plays a role in the latter pathological process, possibly augmented by production of tissue-destructive free oxygen radicals (Rainsford, 1984). However, the volume of gastrointestinal blood loss induced by an NSAID is not a clear predictor of ulcerogenesis in an individual patient. The pharmacological mechanisms which produce the CNS effects of indomethacin are not clearly understood, but the response is dose related and often dose limiting, particularly in the elderly.

The thrombocytopenia associated with parenteral gold therapy (Mettier et al., 1948) and the occurrence of Stevens–Johnson syndrome during administration of various NSAIDs (Levitt and Pearson, 1980; Husain et al., 1981; Sternlieb and Robinson, 1978) constitute Type B reactions. The lack of predictability for these severe adverse effects is characteristic of Type B reactions – even regular monitoring of platelet count during gold therapy usually fails to reduce the morbidity and mortality associated with the precipitous and severe thrombocytopenia. Genetic factors may influence the development of this and other ADRs associated with antirheumatic drugs (see Section 4.6).

4.2   DETECTION OF ADVERSE DRUG REACTIONS

Adverse drug reactions present a polymorphic picture in terms of clinical presentation. Many of them are clinically indistinguishable from aspects of 'natural' disease processes.

Before discussing the process of ADR detection, a definition of what is to be detected is appropriate. Although many forms of words have been used, the definition used by Naranjo et al. (1981) embodies the pivotal information: any noxious, unintended and undesired effect of a drug after doses used in humans for prophylaxis, diagnosis or therapy. However, this and similar definitions imply that a causal relationship has been established. The process of detection should not prejudge causality and Finney (1965) has proposed the concept of an 'adverse event', which does not distinguish between spontaneous and drug-induced effects. Accordingly, an episode of acute gastrointestinal bleeding would represent an adverse event – in a patient receiving NSAID therapy this event could arise from either an adverse reaction to the particular drug or an unrelated pathological process. All adverse events occurring during the course of drug therapy constitute possible ADRs but the process of causality attribution will be considered in a later section. The primary process of detection involves three major tasks:

(a) Patient monitoring;
(b) Documentation of adverse events;
(c) Appropriate reporting and processing of the information collected.

This process is applicable to all phases of a drug's lifespan. There are however important differences in application of the process between the pre-marketing and post-marketing phases.

4.2.1   Pre-marketing phase

The monitoring process represents an integral part of the pre-registration clinical investigation of a new compound. Results from animal studies and/or previous clinical experience with compounds in the same pharmacological class may suggest potential Type A adverse reactions and indicate appropriate emphasis for human safety evaluation. For example, the association of proteinuria with penicillamine (Multicentre Trial Group, 1973) provides a pragmatic rationale for careful urinalysis during evaluation of similar compounds containing thiol groups. Recently the use of the angiotensin I converting enzyme (ACE) inhibitor, captopril, in both hypertension and rheumatoid arthritis has been reported to be associated with proteinuria, (Merlet *et al.*, 1981; Kincaid-Smith, 1981) in line with other thiol compounds which show slow-acting antirheumatic activity (Colamussi and Ciompi, 1981; Drury *et al.*, 1984).

Apart from the direction afforded by such prior knowledge, safety monitoring is based upon general principles – careful clinical observation, recording of symptoms and laboratory monitoring.

However, considerable controversy lies behind such general statements of the process. Should symptomatology be documented by means of check lists or by using non-directed questions ('volunteered symptomatology')? The former approach undoubtedly elicits more symptoms than the latter but may be associated with high 'background noise' level – data arising from the use of check lists in placebo treated or untreated subjects illustrate this point (Green, 1964; Reidenberg and Lowenthal, 1968). My own preference is for 'volunteered symptomatology', except for when one or more symptoms are thought to be of particular interest – for example gastrointestinal symptoms during investigation of a NSAID. Whichever method is used, pre-treatment symptoms should be recorded.

Laboratory monitoring, particularly during the early phases of clinical development, is usually intensive, although it would be difficult to obtain a consensus amongst all investigators and all pharmaceutical companies for a list of 'essential' tests. However, a core group of haematological and clinical

TABLE 4.1

Laboratory tests that are commonly measured during clinical trials

Clinical chemistry	Haematology
* Creatinine and/or urea	* Haemoglobin
* Alanine aminotransferase	Red cell indices (MCHC etc.)
* Aspartate aminotransferase	* Total+differential WBC
* Bilirubin	* Platelet count
* Alkaline phosphatase	Erythrocyte sedimentation rate
Albumin	
Globulin	
Sodium, potassium, chloride	
Bicarbonate	
Calcium, phosphate	
Sugar	
Uric acid	
* Analysis of urine for protein, sugar, blood, bile pigment, ketones urine microscopy as appropriate	

* 'core' measurements

chemistry tests appears quite consistently in publications on new rheumatological drugs (Table 4.1). An inflammatory disease process, such as rheumatoid arthritis, may produce abnormalities in certain clinical chemistry measurements (e. g. glutamyl transpeptidase, alkaline phosphatase (Kendall *et al.,* 1970; Akesson *et al.,* 1980)) and careful documentation of pre-treatment values is therefore particularly important in studies of anti-rheumatic drugs.

(a) *Reporting of adverse reactions*

The responsibilities of both the clinical investigator and sponsoring pharmaceutical company have been laid down by major drug regulatory authorities and in the USA, and failure to comply may result in legal action, of which there have been several recent examples.

In the UK the investigator is responsible for the monitoring process and for reporting to the sponsoring company, which in turn is required to report all possible ADRs arising during clinical trials of drugs subject to a Clinical Trial Certificate (CTC) or to a Clinical Trial Certificate Exemption (CTX); the latter is now the predominant procedure applicable to clinical investigation of new compounds. Speirs and Griffin (1983), in a questionnaire review of experience in the first 12 months operation of the CTX scheme, reported that the frequency of major adverse events during studies of new chemical entities was 1.65%. However, this figure included a significant proportion of events which were almost certainly not drug related. In the context of this section the differentiation of major and minor events merits further comment. In their review, Speirs and Griffin (1983) placed an event in the 'major' category if any of the following criteria were met:

(a) The event was classified as major by the clinical investigator or by the responsible company;
(b) It resulted in a patient dropping out of the trial;
(c) It resulted in the breaking of a double-blind code;
(d) It involved an important physiological disturbance, e. g. any unexplained depression of blood count, any blood dyscrasia, jaundice etc.

The UK licensing authority differentiates between *serious* and *minor* reactions for reporting procedures: for compounds subject either to a CTC or CTX the licence holder is required to report serious reactions immediately on the yellow report form. Minor reactions are however treated differently according to whether a CTC or a CTX applies. For a compound subject to the former, minor reactions are reported in summary format at the conclusion of a study, whereas for CTX compounds, minor reactions follow the yellow form route (Table 4.2).

TABLE 4.2
Guidelines for severity classification of possible adverse drug reactions

Serious reactions	Severe CNS effects
General definition	Severe skin reactions
	Reactions in pregnant women
All fatal, life threatening, disabling or incapacitating reactions.	Unexplained lack of effect or paradoxical effect, e.g. possibility of reduction in efficacy due to drug-interaction, or hypertension with a hypotensive agent
Specific examples	
Anaphylaxis	
Blood dyscrasias	
Congenital abnormalities	
Endocrine disturbances	
Fertility effects	
Haemorrhage from any site	
Jaundice, however mild	
Ophthalmic signs or symptoms	

The licence holder's obligations are not limited to reporting possible ADRs that occur in the UK, but apply to international clinical experience on any drug which is currently under UK pre-registration investigation.

To meet these obligations, a pharmaceutical company must have effective systems, organized on an international basis. However, the quality and timeliness of the investigator's monitoring and reporting to the sponsoring company underpin any internal system, no matter how efficient in terms of electronic data processing.

(b) *Scope of the pre-registration detection process*

The pre-registration phase of clinical investigation presents both advantages and limitations in terms of capability to detect ADRs. The advantages are derived from the intensive monitoring environment of clinical trials, conducted by appropriately experienced investigators.

The limitations relate to the number and type of patients studied in this phase. The total number of patients treated with a new drug before registration usually lies in the range 1000–2000. This number is obviously not adequate to detect 'rare' ADRs. Statistical estimates of patient numbers required for adverse reaction detection have been made and the results of such calculations make sobering reading. In Table 4.3 the numbers required for a 95% detection

TABLE 4.3
The numbers game for ADR detection

Incidence of adverse reaction	Required number of patients for 95% chance of detection		
	one case	two cases	three cases
1 in 100	300	480	650
1 in 200	600	960	1 300
1 in 1 000	3 000	4 800	6 500
1 in 2 200	6 000	9 600	13 000
1 in 10 000	30 000	48 000	65 000

chance are presented, and it can be seen that reactions occurring at frequencies of one per thousand or less require a larger patient population than is usually studied pre-registration. If the reaction in question, for example thrombocytopenia, has a natural incidence then the problem is compounded. As stated earlier, most serious events are not specific to individual drugs. Moreover, data on background frequency are frequently inadequate and because of the protean nature of certain rheumatic diseases, e.g. SLE, the attribution of certain adverse effects (e. g. haematological or renal) between drug and disease presents an intellectual challenge (see Section 4.3).

Patients recruited to pre-registration studies are selected usually on the basis of relatively strict entry criteria. On the one hand, there are scientific pressures in favour of recruiting a relatively homogeneous trial population with typical disease features, reflected by the almost universal statement in RA studies that only patients with 'classical or definite' RA were studied. Similarly, concomitant therapy is restricted or recent treatment with certain drugs excluded. There has also been recent criticism of the age range profile of patients treated before drug registration (Smith et al., 1983), no doubt prompted by the virtual restriction of hepatorenal toxicity from benoxaprofen to 'aged' patients. However, this type of problem will not necessarily be avoided by the inclusion of more fit 70 and 80 year olds in a programme, because general debility/infirmity probably plays a more significant role than age per se. Such potentially high-risk patients do not usually fit into the pattern of outpatient rheumatological clinical studies and require cooperation with departments of geriatric medicine. Nevertheless, an awareness of the potential problems of 'unrestrained' prescribing to the infirm and/or aged must be promoted and efforts made to develop prescribing information, on a sound scientific basis, for high risk populations before marketing. The process for achieving this objective is currently under debate in regulatory, academic and pharmaceutical industry circles. A recent discussion paper from the FDA recognises the inherent problems and suggests one approach, a pharmacokinetic screening process for consideration (FDA 1983). In terms of pre-marketing drug interaction studies, practical considerations must be taken into account and studies of this type are usually directed towards areas indicated either by prior knowledge of similar drugs (e. g. NSAID interactions with anticoagulants, see Chapter 3) or on the basis of preclinical data (e. g. high *in vitro* protein binding).

Despite these limitations the pre-marketing safety evaluation gives a valuable basis for evaluating the balance of safety to efficacy – while recognizing the unexpected may still wait around the corner when a drug emerges into the wider environment of clinical practice.

4.2.2 Post-marketing adverse reaction monitoring

The post-marketing phase presents both quantitative and qualitative differences from the pre-marketing phase. The quantitative differences in terms of patient exposure are considerable. Within months the numbers of patients treated may rise to tens or hundreds of thousands. This order of patient exposure gives an opportunity for detection of less common adverse reactions (<1 in 200–300). As in the premarketing phase, the process of detection involves three primary activities – monitoring, documentation, and reporting. Application of the process, however, differs significantly – no longer is the drug exclusively administered within the framework of clinical trials, subject to supervision by experienced investigators and monitoring by the sponsoring company. The real world of clinical practice lacks effective audit and control mechanisms; clinical freedom is strenuously defended.

Accordingly, it is not surprising that the mainstay of post-marketing ADR detection in the UK has been a voluntary process – the Yellow Card System – which was introduced in 1964. Since its inception, this system has been variously described as the most effective ADR detection in the world and as failing to provide the public with the protection to which it is entitled. In relation to the withdrawal of benoxaprofen, criticism centred on alleged delays in processing Yellow Card reports and in taking regulatory action. The latter criticism is not so much applicable to the detection process as to the subsequent stages of interpretation and evaluation.

The detection capability of the Yellow Card System was strongly criticised by Venning (1983) who claimed that it failed to provide the first indication of a number of serious ADRs that occurred in recent times. This criticism was rebutted by Inman (1983) who pointed out that most of Venning's examples occurred prior to 1964 and also that he had omitted 'successes' such as ibufenac hepatoxicity.

There is no doubt that the Yellow Card System has suffered from chronic under-reporting. The extent of this is difficult to quantitate, but it is probable that less than 10% of many serious ADRs have been reported. Moreover, reporting patterns show variability, often increasing *in response* to publicity of problems; this 'reactive' type of increase occurred for benoxaprofen. Reporting also appears to decrease as a drug becomes 'established' and a survey of seven NSAIDs showed a peak reporting rate at two years post-marketing followed by a steady decline thereafter (Weber, 1984).

Accurate estimation of ADR frequency is therefore impossible because the data relate to a variably incomplete numerator (number of events) divided by a denominator (number of patients treated) that can, at best, be estimated in 'ballpark' terms. The Committee on the Safety of Medicines (CSM) has attempted to increase commitment to the system; for example, recently introduced products are identified by a black triangle in *MIMS*, the *British National Formulary* and the *Data Sheet Compendium*. Guidelines on what to report have also been redefined and publicized in *MIMS* (see also *Drug and Therapeutics Bulletin*, 1983).

There is some evidence that the medical profession is responding positively, although due to the low baseline, a significant preferential increase in reporting level for newly introduced drugs could present problems in comparison of new and established products in the same therapeutic class (e.g. NSAIDs).

Medical journals provide another mechanism for reporting ADRs, and have proved of value for alerting the medical profession, regulatory authority, and pharmaceutical industry to new problems. However, it would seem reasonable to expect that clinicians who are motivated to go into print should, at the same time, use the Yellow Card System. In this respect, the *British Medical Journal* has recently introduced an editorial policy that requires authors of short communications on ADRs to report relevant individual patient information to the CSM and the appropriate pharmaceutical company.

ADR information is also received by the pharmaceutical company from various sources, e. g. from direct clinician contact, from drug information units, and from phase IV clinical studies. Similar reporting obligations as for pre-registration drugs apply in the UK, although reports on minor reactions to established drugs are not required.

Most drugs are marketed on an international basis, and channels exist for transfer of ADR information. Regulatory authorities undoubtedly communicate directly, and the DHSS, for example, requires UK Product Licence holders to report international ADR experience on their drugs. International pharmaceutical companies are committing considerable resources to this complex task, and my own company has a unit within its medical function dedicated to this area.

In addition to the voluntary system, more formalized approaches to post-marketing ADR detection may contribute to the process. In the UK, two main types of prospective monitoring study are presently used:

1. Post-marketing studies, organized by the pharmaceutical company directly or through other agencies.
2. Prescription Event Monitoring (PEM).

The first approach may be viewed as a large clinical survey study in which patients treated with a new drug are monitored at intervals over an appropriate time period (dependent upon the type of drug and therapeutic use). Several studies of this type have been undertaken in recent years, some directly requested by the UK Licensing Authority. One such study monitored ketotifen, an antiasthmatic drug, and another indoprofen, a NSAID. In the former study (Maclay *et al.*, 1984) 19 252 patients were entered by participating doctors, but one year follow-up information was available for only 8291. No new major ADR was detected, although useful data on the frequency of drowsiness, a previously identified ADR, were obtained. In the case of indoprofen, it appears that the data contributed to the withdrawal of the drug from the market, although the study has not yet been published.

The results of another large study highlighted the design problems inherent to this area. A total of 9928 patients taking cimetidine and 9351 controls were studied (Colin-Jones *et al.*, 1983). Excellent follow up (>98%) was achieved over one year, including documentation of death certificates and necropsy reports. The results revealed that mortality in the cimetidine group was almost twice the control group rate, mostly accounted for by deaths from cancer (oesophagus, stomach, colon, lung, lymphatic, and haematopoietic), and from ischaemic heart disease, chronic liver disease, accidents, and poisonings. The authors largely attributed these differences to the use of cimetidine for treating the symptoms of various diseases, either knowingly or unknowingly. The control group had been selected by matching each cimetidine-treated patient with a person of the same sex and similar age, drawn from general practitioner age/sex registers, and obviously constituted a healthier population. Formal randomization of patients, as in controlled clinical trials, is, however, neither feasible nor ethical in the PMS (Post Marketing Surveillance) setting. These problems, together with other aspects of PMS, have been well reviewed elsewhere (Castle *et al.*, 1983).

In relation to the human and financial resources required for post-marketing studies, the amount of new ADR information emerging has been limited. Moreover, much criticism has arisen from certain quarters concerning the possible promotional value of this type of study. The Association of the British Pharmaceutical Industry (ABPI) has recently developed guidelines concerning the ethical aspects of PMS studies, and these are available on request from the

Association (Snell, 1984). Application of these guidelines should negate the criticisms of commercialism in this area.

The PEM scheme (Inman, 1981a, b) offers an alternative approach to 'planned' recruitment of patients and also avoids any criticisms of commercialism. The methodology of this scheme involves identification of patients on a particular drug as prescriptions pass through the Prescription Pricing Authority. Copies of relevant prescriptions are sent, in confidence, to the Drug Surveillance Research Unit, Southampton University, and a simple questionnaire is sent at appropriate intervals to the general practitioner requesting information on new diagnoses, hospital referrals and events. Inman (1981b) believes that this sytem could have identified the practolol syndrome earlier because of increased consultations relating to eyes and skin and resultant hospital referrals.

The difficulties of control group selection have not been solved by this scheme, although patients receiving 'similar' drugs can be identified and monitored. It is of interest that a pilot study of benoxaprofen by Dr Inman's unit identified jaundice as a potential problem in eight of 6000 patients, but in five of these patients benoxaprofen was excluded as a cause. Subsequently, Dr Inman has expanded his benoxaprofen data base to 24 000 patients and concluded that, in this cohort, there was one non-fatal case of jaundice unequivocally due to the drug (Inman, 1984). It is possible that the PEM scheme does not adequately cover 'high risk' patient groups (e. g. elderly infirm patients in long-term hospitalization), and a more general criticism is that PEM is at present inappropriate for drugs that are predominantly used in hospital practice. Dr Inman himself stresses that he views PEM as complementary to the Yellow Card System and not supplanting it.

The 'obvious' conclusion is that no one method for post-marketing ADR detection meets all perceived objectives. The post-marketing study or PEM survey, involving the oft-quoted 10 000 patients, is appropriate for detecting ADRs with a frequency of 1 in 2000–3000 or more, and the Yellow Card System is the only institutionalized system capable of detecting rarer reactions. More use could be made of disease-orientated studies (scrutiny of drug therapy in patients suffering from serious disorders that could be drug related, e. g. aplastic anaemia). Fundamental to all systems are a high standard of patient monitoring, clinical acumen, and motivation to report possible ADRs.

4.3   ATTRIBUTION OF EVENTS

The time has come to address the problem of causality, or the process by which a medical event becomes designated as an adverse reaction to a particular drug. In the course of recent media programmes and articles on this subject, it has often been implied that causality can usually be judged with confidence – or even automatically assumed on the basis of information reported to the CSM via the Yellow Card System (i. e. 'guilty by association'). The reality of the attribution process argues that such confidence is misplaced; as stated by the CSM and reemphasized at the beginning of this chapter, most adverse drug reactions are not unique events and, as such, may occur as part of recognized disease processes or as 'idiopathic' events (e. g. thrombocytopenia). Attribution to an individual drug is also often complicated by the presence of multiple drug therapy, which is particularly common in the population most likely to suffer ADRs – the aged and infirm.

In many respects the 'diagnosis' of causality for possible ADRs is analogous to the diagnosis of a disease process. Consequently, it is not surprising that the algorithm (or decision tree) approach has been proposed for ADRs. One of the longest was developed by Kramer *et al* (1979); this 56-question algorithm gave a high degree of inter-observer reproducibility in the hands of the algorithm developers. When a representative group of clinicians used the algorithm for a set of 30 well documented possible ADRs the between-assessor concurrence improved from that achieved by 'clinical judgement' alone. However, this approach is time-consuming and does not appear to have gained general acceptance, although the advent of microcomputers may revive algorithm usage. A simpler alternative to algorithms has recently been proposed (Castle, 1984), and this 'summary time score method' focuses on time relationships between drug administration/withdrawal/reintroduction and medical events. Further work on this approach would appear to be justified in view of the poor performance of 'clinical judgement'.

In a study designed to measure between-physician variability, Karch *et al.* (1976) asked six physicians (three hospital staff physicians and three clinical pharmacologists) to evaluate independently 60 selected case histories and classify the relationship of events to drug therapy on the following bases: definitely related, probably related, possibly related, unrelated. The clinical pharmacologists reached the same conclusion in 30 cases (50%), and in two-thirds of the cases not agreed the divergence of opinion was major. The level of agreement between staff physicians and individual clinical pharmacologists ranged from 63 to 78%. In a larger study of similar design, Koch-Weser *et al.* (1977) reported a similar level of discordance between clinical pharmacologists.

Nevertheless, it is advisable to make this type of evaluation instead of presenting long lists of events that lack any qualifying comment. In this respect, it is appropriate to bring the reader's attention to notes published by the CSM on interpretation of data from the adverse reactions register (derived from Yellow Card reports). These notes include the sentences . . . 'It is most important to realise that the inclusion of a particular reaction in the Register DOES NOT MEAN THAT IT IS CAUSALLY RELATED TO THE USE OF THE DRUG. The print-out which you have been sent is intended merely as a guide to the pattern of reactions that have been reported, and will include many false associations'. To supplement the individual case-history-based attribution process, it may be appropriate to utilize an analytical epidemiological approach. In the previous section, the descriptive branch of epidemiology was discussed; namely, the process of documenting how often a particular medical event occurs in a group of subjects. Analytical epidemiology sets out to interpret the number of events. If a valid control group has been monitored, then statistical comparisons of event frequency play an important role in the process. However the difficulty of achieving a valid control in PMS studies has been previously highlighted and consequently historical or other controls (e. g. national morbidity/mortality data) are often invoked. The pitfalls of this approach are many; for example, in the rheumatological field, an excess of deaths due to lymphoreticular neoplasms has been reported in rheumatoid arthritis (Isomaki *et al.*, 1982; Symmons *et al.*, 1984). These reports should obviously be taken into account when interpreting cancer incidence data for populations on particular treatments, e. g. immunosuppressive drugs.

Very rarely the interpretation will be apparent without any statistical support, particularly if the background frequency is almost zero. In this situation, less than a handful of events may be of fundamental importance, even though statistical significance either has not been reached or cannot be meaningfully tested.

In the absence of control groups, comparison of the possible ADR data for different dose levels of a drug may assist interpretation, although the 'dose' related placebo response observed by Green (1964) should be taken into account, unless the formulations are matched across dose levels.

If a well-defined clinical event reoccurs on reintroduction of a drug then the causal relationship has the backing of scientific principles. However, a negative result on rechallenge does not necessarily exonerate the putative cause. The ability to rechallenge is often limited by ethical considerations.

In view of the problems highlighted in this section it may be more difficult to establish a cause and effect relationship between the active constituent of a formulation and an adverse effect than between the same constituent and a beneficial effect on a disease process. There are risks if errors are made on one side or other in the interpretive process. The risks if an adverse effect is wrongly attributed to a drug are, first, that the real cause of the effect may be missed with possible detriment to the patient and, second, that an acceptably safe and effective therapy may be unjustly labelled. Conversely, if a causal relationship is missed, unnecessary morbidity will result. Examples of both have occurred in the past, and will no doubt occur again. However, if the medical profession, regulatory authorities, and other interested parties maintain an inquiring but open-minded approach then problems should be minimized.

4.4   ADVERSE REACTION INFORMATION

This topic was touched upon in the section concerned with detection of adverse reactions; a process that involves several information pathways, for example, clinician–pharmaceutical company, clinician–regulatory authority and pharmaceutical company–regulatory authority (or authorities). From the viewpoint of a total information system, it is apparent that other links are required. In broad terms such links are required to provide dissemination of information to parties with a valid interest. Although it is not intended to enter into a philosophical debate on the definition of 'a valid interest', it has become obvious that, in today's society, adverse reactions provide a game for any number of players e. g.

Health care personnel – medical/dental practitioners, nurses, pharmacists *et al.*

Regulatory authorities

Pharmaceutical companies

Patients (and the 'non-patient' general public)

The Media

Politicians

Information sources available for health care personnel are listed in Table 4.4. Dissemination of up-to-date information sources presents considerable difficulties, particularly during early post-marketing on an international basis. At the time of marketing, the product data sheet is derived from the pre-registration clinical trial programme data – a number of journal publications are usually available to provide a more detailed portrayal of ADR information in individual clinical studies. After marketing, clinical trial publications accumulate but the lead-in period of major journals, including those specializing in rheumatology, may exceed a year. The correspondence columns of journals provide a way to cut down such delays but may lead to acrimonious debate instead of useful information dissemination. The *British Medical Jour-*

TABLE 4.4
ADR information sources

Manufacturers data sheets (for brand name products)
Advertisements (particularly in USA journals)
Package inserts (particularly in USA)
Publications with official status (e.g. *British National Formulary*)
Regulatory authority data bases and information letters
Pharmaceutical company adverse reaction or medical information units
Medical textbooks (some deal exclusively with ADR information)
Medical journals (clinical trials; case reports; PMS studies)
Drug information centres (national network in the UK)
'Viewdata' systems (currently under evaluation)
One's colleagues

nal has recently set an interesting example by introducing a section for unrefereed short communications – if such communications concern suspected adverse drug reactions, acceptance is subject to the authors' having reported the information both directly to the pharmaceutical company concerned and to the CSM via the Yellow Card System.

It is of course difficult, if not impossible, for the practitioner to maintain an up-to-date awareness of adverse drug reaction information by personal scrutiny of the journals, and there is a need for central agencies to collate, abstract, interpret, and disseminate information.

The regulatory authorities and the pharmaceutical companies must play central roles in this process. In the UK, it is possible to obtain printouts from the DHSS data base (derived from Yellow Card reporting by practitioners and by companies), but there has been criticism regarding delays in entry to the data base and the lack of interpretation in the information. The CSM, however, has become more proactive in this area by issuing newsletters concerning safety issues that are, in their view, matters of current interest and concern.

An international pharmaceutical company is in a unique position to maintain an overview picture of safety profiles for its drugs and has, as indicated earlier, obligations to report 'international' information to national drug regulatory authorities. As a result of these interactions, appropriate amendments to prescribing information may be made. A company may also need to communicate directly with clinicians in advance of such changes in product literature because of the lead-in time involved in the latter process.

Adverse reaction information also resides in several regularly updated textbooks, and some are solely devoted to adverse reactions, (e. g. *Side Effects of Drugs Annual*), whereas in others admixture with other information occurs (e. g. pharmacokinetic, efficacy in AMA Drug Evaluations). Regional drug information centres in the UK (McNulty, 1983) also provide an invaluable service, particularly to practitioners without ready access to major medical libraries. The era of electronic data processing presents tremendous opportunities for adverse reaction information dissemination (pilot schemes using telephone cable access to data bases have been instituted and offer the advantage of two-way communication) in addition to accessing ADR information. With the appropriate hardware, practitioners will be able to report their own adverse reaction experiences. Although such schemes have tremendous potential, in the UK development may be slow because of funding problems.

Where does the patient fit into this scheme? Or perhaps a better question is – where *should* the patient fit in? There is no doubt that 'patients' are nowadays much more interested in the nature of medical treatment than ever before. In part this derives from laudable changes in educational status and social attitudes. More recently, however, there are signs that the pendulum of change is swinging out of control, largely propelled by media sensation and influence. In particular, credence is given to the postulate that drug safety can be readily defined on an absolute scale. The concept of risk–benefit analysis appears to be virtually ignored in this area, whereas it is accepted in areas such as 'road safety'. The medical profession, drug regulatory authorities, and pharmaceutical companies must enter into this debate in a proactive manner, instead of, for example, suffering at the receiving end of 'trial by television'.

Turning from the general issues to the specific matter of a patient seeking advice for a particular complaint, how should safety issues be approached? In the clinical trial area, this question is relatively easy to answer. The informed consent procedure, by definition, requires that patients are advised of reasonably foreseeable risks associated with the treatments under investigation (in the USA the elements of informed consent are defined by regulatory statute.) Particularly during the early stages of investigation of a new drug there will be risks that cannot be specified; the patient should nevertheless be advised of likely 'class effects', such as gastrointestinal symptoms during treatment with 'classical' cyclo-oxygenase inhibitors.

The relationship of doctor and patient is qualitatively different in the non-trial post-marketing phase. There is more freedom for the doctor to use judgement in transfer of information regarding adverse effects. Nevertheless, due to the increasing public awareness of this area, the issues cannot be avoided as was often done in the not too distant past. The risks associated with different antirheumatic treatments vary considerably – some of these are 'musts' for discussion with patients, for example the risk of ocular side effects during long-term antimalarial therapy; likewise the haematological, cutaneous, and renal adverse effects of sodium aurothiomalate. In addition to specific statements regarding the common/serious effects of individual drugs, general advice for patients to report unexpected events should also be given and a potentially useful leaflet for patients prescribed 'new' drugs (black triangle identification in the *British National Formulary*, *MIMS*, and the *Data Sheet Compendium*) has been suggested by the UK Consumers Association (Drug Therapeutics Bulletin, 1983). Instead of relegating this area to the negative aspects of therapeutics, the clinician is in a unique position to educate positively and to redress the attitudes that may arise out of media sensationalism.

4.5 EVALUATION OF RISK VERSUS BENEFIT

The concept of risk–benefit analysis receives much lip service in therapeutic discussions. There are, however, problems in applying this kind of analysis to drug treatment in general, and particularly to chronic disease areas in which drug therapy is seldom 'life-saving'. As previously discussed, it is seldom possible to accurately measure the risks associated with a particular drug. The Yellow Card System has a generally low but variable reporting rate, thus underestimating the numerator. Valid information on the denominator is equally difficult to obtain, especially for drugs with a significant proportion of hospital usage. A combination of prescription audit data and manufacturers' sales figures may provide a ballpark figure for patient exposure, but subdivision by disease area may be difficult – this information may be of relevance – for example, it appears that proteinuria from captopril occurs predominantly in patients with connective tissue disorders.

Even if it were possible to obtain accurate data for the mortality and serious morbidity caused by a drug, there is at present no accepted methodology for evaluating these negative aspects against the benefits of a drug, for example the pain relief from a NSAID. In such a vacuum, safety tends to be viewed as an absolute issue, particularly outside the medical fraternity.

The basis for recent judgements by the CSM on several rheumatological drugs has not been clearly communicated. The absolute numbers of events associated with, but not necessarily caused by, certain drugs have been given much publicity to the neglect of discussion on the relative risks involved. Inman (Director, Drug Surveillance Research Unit, University of Southampton – see page 136), has criticized the CSM *statement* on its decision to withdraw benoxaprofen on the grounds that it focused on absolute numbers of suspected ADR reports (over 3500) and 'fatal cases' (61) instead of risk evaluation. Dr Inman has recently formulated an original proposal to fill the vacuum referred to earlier in this section (Inman, 1985). According to his proposal, both drugs and diseases would be allocated a risk index (an 8 point scale measuring logarithmically increasing risk from category 8 to category 1). He has also suggested that drugs used to treat potentially lethal diseases should be at least one, and preferably two, orders of magnitude less risky than the disease itself, whereas drugs used for non-lethal conditions should have a three level separation. This framework does not appear to take relative efficacy into account, but nevertheless could represent a major step forward as a process for analysis of this complex area.

Improvements in the analytical process are unlikely without commitment of resources, and it has been suggested that national health authorities should appoint a small group of experts (disease area specialists) for each new drug to provide an authoritative view on safety issues (Brown, 1984).

4.6 CONTROL OF ADVERSE DRUG REACTIONS

My premise for including this section is that a proportion of adverse drug reactions are avoidable, using information that is currently available. For the future, improvements in understanding of ADR pathogenesis and the development of more predictive animal models will no doubt result in 'safer' drugs.

It is well established that adverse drug reactions increase in frequency with age (Seidl et al., 1966; Hurwitz, 1969; Bottiger et al., 1979). A study of 2000 admissions to 42 UK geriatric units showed that about 10% were admitted solely or partly because of adverse drug reactions (Williamson and Chopin,

1980). A Royal College of Physicians working party report (Medication for the Elderly, 1984) attributed this to several factors, including:

(a) Inadequate clinical assessment and supervision;
(b) Excessive prescribing;
(c) Greater intrinsic susceptibility to adverse drug reactions;
(d) Impaired compliance.

The pharmacokinetic contribution to increased ADR susceptibility was highlighted in the report and procedures advocated to reduce ADR frequency included:

(a) The use of nomograms to calculate creatinine clearance in order to make dose adjustments for drugs excreted primarily by the renal route.
(b) Plasma drug level monitoring for drugs with a narrow therapeutic index, such as digoxin or theophylline.

The increasing availability of drug assays can be expected to increase the spectrum of drugs included in the second category. The demonstration that 'chronic inflammatory disease' may alter drug metabolism and/or protein binding (Schneider *et al.*, 1976, 1979) also argues for increased attention to kinetic factors in rheumatological therapeutics, especially during periods of changing disease activity.

Pharmacodynamic changes also occur with increasing years but are less well documented than pharmacokinetic factors. Some drugs with central nervous system actions may produce increased effects for a given blood concentration, and indomethacin appears to fall into this category.

Good prescribing habits and appropriate supervision of medical therapy are of course appropriate to all age groups of patients, but the effects of suboptimae practice will be particularly seen in the elderly. Once initiated, drug therapy for chronic diseases may be continued by, for example, repeat prescriptions. Regular medical review of any drug therapy is advisable and appropriate intervals should be specified in the patient's notes. Specific monitoring procedures for individual drugs could then be superimposed upon the general principles. Monitoring guidelines for parenteral gold, penicillamine, and chloroquine are established, and failure to comply may have medicolegal implications. Patients who fail to keep appointments for such visits should be traced assiduously.

Appropriate patient information on early signs/symptoms of serious adverse reactions should be given. This should be combined with carefully explained dosing instructions, preferably clearly written for the elderly and reinforced by home visits by a member of the primary health care team.

Recent research suggests that genetic factors may predispose to adverse drug reactions (Lunde *et al.*, 1977; Breimer, 1983). The predisposition may in some patients be due to a well-defined metabolic abnormality (e. g. slow acetylators and dapsone toxicity), or, as in the case of gold and penicillamine, currently lack a mechanistic explanation (Wooley et al., 1980; Coblyn et al., 1981). Wider application of this avenue of research can be anticipated as diagnostic methodology (e. g. tissue typing; acetylator phenotyping) becomes more readily available. Earlier research showed that a past history of adverse drug reactions was a risk factor, and this may reflect the genetic factors described above. However, data from rheumatological therapeutic sources are contradictory, at least in respect of gold and penicillamine. Some studies have suggested that a prior adverse reaction to gold or penicillamine predisposes to subsequent problems if the alternative drug is later given (Day and Golding, 1974; Webley and Coomes, 1978; Dodd et al., 1980). Other investigators have not found any such predisposition (Multicentre Trial Group, 1974; Steven et al., 1981).

The recent ADR problems in the rheumatological field have involved both new drugs and new formulations of 'well established' drugs. It is still unclear whether some of these drugs involved were less safe than similar compounds with a longer history of clinical usage. There has been criticism of the pharmaceutical industry for excessive and/or misleading promotion of new market entrants and also of clinicians for poor prescribing habits. It has been proposed that the extent of these ADR problems could be reduced by a conditional approval system which would restrict the usage of a new drug until long-term PMS safety evaluation data became available (Turner, 1984). This proposal is a variation on the earlier theme of monitored release (Dollery and Rawlins, 1977). However, the proponents of such schemes conveniently gloss over the practical implications – patient quotas per clinician, hospital or general practice usage, and further erosion of patent life. Furthermore, the conditional licensing concept has been criticized on scientific grounds by the originator of PEM on the grounds that it would merely delay the recognition of many serious, but rare, adverse reactions instead of avoiding or minimizing such problems (Inman, 1984b). There is obviously a need for constructive discussion between all parties – specialist clinicians, clinical pharmacologists, regulatory authorities, and pharmaceutical companies – if the objective of improved drug safety is to be achieved.

4.7 REFERENCES

Akesson, A., Berglund, K. and Karlsson, M. (1980) Liver function in some common rheumatic disorders. *Scand. J. Rheumatol.*, 9, 81–8.

Bottiger, L. E., Furhoff, A. K. and Holmberg, L. (1979) Drug induced blood dyscrasias. *Acta Med. Scand.*, 205, 457–61.

Breimer, D. D. (1983) Variability in human drug metabolism and its implications. *Int. J. Clin. Pharmacol.*, 3, 399–413.

Brown, P. (1984) Where now for PMS in UK. *Scrip (World Pharmaceutical News)* 902, 2–3.

Castle, W. M. (1984) Assessment of causality in industrial settings. *Drug Information J.*, 18, 297–302.

Castle, W. M., Nicholls, J. T. and Downie, C. C. (1983) Problems of post-marketing surveillance. *Br. J. Clin. Pharmacol.*, 16, 581–5.

Chernish, S. M., Rosenak, B. D., Brunelle, R. L. and Crabtree, R. (1979) Comparison of gastrointestinal effects of aspirin and fenoprofen. *Arthr. Rheum.*, 22, 376–83.

Coblyn, J. S., Weinblatt, B., Holdsworth, D. and Glass, D. (1981) Gold-induced thrombocytopenia. A clinical and immunogenetic study of twenty-three patients. *Ann. Intern. Med.*, 95, 178–81.

Cohen, M. M., Cheung, G. and Lyster, D. M. (1980) Prevention of aspirin-induced faecal blood loss by prostaglandin E_2. *Gut*, 21, 602–6.

Colamussi, V. and Ciompi, M. L. (1981) Dose related side effects of tioprinin in rheumatoid arthritis. *Proc. 15th Int. Congr. Rheumatol.*, Paris, Abstract 0141.

Colin-Jones, D. G., Langman, M. J. S., Lawson, D. H. and Vessey, M. P. (1983) Post-marketing surveillance and the safety of cimetidine: 12 month mortality report. *Br. Med. J.*, 286, 1713–16.

Day, A. T. and Golding, J. R. (1974) Hazards of penicillamine therapy in the treatment of rheumatoid arthritis. *Postgrad. Med. J.*, 50, (Suppl. 2), 71–3.

Del Favero, A. (1983) Side effects to antiinflammatory agents and drugs used in rheumatism and gout. in *Side Effects of Drugs Annual* (ed M. N. G. Dukes), Excerpta Medica Amsterdam, Oxford.

Dodd, M. J., Griffiths, I. D. and Thompson, M. (1980) Adverse reactions to D-penicillamine after gold toxicity. *Br. Med. J.* 280, 1498–500.

Dollery, C. T. and Rawlins, M. D. (1977) Monitoring adverse reactions to drugs. *Br. Med. J.*, 1, 96–7.

Drug and Therapeutics Bulletin (1983) Reporting adverse reactions. The black triangle and the patient. 21, 93–4.

Drury, P. L., Rudge, S. R. and Perret, D. (1984) Structural requirements for activity of certain 'specific' antirheumatic drugs: more than a simple thiol group? *Br. J. Rheumatol.*, 23, 100–6.

FDA Discussion Paper (1983) Discussion paper on the testing of drugs in the elderly. Office of New Drug Evaluation, US Food and Drug Administration.

Finney, D. J. (1965) The design and logic of a monitor of drug use. *J. Chron. Dis.*, 18, 77–98.

Green, D. M. (1964) Pre-existing conditions, placebo reactions and 'side effects'. *Ann. Intern. Med.*, 60, 255–65.

Hurwitz, N. (1969) Predisposing factors in adverse reactions to drugs. *Br. Med. J.*, 1, 536–9.

Husain, Z., Runge, L. A., Jabbs, J. M. and Hyla, J. A. (1981) Sulindac-induced Stevens–Johnson syndrome: report of 3 cases. *J. Rheumatol.*, 8, 176–9.

Inman, W. H. W. (1981a) Postmarketing surveillance of adverse drug reactions in general practice. I Search for new methods. *Br. Med. J.*, 282, 1131–2.

Inman, W. H. W. (1981b) Post marketing surveillance of adverse drug reactions in general practice. II Prescription-event monitoring at the University of Southampton. *Br. Med. J.*, 282, 1216–17.

Inman, W. H. W. (1983) Adverse reactions to new drugs. *Br. Med. J.*, 286, 719–20.

Inman, W. H. W. (1984) Prescription-event monitoring and yellow cards. *Lancet*, i, 130–1.

Inman, W. H. W. (1985) Risk in medical intervention – balancing therapeutic risks and benefits. In *Risk Man-made Hazards to Man* (ed. M. G. Cooper), Oxford Clarendon Press.

Isomaki, H. A., Hakulinen, T. and Joutsenlahtie, V. (1982) Excess risk of lymphomas, leukemia and myeloma in patients with rheumatoid arthritis. *Ann. Rheum. Dis.,* 41 (Suppl. 1), 34–6.

Johansson, C., Kollberg, B., Nordemar, R., Samuelson, K. and Bergstrom, S. (1980) Protective effect of prostaglandin E_2 in the gastrointestinal tract during indomethacin treatment of rheumatic diseases. *Gastroenterology,* 78, 479–83.

Karch, F. E., Smith, C. L., Kerzner, B., Mazzullo, J. M., Weintraub, M. and Lasagna, L. (1976) Commentary: adverse drug reactions – a matter of opinion. *Clin. Pharmacol. Ther.,* 19, 489–92.

Kendall, M. J., Cockel, R., Becker, J. and Hawkins, C. F. (1970) Raised serum alkaline phosphatase in rheumatoid disease. *Ann. Rheum. Dis.,* 29, 537–40.

Kincaid-Smith, P. (1981) Drug induced membranous glomerulonephritis, in cardiovascular medicine in the 80's – angiotensin-converting enzyme inhibition. *Symposium Proceedings.* Biomedical Information, New York.

Koch-Weser, J., Sellers, E. M. and Zacest, R. (1977) The ambiguity of adverse drug reactions. *Eur. J. Clin. Pharmacol.,* 11, 75–8.

Levitt, L. and Pearson, R. W. (1980) Sulindac-induced Stevens–Johnson toxic epidermal necrolysis syndrome. *J. Am. Med. Assoc.,* 243, 1262–3.

Lunde, P. K. M., Frislid, K. and Hansteen, V. (1977) Disease and acetylator polymorphism. *Clin. Pharmacokinet.,* 2, 182–97.

Kramer, M. S., Levanthal, J. M., Hutchinson, T. A. and Feinstein, A. R. (1979) An algorithm for the operational assessment of adverse drug reactions. Background, description and instructions for use. *J. Am. Med. Assoc.,* 242, 623–32.

Maclay, W. P., Crowder, D., Spiro, S., Turner, P. (1984) Postmarketing surveillance: practical experience with ketotifen. *Br. Med. J.,* 288, 911–14.

McNulty, H. (1983) Collaboration and work sharing of drug information services in the United Kingdom. *Drug Information J.,* 17, 95–103.

Medication for the elderly: a report of the Royal College of Physicians (1984) *J. Roy. Coll. Phys. London,* 18, 7–17.

Merlet, C. I., Camus, J-P, Prior, A. and Bergeuin, H. (1981) Captopril in rheumatoid arthritis. *Proc. 15th Int. Congr. Rheumatol.,* Paris. Abstract 1389.

Multicentre Trial Group (1973) Controlled trial of D(–)penicillamine in severe rheumatoid arthritis. *Lancet,* i, 275–80.

Multicentre Trial Group (1974) Absence of toxic or therapeutic interaction between penicillamine and previously administered gold in a trial of penicillamine in rheumatoid disease. *Postgrad. Med. J.,* 50 (Suppl. 2), 77–8.

Naranjo, C. A., Busto, U., Sellers, E. M., Sandor, P., Ruiz, I., Roberts, E. A., Janecek, E., Domecq, C. and Greenblatt, D. J. (1981) A method for estimating the probability of adverse drug reactions. *Clin. Pharmacol. Ther.,* 30, 239–45.

Rainsford, K. D. (1984) Mechanisms of gastrointestinal ulceration by nonsteroidal antiinflammatory/analgesic drugs. In *Advances in Inflammation Research,* Vol. 6, *Side effects of antiinflammatory/analgesic drugs,* Raven Press, New York.

Rainsford, K. D. and Velo, G. (eds) (1984) *Advances in Inflammation Research* Vol. 6, *Side effects of antiinflammatory/analgesic drugs,* Raven Press, New York.

Mettier, S. R., MacBride, A. and Li, J. (1948) Thrombocytopenic purpura complicating gold therapy for rheumatoid arthritis. *Blood,* 3, 1105–11.

Rawlins, M. D. and Thomspon, J. W. (1981) Pathogenesis of adverse drug reactions. In *Textbook of Adverse Drug Reactions* (ed. D. M. Davies), Oxford University Press, Oxford.

Reidenberg, M. M. and Lowenthal, D. T. (1968) Adverse non-drug reactions. *N. Engl. J. Med.,* 279, 678–9.

Rosenheim, M. L. and Moulton, R. (1958) *Sensitivity Reactions to Drugs: A Symposium,* Oxford.

Schneider, R. E., Babb, J., Bishop, H., Mitchard, M., Hoare, A. M. and Hawkins, C. F. (1976) Plasma levels of propranolol in treated patients with coeliac disease and patients with Crohn's disease. *Br. Med. J.*, 2, 794–5.

Schneider, R. E., Bishop, H., Hawkins, C. F. and Kitis, G. (1979) Drug binding to α_1 glycoprotein. *Lancet*, i, 554.

Seidl, L. G., Thornton, G. F., Smith, J. W. and Cluff, L. E. (1966) Studies on the epidemiology of adverse drug reactions. *Bull. Johns Hopkins Hospital*, 119, 299–315.

Smith, C., Ebrahim, S. and Arie, T. (1983) Drug trials, the 'elderly', and the very aged. *Lancet*, ii, 1139.

Snell, E. S. (1984) Post marketing surveillance of adverse reactions to drugs. *Br. Med. J.*, 288, 1156.

Speirs, C. J. and Griffin, J. P. (1983) A survey of the first year of operation of the new procedure affecting the conduct of clinical trials in the United Kingdom. *Br. J. Clin. Pharmacol.*, 15, 649–55.

Sternlieb, P. and Robinson, M. (1978) Stevens–Johnson syndrome plus toxic hepatitis due to ibuprofen. *N. Y. State J. Med.*, 78, 1239–43.

Steven, M., Hunter, J. A., Murdock, R. M., McLaren, A. and Capell, H. A. (1981) The effect of order of second-line drug therapy on the development of side effects in the treatment of rheumatoid arthritis (RA) Abstr. *Ann. Rheum. Dis.*, 40, 204–5.

Symmons, D. P. M., Ahern, M., Bacon, P. A., Hawkins, C. F., Amlot, P. L., Jones, E. L., Prior, P. and Scott, D. L. (1984) Lymphoproliferative malignancy in rheumatoid arthritis a study of 20 cases. *Ann. Rheum. Dis.*, 43, 132–5.

Turner, P. (1984) Food and drugs: why different approaches to their safety? *Lancet*, i, 1116.

Venning, G. R. (1983) Identification of adverse reactions to new drugs III. Alerting processes and early warning systems. *Br. Med. J.*, 286, 458–60.

Weber, J. C. P. (1984) Epidemiology of adverse reactions to nonsteroidal antiinflammatory drugs. In *Advances in Inflammation Research*, Vol. 6, *Side-effects of antiinflammatory/analgesic drugs*. Raven Press, New York.

Webley, M. and Coomes, E. N. (1978) Is penicillamine therapy in rheumatoid arthritis influenced by previous treatment with gold. *Br. Med. J.*, 2, 91.

Williamson, J. and Chopin, J. M. (1980) Adverse reactions to prescribed drugs in the elderly: a multicentre investigation. *Age Ageing*, 9, 73–80.

Wooley, P. H., Griffen, J., Panayi, G. S., Batchelor, J. R., Welsh, K. I. and Gibson, T. J. (1980) HLA-DR antigens and toxic reaction to sodium aurothiomalate and D-penicillamine in patients with rheumatoid arthritis. *N. Engl. J. Med.*, 303, 300–2.

Yeung Laiwah, A. C., Hilditch, T. E., Horton, P. W. and Hunter, J. A. (1981) Antiprostaglandin synthetase activity of non-steroidal anti-inflammatory drugs and gastrointestinal microbleeding: a comparison of flurbiprofen with benoxaprofen. *Ann. Rheum. Dis.*, 40, 455–61.

CHAPTER 5

Evaluation of drug response

R. Madhok and H. A. Capell

5.1 INTRODUCTION

Many of the rheumatic diseases exhibit a number of different clinical signs and symptoms. These are frequently related to multiple anatomical sites and in addition, there may be abnormalities in laboratory tests, on radiographic examination and in other specialized investigations. As a result 'batteries' of assessments have evolved and the reader of clinical trial reports on antirheumatic drugs is usually confronted with a complex array of data, comprising various individual measurements, both subjective and objective. It is thus difficult to obtain a comprehensive evaluation of therapy and even when the individual measurements are combined to produce composite indices the overall picture is often far from clear. This is in sharp contrast with many other disorders; for example, hypertension in which one primary measurement is used, both in clinical trials and clinical practice, to assess response to drug therapy.

In this chapter most emphasis will be placed on the assessment of drug efficacy rather than safety. Both are obviously of considerable importance but the assessment of drug efficacy in rheumatic disorders poses particular problems and, despite the many shortcomings of currently available methodology, deserves detailed scrutiny. Drug safety assessment is also discussed in more depth in Chapter 4 (Adverse Reactions).

In general two categories of systemic drugs are used in the management of patients with rheumatic diseases: first the non-steroidal anti-inflammatory drugs (NSAIDs) and analgesics which offer symptomatic relief from pain and stiffness, and secondly drugs which may have a significant inhibitory action on the underlying disease process, for example gold, penicillamine and immunosuppressive drugs. The second category of drugs is restricted to the chronic, inflammatory diseases, such as rheumatoid arthritis. The inflammatory diseases usually have a greater impact on the health status of the affected individual than is the case for degenerative arthritides. Accordingly, more emphasis will be placed on the assessment of efficacy in inflammatory rather than degenerative disorders.

Evaluation of drug response is important both for evaluating the potential of a new compound and in ascertaining the extent of benefit of an established compound in an individual patient. The assessment of therapy which is purely symptomatic, and may be taken as required, is clearly very different from the assessment of putative disease-modifying drugs, which need to be taken on a regular basis over prolonged periods. Local therapy in the form of intra-articular injection represents another dimension of treatment, which requires careful assessment. In this sphere, as in all other forms of antirheumatic therapy, exclusion of a placebo response is vital.

5.2 GENERAL ASPECTS OF DRUG EVALUATION IN RHEUMATOLOGY

5.2.1 Toxicity

Unfortunately, all drugs used in rheumatology have significant adverse effects and this has to be acknowledged at the outset. Evaluation of the clinical significance of drug toxicity depends both on disease and the type of response that is expected.

(a) NSAIDs

When evaluating these drugs it is clearly important to document the frequency of patient complaints in the form of gastrointestinal upset, rashes, headaches, lightheadedness, or other symptoms that may become immediately apparent, and could be attributable to therapy. Whenever feasible, placebo treated patients should be similarly monitored, although this may only be ethical for short-term studies. Unfortunately something of a hiatus exists in that, in the initial clinical trials, patients with pre-existing gastrointestinal disease tend to be excluded, as do the older age groups, and when the drug is released the most at-risk patients have not been fully evaluated before the launch. This is an aspect of NSAID assessment which requires attention and post-marketing surveillance is currently inadequate. However, from 1985, evidence of drug assessment in the elderly will become mandatory before a product licence is issued. Other problem areas are, first, the detection of toxicity that occurs only after long-term treatment, and, secondly, the identification of rare but potentially serious adverse reactions. Very often, the incidence of the particular event is difficult to assess in the population as a whole and a high index of suspicion is required. When large numbers of similar drugs are available and individual experience of any one preparation is diluted, the problem is compounded. No one system has been shown to be truly foolproof, and vigilance on the part of all prescribing doctors, together with co-ordination of the results by a central body, is the best that we can hope to achieve at present.

No NSAID is free of adverse effects. However, patients with inflammatory joint disease are likely to require medication every day for many years and, while overtly life-threatening adverse effects are clearly unacceptable, rheumatologists acknowledge that some toxicity is at present inevitable. It may be necessary to manage peptic ulceration with appropriate H_2 blockade, while continuing the NSAID (even if dose and preparation are altered). Since gastric and duodenal ulceration are common problems in the 'normal' population, evaluating the excess risk from NSAIDs presents a formidable challenge. The contribution which the stress of pain, immobility, and fatigue of a chronic disease such as RA may make to the tendency towards peptic ulceration is a factor which further complicates drug assessment.

(b) *Second line (disease modifying) drugs*

Again toxicity is currently an inevitable component of such therapy. To some extent, since the anticipated benefit is greater, the level of 'acceptable' toxicity might be higher. However, risk benefit ratios are exceptionally difficult to determine, and have a large subjective element. Evaluation of toxicity in this group in particular needs to be prolonged – early, intermediate and late toxicity may occur, while onset of benefit will be delayed for 2–6 months. Considerable time and resources are directed towards minimizing toxicity for existing drugs in this category. Unfortunately gold levels have proved unhelpful, and penicillamine pharmacokinetics have been difficult to perform. Clinical and laboratory monitoring are therefore restricted, in clinical practice, to early detection rather than prevention of effects such as thrombocytopenia or nephropathy.

(c) *Genetic factors*

The major histocompatibility complex (MHC) on the human leucocyte antigen (HLA) system is encoded for on the short arm of chromosome-6 and determines self-surface antigens of the HLA, A, B, C, D, and DR series, and complement components C2, C4, and Bf. By analogy to the mouse MHC, H_2, it is assumed that the human MHC also contains immune response genes. Several HLA associations are of interest in rheumatoid arthritis. The DR4 haplotype is more prevalent (Stastny, 1978) and affected individuals with the DR4 antigen have higher titres of rheumatoid factor (Stastny, 1980). Of relevance to drug therapy is the association of the DR3 antigen and the occurrence of proteinuria (Wooley *et al.*, 1980) and thrombocytopenia (Coblyn *et al.*, 1981) during chrysotherapy. A similar association probably holds for penicillamine. The extent to which this association can be exploited without withholding potentially useful treatment needs to be more fully determined, since about a third of all patients with RA are HLA DR3 positive and the frequency of proteinuria and thrombocytopenia is low. If, in the present stage of knowledge, DR3 individuals were excluded from therapy, many patients would be denied the potential benefit of gold and penicillamine therapy unnecessarily.

5.2.2 Efficacy

(a) *Osteoarthrosis*

In a disease such as osteoarthrosis, there is much spontaneous variation in symptoms from day to day, and this complicates the assessment of clinical response to any drug therapy. In addition, symptoms will often vary according to the level of activity and this needs to be documented as a background lest changes in symptomatology are attributed to the drug, when in fact a period of enforced rest has contributed. At present, no drug therapy is thought to modify the outcome of osteoarthrosis, and all drugs are given to relieve symptoms.

In general, it is advisable to select one or two joints on which the major impact of the disease has fallen, and apply questions relating to pain and function in relation to these joints. The use of placebo is not as difficult in patients with osteoarthrosis, since they tend to have relatively asymptomatic spells, and it is certainly very important in any assessment because of the spontaneous improvement that may occur. In addition to some of the aspects outlined above, measuring the range of movement in an individual joint, for example the knee, may be helpful, as may documentation of reliance on walking aids.

(b) *Inflammatory arthritides*

In most inflammatory disorders there is the need for daily pain relief, and although there may be some cyclical variation over months or years, stiffness is a fairly constant feature. In rheumatoid arthritis the aims are to provide symptomatic relief (NSAIDs) and to attempt to modify the disease outcome ('second line' or 'disease modifying' drugs), and the evaluation of these aspects differs. In general, 'process' measures are done early and affect mainly anti-inflammatory drugs, whereas 'outcome' measures are used more in 'second-line' or 'disease modifying' drugs. There is, however, much overlap between the two. Certainly in terms of laboratory assessments, beneficial change is not anticipated with anti-inflammatory drugs. In addition, baseline assessment of NSAIDs in a patient with inflammatory joint disease is difficult: most patients tend to be on some form of anti-inflammatory drug and withdrawing treatment tends to be associated with a marked deterioration in symptoms. Thus 'washout' is a difficult procedure which is unpopular with patients and physicians, and evaluation may be clouded by self-medication on the part of the patient who is experiencing a flare. This problem does not arise with second-line drugs where anti-inflammatory preparations are continued, and it is easier to obtain a baseline assessment at the outset.

5.3 EVALUATION IN RHEUMATOID ARTHRITIS

The course that rheumatoid arthritis will follow in any individual patient cannot be predicted with any certainty at the outset. Many patients after an initially relapsing course eventually progress to sustained activity, and several longitudinal studies have suggested that eventually most patients deteriorate despite drug therapy. What is unclear is whether existing drugs alter the natural history of the disease, or whether they only ameliorate symptoms of inflammation, while the disease continues to progress. Essential to answering this question is the availability of meaningful methods of evaluating disease activity and the modification achieved thereof. Superficially, evaluation would appear to be relatively simple, but the problem has continued to baffle rheumatologists, owing to our ignorance of the underlying aetiopathogenesis and the dearth of suitable measures of activity.

The validity, reliability, and reproducibility of some commonly used measures will be discussed later. The mode of application of these measurements complicates evaluation, and individual rheumatologists have diverse policies in assessing changes in disease activity; some may be inconsistent in applying their adopted policy (Kirwan *et al.*, 1983).

TABLE 5.1
Possible assessments for evaluation of NSAIDs

EFFICACY
1.   Pain: visual analogue scale. Patient's own assessment of pain relief.
2.   Morning stiffness: duration rather than severity.
3.   Joint tenderness: Ritchie Articular Index.
              ARA joint count.
              Improvement in signal joints.
4.   Synovial thickening/vasodilatation: Thermography. Technetium scan.
5.   Joint function: grip strength.
6.   Patient preference, 'compliance'.

TOXICITY
1.   Clinical symptoms/signs.
2.   Laboratory tests: urea and electrolytes, hepatic enzymes, full blood count and
              platelets. Urinalysis. Drug levels if relevant.
3.   Post-marketing surveillance.

Methods of assessment and the evaluation of change is therefore a pertinent clinical issue, particularly as more drugs are claimed to have the potential for modifying the disease. Symptomatic relief is the desired end point for NSAIDs, and the patient's own evaluation is thus often satisfactory. Table 5.1 shows a range of suggested assessments for first-line drugs. For potential disease-modifying drugs there is little agreement on methodology or on a therapeutic end point. The suggested possibilities have been:

1. Clinical remission as defined by the American Rheumatism Association (see Table 5.2)
2. Changes in ESR and in the other acute phase proteins
3. Radiological progression
4. Functional status
5. Health status
6. Patient's opinion

TABLE 5.2
American Rheumatism Association criteria for remission (in patients who have met ARA criteria for definite or classical RA in the past)

Five or more of the following features for at least two consecutive weeks
1. Duration of morning stiffness <15 minutes.
2. No fatigue
3. No joint pain (by history)
4. No joint tenderness or pain on motion
5. No soft tissue swelling in joints or tendon sheaths
6. ESR Westergren <30mm/h in female
   <20mm/h in male

Exclusions
Clinical manifestations of vasculitis, pericarditis, pleuritis or myositis, or weight loss or fever attributable to RA.

TABLE 5.3
Process and outcome measures

PROCESS MEASURES
1. Clinical assessment of signs of inflammation.
2. Laboratory tests: CRP; ESR; Viscosity;Rheumatoid factor.
3. Radiology: hands, feet, signal joints.

OUTCOME MEASURES
I   *Functional Index*
1. ARA functional classification.
2. Lee's functional index.

II *Health Status*
1. Health Assessment Questionnaire.
2. Index of wellbeing.
3. McMaster Health Index Questionnaire.

Before considering the merits and shortcomings of each, the distinction between process and outcome measure needs to be drawn (Table 5.3). A process measure is what is done on behalf of the patient to obtain the necessary facts (clinical examination and laboratory tests). Outcome is the health status after intervention, for example, death or disability. Outcome is clearly the more relevant measure. Many extraneous factors may influence outcome measures and complicate reliable interpretation.

5.4   ASSESSMENT METHODOLOGY IN RHEUMATOID ARTHRITIS

5.4.1   Methods of assessing inflammatory disease

Traditionally, methods of assessment have relied on the classical manifestations of inflammation – namely pain, heat, redness, swelling, and loss of function. Efforts directed towards finding a uniform index of disease activity within this framework have met with limited success. Although appropriate, the reliability and reproducibility of some clinical methods are often thought to be suspect, as these measures are either subjective or, at the most, semi-objective. Consequently, there has been a gradual drift towards more objective measures, which are often laboratory based as these provide reproducible, 'hard', numerical data. However, in only a few is there a relationship to subjective measures and therefore their validity in isolation may be considered questionable. It is thus of particular interest that in a recent survey of clinical trial experts, the five most valued end points in rheumatoid arthritis were assessment by the physician, joint count, self report of pain, self report of morning stiffness, and grip strength.

5.4.2   Clinical assessments

(a) *Pain*

Despite a clearer understanding of pain neurophysiology, the assessment of pain remains a formidable problem. This is mainly because of its highly subjective nature and multi-dimensional character, with involvement of both sensory and emotional elements. Precise quantitation of the variation in pain perception between individuals and at various times in one individual has proved elusive. The merits and shortcomings of evaluating pain threshold, pain tolerance and pain relief are acknowledged, and are not peculiar to rheumatology.

Attempts have also been made to measure pain by provocation and ascertaining the effect on body function. So far, no single, simple, objective measurement offers a better assessment than the subjective evaluation of pain.

The most widely used method in clinical trials is a linear visual analogue scale. Personal preference and familiarity govern whether a vertical rather than a horizontal line is used. Similarly, severity may be numerically quantitated or descriptively rated along a 10 cm line. Descriptively rated scales are limited by the number of adjectives that can be chosen, and they are less discriminatory than numerically rated scales. These methods, though apparently simple, are not without pitfalls: some patients may not be able to master the concept, and it is subject to the effects of personality. They are also influenced by the expectations of both the doctor and of the patient, and the immediate sur-roundings. The question of whether or not previous scales should be available to the patient for reference remains unresolved. It seems likely, although there is no direct evidence, that long intervals between assessments magnify the problems inherent in pain evaluation. Memory of type and intensity of pain is notoriously unreliable.

Pain relief is a crucial end point in evaluating NSAIDs. Its inclusion in clinical trials of disease modifying drugs is of rather less importance than other assessments, but evaluation of pain relief should nevertheless feature in the overall study of these agents. In some instances second-line drugs may appear to aggravate pain in the weeks before onset of benefit.

(b) *Morning stiffness*

Stiffness is a characteristic complaint in any inflammatory arthropathy and was suggested as an index of active synovitis by Lansbury in 1956. In active disease it results from both articular and extra-articular tissues (Wright and Johns, 1959). Characteristically it has a diurnal variation. By convention, duration rather than severity of stiffness is assessed. Several sources of error are recognized; estimates of time may be grossly inaccurate, duration is influenced by prior physical activity, patients who are unemployed or retired are likely to view morning stiffness in a different light from those who are struggling out to work, and often the distinction between stiffness and pain is difficult to elucidate. Objective methods of assessing severity of stiffness have been devised; none is entirely satisfactory and most are too cumbersome to use in clinical practice (Wright and Johns, 1960; Backlund and Tiselius, 1967). Despite these limitations it has been shown to be as reliable as the joint count and remains a valuable subjective assessment of disease activity (Eberl, 1980).

(c) *Joint tenderness*

This has been suggested as the most reliable clinical index of joint inflam-mation (Savage, 1958; Copeman, 1964; Deodhar *et al.*, 1973). Initial methods of assessment were fraught with difficulty. Peculiarities of individual joints, lack of standardized exertion of pressure, and of reporting patient response, were recognized sources of error.

TABLE 5.4
Joint score

1. The number of clinically active joints is determined by one of the following:
   (a) tenderness on pressure
   (b) pain on passive movement
   (c) swelling other than bony proliferations

2. The following joints are examined (right and left):
   tempromandibular
   sternoclavicular, acromioclavicular, shoulder, elbow, wrist (one unit)
   MCP (5 units)
   IP joint of thumb, PIP and DIP joints (8 units)
   knee, ankle, tarsus (as one unit)
   MTP (5 units)
   IP of great toe, proximal and distal joints of 4 toes together (4 units)

3. Overall a total of 66 joints (or groups of joints) are assessed.
   (The hip is excluded since swelling in the hip joints cannot usually be determined
   clinically.)

TABLE 5.5
Ritchie Articular Index – summary

1. Each joint/unit is scored 0–3 on firm pressure (except joints marked * below)

   0 – Not tender
   1 – Tender
   2 – Tender and winced
   3 – Tender, winced and withdrew

2. The following joints are treated as a single unit:

   temporomandibular
   * joints of the cervical spine
   sternoclavicular
   acromioclavicular
   metacarpophalangeal and proximal interphalangeal joints of each hand
   metatarsophalangeal joints of each foot.

3. Including a maximum score for each of the above units, and the left and right
   shoulders, elbows, wrists, *hips, knees, ankles, talocalcaneal and tarsal joints, the
   maximum possible score is 78.

   * these joints are assessed by passive movement

   Intra-observer error is low
   Inter-observer error is high

Several methods of assessing joint tenderness have been evaluated but only two have stood the test of time. The American Rheumatism Association Joint Score is in essence a count of inflamed joints (Cooperative Clinics Committee, 1967, 1975), whereas the Ritchie Articular Index (Ritchie *et al.*, 1968) is based on the application of firm pressure to the joint margins, and patient response is scored on a 0–3 scale. For clinical convenience, certain groups of joints are considered together. The Ritchie Index takes only a few minutes to perform, and there is a close correlation with the American Rheumatism Association Joint Score, for details see Tables 5.4 and 5.5. Both indices are widely used. The Ritchie Articular Index has been shown to be one of the most sensitive measures of disease activity and correlates well with objective indices, such as radioisotope scans (Deodhar *et al.*, 1973).

The sensitivity of each method has been substantiated in numerous clinical trials. Both methods of evaluation suffer from a high inter-observer error which limits the value of comparisons between different observers, but the intra-observer variation is small. In clinical trials therefore, assessments should be made by the same observer.

(d) *Measurement of joint swelling*

Assessment of changes in joint circumference in response to drug therapy has proved most disappointing. The jewellers' rings of Hart and Clark, and subsequent modifications of these, have severe limitations (Hart and Clark, 1951). In early, very acute disease there may be a large element of reversible inflammation, and the resultant swelling should respond to anti-inflammatory therapy. However, most patients with inflammatory joint disease will develop chronic synovitis, which shows relatively little capacity to change with either symptom relieving or second-line drugs. Although intra-observer error is small, inter-observer error is surprisingly large. In addition to the requirement for continuity of assessor, 'ring sizes' is a time-consuming way of evaluating therapy and the rewards are small.

(e) *Joint heat*

In active synovitis, this is increased because of vasodilatation and increased vascularity. Subtle temperature changes can be perceived by the human hand, but this sensitivity is difficult to quantitate. Intra-articular temperature recording correlates well with other clinical indices of inflammation (Howarth and Hollander, 1949). It, however, requires the insertion of electrodes into the joint, and is therefore unsuitable for routine use. Thermography and radioisotope scanning are non-invasive techniques that can objectively measure the increased vascularity of joints.

(i) Thermography

The basis of thermography is the recording of infra-red emissions from the body. The emissions may be displayed on an oscilloscope or presented as multicoloured isotherm 'maps'. After appropriate mathematical manipulation, results can be expressed as a thermographic index (Collins *et al.*, 1974). An overall index of activity can be obtained by scanning specified joint areas. The method is sensitive enough to quantitate changes produced by both NSAIDs and second-line agents, but careful attention to environmental conditions is required.

(ii) Radionucleotide scanning

Both the clearance of intra-articularly injected isotopes and the uptake of intravenously injected agents by inflamed joints have been evaluated in rheumatology. The latter is more appropriate for clinical practice (Dick *et al.*, 1970). Several radioisotopes have been evaluated, but technetium salts are the most commonly used because of their short half-life. Currently, interest is focused on technetium pyrophosphate, a bone-seeking agent. Methods of recording and expressing results vary (Dick, 1976; Oka *et al.*, 1971; Huskisson *et al.*, 1976). As with thermography, serial scans are of greater value. A reduction in uptake is seen during effective therapy with second-line agents (Huskisson *et al.*, 1976), but the sensitivity appears to be no better than standard clinical indices.

Each of the two methods of evaluating joint heat provides a reproducible, quantitative, objective measure, but the strict control needed in application, combined with the capital outlay, limits the widespread use of these methods. They remain as novel adjuncts in the evaluation of drug response, and have a limited role in routine practice.

(f) *Functional impairment*

Functional impairment is the most feared outcome of rheumatoid arthritis, and maintaining function has always been a primary goal in the treatment of the disease. It is therefore a sound argument that the response to antirheumatic drugs, particularly disease modifying or second-line therapy, should be evaluated in this way.

The concept of assessment in terms of functional impairment is certainly not new; it was first suggested by Taylor in 1937 and formed the basis of the Steinbrocker functional grades (Steinbrocker *et al.*, 1949). Subsequently a number of other indices have been introduced, differing in the spectrum of disability and weighting used in each. Lee *et al.* (1973), for example, assessed 17 activities of daily living, and used this index to assess outcome in a short-term anti-inflammatory drug trial. Their method was not sensitive enough to detect changes within the study, which is not surprising over the short term that it was used. It has, however, been shown that this index will demonstrate a change after major reconstructive surgery.

Other functional tests are grip strength measurement and 50-feet walking time. Grip strength is a complex assessment of joint, muscle and tendon integrity, and is conventionally measured by recording the pressure that the patient can exert by squeezing a partially inflated bag (at a starting pressure of 20 mmHg). Unfortunately, the maximum recordable pressure is usually restricted to the height of the mercury column in a standard sphygmomanometer (300 mmHg) and this level can be exceeded by a significant proportion of arthritic patients. This limitation could be readily avoided by modern measurement technology but, of course, at a cost. Measurements need to be performed with close attention to detail, particularly concerning standardization of bag size and the position of the patients arm. There are several criticisms that can be made of this assessment; performance can improve with learning and is also dependent on patient motivation. A more fundamental criticism is that it gives little information about the functional level or degree of improvement of the patient in his/her own home environment. Usually the results are presented as the mean of three assessments although the best of three is favoured by some.

The 50-feet walking time has no real value in our hands and is unpopular with the patients. However, some clinicians have found it useful.

The major drawback of all existing methods of functional assessment is that they fail to distinguish between incapacity due to active reversible synovitis and that which occurs as a result of deformity or irreparable cartilaginous/ bony damage. This distinction is of crucial importance to the assessment of drug therapy. The rheumatological literature abounds with trial reports in which, for example, morning stiffness improved dramatically, but grip strength showed little improvement from a low pre-treatment level. This scenario may not so much reflect a relative failure of the study drug as a failure of assessment methodology and patient selection.

Thus, despite many efforts, a satisfactory method of assessing functional impairment is not available. In fact, it is questionable whether a generally accepted measure, applicable to all situations, will be possible in RA. In addition to reversibility considerations which argue for separation of 'early' and 'late' stages of the disease process, functional capacity is dependent on a number of other important variables. Patients with similar levels of disease activity and articular damage react differently. Expectations of outcome, personal goals, age, background, and social support vary and will influence an individual's assessment of functional capacity.

Further, no method can be considered truly representative; this is in part due to the variability of RA. In some patients the major impact of the disease is in the small joints of the hands and feet, while in others the large joints bear the brunt of the disease, making comparison difficult.

(g) Health status and measurement of patient outcome in arthritis

Functional impairment forms only one dimension in the assessment of outcome in RA. The concept of health status covers a wider field of disability, viewing the measure not only as an impairment of physical function but in association with other aspects of health such as discomfort, both physical and psychological, iatrogenic disease, and the mental and social wellbeing of the individual. Such assessments are made by either self-administration or assessor administration of questionnaires.

Several questionnaires have been devised specifically for rheumatic diseases, and most have been tested for validity, reliability, and reproducibility. Examples of health status evaluation are noted below.

(i) The Health Assessment Questionnaire of Fries et al. (1980)

This was published in 1980 and concentrated on five dimensions of patient outcome: death; discomfort; disability; drug (therapeutic toxicity); dollar cost.

Death. This is a self-evident end point, but without a control group mortality data may be difficult to interpret.

Discomfort. A discomfort index was described where pain was evaluated from none (0) to severe (3), and where the trend in pain was evaluated as better = 1, the same = 2, and worse = 3.

Disability. Functional ability was measured by nine general categories which were scored 0–3 being 'able to do without difficulty', 1 'with difficulty', 2 'with some help from another person or device', and 3 'unable to do'. The categories covered included dressing and grooming, arising, eating, walking, personal hygiene, reach, grip, outside activity, and sexual activity.

Drug or therapeutic toxicity. Adverse effects from drugs or surgery were rated from none = 0 to 3 = severe.

Dollar cost. Included are costs of medications, X-rays, surgery, paramedical consultations, devices, laboratory tests, physician's and surgical time, and hospitalization. In addition a social cost was made in terms of changes in employment, income, the need to hire domestic help, and special transportation.

Much emphasis has been put on the assessment of the reliability, validity, and sensitivity of these tests, and the ease with which they can be performed; and certainly work done to date has been useful in eliminating questions from the assessment which simply repeat information obtained from elsewhere, and also excluding those questions which seem to cause confusion. The feasibility of completion by the patient has been demonstrated, and this is a valuable aspect. There are, however, a number of features in this type of assessment questionnaire which are not easily transplanted to other cultures. British patients are unlikely to take kindly to a questionnaire which includes sexual activity, and even North American patients were less likely to respond to this aspect, which has been excluded from recent versions. In addition, differences in socio-economic status would make the relative weighting to be given to inability to drive quite large. Cost is difficult to assess within the National Health Service, and is also less directly relevant to the patient, although obviously it is important to the Health Service finance. Thus, costs within the United Kingdom relate more to changes in employment and income, the need to have domestic help and transportation, and possibly the cost of prescription charges. The other features would not be as relevant.

To date this type of index has not been shown to be a useful way of following response to drug therapy, although its potential is undoubted. The philosophy of outcome assessment is clearly delineated, but its practical application is going to take much time and patience to clarify.

(ii) The Arthritis Impact Measurement Scales

These have been evaluated by Meenan *et al.* (1980). The arthritis impact measurement scales (AIMS) are used to assess various types of arthritis, but again have not really been shown to perform satisfactorily in drug evaluation over a prolonged period. Questions are asked relating to mobility, physical activity, dexterity, household activities, activities of daily living, anxiety, depression, social activity, and pain; and a weighting is given to each. Whether such an assessment would be sensitive enough to show the sort of changes anticipated with drug therapy remains uncertain.

There is little to suggest at present that any one instrument has an advantage over others. However, the choice of questionnaire is not entirely random. Consideration should be given to:

- the population being assessed – expectations are influenced by age, social background, goals etc.

- the nature of intervention, whether surgical, medical or social. The impact of any one may radically alter outcome or patient attitude to daily activities. The purpose and duration of trial also determine choice. At present it is not known whether this approach can meaningfully differentiate between various treatment groups. As experience of these questionnaires increases, their role in evaluating currently available drugs will become clearer.

(h) *Compliance*

Compliance, that is the willingness of patients to continue with their medication, has been suggested as a way of evaluating symptomatic therapies. This method has been used to evaluate the tolerability of a number of NSAIDs (Capell *et al.*, 1979), and has the advantage that it gives a more true-to-life assessment than the intensive, often very contrived, atmosphere of a clinical study. Large groups of patients can be followed very simply, and an idea obtained of how the drug will behave in the community. However, compliance is only a suitable way of assessing symptomatic remedies; it is reasonable to expect that a drug which affords significant symptomatic relief, and does not give intolerable side effects, will be taken. On the other hand, a drug which does not relieve symptoms, or produces side effects greater than the symptoms that are to be treated, will be discarded. In contrast, a second-line drug which takes some time to act, and where the immediate benefit is not apparent to the patient, either in terms of onset as they start therapy, or loss of benefit if they stop it, has to be regarded in a different way and compliance cannot be used as a mode of assessment. In that instance, education about the need for continuing with therapy is vital, and other clinical and laboratory assessments must be made.

5.4.3   Laboratory assessments

Many diverse laboratory tests may be abnormal in patients with rheumatoid arthritis. Some of these have been used to assess therapeutic effect and some have been suggested as end points. Whether we are entirely justified in substituting a laboratory variable as an index of improvement, and particularly as an end point, remains, as yet, an unreconciled point in rheumatological circles. The attraction of laboratory tests has been that hard, numerical, data are obtained, which are not open to patient influence. However, few measures are entirely valid and the reproducibility of some is questionable.

The currently used laboratory tests fall into two broad categories: first, the non-specific responses to any prolonged inflammatory process, for example the ESR and the acute phase reactants; secondly, those presumed to be involved in the pathogenesis of the disease process, such as rheumatoid factor and immune complexes.

(a)   *The erythrocyte sedimentation rate (ESR)*

The ESR is a simple and familiar test, commonly used as a laboratory measure of rheumatoid inflammation. It measures the degree of aggregation of red cells, and is influenced by their shape, size and quantity (haematocrit). It can be considered primarily as an indirect measure of fibrinogen, and to a lesser extent of other acute phase proteins and globulins.

In the absence of other causes, a raised ESR correlates well with clinical indices of activity and a persistent elevation is suggestive of progressive disease. In about 5% of patients, the ESR is normal, despite chronic synovitis; this paradox remains unexplained (Pinnals, 1978). The converse is also true, in that the ESR may remain elevated due to persistent hyperglobulinaemia, when clinically the disease is 'burnt out'. However, in the majority of patients a beneficial clinical response to a second-line agent (but not an NSAID) is followed by a fall in the ESR (McConkey *et al.*, 1973, 1979).

The ESR as an index of activity can be criticized on several grounds; it is influenced by physiological states such as ageing and pregnancy, and account must be taken of these factors; it is a non-specific indicator of disease and changes may be due to either co-existent disease or conditions which are a consequence of rheumatoid disease. A correction factor also needs to be applied for a change in haemocrit, and the method is influenced by many minor, often ignored, technical details. Despite these reservations the ESR remains a useful measure, mainly because it is readily available and familiar (Haataja, 1975). Alternatives to the ESR include the plasma viscosity and acute phase reactants, e. g. CRP.

(b) *Viscosity*

The plasma viscosity is essentially a test of protein changes, independent of the haematocrit, which was first suggested as an index of disease activity by Whittington (1946) and which compares favourably with the ESR, C-reactive protein, and fibrinogen (Crockson and Crockson, 1974; Pickup *et al.*, 1981). It has several advantages over the ESR; values are not affected by sex or age and a normal range is well defined; unlike the ESR, the sample does not have to be processed immediately (Harkness, 1971). The method can be automated and is therefore cheaper. Errors in viscosity measurement are few and arise mainly from sample preparation and inaccuracy of the viscometer, both of which are avoidable if the technique is familiar. This may prove to be a useful measure in the future.

(c) *Acute phase reactants*

The acute phase reaction is a fundamental response to injury and involves in part the release of a number of proteins from the liver. The best studied acute phase proteins are caeruloplasmin, the third component of complement C3, alpha$_1$-glycoprotein, alpha$_1$-antitrypsin, fibrinogen, haptoglobin, C-reactive protein, and serum amyloid A protein. The kinetics of each protein after stimulation differ markedly.

The overall function of these proteins is presumably to contain injury and promote recovery in the period after injury. This is in many ways analogous to the local inflammatory response, and is in part controlled by it.

(d) *C-reactive protein (CRP)*

C-reactive protein is the prototype acute phase reactant, and is present normally in only trace quantities (Claus *et al.*, 1976). Almost immediately after injury the levels increase several hundredfold. The functions of this protein are diverse and may include an immune modulating effect (Kinsella and Fritzier, 1980).

Raised levels are commonly observed in active rheumatoid arthritis, and disease modifying drugs may have a greater effect on CRP levels than ESR. As a single protein, it is less subject to the many variables that affect the ESR and, of the two parameters, CRP has been suggested as a more sensitive index of disease activity (Mallaya *et al.*, 1982).

Measurement of CRP is now done by a quantitative immunological assay but it is not yet widely available.

(e) *Serum amyloid A (SAA)*

SAA protein was initially identified as a serum component reacting to anti-bodies to denatured amyloid fibrils from patients with secondary amyloidosis (Cathcart *et al.*, 1965). It is now known to be a normal plasma protein, secreted by the liver in increased amounts during an acute phase response. The kinetics and structure of SAA are in many ways similar to CRP.

In the presence of active rheumatoid disease, SAA levels are elevated and correlate with subjective and objective indices of disease activity. Persistently raised levels of SAA may predispose to the development of amyloidosis. It is not yet established if disease modifying drugs will lower SAA levels and thereby prevent this invariably fatal complication. Assays are not widely available, and in terms of evaluation of drug effect, the use of SAA is at present limited.

(f) *Haematological indices*

A mild normochromic, normocytic anaemia is a frequent accompaniment of active rheumatoid disease and, in the absence of iron deficiency, the anaemia corrects with the improvement which occurs with successful 'second line' therapy.

Another long recognized but somewhat variable feature of active disease is a neutrophilia resulting initially from increased release from the marrow, and subsequently increased marrow production.

Thrombocytosis is also recognized in active disease. It has been suggested as an index of disease activity, but platelet changes secondary to chronic gastroin-testinal blood loss may complicate the picture.

A routine haematological count is probably of more benefit for detecting systemic complications and in monitoring drug toxicity than evaluating drug response. Nevertheless, an increase in haemoglobin and a fall in platelet count to within the normal range provide supportive evidence of a 'second-line' beneficial effect.

(g) *Liver function tests*

In response to inflammation, the liver undergoes several ultrastructural and metabolic changes, with a change in the activities of a large number of enzymes. In active rheumatoid arthritis it is common to find raised levels of gamma glutamyl transpeptidase (gamma GT) (Lowe *et al.*, 1978), and hepatic alkaline phosphatase. Raised levels of gamma GT are probably a reflection of increased hepatic protein synthesis, rather than due to hepatocyte injury. Raised levels may also be due to drug toxicity.

Plasma albumin levels may be low in persistently active disease, and it is not clear to what extent this is due to decreased synthesis or increased catabolism. A polyclonal hyperglobulinaemia is frequent, but correlation with disease activity is poor. These changes tend to return to normal with control of disease activity. Although these tests are routinely available, their non-specific nature and/or the relatively low frequency of abnormality in RA renders them less useful as measures of activity in clinical trials.

(h) *Complement*

Complement levels may be slightly raised in rheumatoid arthritis, behaving as acute phase reactants. However, in about 5% of patients, CH_{50}, C_4 and C_3 levels are low and imply systemic disease, particularly vasculitis (Franco and Schur, 1971; Hunder and McDuttie, 1973; Scott *et al.*, 1981). With successful therapy, levels tend to return to normal (Abel *et al.*, 1980). In this small subset, serial complement levels are helpful in assessing systemic disease activity, but in most cases their contribution to drug evaluation is minimal.

(i) *Rheumatoid factors*

The presence of serum IgM rheumatoid factor (RF) within the first year of the onset of rheumatoid arthritis is associated with a poorer prognosis (Stage and Mannik, 1973), although the titre does not correlate with disease activity at any particular point. The ability of 'disease modifying' drugs to lower the RF titre is established, but to what extent this signifies benefit is unclear. Gold and penicillamine have been shown to lower synovial fluid RF titres (Pritchard and Nuki, 1978), and a similar fall in serum IgM rheumatoid factor titre is seen with gold, penicillamine, and some cytotoxics (Popert *et al.*, 1961; Multicentre Trial Group, 1973; Huskisson *et al.*, 1974; Amor and Mery, 1980). The fall in titre, however, is not seen in all patients who improve and often clinical improvement is seen before there is a fall in RF titre. Moreover comparable benefit occurs in RA patients who do not have serum IgM RF. In seropositive patients, serum IgM RF titres may be of some value in assessing the antirheumatic effect of new drugs, although it appears that not all drugs that have typical disease modifying profiles in terms of ESR, APP and clinical responses, lower IgM RF levels (Bird *et al.*, 1983).

IgG RF is of potentially greater pathogenetic significance than IgM RF since it shows better correlation with disease activity (Munthe and Pahle, 1976; Hay *et al.*, 1979; Allen *et al.*, 1981). Further, a number of IgM sero-negative patients are IgG RF positive. Systemic complications, particularly vasculitis, are associated with IgG RF. However, its role in assessing drug effect remains to be determined. Preliminary reports on the effect of penicillamine on IgG RF show no additional advantage in monitoring response.

(j) Immune complexes

In RA, immune complexes have been found both intra-articularly and in the circulation, and appear to be involved in the pathogenesis of the disease (Zubler *et al.*, 1976). Many immune complex assays are now available. The performance of these assays as laboratory markers of disease activity has been disappointing (Plotz, 1982), and whether high levels predict poorer outcome at the onset of disease remains to be substantiated. The presence of circulating immune complexes, measured by the Clq binding method, is associated with extra-articular disease (Zubler *et al.*, 1976). However, the role of these more expensive laboratory tests needs to be clarified further before they can be advocated as useful measures.

(k) Free oxygen radicals (redox imbalance)

Much evidence has accumulated implicating oxygen-derived free radicals (ODFR – O^-_2, H_2O_2, OH·) as propagators of inflammation and subsequent participants in cellular damage. These potentially toxic agents are generated by stimulated inflammatory cells – polymorphonuclear cells, macrophages, and monocytes – undergoing a respiratory burst, characterized by the consumption of oxygen (O_2) (Goldstein *et al.*, 1975).

The O_2 is not used for oxidative phosphorylation, but is catalysed by a membrane-associated oxidase to yield the superoxide radical O^-_2, which then undergoes a spontaneous self-reaction to produce hydrogen peroxide (H_2O_2), with concomitant reduction of the ferric ion to ferrous.

$$2O_2 + NADPH \rightarrow 2O^-_2 + NADPH^+ + H^+$$
$$O^-_2 + O^-_2 + 2H^+ \rightarrow H_2O_2 + O_2$$
$$Fe^{3+} + O^-_2 \rightarrow Fe^{2+} + O_2$$

A reaction between the intermediate products, ferrous ions and H_2O_2, yields a hydroxyl anion and the OH radical.

$$Fe^{2+} + O_2 \ Fe^{2+} + H_2O_2 \rightarrow Fe^{3+} + OH· + OH^-$$

Once generated, these radicals may cause peroxidative injury to unsaturated cell membrane fats with resultant loss of membrane integrity (Salin and McCord, 1975; Lynch and Fridovich, 1978).

Several protective mechanisms against ODFR exist and include both intra- and extracellular scavengers. Important extracellular antioxidants are sulphydryl groups (Brown *et al.*, 1981), caeruloplasmin oxidase (Goldstein *et al.*, 1979) and copper ions. Superoxide dismutase (SOD), catalase and glutathione peroxidase are intracellular counterparts (Chance *et al.*, 1979). Their role in the tissue damage associated with rheumatoid arthritis is suggested by a number of *in vivo* and *in vitro* observations; the ability of O^-_2 to degrade bovine synovial fluid, the ability to depolymerize purified hyaluronic acid (McCord, 1974), the presence of lipid peroxidation products in rheumatoid synovial fluid (Lunec and Dormandy, 1979), and reduced leucocyte (Rister *et al.*, 1978) and erythrocyte SOD levels (Banford *et al.*, 1982a), and increased glutathione concentration (Voetman *et al.*, 1980; Banford *et al.*, 1982b). It has been suggested in rheumatoid arthritis that there is an impaired ability to handle the oxygen-derived free radicals and the equilibrium between oxidative processes and anti-oxidative mechanisms is upset. Various observations support this hypothesis: caeruloplasmin, serum anti-oxidant and glutathione levels are raised in rheumatoid arthritis, while plasma thiols and superoxide dismutase levels in erythrocytes and leucocytes are low. Of interest are the changes towards normal seen in some of these variables once a clinical response to disease-modifying drugs is apparent. There have also been several attempts to use free radical scavengers such as bovine superoxide dismutase ('Orgotein') for therapeutic purposes, but controlled studies of their efficacy are lacking. At present these measurements should still be regarded as experimental.

5.4.4 Radiology

Recently, in a provocative article (Ianuzzi *et al.*, 1983), the question was again asked 'Does drug therapy slow radiographic deterioration in rheumatoid arthritis?'. This is a crucial question in RA and indeed in any destructive arthritis, but it is only in RA that there is some evidence that slowing of erosive change may be possible. This article was highly critical of the inadequacy of studies conducted to date, but perhaps did not acknowledge sufficiently the considerable practical problems associated with radiological assessment in a disease such as rheumatoid arthritis. In the first instance, the various proposed methods for scoring radiological change in rheumatoid arthritis will be reviewed, and then the practical problems which arise with the application of any or all of these will be summarized. Whatever the actual method used to read the films, it is obviously necessary that there should be uniformity in the taking of the films at various time points. Standardization may be difficult if a study is conducted over a number of years or involves more than one centre.

(a) *The Sharp method (Sharp et al., 1971)*

After evaluating various methods of reading X-ray films, Sharp has concentrated on reading the radiological severity in each patient as functions of two scores:

(i)   Defects and destruction
(ii) Joint space narrowing and ankylosis.

(i) Erosive changes

Twenty-nine areas in each hand and wrist (14 finger-joints, 5 metacarpal bases, 8 carpal bones, and the radius and ulna) are read for erosive changes. Individual lesions up to a maximum of four are counted since it is felt that more than this cannot be distinguished with certainty. A point is given for each erosion without attempting to judge the size of the lesion, and if the articular surface or juxta-articular area show loss of bone substance, it is considered to be destroyed and the score of 5 is given for this area. The total defect score for the two hands is 290 using this method.

(ii) Evaluation of joint space narrowing

Twenty-seven articulations in each hand and wrist are read (14 finger joints, 5 carpo/metacarpal, and the trapezium-navicular, navicular-lunate, lunate-tri-quetrum, triquetrum-hamate, hamate-capitate, capitate-navicular-lunate, radiocarpals, and radio-ulnar joints). The highest possible joint space narrowing score is 216, and joints that are ankylosed are given an individual score of 4.

The method is time consuming, and is open to some criticism. However, it is reproducible and films can be read randomly, blindly and repeatedly, and give a standardized permanent result.

(b) *The Larsen method (Larsen et al., 1977)*

This method utilizes standard reference films for arthritis, graded for severity. All the standard projections are AP films except the tarsus which is seen in the lateral projection, and all joints are exposed without weight bearing. In the standard series, Larson has included the DIP joint, PIP joint, and MCP joints in the hands, wrist, elbow, shoulder, hip, knee, ankle, tarsus, first MTP joint and other MTP joints (2–5), and the interphalangeal joints of the great toe. Gradings are as follows:

Grade 0 – a normal film apart from abnormalities which are not related to an inflammatory arthritis
Grade 1 – a slight abnormality, i. e. there may be periarticular soft tissue swelling, periarticular osteoporosis or slight joint space narrowing, or a

combination of these features. These changes of course could be seen after simple trauma and do not necessarily imply an erosive arthritis.

Grade 2 – definite early erosion, except in weight-bearing joints.

Grade 3 – medium destructive abnormality.

Grade 4 – severe destruction.

Grade 5 – mutilating destruction.

Whereas this system has been used quite extensively by its originator, it is more difficult to apply than the Sharp method, and is perhaps more appropriate for epidemiological assessment than for serial evaluation during drug therapy.

(c) *Steinbrocker*

This method was suggested by Steinbrocker *et al.* in 1949, and again is more appropriate for epidemiological assessment than for routine clinical monitoring. The stages involved in this classification are:

1. Osteoporosis, no erosions.
2. Osteoporosis with slight cartilage or subchondral bony erosion.
3. Osteoporosis, cartilage and bone destruction.
4. As stage 3, but with the addition of bony ankylosis.

No currently available drug is likely to alter the course of the disease sufficiently for such a coarse assessment to show a change.

(d) *Microfocal radiography (Buckland-Wright, 1983)*

This type of X-ray technique overcomes the limitations of current X-ray assessment, and gives excellent resolution of a small area. A three-dimensional assessment of bone is possible, and the radiographs obtained are termed stereo-microradiographs. This is a sophisticated method available in only a few centres at present.

(e) *Which method to use?*

It is unfortunate that radiological assessment remains so difficult. From a theoretical point of view, X-rays would appear to be truly attractive in that they can be read independently of observer bias, and provide a permanent and reproducible record which can be re-examined many times. Why then has radiology proved so disappointing? The major obstacle is that it is not known what the rate of destruction would have been without the given treatment. The answer to the question 'Does the therapy slow the rate of radiological progression?' cannot be readily obtained since a control group is so difficult to keep on any one therapy for prolonged periods, and those patients who do manage to stay on placebo are likely to be atypical of the group as a whole.

It is in this respect that the undoubted technical advances that are being made are of relatively limited benefit. If one looks at the X-ray progression over the first year of a second-line drug, it is likely that deterioration will continue for the first three months, and possibly even up to six months. Placebo groups tend to be very small beyond six months, and thus at the crucial time when evidence could be gathered from an active drug, the placebo group is falling off. The numbers in the studies which are widely quoted, such as Sigler et al. (1974) comparing gold and control, were very small and included only a handful of patients who remained without gold therapy for the two-year period. The rate method is notoriously unreliable, and cannot be utilized in major studies. It is unusual to see the healing of erosions; and most second-line drug studies that have dealt with definite or classical disease rather than very early possible or probable disease, have shown deterioration of X-ray appearance in most instances. Radiology may only achieve a firm place in evaluation of therapy when a drug is produced which will not slow but will actually halt and reverse erosive change. In that instance the knowledge of what a control group might have done will seem less essential.

5.5   INTRA-ARTICULAR THERAPY

Intra-articular therapy is appropriate where only a few joints are involved in a truly active process. The goals of intra-articular therapy tend to be rather different from those of systemic treatments with non-steroidal anti-inflammatory drugs or second-line agents.

5.5.1   Corticosteroid preparations

The aim of these is purely to provide symptomatic relief and they are best regarded as an adjunct to other treatments.

5.5.2   Medical synovectomy

This has been attempted with radioactive colloids such as yttrium.

Both these methods have their drawbacks, corticosteroids are associated with a small risk of infection, and medical synovectomy has the disadvantages of handling radioactive material and a potential problem with leakage. In the long term, the effect of the use of these drugs is not fully elucidated. Assessments in all these should thus aim to evaluate immediate, medium, and long-term outcome. In the immediate period after therapy, assessment such as pain score, range of movement of an individual joint, swelling, heat, and objective measurements of radioisotopes or thermography may all be useful. It is difficult, however, to perform a controlled study of this treatment (ARC Radiosynoviorthesis Trial Group, 1984), since there is some evidence to suggest that even the needling of a joint and the use of local anaesthetic at the time of doing this will provide some symptomatic benefit. Perhaps the best chance for objective evaluation is where two knees are considered to be equally involved and one is treated and the other not. Surprisingly few controlled studies have been carried out, and in some that have been reported, the results have been at variance with current clinical thinking (Chalmers *et al.*, 1980). In the medium term, assessments again need to be carried out in terms of pain, range of movement and radioisotope or thermographic assessment. As has been described elsewhere, patients' memory of pain might be unreliable, especially over a period of some months or years. Long-term evaluation should include radiology of affected joints with assessment of morbidity, pain and functional outcome.

5.6 EVALUATION IN OSTEOARTHROSIS (OA)

In contrast to rheumatoid arthritis, osteoarthrosis does not provoke controversy with regard to disease modifying therapy – it is generally accepted that no existing drugs inhibit the progression of osteoarthrosis. However, one of the mainstays of treatment in the past, indomethacin, may accelerate the development and progression of articular damage in the hip (Rønningen and Langeland, 1979).

In practice, the assessment of drug efficacy in OA is restricted to symptomatic measures, of which pain predominates. Pain assessment methodology is analogous to RA although, as previously indicated in Section 5.2.2, it may be appropriate to restrict the measurement to a few joints, instead of the usual 'whole body' approach. Stiffness is also measured, although inactivity stiffness is more relevant to osteoarthrosis than morning stiffness.

The significance of inflammatory mechanisms in OA has been debated for some considerable time. By analogy to the assessment of RA, an articular index for OA has been developed by proponents of the inflammatory 'school' (Doyle *et al.*, 1981). This index is capable of differentiating between NSAIDs and analgesics but its utility has not as yet been evaluated on a wider basis.

The difficulties of functional and outcome measurement previously discussed in Section 5.4.2 in relation to RA, are equally applicable to OA. Range of movement measurement, either using a goniometer, or by clinical grading has been used more in OA than RA, perhaps because of the ability to limit assessment to large joints (e. g. knees and hips).

Laboratory tests have hardly featured in assessment of drug response but measures of cartilage degradation have recently been developed for assessing animal models of OA (Friman *et al.*, 1982). These may also be applicable to human disease and will assume greater relevance as and when 'disease modifying' OA drugs become available. Similar considerations apply to radiology and imaging techniques.

5.7   EVALUATION IN OTHER RHEUMATIC DISORDERS

The wide spectrum of rheumatic disorders precludes in depth individual coverage of assessment methodology in this chapter. Fortunately, it is possible to draw heavily upon the measurements described for rheumatoid arthritis. For example, evaluation of drug response in acute gout centres on pain assessment by the patient, by means of visual analogue or rating scales. This methodology is also applicable to painful conditions such as 'tennis elbow' and 'frozen shoulder', supplemented, as for OA involving large joints, by range of movement measurement. However, it should be recognized that 'objective' measurement of joint mobility may not correlate well with functional status as expressed by the patient (Binder *et al.*, 1984).

In addition to the above 'universal' aspects of rheumatic disease assessment, certain disorders have 'individualistic' measurements that merit further comment.

5.7.1   Ankylosing spondylitis and related spondyloarthropathies

Considerable emphasis has been placed on the measurement of spinal mobility: flexion, by Schober's test (Moll and Wright, 1971), loss of extension by wall-occiput distance. Chest expansion and tests of respiratory function are also relevant measures. However, as ankylosis progresses, these measures lose their usefulness for assessment of drug response and subjective assessments (pain, stiffness, patient drug preference) assume pre-eminence. Assessment of sacroiliitis likewise relies heavily on subjective methods, although quantitative sacroiliac scintigraphy has been claimed to detect improvement during NSAID therapy (Chalmers *et al.*, 1979; Rothwell *et al.*, 1981).

The value of laboratory measurements (ESR, acute phase proteins) in the assessment of drug response is currently uncertain. There have been conflicting reports on the frequency and severity of abnormalities in AS (Cowling *et al.*, 1980; Laurent and Panayi, 1983). The former report described abnormalities comparable in degree to RA whereas in the latter, ESR and APP elevations were minor in patients with pelvospondylitis alone, and higher levels were associated with iritis and/or peripheral arthritis.

5.7.2   Systemic lupus erythematosus (SLE)

The protean nature of this disease has resulted in the development of numerous measurements relating to the major organs/systems that are involved. Clinical assessments may be used for arthritis/arthralgia (clinical measures used in RA), pleurisy/pericarditis, and skin changes. Haematological monitoring is relatively straightforward but renal and neurological disease require more specialized techniques and also present problems of test interpretation. For example, the absence of red cell and granular casts in the urine does not exclude active renal disease (Ropes, 1976).

By analogy to RA, various laboratory tests have been proposed as 'overall' indicators of disease activity. These include complement levels (CH_{50}, C_3C_4) anti-ds DNA antibody (ADA), DNA immune complexes (DNA-IC). In a long-term (30 month) study, Klemp *et al.* (1983) found that CH_{50} reduction showed the best correlation with clinical flares of the disease, followed by DNA-IC and ADA. In contrast IC measurement by the Clq binding assay gave disappointing clinical correlations (Inman *et al.*, 1980).

Tests such as ADA and complement levels, used in conjunction with organ specific measures may be of value in monitoring response to drug therapy, particularly corticosteroids and immunosuppressive drugs.

Although high ESR levels are common in SLE, this measure is not a good index of disease activity (Hughes, 1977). In view of the tissue damage that can occur in SLE, it is surprising that only mild to moderate increases in CRP are usually seen, even in very active disease. However, high CRP levels (>60 mg l^{-1}) have been reported in SLE patients suffering from microbial infections (Becker *et al.*, 1980) and may be of diagnostic value in febrile patients. In contrast to RA, the ESR and APP are of limited value for drug assessment in SLE.

5.8   THE THIRTEEN MORTAL SINS OF CLINICAL ASSESSMENT

These were referred to by Hart and Huskisson in an occasional survey in the *Lancet* in 1972. They have lost little of their relevance in the ensuing decade. They range from showing undue enthusiasm or scepticism about any drug, to the importance of having a constant assessor and a constant time of day for the assessment, not rushing or bullying the patient, or anticipating the outcome, and not performing the work simply to achieve a publication, being careful to be impartial and not enrolling patients who do not satisfy the admission criteria, balancing the study where entry factors are relevant, and being meticulous about statistical interpretation.

5.9   CONCLUSION

In our present state of knowledge, there is no single ideal test, either clinical or laboratory, that can be used as a universal way of evaluating drug therapy in rheumatology. Of those described above, simple pain score or ESR can yield useful information, but in order to gain a comprehensive picture a combination of several tests is usually required – some clinical and some laboratory.

Functional assessment provides a further dimension. Tables 5.1, 5.6 and 5.7 are suggested assessments for evaluation of drugs in rheumatoid arthritis. Pure scientists regard with horror the imprecision of these available tests, and it is to be hoped that in the future better methods of assessment will evolve. Until they do, however, it must be acknowledged that much clinical evaluation remains more in the realms of art than science.

TABLE 5.6
Evaluation of a new compound for a second-line effect
(duration 6 months – 1 year)

EFFICACY
 1. Pain: visual analogue scale
 2. Morning stiffness: duration rather than severity
 3. Joint tenderness: Ritchie Articular Index. ARA joint count
 4. Joint function: grip strength
 5. Laboratory tests:
    Acute phase reactants: ESR (or CRP, viscosity)
    Rheumatoid factor: IgM RF

TOXICITY
 1. Clinical symptoms/signs
 2. Laboratory – Renal, haematological, hepatic
                 Drug levels if relevant
                 Urinalysis

TABLE 5.7
Suggested assessments for evaluation of established disease modifying drugs –
duration ≥1 year

EFFICACY
 1. Pain: visual analogue scale
           Patients own assessment
 2. Joint tenderness: Ritchie Articular Index, ARA joint count
 3. Functional Index or Health status: Lee Functional Index, HAQ
 4. Radiology: Hands and wrists, signal joints
 5. Laboratory
    Acute phase reactants: CRP, ESR, Viscosity (governed by availability)
    Rheumatoid factor: IgM RF

TOXICITY
 1. Clinical symptoms/signs
 2. Laboratory: Renal, haematological, hepatic, urinalysis, HLA status,
                 sulphoxidation status, acetylator status
 3. Continued surveillance for long term toxicity, e.g. malignancy

5.10   REFERENCES

Abel, T., Andrews, B. S., Cunningham, P. H. *et al.* (1980) Rheumatoid vasculitis: Effect of cyclophosphamide on the clinical course and levels of circulating immune complexes. *Ann. Intern. Med.,* 93, 407–13.

Allen, C., Elson, C. J., Scott, D. G. I. *et al.* (1981) IgG antiglobulins in rheumatoid arthritis and other arthritides: relationship with features and other features. *Ann. Rheum. Dis.,* 40, 127–31.

Amor, B. and Mery, C. (1980) Chlorambucil in rheumatoid arthritis. *Clin. Rheum. Dis.,* 6, 567–84.

Arthritis and Rheumatism Council Multicentre Radiosynoviorthesis Trial Group (1984) Intra-articular radioactive yttrium and triamine hexacetomide: an inconclusive trial. *Ann. Rheum. Dis.,* 43, 620–3.

Backlund, L. and Tiselius, P. (1967) Objective measurements of joint stiffness in rheumatoid arthritis. *Acta Rheumatol. Scand.,* 13, 275–88.

Banford, J. C., Brown, D. H., Hazelton, R. D., Sturrock, R. D. and Smith, W. E. (1982a) Serum copper and erythrocyte superoxide dismutase in rheumatoid arthritis. *Ann. Rheum. Dis.,* 41, 458–62.

Banford, J. C., Brown, D. H., Hazelton, R. D. and Sturrock, R. D. (1982b) Altered thiol status in patients with rheumatoid arthritis. *Rheumat. Int.,* 2, 107–11.

Becker, G. J., Waldburger, M., Hughes, G. R. and Pepys, M. B. (1980) Value of serum c-reactive protein in the investigation of fever in systemic lupus erythematosus. *Ann. Rheum. Dis.,* 39, 50–2.

Binder, A. I., Bulgen, D. Y., Hazleman, B. L. and Roberts, S. (1984) Frozen shoulder: a long-term prospective study. *Ann. Rheum. Dis.,* 43, 361–4.

Bird, H. A., Dixon, J. S., Finney, P. L., Leatham, P. A., Lower, J. R., Pickup, M. E., Rhind, V. M., Rushton, A., Sitton, N. G. and Wright, V. (1983) A clinical and biochemical evaluation of Clozic, a novel disease modifying drug in rheumatoid arthritis. *Clin. Exp. Rheumatol.,* 1, 93–9.

Brown, D. H., Dunlop, J. and Smith, W. E. (1981) *Trace Elements in the Pathogenesis and Treatment of Inflammation* (Ed. K. D. Rainsford, K. Brune and M. W. Whitehouse), Brokhauser, Stuttgart, pp. 199–207.

Buckland-Wright, J. C. (1983) Advances in radiological assessment of rheumatoid arthritis. *Br. J. Rheumatol.,* 22 (Suppl.), 18–23.

Capell, H., Rennie, J. A. N., Rooney, P. J. *et al.* (1979) Patient compliance: a novel method of testing non-steroidal anti-inflammatory analgesics in rheumatoid arthritis. *J. Rheumatol.,* 6, 584–95.

Cathcart, E. S., Comerford, F. R. and Cohen A. S. (1965) Immunological studies on a protein extracted from human secondary amyloid. *N. Engl. J. Med.,* 273, 143–6.

Chalmers, I. M., Lentle, B. C., Percy, J. S. and Russell, A. S. (1979) Sacroiliitis detected by bone scintiscanning: a clinical, radiological and scintigraphic follow-up study. *Ann. Rheum. Dis.,* 38, 112–17.

Chalmers, I. M., Rylance, H. J. and Elton, R. A. (1980) Clinical trials of intra-articular aspirin in rheumatoid arthritis. *Lancet,* ii, 1099–102.

Chance, B., Sies, H. and Boreris, A. (1979) Hyperoxide metabolism in mammalian organs. *Physiol. Rev.,* 59, 527–606.

Claus, D. R., Osmand, A. P. and Gewurz, H. (1976) Radioimmunoassay of human C-reactive protein and levels in normal sera. *J. Lab. Clin. Med.,* 87, 120–8.

Coblyn, J. S., Weinbiatt, M., Holdsworth, D. and Glass, D. (1981) Gold induced thrombocytopenia, a clinical and immunogenetic study of twenty three patients. *Ann. Intern. Med.,* 95, 178–81.

Collins, A. J., Ring, E. F. J., Cosh, J. A. and Bacon, P. A. (1974) Quantitation of thermography in arthritis using Multi A Analysis, In the thermographic index. *Ann. Rheum. Dis.*, 33, 113–15.

Co-operating Clinics Committee of the American Rheumatism Association (1967) A three month trial of indomethacin in rheumatoid arthritis with special reference to analysis and inference. *Clin. Pharmacol. Ther.*, 8, 11–38.

Co-operating Clinics Committee of the American Rheumatism Association (1975) A seven day variability study of 499 patients with peripheral rheumatoid arthritis. *Arthr. Rheum.*, 8, 302–34.

Copeman (1964) *Textbook of the Rheumatic Diseases*, 3rd ed., E & S Livingstone, Edinburgh and London.

Cowling, P., Ebringer, R., Cawdell, D., Ishii, M. and Ebringer, A. (1980) C-reactive protein ESR and klebsiella in ankylosing spondylitis. *Ann. Rheum. Dis.*, 39, 45–9.

Crockson, R. A. and Crockson, A. P. (1974) Relationship of the erythrocyte sedimentation rate to viscosity and plasma proteins in rheumatoid arthritis. *Ann. Rheum. Dis.*, 33, 53–6.

Deodhar, S. D., Dick, W. C., Hodgkinson, R. and Buchanan, W. W. (1973) Measurement of clinical response to anti-inflammatory drug therapy in rheumatoid arthritis. *Q. J. Med.*, 42, 387–401.

Dick, W. C. and Grennan, D. M. (1976) Radioisotopes in the study of normal and inflamed joints. *Clin. Rheum. Dis.*, 2, 67–76.

Dick, W. C., Neufield, R. R., Prentice, A. G., Woodburn, A., Whaley, K., Nuki, G. and Watson-Buchanan, W. (1970) Measurement of joint inflammation. A radio isotopic method. *Ann. Rheum. Dis.*, 29, 135–7.

Doyle, D. V., Dieppe, P. A., Scott, J. and Huskisson, E. C. (1981) An articular index for the assessment of osteoarthritis. *Ann. Rheum. Dis.*, 40, 75–8.

Eberl, R. (1980) *Controversies in the Clinical Evaluation of Analgesic, Anti-inflammatory and Anti-rheumatic Drugs: Symposium Santa Barbara, USA.* (ed. H. H. Paulus, G. E. Erlich and E. Lindenbaub), F. K. Schawer–Verlag, Stuttgart, pp. 114–17.

Franco, A. E. and Schur, P. H. (1971) Hypocomplementemia in rheumatoid arthritis. *Arthr. Rheum.*, 14, 231–8.

Fries, J. F., Spitz, P., Kraines, R. G. and Holmen, H. R. (1980) Measurement of patient outcome in arthritis. *Arthr. Rheum.*, 23, 137–45.

Friman, C., Eronen, I. and Videman, T. (1982) Plasma glycosaminoglycans in experimental osteoarthritis caused by immobilization. *J. Rheum.*, 9, 292–4.

Goldstein, I. M., Kaplen, H. E., Edelson, H. S. (1979) Caeruloplasmin. A scavenger of superoxide anion radicals. *J. Biol. Chem.*, 254, 4040–5.

Goldstein, I. M., Roos, D., Weissman, G. *et al.* (1975) Complement and immunoglobulins stimulate superoxide production by human leucocytes independently of phagocytosis. *J. Clin. Invest.*, 56, 1155–63.

Haataja, M. (1975) Evaluation of the acitivity of rheumatoid arthritis: A comparative study on clinical symptoms and laboratory tests with special reference to serum sulphydryl groups. *Scand. J. Rheumatol.*, 7 (Suppl.), 6–54.

Harkness, J. (1971) The viscosity of human plasma: its measurement in health and disease. *Biorheology*, 8, 171–93.

Hart, F. D. and Clark, C. J. M. (1951) Measurement of digital swelling in rheumatoid arthritis. *Lancet*, i, 775.

Hart, F. D. and Huskisson, E. C. (1972) Measurement in rheumatoid arthritis. *Lancet*, i, 28–30.

Hay, F. C., Nineham, L. J. and Roitt, I. M. (1979) Routine assay for detection of IgG and IgM antiglobulins in seronegative and seropositive rheumatoid arthritis. *Br. Med. J.*, iii, 203–4.

Howarth, S. M. and Hollander, J. L. (1949) Intra-articular temperature as a measure of joint reaction. *J. Clin. Invest.*, 28, 469–73.

Hughes, G. R. V. (1977) in *Connective Tissue Diseases*. Blackwell Scientific Publications, Oxford.

Hunder, H. and McDuttie, F. (1973) Hypocomplementia in rheumatoid arthritis. *Am. J. Med.*, 54, 461–72.

Huskisson, E. C., Gibson, T. J. and Balone, H. W. (1974) Trial comparing D-penicillamine and gold in rheumatoid arthritis, preliminary report. *Ann. Rheum. Dis.*, 33, 532–5.

Huskisson, E. C., Scott, J. and Balone, G. W. (1976) Objective measurement of rheumatoid arthritis using a technetium index. *Ann. Rheum. Dis.*, 35, 81–2.

Ianuzzi, L., Dawson, N., Zein, N. and Kushner, I. (1983) Does drug therapy slow radiographic progression in rheumatoid arthritis. *N. Engl. J. Med.*, 309, 1023–8.

Inman, R. B., Fong, J. K. K., Pussell, B. A., Ryan, P. J. and Hughes, G. R. V. (1980) The Clq binding assay in systemic lupus erythematosis: discordance with disease activity. *Arthr. Rheum.*, 23, 1282–8.

Kinsella, T. D. and Fritzier, M. J. (1980) CRP – An immunoregulatory protein. *J. Rheumatol.*, 7, 272–4.

Kirwan, J. R., De Saintonge, O., Joyce, C. R. B. and Currey, H. L. F. (1983) Clinical judgement analysis – practical application in rheumatoid arthritis. *Br. J. Rheumatol.*, 2 (Suppl.), 18–23.

Klemp, P., Meyers, O. L. and Harley, E. H. (1983) A new specific assay for the detection of DNA immune complexes: its relevance in SLE. *Ann. Rheum. Dis.*, 42, 317–22.

Lansbury, J. (1956) Quantification of the activity of rheumatoid arthritis. *Am. J. Med. Sci.*, 232, 300–10.

Larsen, A., Dale, K. and Eck, M. (1977) Radiographic evaluation of rheumatoid arthritis and related conditions by standard reference films. *Acta Radiol. Diag.*, 18, 481–91.

Laurent, M. R. and Panayi, G. S. (1983) Acute-phase proteins and serum immunoglobulins in ankylosing spondylitis. *Ann. Rheum. Dis.*, 42, 524–8.

Lee, P., Jasani, M. K., Dick, W. C. and Buchanan, W. W. (1973) The evaluation of a functional index in rheumatoid arthritis. *Scand. J. Rheumatol.*, 2, 71–7.

Lowe, J. R., Pickup, M. E. and Dixon, J. S. et al. (1978) Gamma glutamyl peptidase levels in arthritis: a correlation with chemical and laboratory indices of disease activity. *Ann. Rheum. Dis.*, 37, 428–31.

Lunec, J. and Dormandy, T. C. (1979) Lipid peroxidation products in synovial fluid. *Clin. Sci.*, 56, 53–9.

Lynch, R. E. and Fridovich, E. (1978) Effects of superoxide on erythrocyte membrane. *J. Biol. Chem.*, 253, 1845–8.

Mallaya, R. K., de Beer, F. C., Berry, H., Hamilton, E. D. B., Mace, B. E. M. and Pepys, M. B. (1982) Correlation of clinical parameters of disease activity in rheumatoid arthritis with serum concentration of c-reactive protein and erythrocyte sedimentation rate. *J. Rheumatol.*, 9, 224–8.

McConkey, B., Crockson, R. A., Crockson, A. P. and Wilkinson, A. R. (1973) The effects of some anti-inflammatory drugs on the acute phase proteins in rheumatoid arthritis. *Q. J. Med.*, New Series XLII, 168, 785–91.

McConkey, B., Davies, P., Crockson, R. A., Crockson, A. P., Butler, M., Constable, T. J. and Amos, R. S. (1979) Effects of gold, dapsone, and prednisone on serum c-reactive protein and the erythrocyte sedimentation rate in rheumatoid arthritis. *Ann. Rheum. Dis.*, 38, 141–4.

McCord, J. M. (1974) Free radicals and inflammation: protection of synovial fluid by superoxide dismutase. *Science*, 185, 529–31.

Meenan, R. F., Gertman, P. M. and Mason, J. H. (1980) Measuring health status in rheumatoid arthritis. *Arthr. Rheum.*, 23, 146–52.

Moll, J. M. H. and Wright, V. (1971) Normal range of spinal mobility: an objective clinical study. *Ann. Rheum. Dis.*, 30, 381–6.

Multicentre Trial Group (1973) Controlled trials of D-penicillamine in severe rheumatoid arthritis. *Lancet*, ii, 275–80.

Munthe, E. and Pahle, J. (1976) Value of immunological studies of synovial membranes in forseeing destruction and deformity in juvenile rheumatoid arthritis. In *Still's Disease: Juvenile Chronic Polyarthritis* (ed. M. I. V. Jayson), Academic Press, London, pp. 161–75.

Oka, M., Rekonen, A. and Ruotsi, A. (1971) ^{99}Tc in the study of systemic inflammatory activity in rheumatoid arthritis. *Acta Rheumatol. Scand.*, 17, 27–30.

Pickup, M. E., Dixon, J. S., Hallet, C., Bird, H. A. and Wright, V. (1981) Plasma viscosity – a new appraisal of its use as an index of disease activity in rheumatoid arthritis. *Ann. Rheum. Dis.*, 40, 272–5.

Pinnals, R. S. (1978) Rheumatoid arthritis with a normal ESR. *J. Rheumatol.*, 5, 272–4.

Plotz, P. (1982) Studies on immune complexes. *Arthr. Rheum.*, 25, 1151–5.

Popert, A. J., Meijers, K. A. E., Sharp, J. and Bier, F. (1961) Chloroquine diphosphate in rheumatoid arthritis. *Ann. Rheum. Dis.*, 20, 18–33.

Pritchard, M. H. and Nuki, G. (1978) Gold and penicillamine: a proposed mode of action in rheumatoid arthritis, based on synovial fluid analysis. *Ann. Rheum. Dis.*, 37, 493–503.

Rister, M., Vauermeister, K., Gravert, V. *et al.* (1978) Superoxide dismutase deficiency in rheumatoid arthritis. *Lancet*, i, 1094.

Ritchie, D. M., Boyle, J. A., McInnes, J. M., Jasani, M. K., Dalakos, T. G., Grieveson, P. and Buchanan, W. W. (1968) Clinical studies with an articular index for assessment of joint tenderness in patients with rheumatoid arthritis. *Q. J. Med.*, 37, 393–406.

Rønningen, H. and Langeland, N. (1979) Indomethacin treatment in osteoarthritis of the hip joint. Does the treatment interfere with the natural course of the disease? *Acta Orthop. Scand.*, 50, 169–74.

Ropes, M. W. (1976) *Systemic Lupus Erythematosus*, Harvard University Press, Cambridge, Massachusetts and London, pp. 1–12.

Rothwell, R. S., Davis, P. and Lentle, B. C. (1981) Radionuclide bone scanning in females with chronic low back pain. *Ann. Rheum. Dis.*, 40, 79–82.

Salin, M. L. and McCord, J. M. (1975) Free radicals and inflammation; protection of phagocytosing leucocytes by superoxide dismutase. *J. Clin. Invest.*, 56, 1319–23.

Savage, O. (1958) Criteria for measurement in chronic disease. *Report of a Symposium on Clinical Trials*, Kent, Pfizer.

Scott, D. G. I., Bacon, P. A. and Tribe, C. R. (1981) Systemic rheumatoid vasculitis: a clinical and laboratory study of 50 cases. *Medicine*, 60, 288–97.

Sharp, J. T., Lidsky, M. D., Collins, L. C. and Moreland, J. (1971) Methods of scoring the progression of pathologic changes in rheumatoid arthritis. *Arthr. Rheum.*, 14, 706–20.

Sigler, J. W., Bluhm, G. B., Duncan, H., Sharp, J. T., Ensign, D. C. and McCrum, W. R. (1974) Gold salts in the treatment of rheumatoid arthritis – a double blind study. *Ann. Intern. Med.*, 80, 21–6.

Stage, D. E. and Mannik, M. (1973) Rheumatoid factors in rheumatoid arthritis. *Bull. Rheum. Dis.*, 23, 720–5.

Stastny, P. (1978) Association of the B cell alloantigen DRW4 with rheumatoid arthritis. *N. Engl. J. Med.*, 298, 868–71.

Stastny, P. (1980) *Rheumatoid Arthritis: Joint Report In Histocompatibility Testing* (ed. P. I. Terasaki), UCLA Tissue Typing Laboratories, Los Angeles CA, pp. 681–6.

Steinbrocker, O., Traeger, C. H. and Bateerman, R. C. (1949) Therapeutic criteria in rheumatoid arthritis. *J. Am. Med. Assoc.*, 140, 659–65.

Taylor, S. (1937) Table for degree of involvement in chronic arthritis. *Can. Med. Assoc. J.*, 36, 608–10.

Voetman, A. A., Loos, J. A. and Roos, D. (1980) Changes in the levels of glutathione in phagocytosing human neutrophils. *Blood*, 5, 741–7.

Whittington, R. B. (1946) Plasma viscosity – a clinical index. *Br. J. Phys. Med. Industr. Invg.*, 9, 184.

Wright, V. and Johns, R. J. (1960) Physical factors concerned with the stiffness of normal and diseased joints. *Bull. Johns Hopkins Hosp.*, 106, 215–31.

Wright, V. and Johns, R. J. (1960) Observations on the measurement of joint stiffness. *Arthr. Rheum.*, 3, 328–40.

Wooley, P. H., Grifeen, J., Panayi, G. S., Batchelor, J. R., Welsh, K. I. and Gibson, T. J. (1980) HLA-DR antigens and toxic reactions to sodium aurothiomalate and D-penicillamine in patients with rheumatoid arthritis. *N. Engl. J. Med.*, 303, 300–2.

Zubler, R. H., Nydegger, V. and Perrin, L. H. (1976) Circulating and intra-articular immune complexes in patients with rheumatoid arthritis. Correlation of 125/-Clq binding activity with clinical and biological features of the disease. *J. Clin. Invest.*, 57, 1308–19.

SECTION II

The rheumatological pharmacopoeia

INTRODUCTION

H. A. Bird

Although this section of the book is devoted to the rheumatological pharmaco-poeia, the reader should not lose sight of the fact that all drugs have side effects and alternative means of treatment may be equally as effective. This has also been stressed in the next section. Once attention has been given to simple general measures, drug therapy of the arthritis can start in earnest. Although inflammation may be fundamental to the pathogenesis of most arthritic condi-tions, the main problem experienced by patients is *pain*. *Pure pain killers* are often as effective as anti-inflammatory agents, and Chapter 6 deals with the pathophysiology of pain in addition to reviewing drugs that might relieve it. Although analgesics available are few, the NSAIDs available are legion. These are fully reviewed in Chapter 7. Oral corticosteroids have undoubtedly revolu-tionized the treatment of polymyalgia rheumatica and giant cell arteritis; their role in the management of other rheumatic conditions may have been under-played and their use, together with the use of intra-articular treatment, is reviewed in Chapter 8. Chapter 9 considers drugs that alter the course of rheumatoid arthritis – *anti-rheumatoid agents* – though the use of these will only be relevant to a very small proportion of the total number of patients suffering from 'arthritis and rheumatism'. Many physicians feel that super-vision of these drugs should be restricted to specialist hospital clinics. Chapter 10, which is speculative, reviews the most recent drugs to have percolated through the intricacies of the registration authorities. It discusses new ways of treatment, either with completely novel compounds, or by reappraisal of existing compounds already safely established in the pharmacopoeia, but for uses other than the conventional treatment of arthritis.

CHAPTER 6

Simple analgesics and pain

D. E. Caughey

6.1 PAIN AS A SYMPTOM

Pain is the major symptom of patients with disorders of the musculoskeletal system. Depending upon the structures involved, the pathophysiological basis for it, and the modulating influences, the severity and quality of the pain may change. Because of differences in pathophysiology, the varying role of psychological factors, and the different approaches to management, it is useful to divide pain into acute and chronic.

Acute musculoskeletal pain, although most commonly caused by injury, either direct or due to overuse, may also occur in acute inflammation secondary to a wide variety of events. These include the deposition and phagocytosis of crystals, acute viral or bacterial infections, rupture of inflamed synovial cavities, and vasculitis. It may also occur in palindromic rheumatism and muscle cramps for reasons unknown, in collapse of porotic vertebrae, or as an episode in chronic inflammatory arthritis when the acute inflammation may in part be immunologically mediated.

In the management of patients with musculoskeletal pain, simple analgesics are but one way of treating the pain and, while important, should be seen in the context of other effective forms of treatment with which they may be used in combination.

6.1.1 Pathophysiology of pain

Direct mechanical stimulation of nerve endings, the distension or stretching of tissues by oedema, e.g. the lifting of periosteum in bone infection or fracture, or the distension of the tissues of an inflamed bursa, may give rise to pain.

Well-innervated tissues commonly involved in causing musculoskeletal pain are periosteum, ligaments, fascia and joint capsules, but not synovium or cartilage (Wyke, 1980, 1981a). The nociceptive receptors in these tissues take the form of a plexus of unmyelinated nerve fibres which is interwoven in the tissue. A similar plexus is to be found in the adventitial sheaths of arterioles, arteries, venules and veins, but not in the capillaries.

Three types of articular mechano-receptors have been described. Sensory input from these receptors probably plays an important part in the modulation of pain from nociceptors (Wyke, 1981b).

In osteoarthrosis with its variable and usually minor inflammatory component within the joint, much of the pain arises in the extra-articular tissues.

6.1.2   Release of chemical mediators

Pain may arise from inflammatory or mechanical tissue injury secondary to the release of chemical mediators, several of which cause pain by directly stimulating nerve fibres (histamine, serotonin, and bradykinin). These mediators are primarily there to initiate the histological and chemical events of the inflammatory process. More are released by white cells migrating to the area. They include the kinins, such as bradykinin, complement components, and vasoactive amines such as histamine and prostaglandins.

Prostaglandins, rather than activating pain fibres directly, seem to sensitize pain receptors to mechanical stimuli and to low concentrations of chemical stimulants such as lactic acid, K^+ ions, as well as those substances already mentioned (Bond, 1979). This explains the efficacy of NSAIDs in relieving pain. Cells of ischaemic tissues release K^+ and lactic acid which probably accounts for some muscle pain.

Pain that is provoked by chemical mediators is usually burning, as opposed to pressing, pricking, bursting, throbbing or stabbing; the adjectives often applied to pain from a mechanical stimulus.

6.2   PAIN PATHWAYS

Pain stimuli received by peripheral nociceptors are transmitted to the dorsal horn of the spinal cord by A-delta and C nerve fibres. These fibres synapse across the cord and are transmitted to the thalamus by way of the ventral spinothalamic tract. From the thalamus, stimuli are relayed to the cerebral cortex.

6.3   NEUROTRANSMITTERS

Research into the effects of opiate analgesics has revealed specific opiate receptors in limbic and periaqueductal structures within the nervous system and the production of endogenous opioids or endorphins that act as neuro-transmitters. They include endorphin and at least two enkephalins.

In the interneurones, encephalin is thought to exert an inhibitory effect that reduces pain transmission. Enkephalin may also reduce the release of another transmitter, substance P, found in the terminals of the primary afferent neurons and which is one of the chemical messengers for nociception (Fig. 6.1).

β-endorphin is found in the hypothalamus, the pituitary gland, the reticular formation of the periaqueductal area, pons and medulla. Enkephalins are more widely distributed in axons and nerve terminal interneurons in the lamina of the dorsal horn, in the medulla, pons, periaqueductal grey matter, thalamus

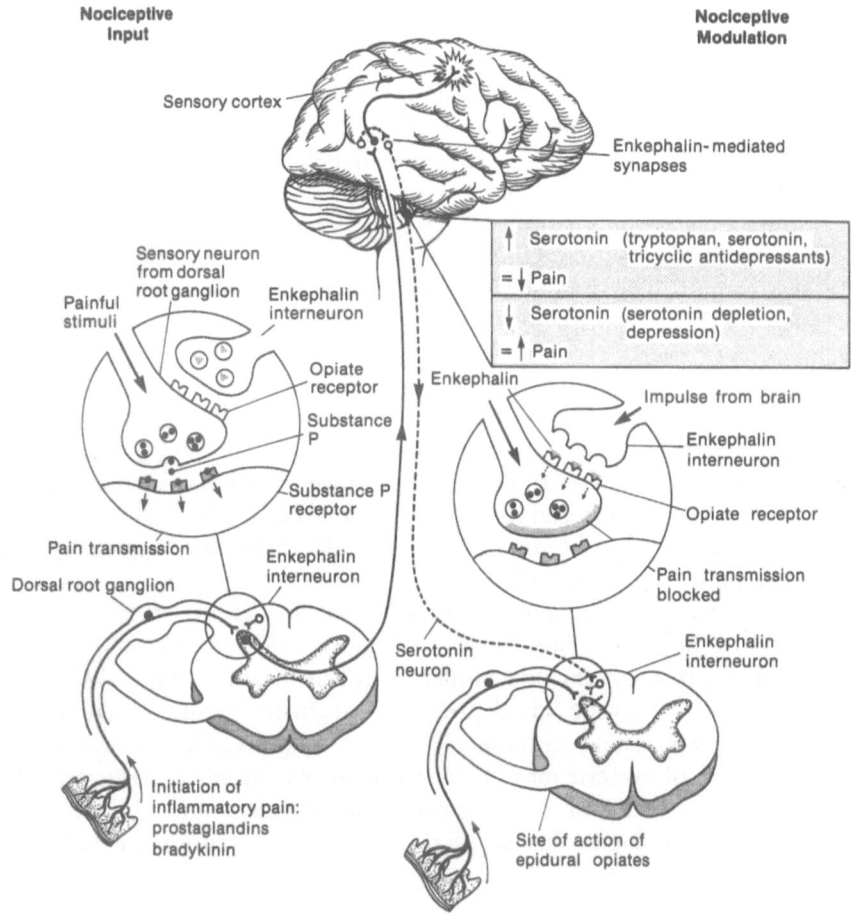

Figure 6.1 Pain stimuli travel to the brain via the spinothalmic tract (shown on the left). Pain modulation occurs in the brain, the spinal cord and to some extent at peripheral receptors. In the pain modulation pathway (shown on the right) descending sero-tonergic neurons stimulate enkephalin interneurons. Pain stimuli are blocked when enkephalin inhibits secretion of the neurotransmitter substance P.

and other nuclei, and in the autonomic nervous system. Concentrations of β-endorphin in the CSF are increased after acupuncture (Clement Jones *et al.*, 1980) and transcutaneous electrical nerve stimulation (TENS) (Goodman, 1983).

Serotonin or 5-hydroxytryptamine is a monoamine neurotransmitter that is widely distributed in the body and, in addition to its involvement in the descending inhibitory system, it probably plays a role in the establishment of normal sleep patterns (Seltzer *et al.*, 1981). Dopamine, a precursor of the neurotransmitter substance noradrenaline, may be the neurotransmitter for ascending pathways (Bond, 1979).

6.4   PAIN MODULATION

The concept of modulation of incoming pain impulses in the peripheral nervous system by stimulatory and inhibitory pathways was put forward by Melzack and Wall (1965). They suggested that the pain stimulus was carried by slow conducting C fibres and more rapidly conducting A delta fibres. A delta fibres triggered mechanisms in the spinal cord, blocking transmission by C fibres to higher centres, i.e. the A delta fibres closed the gate to lower intensity stimuli. This inhibition could be overcome by stimuli of greater intensity which could then pass by way of the spinothalamic tracts to the thalamus and cortex.

Modulation at the spinal level depends on producing an intense sensory input, such as is produced by transcutaneous electrical nerve stimulation, acupuncture, acupressure, massage, vibration, cold and heat, and dorsal column stimulation. These stimuli produce sensations carried by the A fibres, which inhibit nociceptors and the pain sensations carried by C fibres.

At the level of the mid-brain and medulla, electrical stimulation may produce endorphins and enkephalins.

The third site of pain modulation is at the cortical level where pain can be influenced by behaviour modification, hypnosis, biofeedback, and psychotherapy. The latter may include antidepressant medication. Some of the antidepressants, e.g. tricyclic antidepressants, augment natural pain control mechanisms by blocking serotonin re-uptake in the CNS. The observable mood elevation of exercise may be due to enhancement of aminergic synaptic transmission in the CNS or increased endorphin production, in addition to the physical and psychological benefits that exercise gives (Ransford, 1982).

6.5   QUALITY, LOCALIZATION AND REFERRAL OF MUSCULOSKELETAL PAIN

Pain arising from the deeper structures is usually diffusely felt, has an aching quality, is poorly localized, and is often felt at some distance from the point of origin. These qualities are more pronounced the deeper the origin of the pain. With increasing severity of the stimulus, pain referral may be more distant from the site of origin. Although usually this referral is distal, it may occasionally be proximal. Deep pain is made worse by cold. This was shown by Kellgren (1939) in his study of the distribution of pain from structures around the knee.

Kellgren *et al.* (1948) showed that the areas of pain referral from deep structures do not follow the segmental dermatomes, determined either by demonstrating hypoalgesia from compression of single nerve roots or by the method of remaining sensibility after injecting nerve roots.

6.5.1 Referred tenderness

In the same area of pain referral, there may be referred tenderness, redness and sweating of the skin, and muscle spasm. The referred tenderness, as well as pain, is often thought to be justification for the local injection of steroids at such points when the cause of the pain lies elsewhere. In fact, brief respite from pain and tenderness may occur after injection of a site of *referred* pain and tenderness.

6.5.2 Myofascial trigger points

These have been defined as hyperirritable spots (Travell and Simons, 1983), usually within a taut band of skeletal muscle or in the muscle's fascia, that are painful on compression and can give rise to characteristic referred pain, tenderness, and autonomic phenomena. Trigger points may also be found in cutaneous, ligamentous, periosteal and other non-muscular or fascial tissues. These trigger points are activated directly by acute overload, overwork, fatigue, direct trauma, and by chilling. Some correspond to the referred deep tenderness of Kellgren *et al.* (1948), and some to the tender points described by Smythe (1979) which may become apparent after deprivation of delta wave or non-REM sleep.

6.5.3 Psychological pain in musculoskeletal tissues

Pain influenced or caused by the psychological state of the patient is often diffusely felt, the description is usually out of keeping with the impairment of function, and it commonly does not fit disorder of one structure. It is uninfluenced by any medication, but occasionally by physical therapy such as massage, and is unaccompanied by signs of inflammation. It may disappear with distraction, such as a holiday. It may worsen at times of tension, anxiety or depression, fatigue, or in women at times of fluid retention.

6.6   PAIN THRESHOLDS AND THE MEASUREMENT OF PAIN

When a noxious stimulus such as heat or pressure is applied, there is a threshold at which a change of feeling is first noted – the *sensation threshold* – and a threshold when the sensation becomes painful rather than heat or pressure – the *pain perception threshold*. *Severe pain threshold* or threshold of reaction occurs as the pain becomes unbearable with increase in strength of the stimulus. Many methods have been devised for measuring pain threshold and several devices made to record pain in joints (Orloff, 1979).

Bond (1979) states that both pain perception and severe pain thresholds are lower in women and in more emotional people of either sex. They are also lower in those suffering from anxiety, depression, or who are introspective about their health. The presence of physical disease does not have a constant effect. Thresholds tend to be higher in heavy manual workers compared with clerical workers. Thresholds are increased by analgesic drugs and by tranquillizers, if anxiety is a prominent feature.

The sensation threshold is similar for people of different social and ethnic groups, but pain perception threshold and thresholds of reaction vary widely due to a combination of social and cultural factors. The difference between the two thresholds is a measure of the degree of an individual's *tolerance* of pain. Tolerance is less in Latin and Southern European races than in Northern and Western European races. Cultural patterns may lead to the seeking of sympathy early, with relief of emotional tension and thus pain. Appreciation of the different patterns of pain behaviour is necessary in understanding how to manage the patient's pain.

6.6.1   Change of function

Because many factors modulate pain, it is useful to assess pain in terms of the limitation it places on the patient's function. The progress of the disease can also be followed in this way. Osteoarthrosis of the hip may first limit walking at 100 metres, but it may later limit the time of standing, occur at rest, and eventually cause the patient to wake from sleep. Knowledge of this sort helps the surgeon decide when to operate.

Measurement of grip strength with a sphygmomanometer cuff assesses pain in finger joints, but also reflects changes in integrity and inflammation of other joints, muscles, tendons, ligaments, and nerves.

6.6.2   Analgesic score

The number of analgesic tablets required daily to control the pain is another useful method to determine change of pain intensity. It is useful for trials of NSAIDs used for musculoskeletal conditions. Paracetamol, with its negligible anti-inflammatory effect and few side effects, is commonly used.

6.6.3   Verbal rating scale

A scale can be devised from 'No pain' to 'My pain could not be worse', but this does not give fine grading. The language of pain is being studied in detail (Melzack and Wall, 1982).

6.6.4   The visual analogue scale

This records on a 10 cm line, from no pain to intolerable pain, the intensity of pain the patient feels at a given time (Bond, 1979). The patient may mark a vertical line differently from a horizontal line and be influenced differently by knowing where he placed his last mark. Such a method of measurement is influenced by the personality of the patient, and is best recorded in the presence of someone not involved in treating the patient.

6.6.5   Establishing a base line

In examination, pressure over a bony point such as the clavicle will give a base line of tenderness of the subcutaneous tissues with which to compare pain at pressure over tendon, ligamentous bony attachment, muscle or joint.

Overreaction to such testing may be because of anxiety, fatigue or because they have previously been hurt by an examiner. Other reasons for a low threshold of reaction to pain are discussed below.

The tenderness of subcutaneous tissues (particularly of the lower leg) in patients treated with steroids and in many women not on steroids, over the lumbosacral region and beneath the iliac crests, often with palpable nodules in the subcutaneous tissue, is unexplained.

6.7   CHRONIC MUSCULOSKELETAL PAIN

This may arise on the basis of injury from organic disease, from emotional stress or psychosis (Bond, 1979). Once established, it may be influenced by many factors such as learnt behaviour, environmental factors, personality traits, and the meaning of pain for the patient. In musculoskeletal medicine, chronic pain most commonly involves the neck and low back, attachments of muscle and ligaments to bone, and of central and peripheral joints which are arthritic.

A multidisciplinary approach to patients with difficult pain to manage is now common practice. The team may include psychologists, psychiatrists, anaesthetists, and therapists, as well as physicians and surgeons. Rheumatologists, although early into the field of research into inflammatory mechanisms, and anti-inflammatory drugs, have been slow to become involved in the study of pain.

6.7.1 Meaning of pain

The patient in chronic pain may feel that its presence implies progressive physical damage, loss of mobility or other function, or of independence in the future which he is powerless to prevent. This sense of helplessness, coupled with the fatigue, stiffness, unpredictability of pain, and the side effects of drugs, generates anxiety. This is sometimes to the point of panic or depression, which in turn may lower the threshold of reaction to pain. It is important to recognize these factors in the generation of pain, for most are better handled by counselling and, less often, by a change or addition of drugs.

Pain to the patient may be a means of expressing hostility or of relieving guilt. In these circumstances, medication may not be helpful.

Pain may also be a means of communication. This may be seen in the chronic arthritis sufferer who feels the only way to capture his doctor's attention is by complaint of pain, when in fact it is fatigue, stiffness, anxiety about the future, or about another family member that is troubling him.

6.7.2 Pain behaviour

Pain behaviour may be modelled on observation of how members of the family or race react to or use pain (see Section 6.7.4). Pain communicated verbally or non-verbally may be used to control the behaviour of others, may gratify the patient's dependency needs, and punish others by depriving them of the attention of another.

It allows the patient to withdraw from the company of those he would avoid, and may permit irritability and rudeness which would not usually be tolerated by others. It may also allow the covert gratification of sexual drives in the physical contact allowed in medical and nursing care. Those who provide care may have negative feelings of anger, guilt, and vicarious gratification by identifying with the patient needing support. The type of care given the patient may encourage invalidism.

When the patient continues to occupy the sick role without genuine physical basis for it, he is said to be exhibiting abnormal illness behaviour.

6.7.3 Personality and chronic pain

Psychiatric patients with pain were found by Woodford and Merskey (1972) to have slightly lower neuroticism scores than those with pain of physical origin. The latter were more anxious, more depressed, and more subject to signs of neuroticism.

Bond (1976) found pain complainers had higher extroversion scores.

Anxiety and depressive traits contribute to, and increase, the patient's pain. These traits in turn are often more manifest in the presence of pain. Those with hysterical traits usually exaggerate pain and those with hypochondriacal traits may need constant reassurance rather than medication.

Obsessional patients, although not complaining of more pain, may make demands of their doctor about causes and treatment of pain, which are often difficult to meet and which may lead to tension and hostility.

Denial of pain is common in young patients developing arthritis. It may be followed by anxiety and by the hysterical pursuit of pain relief cures from many doctors and others who promise relief. They find difficulty coping with uncertainty and the time it takes to try each drug. They are often given corticosteroid therapy, leading to problems with side effects in the long term, if spontaneous remission does not rescue them.

6.7.4   Pain prone people

Engel (1959) has described a group of people in whom pain is essential to relieve emotional turmoil and in whom usually no cause can be found for the pain. They are usually pessimistic, gloomy, and depressive. In the past, they have often had feelings of aggression and suffering, and have felt resentment towards doctors.

6.7.5   Personality profiles

Measurement of personality profiles is routine in many clinics coping with large numbers of patients with chronic low back pain. The personality profiles of chronic pain patients can not always be generalized to all patients with chronic pain (Moldofsky *et al.*, 1975).

6.8   OTHER FACTORS INFLUENCING PAIN

6.8.1   Sleep deprivation

Deprivation of stage 4 sleep in normal males has been found to lead to stiff, sore muscles, a lower pain threshold, and mood disturbance (Nachemson, 1980).

6.8.2   Posture and pain

Posture plays an important role in the genesis of musculoskeletal pain. Advice about posture (driving, reading, watching television, and doing handcrafts) and pillow size and filling may be of particular importance in managing painful cervical spondylosis. A feather-filled, thin pillow should be used where possible.

The shoulder may become a weight-bearing joint at night, and active synovitis of the glenohumeral joint in rheumatoid arthritis or a rotator cuff lesion may be causes of recurrent broken nights' sleep and secondary fibromyalgia (Smythe, 1979).

Spinal lesions are usually worse standing, doubtless because of the extra loading of the spine in this condition (Nachemson, 1980). In osteoporosis with vertebral collapse, the balance between keeping the patient on his feet to prevent further bone absorption must be weighed against the freedom from pain lying in bed.

Congestion in a dependent injured limb leads to pain.

Joints containing effusions are least painful when supported in the position in which volume is maximal and pressure low (Farreau and Laurin, 1963).

6.8.3 Night pain

Night pain leading to loss of sleep, fatigue, and a fall in pain tolerance is a problem in rheumatoid arthritis, particularly of the shoulders and neck. It requires prompt treatment with local steroid injections, the use of a soft rubber collar, advice about posture and pillows, or night sedation. Stiffness and pain at night in the patient with spondylitis or peripheral synovitis requires slow-acting NSAIDs that are slowly released in the gastrointestinal tract or slowly metabolized.

The role of sedation in painful musculoskeletal pain is not well understood despite the absence of analgesic effect. Many sedative drugs seem to enable patients who have been kept awake by musculoskeletal pain to sleep. This remains unexplained unless it is that patients wrongly attribute their sleeplessness to pain.

It is important for the patient to sleep by night rather than by day, largely because distractions by day lessen pain and the analgesic therapy required.

6.8.4 Muscle tension

Muscle tension has also been shown to be increased in those with muscle contraction headaches (Vaughan *et al.*, 1977), and is a common clinical observation in those with chronic pain.

6.9 THE MANAGEMENT OF PAINFUL MUSCULOSKELETAL CONDITIONS

This is best done by treatment of the source of the pain. This avoids parenteral medication with its attendant risks of side effects, and has a compelling logic for the patient. Three problems arise. First, localization of the deep structure (deep to the deep fascia) producing pain is made difficult by the distant referral from the structure of both pain and tenderness. Secondly, not all patterns of referral are well understood, and third, the relationship of trigger points to tissues, and to the diseased structure causing them, is far from clear and the treatment of trigger points remains empirical. The diagnostic use of local anaesthetic injections may be helpful, but injections and splinting or bandaging a joint may all work, at least in part, by causing distraction.

6.9.1 Acute pain

This often responds well to physical methods of treatment. The patient doing something for himself, and with the information that the pain is for a defined period, often copes well and does not require drugs. Better knowledge of the natural history of sporting injuries will reduce the need for pain medication. Prompt treatment, with elevation, ice and compression for sports injuries, with anti-inflammatories for acute gout or wherever inflammation is contributing, and with local steroid injections (e.g. in acute rotator cuff lesions), usually shortens the period of pain and disability.

Local treatment may relieve temporarily a referred pain in the region of tenderness without improving the primary lesion, e.g. injecting the insertion of the deltoid muscle, the site of pain and tenderness referred from a rotator cuff lesion of the shoulder. Local pain treatment, unless it immobilizes and allows healing, counters the protective aspect of pain which is to immobilize. With movement, an inflammatory process may be slower to resolve. Wherever possible, the management of pain should be with a method that promotes healing or the resolution of inflammation.

Thus, a sprained ankle is best treated initially by ice compresses, elevation, and a compression bandage – rather than with analgesic and anti-inflammatory drugs to enable a sportsman to stand at the bar after the game and produce inflammatory oedema from alcohol dilated vessels and the effect of gravity!

6.9.2 The placebo effect

A placebo effect is most likely to occur in acute disorders where there is a high level of emotional stress and anxiety. However, it may also occur in chronic illness of unknown aetiology whose natural course fluctuates in intensity and in which there is a close relationship between doctor and patient and a high expectation of the patient from the doctor. In musculoskeletal disorders, injections and tablets are given and may have powerful placebo effects, as do many physiotherapeutic forms of treatment, including manipulation. This effect makes assessment of any treatment for pain difficult.

Beecher (1959) noted the level of effectiveness of placebo to be about 35 per cent. He found younger women and those of lower intelligence, together with those of a stable and extroverted temperament, to respond well to placebos, but this was not found in those with neurotic traits.

6.9.3 Chronic pain

This is a feature of most chronic arthritides and is particularly difficult to manage in mechanical derangements of the spine with or without degenerative changes (see Chapter 13). It is also a feature of the fibromyalgic syndrome (Smythe, 1979) and may be a feature of depression. In certain patients chronic pain may lead to patterns of behaviour which become complex to manage. They may require withdrawal of analgesic medication, psychological assessment and counselling of the patient and his family (Pilowsky, 1981).

6.9.4 Variability of chronic pain

Especially in rheumatoid disease the variability of chronic pain is ill-understood once one has excluded such factors as fluid retention, anxiety, depression, the approach of bad weather, or sudden changes of therapy as the factors responsible. Sudden worsening of pain in *all* joints with little objective change usually indicates anxiety or depression.

The unpredictable and inexplicable variability of pain is difficult for patients and their relatives to cope with. It is best handled by understanding and acceptance that it happens, analgesic medication that the patient can control, and baseline anti-inflammatory therapy.

The patient with chronic pain may need to be taught his role in the management of his pain by attention to posture in work and relaxation, the use of splints, rest, the application of heat or cold, local massage, the use of TNS, and, as Hart (1982) has stressed, as powerful as any analgesic is a distracting activity that occupies the mind.

6.9.5 Analgesic drugs

These may act by affecting perceptual mechanisms or on the emotional response to pain. They may interfere with the formation and breakdown of peripheral pain producing substances such as kinins or prostaglandins, as happens when antipyretics and vasodilators are used to improve the blood flow to ischaemic tissue. Analgesic action may also be produced by influencing the levels of neurotransmitters that affect the modulation of pain, e.g. antidepressant drugs, which increase the level of serotonin in the brain and which are thought to increase inhibitory mechanisms in the descending controls.

Bond (1979) described the ideal analgesic as:

Reducing early perception of pain, producing analgesia over a wide range of pain levels, acting satisfactorily whether given by mouth or parenterally, being effective at all ages and in all disorders giving rise to pain, producing few and minor side-effects, and being free from any tendency to produce tolerance and drug dependence.

Low-dose soluble aspirin and paracetamol are probably the most useful choices for rheumatic conditions (Georgetown Symposium, 1981; Hardin and Kirk, 1978). They are useful too in early rheumatic disease when symptoms may be episodic and regular NSAIDs have not been begun. They should be given with careful instruction as to how they should be taken. For example, they should be taken before painful activities, dissolved if the preparation is soluble, not with alcohol, and preferably with food. It is wise to advise all patients to regard any new symptoms as due to medication and to report them.

One can make an argument for various pain-killing cocktails once certain factors are known. These include: the site of action of each analgesic, and the relative contributions to pain made by substances and mechanisms in different pathophysiological processes at different stages of their evolution. We are some way from this but a combination of a simple analgesic, a NSAID, and a muscle relaxant, e.g. diazepam, is a reasonable cocktail for acute low back pain.

6.9.6   Analgesic abuse

The analgesic syndrome seen in patients who abuse analgesics has been reported from many countries and Nanra (1980) has stressed the consequence to the kidney.

6.9.7   Analgesia for children, pregnant and lactating women, and the elderly

Despite the fact that studies are few, there is little evidence that in any such patient where pain is an important symptom, and cannot be relieved by physical means or local injection, the drugs listed below can be given without danger. In particular notice must be taken of warnings, e.g. caution in those with organ failure. Avoidance of all drugs at the time of conception would still seem to be good advice, although there is no proof of congenital abnormalities with use of the following drugs in recommended dosage. The list of available drugs and combinations varies in different countries and the following list may not be complete.

6.10   DETAILS OF ANALGESIC DRUGS

6.10.1   Aspirin

At low dosage, i.e. 2 g or less daily, the action of aspirin is largely analgesic. For quick effective action, it should be taken in a soluble form which is rapidly absorbed. See Chapter 7 for detailed pharmacology and preparations available.

Cautions

Aspirin is probably best avoided for the last weeks of pregnancy because of the possibility of producing bleeding post partum and in the new born (Stuart *et al.*, 1982), although this work has been questioned.

The role of salicylates in causing abnormal liver function tests or in possibly causing Reye's syndrome is probably nil at dosages used for pain relief. Reye's syndrome (Reye *et al.*, 1963) is a combination of encephalopathy, hepatitis and fatty accumulations in the viscera. It is often fatal in children and probably related to some viral infections.

Repeated doses should be avoided in children under one year to avoid metabolic acidosis.

6.10.2 Paracetamol

Paracetamol has analgesic and antipyretic properties, but little or no anti-inflammatory action. It is the major active metabolite of phenacetin and acetanilide, now largely discarded because of their toxic side effects. Paracetamol is only a weak inhibitor of prostaglandin biosynthesis.

Paracetamol is rapidly and almost completely absorbed from the gastrointestinal tract, plasma concentrations reaching a maximum in 30 to 60 minutes. The plasma half-life is 1–3 hours. Paracetamol is distributed throughout most body fluids relatively evenly, binding to plasma proteins being very variable. At 24 hours after therapeutic doses 90–100% of the drug may be recovered in the urine but less than 3% is excreted unchanged, some 80% being conjugated in the liver. Hydroxylated metabolites are responsible for methaemoglobin formation and liver toxicity. With impaired renal function, only small amounts of unchanged paracetamol are found in the plasma but a larger amount of the conjugated form.

(a) *Drug interactions*

Induction of hepatic microsomal drug metabolizing enzymes and potentiation of oral anticoagulants at the usual dosage is negligible, although heavy continuous dosage may affect both processes.

(b) *Side effects*

Paracetamol is usually well tolerated. Acute overdosage, however, may produce fatal hepatic necrosis. Reports of chronic overdosage causing liver damage are exceedingly rare. Thrombocytopenia has been reported; rashes and allergic reactions are rare.

(c) *Clinical use*

In the rheumatic disorders, paracetamol is used as required to relieve pain, usually in addition to regular administration of non-steroidal anti-inflammatory agents and often as required to cope with variable pain. Fever may be reduced in febrile rheumatic disorders.

(d) *Preparations and dosage*

Tablets contain 500 mg, and the usual dose is 2 tablets, taken as required, up to 3–4 g daily. Soluble forms, elixirs and many compound tablets are available. The elixirs are useful for children.

(e) *Cautions*

Paracetamol must be used with caution in patients with liver disease. Over 7 g daily may cause liver damage and larger regular dosage irreversible hepatic necrosis (Prescott, 1980). In suicidal overdosage, death from hepatic necrosis may be delayed several hours or days, the patient having apparently recovered from the suicidal gesture. A single dose of 25 g or more is potentially lethal, concurrent ingestion of alcohol enhancing the toxic effect.

6.10.3 Pentazocine

Pentazocine has analgesic but no anti-inflammatory action, its main action being on the central nervous system and smooth muscle.

Pentazocine is well absorbed from the gastrointestinal tract and from subcutaneous and intramuscular injection sites, peak plasma levels occurring 1–3 hours after oral administration and 15–60 minutes after intramuscular administration. The plasma half-life is about 2 hours after intramuscular administration.

Duration of action after oral administration is usually 2 to 6 hours. Most of the drug is metabolized in the liver, the metabolites being excreted in the urine along with a small and variable amount of unchanged pentazocine. About 60% of the total dose is excreted within 24 hours.

(a) *Side effects*

Side effects are uncommon but include nausea, sedation, sweating, dizziness and, rarely, hallucinations. High dosage may produce respiratory depression (reversible by naloxone but not nalorphine), tachycardia, and hypertension. In some patients with repeated and frequent use, the analgesic action diminishes, but addiction is rare, whether given by mouth or injection. Injections may sometimes be painful and cause soft tissue induration and nodule formation.

(b) *Clinical use*

Pentazocine is a mild analgesic when given orally but is more potent when given by subcutaneous or intramuscular injection.

(c) *Preparations and dosage*

Pentazocine is available as tablets of 25 mg and capsules of 50 mg, also as ampoules of 30 and 60 mg (1 and 2 ml) for subcutaneous or intramuscular injection. Oral adult dosage is 25–100 mg 3 to 4 hourly after meals, as required. Suppositories containing 50 mg are also available.

(d) *Cautions*

There is much individual variation in the extent of hepatic metabolism and therapeutic effect. Addiction, though rare, may occur in certain individuals, often previously addicted to other drugs; this occurs largely with the use of parenteral preparations. Pentazocine should be used with great care in pregnancy, in patients with impaired renal, hepatic or respiratory function, or with monoamine oxidase inhibitors or alcohol, or after large doses of narcotic analgesics.

Pentazocine is contraindicated in narcotic addicts, respiratory depression, raised intracranial pressure, head injury or pathological conditions of the brain, or after coronary occlusion where it may cause a rise in pulmonary artery pressure.

When given repeatedly intramuscularly, the site of injection should be varied.

6.10.4   Dextropropoxyphene

Dextropropoxyphene has a central analgesic, but no antipyretic or anti-inflammatory action. It is readily absorbed from the gastrointestinal tract; plasma levels are apparent at 1 hour, maximal at about 2 hours, thereafter slowly declining over a further 3–4 hours, but there is considerable individual variability. It is partly demethylated in the liver. It has a plasma half-life of 12 hours. The major route of metabolism in man is N-demethylation to yield norpropoxyphene, which is excreted in the urine. About 25% of the drug is excreted unchanged, mostly within the first 6 hours.

(a) *Side effects*

Toxicity is negligible at therapeutic dosage. However, at excessive dosage, central nervous system, cardiac and respiratory depression may occur and sometimes convulsions. Combinations with paracetamol cause major treatment problems on overdosage (Editorial, 1977). Continued administration of 800 mg or more daily may cause toxic psychoses or convulsions.

(b) *Clinical use*

Dextropropoxyphene is used in the rheumatic diseases as required; up to 260 mg of the hydrochloride or 400 mg of the napsylate daily in divided dosage.

(c) *Preparations*

Capsules of dextropropoxyphene napsylate 100 mg (equivalent to 65 mg of the hydrochloride). There are also available many combinations with aspirin, paracetamol, and other preparations, and also a sustained-release capsule containing 150 mg dextropropoxyphene for use 8 to 12 hourly as required.

(d) *Cautions*

Dextropropoxyphene only rarely causes tolerance, euphoria or drug dependence. Nevertheless, it is a narcotic analgesic and its depressant effect may be additive if given with other central nervous depressants, impairing mental and/ or physical abilities for the performance of tasks such as driving a car or operating machinery.

6.10.5   Codeine

Codeine has a mild analgesic action and causes constipation. It has a plasma half-life of 2 hours and a duration of action of 4–6 hours. Once absorbed, codeine is metabolized by the liver to morphine (about 10% of a given dose) and norcodeine, which with codeine are excreted in the urine, partly as conjugates with glucuronic acid. Most of the excretion products appear in the urine within 6 hours and up to 86% of the dose is excreted within 24 hours. Only traces are excreted in the faeces.

(a) *Side effects*

Codeine constipates at ordinary dose levels and at high levels causes respiratory depression.

(b) *Clinical use*

Codeine is used in the rheumatic disorders as a mild analgesic (usually in combination with other more effective analgesics such as aspirin) and to control diarrhoea. It is useful in those arthropathies associated with diarrhoea (e.g. colitic arthropathies).

(c) *Preparations and dosage*

Codeine is available as the phosphate in tablets. The dosage ranges from 10 to 60 mg daily in divided doses. The dose in compound analgesic tablets is usually 5–10 mg per tablet. If high doses of 60 mg every 4 to 6 hours fail to relieve pain, larger doses rarely succeed and may cause restlessness and excitement.

(d) *Cautions*

Use with caution in patients with constipation and in the elderly.

6.10.6 Dihydrocodeine

Dihydrocodeine tartrate is an analgesic of greater potency than codeine but less than morphine. Sedation is less than with morphine. It is readily absorbed from the gastrointestinal tract and after intramuscular injection, excretion being mostly via the kidneys within 24 hours of administration. Duration of therapeutic action is about 4–6 hours.

(a) *Side effects*

Taken by mouth there is little risk of addiction; by intramuscular injection dihydrocodeine is potentially addictive and is controlled under the *Misuse of Drugs Act* in Great Britain. It is slightly constipating.

(b) *Clinical use*

Dihydrocodeine is used in the rheumatic disorders as an analgesic with mild sedative and constipating properties. It is much more effective given by intramuscular injection when it is considered to be potentially addictive.

(c) *Preparations and dosage*

Tablets of dihydrocodeine tartrate 30 mg, 1 to 2 as required, or as a sterile solution 50 mg of dihydrocodeine tartrate in 1 ml with 0.1% of sodium metabisulphite for intramuscular injection. An elixir (syrup) containing 10 mg per 5 ml is also available in some countries. In Great Britain, dihydrocodeine by intramuscular injection is controlled under the *Misuse of Drugs Act*, while pentazocine and buprenorphine (see below) are·not.

(d) *Cautions*

Use with caution in patients with constipation, asthma or liver disease. There is a risk of addiction with parenteral administration. Dihydrocodeine should therefore not be used intramuscularly in individuals considered to be potential addicts.

6.10.7 Nefopam

Nefopam is a non-narcotic analgesic, its exact mode of action being uncertain. It is a cyclized analogue or orphenadrine, chemically unrelated to other analgesics. It is rapidly absorbed in 15–30 minutes after oral administration, producing pain relief within an hour, its action lasting about 4–5 hours. The plasma half-life for unchanged nefopam is 4 to 8 hours. The drug is excreted mostly (90%) in the urine as metabolites, about 6% in the faeces, most of this excretion (82%) occurring within 24 hours of administration.

(a) *Side effects*

Dry mouth, insomnia, anorexia, nausea, drowsiness, dizziness, and sweating have been reported, as well as hypothermia, which is sometimes persistent.

(b) *Clinical uses*

To relieve pain uncontrolled by simple analgesics in acute or chronic rheumatic conditions or after operations (Campos and Solis, 1980). It is not indicated for the treatment of minor aches and pains. It does not cause respiratory depression as does morphine or pethidine and so far has shown no tendency to cause habituation or tolerance. It may be more effective given parenterally.

(c) *Preparations and dosage*

Tablets containing 30 mg nefopam hydrochloride, initially one, thrice daily, to a maximum of 9 tablets daily (270 mg). Not recommended for children under 12 years of age. Also 20 mg (1 ml) by intramuscular or slow intravenous injection repeated after 6 hours if necessary. In Great Britain it does not come under the *Misuse of Drugs Act*.

(d) *Cautions*

Nefopam is contraindicated in myocardial infarction and if there is a history of convulsions. Special care is indicated if anticholinergic or sympathomimetic drugs are being used concurrently.

6.10.8 Buprenorphine

Buprenorphine, a derivative of the morphine alkaloid thebaine, is a strong analgesic with marked narcotic antagonist activity (Heel *et al.*, 1979). It is given by intramuscular or slow intravenous injection for severe pain. Oral preparations are not yet available and it is not recommended for use in childhood. Pain relief is usually apparent within minutes of intravenous or 20 to 30 minutes of intramuscular injection and lasts 6 hours or more.

(a) Side effects

Drowsiness, nausea, vomiting, dizziness, and sweating; occasionally mild euphoria, rarely respiratory depression. Human and animal work does not so far suggest a high dependency risk and it does not come under the *Misuse of Drugs Act* in Great Britain.

(b) Clinical use

To control episodes of severe pain in acute painful crises or after surgical operations or at night when sleep is prevented by severe pain.

(c) Preparations and dosage

Buprenorphine is available in ampoules containing 0.3 mg/ml for intramuscular use and as the hydrochloride in 5% dextrose containing 1 ml (0.3 mg) or 2 ml (0.6 mg). It may be given 6 to 8 hourly as required. A sublingual 0.2 mg preparation is now available in Great Britain.

(d) Cautions

Use with care if respiratory or hepatic function is impaired. Until further information is forthcoming, buprenorphine should be used with caution in patients receiving monoamine oxidase inhibitors and it is not recommended in pregnancy. As it has antagonist properties it may precipitate mild withdrawal symptoms in narcotic addicts or patients previously treated with narcotics.

6.11 ANALGESICS IN COMBINATION

Different combinations of the above are available either by prescription or direct from the pharmacist in different countries. Theoretically, the lower dosage of each component reduces the chance of dangerous overdosage, and if the components act at different points in the elaboration of pain, there might be summation of effect. Such combinations are widely used and appear to be effective, but because of difficulties in methodology, there are few good studies that show combinations to be better than adequate dosage of soluble aspirin or paracetamol. However, work by Beaver (1981) is noteworthy.

6.12 LOCAL ANAESTHETICS

6.12.1 Lignocaine

Local anaesthetic drugs act by causing a reversible block to conduction along nerve fibres. Smaller fibres carrying pain sensation and autonomic impulses are more sensitive, and local anaesthesia blocks them while sparing coarse touch and movement. There is a wide range of potency, toxicity, duration of action, and ability to penetrate mucous membranes.

Effect is determined by age, height, weight, and physical condition, but particularly by the vascularity of the region (*British National Formulary*, 1982).

Lignocaine is rapidly absorbed and lasts for 1–2 hours, while bupivacaine is absorbed over half an hour and last up to 8 hours.

(a) *Clinical uses and side effects*

For injection with or without steroid preparations into trigger points and around painful ligaments and their attachments in a dose of 1–2 ml at each site.

At the dosage used in relieving musculoskeletal pain, 1–3 ml of lignocaine or bupivacaine into one site, complications are rare although barbitizing is advisable. The use of adrenaline in combination is not usually necessary and should be avoided in the fingers.

(b) *Cautions*

Hypersensitivity is unusual with lignocaine and bupivacaine. Only in large dosage is the cardiovascular system depressed or the central nervous system excited.

6.13 REFERENCES

Beaver, W. T. (1981) Aspirin and acetominophen as constituents of analgesic combinations. *Arch. Intern. Med.*, **141**, 293–300.

Beaver, W. T. and McMillan, D. (1980) Methodological considerations in the evaluation of analgesic combinations: acetaminophen and hydrocodeine in post partum pain. *Br. J. Clin. Pharmacol.*, **10**, 215S–223S.

Beecher, H. K. (1959) *Measurement of Subjective Responses.* Oxford University Press, New York.

Bond, M. R. (1976) Pain and personality in cancer patients. *Advances in Pain Research and Therapy* (eds J. J. Bonica and D. Albe-Fissard), Raven Press, New York.

Bond, M. R. (1979) *Pain, Its Nature, Analysis and Treatment*, Churchill Livingstone, Edinburgh and London.

British National Formulary (1982) British Medical Association and Pharmaceutical Society of Great Britain.

Campos, Y. M. and Solis, E. L. (1980) The analgesic and hypothermic effects of nefopam morphine, aspirin, diphenhydramine and placebo. *J. Clin. Pharmacol.,* 20, 42.

Clement Jones, V., Tomlin, S., Rees, L. H. *et al.* (1980) Increased β endorphine but not met-encephalin levels in human cerebrospinal fluid after acupuncture for recurrent pain. *Lancet,* ii, 946–9.

Editorial (1977) Dangers of dextropropoxyphene. *Br. Med. J.,* 1, 668.

Engel, G. L. (1959) 'Psychogenic' pain and the pain prone patient. *Am. J. Med.,* 26, 899–918.

Farreau, J. C. and Laurin, C. A. (1963) Joint effusions and flexion deformities. *Can. Med. Assoc. J.,* 88, 575–6.

Georgetown University Symposium on Analgesics (1981) Aspirin and acetaminophen. *Arch. Intern. Med.,* 141, 273–406.

Goodman, C. E. (1983) Pathophysiology of pain. *Arch. Intern. Med.,* 143, 527–30.

Hardin, J. G. and Kirk, K. A. (1978) Comparative effectiveness of five analgesics for the pain of rheumatoid synovitis. *Arthr. Rheum.,* 21, 564.

Hart, F. D. (1982) *Drug Treatment of the Rheumatic Diseases,* Adis Press, Australasia.

Heel, R. C., Brogden, R. N., Speight, F. M. and Avery, G. S. (1979) Buprenorphine, a review of its pharmacological properties and therapeutic efficacy. *Drugs,* 17, 81.

Kellgren, J. H. (1939) On distribution of pain arising from deep somatic structures with charts of segmented pain areas. *Clin. Sci.,* 4, 35–46.

Kellgren, J. H., McGowan, A. M. and Hughes, G. R. (1948) On deep hyperalgesia and cold pain. *Clin. Sci.,* 7, 13–27.

Melzack, R. and Wall, P. D. (1965) Pain mechanisms: a new theory. *Science,* 150, 971–9.

Melzack, R. and Wall, P. (1982) *The Challenge of Pain,* Penguin Books, The Chaucer Press.

Moldofsky, H., Scarisbrick, P., England, R. and Smythe, H. A. (1975) Musculoskeletal symptoms and non REM sleep disturbance in patients with 'fibrositis syndrome' and healthy subjects. *Psychosom. Med.,* 37, 341.

Nachemson, A. (1980) Lumbar intradiscal pressure, in *The Lumbar Spine and Back Pain,* (ed. M. I. V. Jayson), Pitman Medical, Bath, pp. 341–58.

Nanra, R. S. (1980) Clinical and pathological aspects of analgesic nephropathy. *Br. J. Clin. Pharmacol.,* 10, 359S–368S.

Orloff, S. (1979) Pain perception and pain tolerance thresholds in clinical and experimental studies. *Clinics Rheum. Dis.,* 5, 755–73.

Pilowsky, I. (1981) Current views on the role of the psychiatrist in the management of chronic pain, in *The Therapy of Pain* (ed. M. Swerdlow), (*Current Status of Modern Therapy* vol. 6) MTP Press, Lancaster, pp. 31–60.

Prescott, L. F. (1980) Kinetics and metabolism of paracetamol and phenacetin. *Br. J. Clin. Pharmacol.,* 10, 291S–8S.

Ransford, C. P. (1982) A role of amines in the antidepressant effect of exercise: a review. *Med. Sci. Sports Exercise,* 14, 1–10.

Reye, R. D., Morgan, G. and Baral, J. (1963) Encephalopathy and fatty degeneration of the viscera. *Lancet,* ii, 749–52.

Seltzer, S., Marcus, R. and Stock, R. (1981) Perspectives in the control of chronic pain by nutritional manipulation. *Pain,* 11, 141–8.

Smythe, H. A. (1979) 'Fibrositis' as a disorder of pain modulation. *Clinics Rheum. Dis.,* 5, 823–32.

Stuart, M. J., Gross, S. J., Elrad, H. and Card Graeber, J. E. (1982) Effects of acetyl-salicylic acid ingestion on maternal and neonatal haemostasis. *N. Engl. J. Med.*, 307, 909.

Travell, J. G. and Simons, D. G. (1983) *Myofascial Pain and Dysfunction. The Trigger Point Manual*. Williams and Wilkins, Baltimore, London.

Update: Reye Syndrome Pilot Study – United States (1984) *JAMA* (1985), 253, 1707.

Vaughan, R., Pall, M. L. and Haynes, S. N. (1977) Frontalis E.M.G. response to stress in subjects with frequent muscle contraction headaches. *Headache*, 16, 313.

Woodford, J. M. and Merskey, H. (1972) Personality traits of psychiatric patients with chronic pain. *J. Psychosom. Res.*, 16, 167–72.

Wyke, B. D. (1980) The neurology of low back pain, in *The Lumbar Spine and Back Pain* (ed. M. I. V. Jayson), Pitman Medical Ltd., Bath, pp. 265–339.

Wyke, B. D. (1981b) Neurological aspects of pain therapy, in *The Therapy of Pain* (ed. M. Severdlow), MTP Press, Lancaster, pp. 1–30.

Wyke, B. D. (1981a) The neurology of joints: a review of general principles. *Clinics Rheum. Dis.*, 7, 223–39.

CHAPTER 7

Non-steroidal
anti-inflammatory drugs

David M. Grennan and
Carol Higham

7.1 GENERAL COMMENT

This is a group of drugs with analgesic, antipyretic and anti-inflammatory properties whose main role is to provide symptomatic relief of pain and stiffness in various rheumatic and other conditions. In 1980 these drugs accounted for 5% of all patient prescriptions and around 10% of the total ingredient cost of all drugs (McLean, 1983). With such a potential market it is not surprising that the pharmaceutical industry has responded by producing a vast range of different NSAIDs, although these all tend to have comparable efficacies and indications. Release of new NSAIDs is continuing and this chapter will confine discussion to those marketed in the United Kingdom recently.

Indications for prescribing NSAIDs include the following:

(a) The main indication is to provide symptomatic relief of pain and stiffness in inflammatory joint disorders not associated with bacterial or fungal infection. This includes the polyarthritides of rheumatoid arthritis, viral arthritis, SLE, gout or pseudogout, as well as both peripheral and axial inflammation of the seronegative arthritides (ankylosing spondylitis, psoriatic arthritis, Reiter's disease and enteropathic arthritis).

(b) Simple analgesics are the first choice for the relief of the pain in osteoarthrosis, and in cervical or lumbar spondylosis. NSAIDs are indicated if simple analgesics do not relieve pain adequately, and particularly if there is an inflammatory element to the disease (Doyle, 1981).

(c) NSAIDs have been used in obstetrics and gynaecology for relieving menstrual pain, inhibiting pre-term labour, and promoting closure of a patent ductus arteriosus in the unborn (Editorial, 1980). These effects of NSAIDs are related to their abilities to inhibit prostaglandin synthesis.

(d) NSAIDs may relieve bone pain associated with bone metastases. Prostaglandin release is thought to mediate some of the effects of bone secondaries (Editorial, 1979).

(e) Low dosages of aspirin inhibit thromboxane (TXA_2) synthesis by platelets (O'Grady and Moncada, 1978), and have been used for their antithrombotic effect in the prevention of deep vein thrombosis after hip surgery (Kakkar, 1980). Aspirin has also been used with varying success to try to prevent strokes after recurrent transient cerebral ischaemic episodes and further attacks after a myocardial infarction (Fields et al., 1980). Its exact role for both these indications remains uncertain.

(f) NSAIDs may relieve the symptoms of a rare illness called Bartter's syndrome which is associated with hypokalaemic alkalosis and primary potassium loss. Many of the features of Bartter's syndrome are caused by overproduction of prostaglandins which are inhibited by NSAIDs.

As mentioned above (f), the role of NSAIDs has recently been extended beyond rheumatology, in the treatment of Bartter's syndrome (Bartter et al., 1962; Bartter and Schwartz, 1967; Vaisrub, 1978). This is a syndrome of secondary hyperaldosteronism, characterized by juxtaglomerular hyperplasia and, paradoxically, by the absence of hypertension that would be expected with such pathology. Many pathogenetic theories have been considered, but the most recent implicates prostaglandins. There is a possibility that prostaglandins could be involved through their stimulating effect on renin release and their inhibiting effect on renal sodium reabsorption. Indomethacin, a prostaglandin synthetase inhibitor reduces plasma aldosterone and renin concentrates and also improves potassium balance and reversed vascular insensitivity to infused angiotensin. Norby et al. (1976) reported similar results with aspirin, and other workers have extended these observations to other NSAIDs such as ibuprofen, as well as confirming the effects induced by indomethacin and aspirin (Bowden et al., 1978). However, of all NSAIDs, indomethacin is probably the most widely used for this therapeutic purpose, and for fuller pharmacological explanations of its action the reader is referred to the report by McGiff (1977).

7.2 MECHANISMS OF ACTION

All the NSAIDs are weak acids which are strongly bound to albumin in vivo. This property may be important for penetration and concentration at sites of inflammation. Synovial fluid levels of NSAIDs peak later and remain raised longer than plasma levels (Mitchell *et al.*, 1975). The NSAIDs have been shown to have numerous effects on various experimental systems *in vitro*. These include inhibiting oxidative phosphorylation, leucocyte migration and lysosomal enzyme release. However, most of these effects are produced by drug concentrations which are unrealistically high and are unlikely to be achieved therapeutically *in vivo*.

On the other hand, prostaglandin synthesis is inhibited by concentrations of NSAIDs achieved *in vivo* (Flower *et al.*, 1972). This effect is due to inhibiting the enzyme cyclo-oxygenase, which catalyses the production of endoperoxides from fatty acid precursors. Inhibiting cyclo-oxygenase decreases production of prostacyclin and thromboxanes as well as decreasing the E series of prostaglandins, and all these substances may be pro-inflammatory. Fatty acids may also be metabolized via the lipoxygenase enzyme pathway to the highly chemotactic leukotrienes (Higgs and Vane, 1983). Most NSAIDs do not inhibit leukotriene synthesis, although the drug benoxaprofen does (Higgs and Vane, 1983). Inhibiting prostaglandin synthesis may also mediate many of the side effects of NSAIDs. Thus local inhibition of PGE_2 production may contribute to gastrointestinal ulceration.

In chronic diseases inhibiting prostaglandin synthesis may not be wholly beneficial. This is because several fatty acid metabolites may have immunoregulatory properties, so that inhibiting prostaglandin synthesis may augment some lymphocytic functions and actually promote some aspects of inflammation (Lewis, 1983). On long-term treatment these drugs provide symptomatic relief in rheumatoid arthritis, but do little if any good in retarding progression of disease. *In vitro* NSAIDs have been shown to inhibit rheumatoid factor production by cultured lymphocytes via inhibition of PGE_2 synthesis (Ceuppens *et al.*, 1982). There is little evidence that a similar effect on rheumatoid factor production occurs *in vivo*.

7.3 SIDE EFFECTS

Gastrointestinal problems are the most frequent side effects of NSAIDs, and all NSAIDs have a tendency to cause gastrointestinal ulceration and bleeding. These problems are related to the inhibition of local synthesis of PGE_2 which has a cyto-protective role to the gastric mucosa. There is much inter-individual variation in susceptibility to gastrointestinal side effects as there is to other toxic effects. Symptoms such as abdominal pain, nausea and indigestion are common with NSAIDs, but there is a poor correlation between the presence or absence of symptoms and mucosal abnormalities found on gastroscopy. In general, the risk of gastrointestinal toxicity is highest with indomethacin, phenylbutazone and ordinary aspirin. An increase in faecal loss of ^{51}Cr-labelled red blood cells is a predictable effect of NSAIDs in most patients, and most of the newer NSAIDs produce less bleeding than aspirin. However, the use of ^{51}Cr-labelled red cells as an index of gastrointestinal micro-bleeding has been criticized, as salicylates may stimulate biliary reaction of ^{51}Cr so that an increased faecal count may relate to this property rather than to a measure of gastrointestinal bleeding (Rees and Turnberg, 1980).

Despite the elapse of over 40 years since the first reports (Douthwaite and Lintott, 1938; Hurst and Lintott, 1939) of an 'association' between aspirin ingestion and gastric haemorrhage, the exact relationship between NSAID therapy and *clinically significant* intestinal bleeding remains unclear (Henry and Langman, 1981). However, it is not disputed that some degree of gastro-intestinal micro-bleeding occurs with aspirin and to a lesser extent with other NSAIDs, notably indomethacin, and that acute gastrointestinal lesions can be readily induced by NSAIDs given in high doses to experimental animals (Kent *et al.*, 1969; Wax *et al.*, 1970). Major gastrointestinal bleeding is a less common side effect of NSAIDs. Factors such as rheumatoid arthritis, concurrent alcohol intake or vitamin C deficiency may increase the risk of a major bleed.

Indomethacin may cause pre-pyloric peptic ulceration, but the evidence linking other NSAIDs to peptic ulcer formation is less well documented.

Non-specific rashes are also a common side effect of NSAIDs. Uncommonly they may represent a generalized drug-induced vasculitis. Other uncommon side effects include blood dyscrasias such as thrombocytopenia and leuco-penia, hepatotoxicity, acute anaphylactoid reaction, and peripheral oedema and fluid retention. Hepatotoxicity occurs particularly in SLE patients and in children. Renal toxicity from individual NSAIDs is uncommon in rheumatolo-gical practice, but is being more frequently reported by nephrologists as a cause of renal disease (Herrich, 1983). Renal side effects include renal insuffi-ciency, interstitial nephritis, hyperkalaemia, and sodium and fluid retention. Renal failure is particularly likely in patients who are dependent on renal prostaglandins to maintain renal bloodflow, as in low output cardiac states and cirrhosis of the liver. Interstitial nephritis has been recorded with most of the propionic acid derivatives. Although the risk of either renal or hepatic side effects in an individual patient treated with an NSAID is relatively low, it is still wisest to check both urea and electrolytes, and liver function occasionally, in all patients receiving these drugs long term.

7.4 CLASSIFICATION

A classification of NSAIDs concurrently available in the UK is shown in Table 7.1. The salicylates are the prototype of this group of drugs and none of the more recently introduced drugs is much more effective than aspirin, although some may be better tolerated than non-enteric coated or delayed-release forms of aspirin.

TABLE 7.1
Classification of NSAIDs

SALICYLATES	acetylsalicylic acid (aspirin)
	salicylsalicylic acid
	aloxiprin
	benorylate
	diflunisal
	choline magnesium trisalicylate
PROPIONIC ACIDS	ibuprofen
	flurbiprofen
	ketoprofen
	naproxen
	fenoprofen
	fenbufen
	tiaprofenic acid
	(indoprofen)
	(benoxaprofen)
ANTHRANILIC ACIDS	phenylbutazone
	oxyphenbutazone
	azapropazone
	feprazone
PHENYLACETIC ACIDS	fenclofenac
	diclofenac
INDOMETHACIN AND RELATED DRUGS	indomethacin
	sulindac
	tolmetin
OXICAMS	piroxicam

7.5 SALICYLATES

The structures of various salicylates are shown in Fig. 7.1. Aspirin (acetylsali-cylic acid) is the standard. Sodium salicylate has anti-inflammatory properties but is less effective in experimental models of inflammation than aspirin, and on anecdotal evidence is said to be less effective than aspirin clinically (Lasagna, 1961). It is not used as an anti-inflammatory drug in the UK.

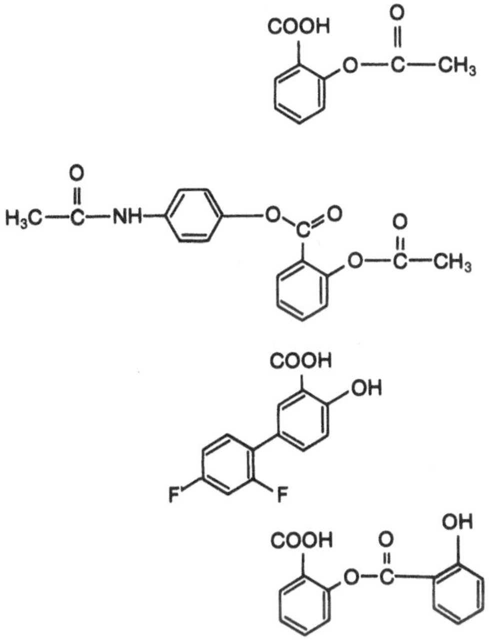

Acetylsalicylic acid (Aspirin)

Paracetamol ester of acetylsalicylic acid (Benorylate)

Diflunisal

Salicyl salicylic acid (Salsalate)

Figure 7.1 Salicylates.

7.5.1 Aspirin

Aspirin is usually prescribed as either soluble aspirin or as one of a number of delayed-release preparations. The latter have been designed to reduce gastrointestinal toxicity, but are more expensive than soluble aspirin. These preparations include enteric-coated aspirin, micro-encapsulated aspirin (Levius) and aloxiprin, a polymeric condensate of aspirin and aluminium oxide.

(a) *Pharmacokinetics*

Aspirin is a weak acid with p*K*a of 3.0. At alkaline pH aspirin becomes more ionized and less lipid soluble, and the reverse occurs at acid pH. Although the theoretical optimum pH for absorption is thus equivalent to the lower pH likely to be found in the stomach, maximal absorption of soluble aspirin occurs from the small intestine because of its proportionately larger absorbing area. After absorption aspirin is rapidly hydrolysed to salicylic acid, and the plasma half-life of aspirin is only 15–20 minutes (Levy, 1974). Peak salicylate levels are achieved around 2 hours after ingesting soluble aspirin. Salicylic acid is metabolized by conjugation with glucuronic acid to salicyl phenolic glucuronide and salicyl acyl glucuronide, and by conjugation with glycine to salicyluric acid. Both these enzymes processes are saturable at plasma levels around

5 mg per 100 ml, so that further dosage increments produce disproportionate increases in plasma salicylate (Davison, 1971). Small amounts of salicylate are metabolized by hydroxylation to gentisic acid and the rest is excreted as salicylic acid itself by glomerular filtration and tubular secretion. Renal elimination is increased by alkalinization of urine. With low dosages of soluble aspirin (300–600 mg), the plasma half-life is around 4 hours; with high dosages of around 4 g daily, the plasma half-life is 15–20 hours (Paulus and Furst, 1979). There is much inter-individual variation in the plasma levels achieved by a particular aspirin dose, and some monitoring of plasma level is usually necessary to optimize therapy. Plasma levels of 15 mg per 100 ml are thought to be necessary for an anti-inflammatory effect.

Like other NSAIDs, circulating salicylate is highly albumin bound. At plasma concentrations of around 10 mg per 100 ml and less, 92% of the drug is protein bound, whereas at concentrations of 30 mg per 100 ml only 80% of the drug is protein bound.

(b) *Efficacy*

Aspirin was the forerunner of the whole group of NSAIDs, and in high dosage is as effective as any of its successors. Low doses of soluble aspirin (300–600 mg) provide a rapid analgesic effect, but are not very effective in providing pain relief in patients with rheumatoid arthritis. Higher doses from 3–5 g daily are required for an anti-inflammatory effect (Boardman and Hart, 1967), but these produce a high frequency of side effects.

Anti-inflammatory doses of aspirin are used in the treatment of rheumatoid arthritis in adults and, in paediatric practice, for the treatment of Still's disease (particularly the systemic type) and rheumatic fever.

(c) *Side effects*

Gastrointestinal side effects are the main factor limiting the prescription of anti-inflammatory doses of aspirin. About one in fifteen patients receiving salicylates develops dyspepsia (Muir, 1963). Micro-bleeding into the gut lumen is very common and is reduced, but not completely prevented, by using enteric-coated preparations. Soluble aspirin is better tolerated than the older insoluble, ordinary aspirin preparations (Muir, 1963). Major bleeding does occur with aspirin, but is probably uncommon when related to the total number of users of the drug (Levy, 1974). The risk of gastric, but probably not duodenal, ulcer formation is increased by salicylate therapy (Levy, 1974).

Salicylates are thought to damage the gastrointestinal tract both by destroying the mucus barrier, which allows back diffusion of gastric acid into the mucosal cells, and by inhibiting local prostaglandin production (Rees and Turnberg, 1980). Aspirin inhibits platelet aggregation probably by inhibiting thromboxane synthesis, and this may contribute to gastrointestinal blood loss. Acetylation of platelet cyclo-oxygenase contributes to this effect, and non-acetylated salicylate derivatives have less or no effects on platelets (Buchanan *et al.*, 1979).

Intravenous and enteric-coated salicylates also produce gastrointestinal bleeding (albeit less than do oral salicylates), and this effect correlates with circulating salicylate levels (Mielants *et al.*, 1979).

Tinnitus is a common side effect, particularly of high salicylate doses, and does not correlate well with plasma salicylate levels. Acute overdosage produces metabolic acidosis in children, but usually alkalosis in adults.

Salicylates alone are an uncommon cause of clinically important renal disease (New Zealand Rheumatism Association, 1974), unlike salicylate/phenacetin combinations which were a more frequent cause of renal papillary necrosis. In low doses, salicylates produce urate retention by the kidney but in high dosage are uricosuric. Hepatotoxicity may occur with high dosages of salicylates, particularly in SLE (Seaman *et al.*, 1974). Hypersensitivity reactions to aspirin occur in 0.2% of patients and features include shock, asthma, urticaria and angioneurotic oedema.

(d) *Dosage and preparations*

There is much variation in absorption and metabolism of aspirin, so that dosage is tailored to a particular patient response. Total serum salicylate levels of over 15 mg per 100 ml are required for an anti-inflammatory effect, whereas levels of 35 mg per 100 ml and over are usually associated with toxicity. In 'normal' adults, daily dosages of soluble aspirin of 3.6 g or higher (up to 5 g daily), given in a four times daily regime, are usually required. Enteric-coated and delayed-release preparations are better tolerated than soluble aspirin, but are associated with greater variability in absorption, so that monitoring circulating drug levels is helpful. There is a delay in absorption of these other preparations of aspirin, so that they are not suitable for 'on demand analgesia', where a rapid onset of action is required.

7.5.2 Benorylate

Benorylate is an ester of paracetamol and aspirin available as suspension or granules. Benorylate is hydrolysed in the bloodstream to salicylic acid and paracetamol. Both paracetamol metabolites and salicylates may contribute to drug efficacy. A dose of 8.0 g of benorylate daily (given as 4.0 g twice daily) is equivalent therapeutically to 4.8 g daily of soluble aspirin (Sasisekhar *et al.*, 1973). Benorylate is more expensive than soluble aspirin and enteric-coated aspirin, and may be useful in younger children when palatability is particularly important.

7.5.3 Diflunisal

Diflunisal is a fluorinated derivative of salicylate which is well absorbed orally. The drug is not metabolized to salicylic acid, and peak blood levels occur at 2 hours. The plasma half-life is around 10–12 hours in individuals with normal renal function (Brodgen *et al.*, 1980). Diflunisal is metabolized to the phenolic glucuronide and subsequent elimination is mainly renal.

Diflunisal is better tolerated than soluble aspirin, produces less gastro-intestinal bleeding, and has little or no effect on platelets. Diflunisal is prescribed as 250–500 mg twice daily. In osteoarthrosis a dosage of 500–750 mg of diflunisal has been shown to have equivalent efficacy to 2–3 g of aspirin daily. Although mainly promoted as an analgesic for osteoarthrosis and soft tissue injuries (Brodgen *et al.*, 1980), 750 mg daily of diflunisal has been shown to be as effective as 1600 mg daily of ibuprofen in rheumatoid arthritis (Palmer *et al.*, 1981).

7.5.4 Salsalate

Salsalate is an insoluble ester of salicylic acid which is absorbed from the small intestine and hydrolysed after absorption to salicylic acid. The plasma half-life is about 8 hours and the adult dosage is 1 g twice or three times daily. Salsalate produces less gastrointestinal blood loss than aspirin in healthy volunteers (Cohen, 1979) and appears to have comparative efficacy to other NSAIDs (Deodhar *et al.*, 1977).

7.5.5 Choline magnesium trisalicylate

This drug has similar properties to diflunisal and salsalate and produces little or no gastrointestinal blood loss in short-term studies in normal volunteers. A daily dosage of 3 g of choline magnesium trisalicylate has been shown to have equivalent efficacy to daily dosages of 3 g of aspirin and 2.4 g of ibuprofen in the treatment of rheumatoid arthritis (Blackman and Leckner, 1979; Ehrlich *et al.*, 1980).

7.6 PROPIONIC ACID DERIVATIVES

The structures of the propionic acid derivatives are summarized in Fig. 7.2. The prototype, ibufenac, was first marketed in 1964 and withdrawn from the UK market in 1967 because of hepatocellular toxicity. Two recently introduced propionic acid derivatives, benoxaprofen and indoprofen, have already been withdrawn from the UK market because of excessive toxicity, but their structures are included for interest.

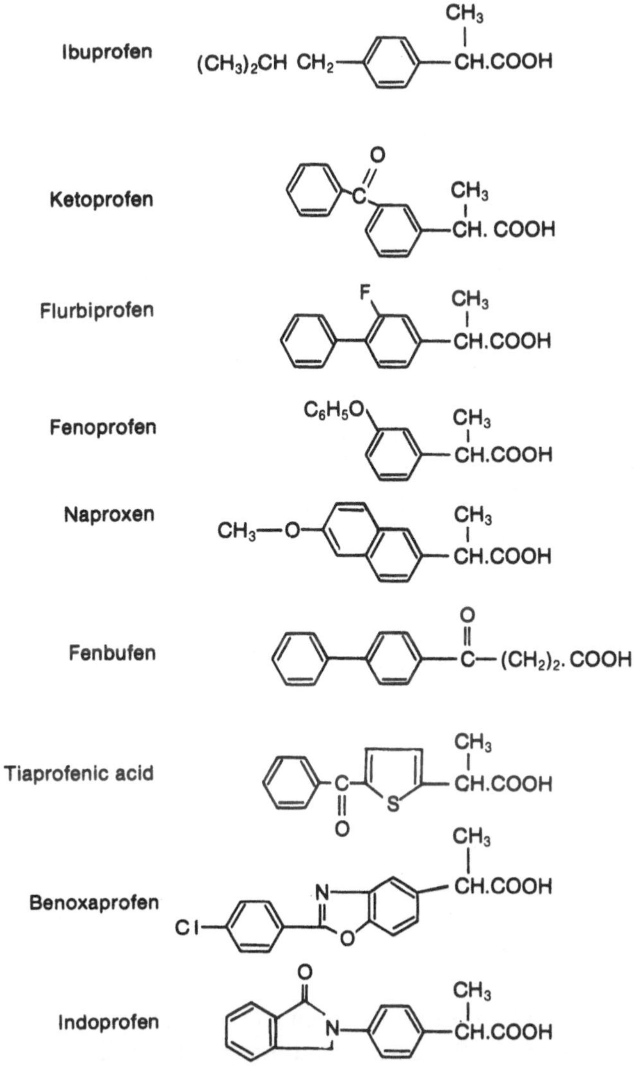

Figure 7.2 Propionic acid derivatives.

7.6.1 Ibuprofen

Ibuprofen was introduced to the UK market in 1969 and was the first of the currently available propionic acid derivatives (Hart and Boardman, 1975). Since August 1983 ibuprofen has been available over the counter in Great Britain.

(a) *Pharmacokinetics*

Ibuprofen is readily absorbed, and peak plasma levels are achieved 1–2 hours after oral dosage. The plasma half-life of the drug is around 2 hours, and most of an oral dose is excreted in the urine within 24 hours. The drug is metabolized in the liver, and over 90% of the administered drug is excreted as hydroxy or carboxy metabolites (Adams and Buckler, 1979). There is a tendency for dose-normalized plasma levels to fall with increasing dosage from 800 mg to 2400 mg daily due to an increase in the non-protein bound drug fraction (Grennan *et al.*, 1983).

(b) *Interaction*

Ibuprofen does not interfere with antipyrine metabolism nor does it displace warfarin from protein binding. Concurrent salicylate therapy roughly halves plasma ibuprofen levels via a displacement effect on plasma protein binding of ibuprofen (Grennan *et al.*, 1979b).

(c) *Efficacy*

A daily dosage of 1200–1600 mg of ibuprofen is about as effective as salicylates and other NSAIDs in the treatment of rheumatoid arthritis and osteoarthrosis (Adams and Buckler, 1979). Ibuprofen was initially prescribed in a dosage of 600–900 mg daily, which is less effective in the treatment of rheumatoid arthritis (Grennan *et al.*, 1983). High daily dosages of up to 2400 mg daily have been used in the treatment of rheumatoid arthritis (Godfrey and De La Cruz, 1975). Ibuprofen is also used in the treatment of juvenile polyarthritis (Adams and Buckler, 1979).

(d) *Side effects*

A major advantage of ibuprofen has been its relatively low toxicity in conventional dosages (up to 1600 mg daily) and the drug has had a low frequency of adverse reactions reported to the Committee on Safety of Medicines over a 15-year period. Like all NSAIDs, ibuprofen may cause gastrointestinal side effects such as indigestion, nausea and bleeding in susceptible individuals. Uncommonly, hepatotoxicity occurs and rare cases of toxic amblyopia and bone marrow depression have been recorded (Adams and Buckler, 1979).

(e) *Dosage*

The adult dosage is 200–400 mg three to four times daily.

7.6.2   Flurbiprofen

Flurbiprofen was launched in 1977. *In vitro* flurbiprofen is a particularly potent inhibitor of prostaglandin synthesis and has a slightly different spectrum of activity in standard pharmacological assays compared with ibuprofen (Adams and Buckler, 1979).

(a) *Pharmacokinetics*

Peak plasma levels are achieved 1.5 hours after ingestion and the plasma half-life is about 4 hours. Nearly all an oral dose is excreted via the urine, either as unchanged drug (20%) or as metabolites (80%). About 99.9% of flurbiprofen in plasma is protein bound.

(b) *Efficacy*

Flurbiprofen has been shown to provide relief of symptoms in rheumatoid arthritis, osteoarthrosis and ankylosing spondylitis (reviewed by Brogden *et al.*, 1979). In rheumatoid arthritis 100 mg of flurbiprofen was found to be about as effective as 3–4 g of aspirin daily, and doses of 200 mg of flurbiprofen daily as effective as 100 mg of indomethacin (Brewis, 1977). Daily flurbiprofen dosages of 120–150 mg daily have provided equivalent efficacy to daily dosages of 150 mg of sulindac, 1500 mg of mefenamic acid and 2400 mg of ibuprofen. In ankylosing spondylitis, 150–200 mg of flurbiprofen has been shown to be about as effective as 75–100 mg of indomethacin (Good and Mena, 1977) and 300–400 mg of phenylbutazone (Brogden *et al.*, 1979).

(c) *Toxicity*

In healthy volunteers, 150 mg daily of flurbiprofen produced less gastrointestinal bleeding than 2.1 g of aspirin daily (Vakil *et al.*, 1977). Of patients receiving flurbiprofen long-term 50% develop some form of side effect, usually gastrointestinal (Sheldrake *et al.*, 1977).

(d) *Interactions*

In patients receiving oral anticoagulants, concurrent flurbiprofen produces up to 25% lowering of the prothrombin time (Marbet *et al.*, 1977).

(e) *Dosage*

The usual oral dosage of flurbiprofen is 50–100 mg twice daily.

7.6.3 Ketoprofen

Ketoprofen was first marketed in November 1973 and is a short plasma half-life NSAID, with similar clinical efficacy and overall toxicity to ibuprofen and flurbiprofen.

(a) Pharmacokinetics

Peak blood levels are achieved at 1–1.5 hours after oral dosage and 45 minutes to 1 hour after administration of a ketoprofen suppository. The plasma half-life is 1.5–2 hours after oral dosage. Ketoprofen is excreted mainly in the urine, and more than 50% is in the form of metabolites, mainly glucuronides (Tamisier, 1979).

(b) Efficacy

Ketoprofen has been shown to be more effective than placebo in the treatment of rheumatoid arthritis. In this disorder dosages of 75–300 mg daily have equivalent efficacy to daily dosages of 3.6–4 g of aspirin, 150–600 mg of phenylbutazone, 75–150 mg of indomethacin and 1200–2400 mg of ibuprofen (Mitchell *et al.*, 1975; Tamisier, 1979). Ketoprofen has also been shown to be effective in the treatment of ankylosing spondylitis, gout and osteoarthrosis.

(c) Toxicity

Ketoprofen is better tolerated than aspirin and has gastrointestinal toxicity equivalent to other propionic acid derivatives.

(d) Dosage and preparations

Oral ketoprofen is prescribed in a daily dosage of 100–300 mg daily, either in a twice or three times daily dosage. Ketoprofen is also available in suppository and sustained-release preparations. The sustained-release preparation was introduced in 1982 and depends on a novel pH-sensitive semi-permeable membrane to release ketoprofen in the alkaline milieu of the small intestine. The manufacturers claim that this preparation should have less toxicity by producing a sustained plasma drug profile with fewer peaks and troughs than standard oral capsules. Both oral ketoprofen and the sustained-release preparation produce less faecal blood loss in normal volunteers than soluble aspirin (Ranlov *et al.*, 1983). Whether the sustained-release preparation is really better tolerated than the cheaper standard ketoprofen in arthritic patients is still to be proven.

7.6.4   Naproxen

Naproxen is a long plasma half-life propionic acid which was first marketed in the UK in 1973.

(a) *Pharmacokinetics*

Peak blood levels are achieved between one and two hours after ingestion of naproxen on an empty stomach. The plasma half-life in normal volunteers is 11–20 hours (Segre, 1979). The pharmacokinetics of naproxen are dose dependent, and increasing the daily dosage above 1 g daily produces less than proportionate increases in plasma levels (Segre, 1979). This is probably due to an increase in the unbound drug fraction in the plasma with higher doses, which in turn increases renal clearance. In patients with impaired renal function, a similar protein-binding effect and increased elimination of naproxen also occurs, so that an oral dose of 250 mg of naproxen may be given to patients with a creatinine clearance as low as 3 ml per minute (Antilla *et al.*, 1980).

Excretion of naproxen is almost completely renal, with about 10% of the drug excreted unchanged, 60% as the glucuronide conjugate, and the rest as the 6-desmethyl-naproxen metabolite.

(b) *Efficacy*

Naproxen has been shown to provide symptomatic relief in the treatment of rheumatoid arthritis, ankylosing spondylitis, gout, osteoarthrosis, soft tissue injuries, and juvenile arthritis (Segre, 1979). In the treatment of rheumatoid arthritis an oral dose of 500 mg naproxen daily has equivalent efficacy to daily dosages of 4 g aspirin (Mowat *et al.*, 1979) and 2.4 g fenoprofen (Huskisson *et al.*, 1979). In this later study, 500 mg of naproxen daily in rheumatoid arthritis was slightly more effective overall than 1200 mg ibuprofen or 150 mg ketoprofen, and equivalent to 2.4 g of fenoprofen daily (Huskisson *et al.*, 1979). However, there were subgroups of patients who preferred each of the four drugs tested – ibuprofen, ketoprofen, naproxen, and fenoprofen.

(c) *Side effects*

Naproxen, like other propionic acid derivatives, is better tolerated and produces less gastrointestinal bleeding than high doses of aspirin. Other uncommon but serious side effects of naproxen include interstitial nephritis and renal failure (Cartwright *et al.*, 1979), generalized vasculitis (Grennan *et al.*, 1979a), thrombocytopenia and agranulocytosis (Segre, 1979). When prescribed in patients receiving oral anticoagulants, naproxen increases the non-protein bound fraction of warfarin but usually produces either no (or clinically insignificant) changes in the prothrombin time (Petersen *et al.*, 1979; Segre, 1979).

(d) *Dosage*

The adult dose of naproxen is 250–500 mg twice daily. A higher single loading dose is sometimes given when rapid effect is required as in patients with acute gout. Naproxen suppositories (500 mg) are available.

7.6.5 Fenoprofen

Fenoprofen is a short plasma half-life propionic acid derivative.

(a) *Pharmacokinetics*

Peak plasma levels are achieved about 60 minutes after oral administration of fenoprofen, and the plasma half-life is between 150 and 190 minutes. Plasma levels rise linearly with oral dosage up to 3200 mg daily (Ridolfo *et al.*, 1979). Fenoprofen is mainly excreted in the urine as fenoprofen glucuronide or hydroxy-fenoprofen-glucuronide, and less than 5% of the drug in the urine is unchanged (Brogden *et al.*, 1979).

(b) *Efficacy*

Fenoprofen has been shown to relieve symptoms in rheumatoid arthritis and osteoarthrosis. In rheumatoid arthritis 2.4 g fenoprofen daily is about as effective as 3.9–6 g of aspirin daily (Brogden *et al.*, 1977) and 500 mg naproxen daily (Huskisson *et al.*, 1979).

(c) *Toxicity*

Like other propionic acid derivatives, fenoprofen is better tolerated than ordinary or soluble aspirin, and uncommonly may cause interstitial nephritis and renal failure (Brezin *et al.*, 1979).

(d) *Dosage*

Fenoprofen is prescribed as 300–600 mg four times daily by mouth.

7.6.6 Fenbufen

Fenbufen was launched in the UK in 1980. It is a prodrug which becomes active after metabolism to *p*-biphenyl acetic acid.

(a) *Pharmacokinetics*

Peak blood levels are achieved about 2 hours after oral administration of fenbufen. Steady-state levels are achieved in 3 days. Fenbufen is metabolized to γ-hydroxyphenylbutanoic acid and to *p*-biphenylacetic acid. *p*-biphenylacetic acid is anti-inflammatory and inhibits prostaglandin synthesis, but neither the parent compound nor γ-hydroxyphenylbutanoic acid is anti-inflammatory (Mawdsley, 1979).

(b) *Efficacy*

In a daily dosage of 600–1000 mg, fenbufen has been shown to provide symptomatic relief in the treatment of both rheumatoid arthritis and osteoarthrosis (Mawdsley, 1979). In rheumatoid arthritis 600 mg of fenbufen has been shown to have equivalent efficacy to 3600 mg of aspirin, and in one study was more effective than 75 mg of indomethacin daily (Vergara-Castro *et al.*, 1976). In a double-blind study in osteoarthrosis 75 mg of indomethacin was found to be more effective overall than 600 mg daily of fenbufen (Buxton *et al.*, 1978).

(c) *Side effects*

Fenbufen produces fewer gastrointestinal side effects than non-enteric-coated forms of aspirin and indomethacin (Mawdsley, 1979). Particularly in high dosage (over 1000 mg daily), but also in lower dosages (600 mg daily), fenbufen may produce liver function test abnormalities that are reversible when the drug is stopped (Buxton *et al.*, 1978).

(d) *Dosage*

Fenbufen is prescribed as 600–900 mg daily, either as a single night time dose of 600 mg, or as a twice daily dosage.

7.6.7 Tiaprofenic acid

Tiaprofenic acid was first marketed in the UK in 1982 and is a short plasma half-life drug with similar properties to ibuprofen.

(a) *Pharmacokinetics*

Peak plasma levels are achieved 1–2 hours after ingestion of the drug and the plasma half-life is about 1.5 hours. About 60% of the drug is excreted in the urine, mainly as unchanged drug either before or after conjugation to the acylglucuronide (Pottier *et al.*, 1977). A small proportion of the drug is excreted as hydroxylated metabolites.

(b) *Efficacy*

Tiaprofenic acid is effective in both rheumatoid arthritis and osteoarthrosis. A daily dose of 600 mg of tiaprofenic acid is as effective as 1200 mg daily of ibuprofen in rheumatoid arthritis (Daymond *et al.*, 1979) and as 75 mg of indomethacin in osteoarthrosis (Wojtulewski *et al.*, 1981).

(c) *Dosage*

Tiaprofenic acid is prescribed as 200 mg twice daily.

7.6.8 Indoprofen

Indoprofen was first marketed in the UK in September 1982 but was withdrawn in December 1983 because of a high frequency of adverse reactions, particularly gastrointestinal, reported to the Committee on Safety of Medicines.

7.6.9 Benoxaprofen

Benoxaprofen was launched in 1980 and was interesting pharmacologically in that although it had definite anti-inflammatory properties, it was only a weak inhibitor of the cyclo-oxygenase enzyme of prostaglandin synthesis, but a strong inhibitor of the lipoxygenase pathway involved in leukotriene synthesis (Higgs and Vane, 1983). As a poor inhibitor of prostaglandin synthesis, benoxaprofen was expected to produce fewer gastrointestinal side effects than standard NSAIDs. *Benoxaprofen was withdrawn from the market in the UK in 1982* after more than 3500 adverse reactions, including 61 deaths, had been reported to the Committee on Safety of Medicine (Editorial, 1982). The deaths were mainly due to hepatotoxicity and the elderly appeared particularly vulnerable. Other side effects, unusual for an NSAID, were photosensitivity skin eruptions and onycholysis.

7.7 ANTHRANILIC ACID DERIVATIVES

Two anthranilic acid derivatives (Fig. 7.3), flufenamic acid and mefenamic acid, are marketed as NSAIDs in the UK. A third anthranilic acid derivative, sodium meclofenamate, has also been shown to be effective in the treatment of rheumatoid arthritis in short-term studies (Rennie *et al.*, 1977; Palmer *et al.*,

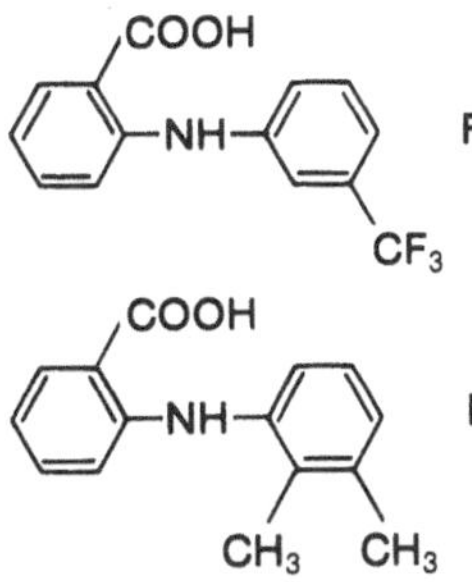

Figure 7.3 Anthranilic acid derivatives.

1981), but is a frequent cause of diarrhoea and is not currently marketed in the UK. Flufenamic acid and mefenamic acid will be considered together here (note that flufenamic acid was withdrawn in 1985).

(a) *Pharmacokinetics*

Both drugs are well absorbed from the gastrointestinal tract, with peak blood levels of flufenamic acid being reached about 6 hours and of mefenamic acid about 2 hours post ingestion (Winder *et al.*, 1967). Both drugs are highly protein bound. About 50% is eliminated in the urine and the rest in the faeces. Flufenamic acid is partly metabolized to hydroxyl derivatives and excreted as unchanged drug, glucuronide conjugate, and conjugated metabolite. Mefenamic acid is metabolized to 3-hydroxymethyl and 3-carboxyl derivatives and excreted both as conjugated mefenamic acid and as either metabolite.

(b) *Efficacy*

Both flufenamic acid (in a daily dose of 300–400 mg) and mefenamic acid (in a daily dose of 1500 mg) have been shown to relieve symptoms in rheumatoid arthritis (Sydnes, 1969; Mavrikakis *et al.*, 1977). In rheumatoid arthritis 1500 mg daily of mefenamic acid was found to be as effective as 75 mg daily of indomethacin in a short-term study in rheumatoid arthritis (Mavrikakis *et al.*, 1977).

(c) *Side effects*

There is very little information on either long-term or short-term side effects of flufenamic acid and mefenamic acid. In a 7-day study, 600 mg daily of flufenamic acid produced insignificant gastrointestinal blood loss as measured by the ^{51}Cr-labelled red blood cell technique (Tudhope, 1967). Diarrhoea is a more frequent side effect with these drugs than with other NSAIDs, and the frequency of this side effect often appears dose related (Winder *et al.*, 1967).

7.8 PYRAZOLE DERIVATIVES

The structures of the pyrazoles are shown in Fig. 7.4.

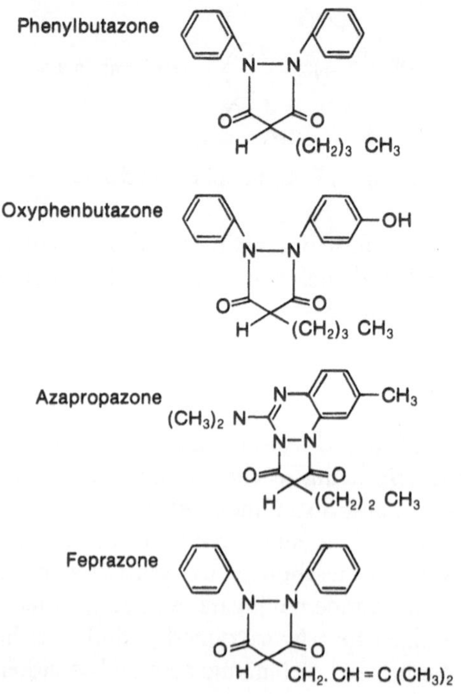

Figure 7.4 Pyrazole derivatives. Feprazone has now been withdrawn from the UK market.

7.8.1 Phenylbutazone and oxyphenbutazone

These drugs have been used as anti-inflammatory agents since the 1950s. Their usefulness is limited by their potential haematological side effects.

(a) *Pharmacokinetics*

Phenylbutazone is absorbed rapidly from the gut and produces peak blood levels about 2 hours after ingestion. The plasma half-life is about 72 hours and steady-state levels are achieved after 3–4 hours. Phenylbutazone is extensively metabolized to either oxyphenbutazone or γ-hydroxyphenylbutazone (Higham *et al.*, 1981). Both metabolites are pharmacologically active. The total plasma concentration of phenylbutazone increases less than proportionately with increasing dosage from 200–400 mg daily. This is due to a progressive decrease in plasma protein binding as the dosage increases (Higham *et al.*, 1981).

Oxyphenbutazone is absorbed more slowly from the gut than phenylbutazone, but its plasma half-life is of similar duration (Brooks and Buchanan, 1976).

(b) Efficacy

Both phenylbutazone in a dosage of 300 mg daily, and oxyphenbutazone have been shown to have an anti-inflammatory effect in the treatment of rheumatoid arthritis (Brooks et al., 1975; Brooks and Buchanan, 1976).

(c) Side effects

The most important problem with phenylbutazone and oxyphenbutazone is the risk of potentially fatal haematological side effects. The mortality rate in users of these drugs has been estimated as 2.2 per 100 000 users for phenylbutazone and 3.8 per 100 000 users for oxyphenbutazone (Inman, 1977). Aplastic anaemia is the most frequent cause of death, but thrombocytopenia, agranulocytosis and leucopenia also occur. Elderly women seem at particular risk of haematological toxicity (Inman, 1977). Phenylbutazone and oxyphenbutazone appear to be just as likely to cause gastrointestinal bleeding as indomethacin and other NSAIDs (Cuthbert, 1974).

In view of the potential toxicity of these drugs and the large number of alternatives now available, the Committee on Safety of Medicines withdrew the licence for oxyphenbutazone in 1984 and restricted phenylbutazone to hospital use for the treatment of ankylosing spondylitis only.

(d) Interactions

Phenylbutazone enhances the activities of oral anticoagulants, anticonvulsants and oral hypoglycaemics by inhibition of metabolism and displacement from plasma protein binding.

7.8.2 Azapropazone

Azapropazone was introduced into clinical practice in 1976. Structurally it has a pyrazolidine ring in common with phenylbutazone from which it differs by also having a benzotriazine ring (Fig. 7.4). It does not have the haematological toxicity of phenylbutazone.

(a) Pharmacokinetics

Azapropazone is absorbed from the gastrointestinal tract and produces peak blood levels about 4 hours after ingestion. In man, the plasma half-life varies from 4 to 16 hours, with a mean of 8.5 hours (Jones, 1976). Unlike phenylbutazone, azapropazone is not extensively metabolized, and only unchanged drug is found in plasma. Sixty per cent of an ingested dose is excreted in the urine, of which 60% consists of unchanged azapropazone, about 20% is the pharmacologically inactive 6-hydroxyazapropazone, and the rest consists of several metabolites of unknown structures (Jones, 1976). The elimination of azapropazone in the elderly may be reduced and is related to creatinine clearance (Ritch et al., 1982). The starting dose in the elderly should not be above 600 mg daily instead of the usual adult dose of 1200 mg daily.

(b) Efficacy

Azapropazone has been shown to be effective in rheumatoid arthritis in a daily dose of 1200 mg daily, which is at least as effective as a daily dose of 3.9 g of aspirin (Grennan et al., 1976; Brooks et al., 1976a). In psoriatic arthritis and Reiter's disease, 1200 mg daily of azapropazone was found to be as effective as 100 mg daily of indomethacin (Lassus, 1976). Azapropazone has also been shown to provide an analgesic effect in the treatment of osteoarthrosis (Brooks and Buchanan, 1976a). Azapropazone has been shown to be effective as an anti-inflammatory drug in the treatment of acute gout and has a uricosuric effect which may be useful in the treatment of chronic gout (Dieppe et al., 1981).

(c) Side effects

In a daily dose of 1200 mg azapropazone is tolerated as well as other NSAIDs and did not increase gastrointestinal bleeding in 20 rheumatoid patients investigated using the ^{51}Cr-labelled red blood cell technique (Mintz and Fraga, 1976).

(d) Interactions

Azapropazone inhibits the elimination and enhances the effect of oral hypoglycaemics and phenytoin (Andreasen et al., 1981; Geaney et al., 1982). Azapropazone like phenylbutazone, potentiates the effects of warfarin by displacing warfarin from plasma protein binding and inhibiting metabolism.

Like phenylbutazone, azapropazone enhances the effects of oral anticoagulants, hypoglycaemics and anticonvulsants (Andreasen et al., 1981; Geaney et al., 1982).

(e) Dosage

Azapropazone is prescribed in a dosage of 300 mg four times daily or 600 mg twice daily in adults (Templeton, 1981). A reduced starting dose of 600 mg daily is used in the elderly.

7.9   PHENYLACETIC ACID DERIVATIVES

The structures of two phenylacetic acids derivatives are shown in Fig. 7.5. Alclofenac, a third phenylacetic acid derivative was effective as an anti-inflammatory drug but was withdrawn because of a high incidence of drug-related skin rashes and vasculitis.

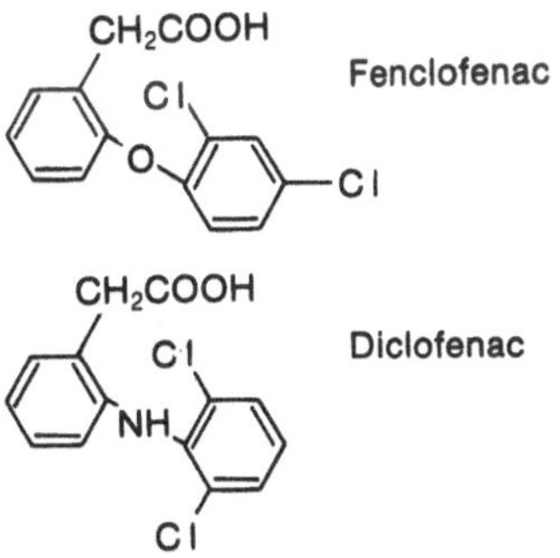

Figure 7.5 Phenylacetic acids.

7.9.1   Fenclofenac

The licence for fenclofenac was withdrawn by the Committee on Safety of Medicines in 1984. Fenclofenac was a relatively effective anti-inflammatory drug but controversially was also suggested to have disease-suppressing pro-perties similar to gold and penicillamine. The case for this statement rested firstly on the observation that in several studies a fall in the ESR was noted in patients treated with fenclofenac (Goldberg and Godfrey, 1980). Secondly, in a 6-month study of rheumatoid arthritis, the patients treated with either fenclo-fenac (16 patients), or D-penicillamine (16 patients) showed significant improvement in standard clinical measurements of joint pain and tenderness as compared with those treated with placebo in addition to their previous NSAID therapy (Berry *et al.*, 1980). In a similar 1-year comparison of fenclofenac with chrysotherapy in rheumatoid arthritis both groups of patients showed an improvement in clinical measurement of disease activity and in ESR although there was a trend for gold-treated patients to improve more than the fenclo-fenac group (Bach-Andersen *et al.*, 1982). We regard the case for fenclofenac having second-line antirheumatic properties as 'unproven'.

7.9.2   Diclofenac

Diclofenac is a short plasma half-life drug with similar efficacy to other NSAIDs.

(a) *Pharmacokinetics*

Diclofenac is well absorbed orally, and peak blood levels are achieved within 2 hours of ingestion. The plasma half-life is 1.2–2 hours. About 60% of an administered dose is excreted in the urine and the rest in the faeces. Excretion is either as a hydroxy metabolite or as a diclofenac conjugate (Fowler, 1979). Elimination of the drug does not fall with age.

(b) *Efficacy*

Diclofenac has been shown to relieve symptoms in rheumatoid arthritis, osteoarthrosis and gout (Brogden *et al.*, 1980). In rheumatoid arthritis diclofenac in a daily dosage of 75–150 mg was as effective as 75–150 mg of indomethacin; and 100 mg of diclofenac daily was as effective as 500 mg of naproxen, 1600 mg daily of ibuprofen and 300 mg daily of phenylbutazone. In acute gout, intramuscular diclofenac was of equivalent efficacy to intramuscular phenylbutazone.

(c) *Side effects*

Gastrointestinal side effects are the most frequent and oral diclofenac is better tolerated than non-enteric-coated aspirin. Other side effects include rashes, headaches and dizziness. Although uncommon, blood dyscrasias and liver function test abnormalities have been reported (Fowler, 1979).

(d) *Interactions*

Diclofenac has no pharmacokinetic interactions with oral hypolycaemic drugs nor with oral anticoagulants.

(e) *Dosage and preparations*

The standard diclofenac tablet is enteric coated and the usual adult dosage is 25–50 mg three times daily. Diclofenac suppositories and slow-release and intramuscular preparations are available.

7.10 INDENE ACETIC ACID DERIVATIVES AND RELATED DRUGS

The structures of indomethacin, sulindac and tolmetin are shown in Fig. 7.6. Indomethacin and sulindac are indoles or indene acetic acid derivatives, whereas tolmetin is a pyrrole.

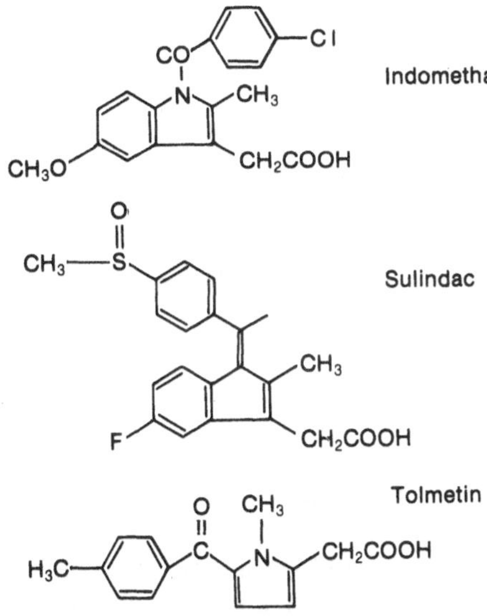

Figure 7.6 Indomethacin and related drugs.

7.10.1 Indomethacin

Indomethacin was launched as an NSAID in the UK in December 1964. It is used in the treatment of rheumatoid arthritis, ankylosing spondylitis, gout and osteoarthrosis.

(a) *Pharmacokinetics*

Indomethacin is well absorbed orally and produces peak blood levels 1–2 hours after ingestion on an empty stomach (Helberg, 1981). Food delays absorption of the drug. The plasma half-life is usually 5–6 hours, but there is enterohepatic recirculation and the half-life may be longer. Indomethacin is metabolized to O-desmethyl, N-deschlorobenzoyl and O-demethyl-N-deschlorobenzoyl derivatives. About 60% of an oral dose is excreted in the urine predominantly in glucuronidated form and the rest is excreted in the faeces after bilary secretion (Helberg, 1981). The elimination of indomethacin is decreased by concurrent administration of probenecid and increased by concurrent frusemide therapy (Brooks et al., 1974a, b).

(b) *Efficacy*

Indomethacin has been confirmed as effective in the treatment of rheumatoid arthritis in double-blind controlled trials versus placebo (Brooks and Buchanan, 1976). Earlier studies that failed to find differences between indomethacin and placebo were complicated by the use of salicylates in 'control' and active treatment groups (Co-operating Clinics, 1967; Donnelly *et al.*, 1967). Indomethacin is often considered by clinicians as being particularly useful in the treatment of ankylosing spondylitis, although there are few clinical trial data to demonstrate its superiority over other NSAIDs in this condition (Rhymer and Gengos, 1979). Indomethacin is also useful in the treatment of acute gout, in which it is used in dosages up to 400 mg in the first 24 hours (Rhymer and Gengos, 1979). Indomethacin is used in the treatment of osteoarthrosis usually in lower dosages of around 75 mg daily.

(c) Side effects

The most frequent side effects are gastrointestinal or related to the central nervous system. Gastrointestinal side effects include indigestion, nausea and vomiting, haemorrhage, and prepyloric gastric ulceration (Brooks and Buchanan, 1976). Headache, dizziness and vertigo are also common and thought to be related to vasoconstriction of the cerebral vasculature (Brooks and Buchanan, 1976). Uncommon side effects of indomethacin include perforation of stomach or small bowel, hepatitis, peripheral neuropathy, oedema and blood dyscrasias. The last include aplastic anaemia, agranulocytosis and leucopenia (Rhymer and Gengos, 1979).

(d) Interactions

Concurrent indomethacin therapy can decrease the antihypertensive effects of beta-blockers and thiazide diuretics in patients established on an antihypertensive regime (Donnelly *et al.*, 1967). Indomethacin does not significantly displace warfarin from protein binding (Rhymer and Gengos, 1976).

(e) Dosage and preparations

The usual oral dosage in adults with inflammatory joint disease is 25–50 mg three times daily. In acute gout up to 600 mg may be given in the first 24 hours of an attack.

Indomethacin suppositories are available and produce an earlier but lower peak blood level than the equivalent dose given orally (Baker *et al.*, 1980). They are usually prescribed in a 100 mg night time dosage, but the equivalent dose given orally is just as effective in relieving morning stiffness.

Slow-release capsules (75 mg) of indomethacin (Indocid R) are also available and are prescribed once to twice daily. They are more expensive than the standard 25 or 50 mg capsules and as levels of drug within the synovial fluid persist longer than plasma levels (Emori *et al.*, 1976), slow-release preparations probably have little clinical advantage.

Osmosin was another delayed-release form of indomethacin in which the drug was enclosed in a rigid, semi-permeable membrane. Drug release occurred by an osmotic pump action as the capsule passed through the gut. Osmosin was advertized as having fewer side-effects than standard indomethacin preparations, but was withdrawn from the market in August 1983 after 200 reports of adverse reactions, including gastrointestinal haemorrhage and perforations.

7.10.2 Sulindac

Sulindac was launched on the UK market in 1977. Sulindac is a prodrug and depends on metabolism to its sulphide derivative for pharmacological activity.

(a) *Pharmacokinetics*

After a single oral dose of 200 mg of sulindac, plasma levels peak at about 1 hour and then decrease with a plasma half-life of about 8 hours (Rhymer, 1979). The methyl sulphinyl group of sulindac is reversibly reduced to the sulphide ($-S-CH_3$), the active metabolite, and irreversibly oxidized to the sulphone ($-SO_2-CH_3$), an inactive metabolite. The plasma levels of the sulphide peak at about 2 hours and then decrease slowly with a plasma half-life of about 16 hours. Sulindac and the sulphone are both partially excreted in the urine, either unchanged or after conjugation to glucuronides. The sulphide is only present in the urine in small amounts. Sulindac and both metabolites undergo enterohepatic recirculation, and all three compounds appear in the faeces. The sulphide is thus partly eliminated in the faeces and partly eliminated by reoxidation to sulindac. Steady-state levels of sulindac and the sulphide are reached within 5 days of treatment on a twice-daily dosage (Huskisson, 1978).

(b) *Efficacy*

Sulindac has been used in the treatment of rheumatoid arthritis, osteoarthrosis and gout. In rheumatoid arthritis, a dose of 200 mg of sulindac twice daily has been found to be as effective as 3.6 g of aspirin daily (Huskisson, 1978). In osteoarthrosis, sulindac in a daily dosage of 200 mg or 300 mg was as effective as aspirin and ibuprofen (Andrade and Fernandez, 1978; Huskisson, 1978). In acute gout, a dose of 400 mg daily of sulindac may be of equivalent efficacy to 600 mg daily of phenylbutazone (Calabro, 1978).

(c) *Side effects*

Despite its 'pro-drug status', gastrointestinal side effects are still relatively common with sulindac as with other NSAIDs. Sulindac produces less gastrointestinal toxicity but more headaches and nervous system side effects than equivalent doses of non-enteric-coated forms of aspirin.

(d) Dosage

The usual dosage of sulindac in patients with rheumatoid arthritis is 200 mg twice daily, and in osteoarthosis lower dosages of 100 mg twice daily are usual.

7.10.3   Tolmetin

Tolmetin is a recently introduced drug with similar clinical properties to indomethacin.

(a) Pharmacokinetics

Tolmetin is rapidly absorbed after an oral dose, and peak blood levels are achieved about 30 minutes after ingestion (Ehrlich, 1979). The plasma half-life has been calculated at around 1 hour or 4.5–6 hours depending on whether a linear or non-linear pharmacokinetic model is used. Tolmetin is rapidly cleared from plasma, mainly by metabolism to the decarboxylic acid metabolite. Most of an administered dose is excreted via the urine, about 70% as the decarboxylic acid metabolite and the rest as other metabolites and unchanged drug (Ehrlich, 1979).

(b) Efficacy

Tolmetin has been shown to produce relief in the treatment of rheumatoid arthritis, osteoarthrosis, ankylosing spondylitis and Still's disease (Brogden et al., 1978). In rheumatoid arthritis tolmetin in a dose of 1200–1500 mg daily has been shown to be as effective as daily dosages of 4.5 g of aspirin, 100–150 mg of indomethacin and 400 mg of phenylbutazone (Brogden et al., 1978). In ankylosing spondylitis, 800 mg daily of tolmetin was as effective as 100 mg daily of indomethacin.

(c) Side effects

As with indomethacin, the main side effects of tolmetin are gastrointestinal, and headaches and dizziness. In general, tolmetin causes less gastrointestinal side effects than equivalent dosages of non-enteric-coated forms of aspirin, and less central nervous system side effects than equivalent dosages of indomethacin. Other uncommon side effects of tolmetin include peripheral oedema, rashes and interstitial nephritis.

(d) *Interaction*

There is no evidence for a pharmacokinetic interaction between tolmetin and oral anticoagulants when the two are prescribed concurrently (Ruest *et al.*, 1975).

(e) *Dosage*

The usual adult dosage of tolmetin is 200–400 mg three times daily.

7.11 OXICAMS

7.11.1 Piroxicam

This is the first oxicam to be marketed in the UK. The structure is given in Fig. 7.7.

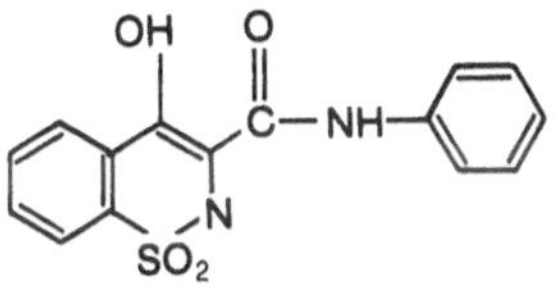

Figure 7.7 Piroxicam.

(a) *Pharmacokinetics*

Piroxicam is well absorbed from the gastrointestinal tract and produces peak blood levels at 4 hours. The plasma half-life is around 58 hours (Rogers *et al.*, 1981). Piroxicam is extensively metabolized, mainly to hydroxyl derivatives. These are excreted in urine or faeces either free or conjugated to glucuronic acid. The long plasma half-life of piroxicam means that a once daily dosage is adequate to maintain therapeutic blood levels over a full 24-hour period.

(b) *Efficacy*

Piroxicam has been shown to relieve symptoms of rheumatoid arthritis and osteoarthrosis (Wiseman and Boyle, 1980). In rheumatoid arthritis, one short-term study showed that 20 mg of piroxicam daily was as effective as daily dosages of 75 mg of indomethacin and 1200 mg of ibuprofen (Balogh *et al.*, 1979). In other studies in rheumatoid arthritis a dosage of 20 mg of piroxicam has been found to be more effective than either 500 mg of naproxen daily or 75 mg of indomethacin daily (Davies *et al.*, 1981; Sydnes, 1981). In osteoarthrosis, 20 mg of piroxicam daily was equivalent to 75 mg of indomethacin daily (Wiseman and Boyle, 1980).

In uncontrolled studies, piroxicam has been effective in the treatment of acute gout and ankylosing spondylitis (Widmark, 1978; Wiseman and Boyle, 1980).

(c) Side effects

Gastrointestinal symptoms are the most frequent forms of adverse reaction to piroxicam, but in general piroxicam seems better tolerated than indomethacin, phenylbutazone or aspirin and about as well tolerated as naproxen or ibuprofen (Wiseman and Boyle, 1980).

(d) Dosage

The usual adult dosage in rheumatoid arthritis and osteoarthrosis is 20 mg daily. In acute gout, a dosage of 40 mg daily has been used for the first 4–6 days of an attack.

7.12   WHICH NSAID?

Choice between the different NSAIDs should be considered mainly in terms of clinical efficacy and safety, and, where these are equal, also in terms of cost.

7.12.1   Clinical efficacy

It is difficult to make an overall grading of the NSAIDs in terms of clinical efficacy. Interpretation of the results of the many comparative studies that have been carried out in various centres is complicated by the different dosage regimes chosen for each drug, and by the different populations studied. Furthermore, there is always a possibility that in some studies different pharmaceutical preparations of particular NSAIDs, made up to enable double-blind comparisons, may not have the same bioavailability and efficacy as the standard pharmaceutical preparation. There is inter-individual variation in response as well as tolerance to different NSAIDs (Huskisson et al., 1979), so that drug B may relieve symptoms in particular patients when drug A has failed. Furthermore, certain drugs or groups of drugs may be more effective in particular inflammatory diseases. Thus, many clinicians consider indomethacin the drug of choice for ankylosing spondylitis. However, in general, usually all the NSAIDs now available have been shown to relieve symptoms in some patients with most forms of arthritis, and at optimum dosages have roughly similar efficacies.

TABLE 7.2
Relative costs of NSAIDs in the UK

Weekly cost for standard adult dosage

£1 or less	More than £1 £2 or less	More than £2 £3 or less	More than £3 £4 or less	More than £4
Soluble aspirin	Aspirin (enteric coated)	Benorylate suspension	Salsalate	Fenoprofen
Aloxiprin	Diflunisal	Flurbiprofen	Choline magnesium	Tolmetin
Microencapsulated aspirin	Ketoprofen	Fenbufen	trisalicylate	
Ibuprofen	Tiaprofenic acid	Mefenamic acid	Naproxen	
Phenylbutazone*		Azapropazone	Slow-release indomethacin	
Indomethacin		Diclofenac		
		Sulindac		
		Piroxicam		

* Prescription restricted to ankylosing spondylitis treated from hospital

7.12.2   Tolerance

Most of the newer NSAIDs are better tolerated and produce fewer gastrointestinal side effects than non-enteric-coated forms of aspirin and indomethacin, phenylbutazone and oxyphenbutazone. However, they have less often been compared with the better tolerated enteric-coated and various delayed-release forms of aspirin. The problem in the assessment of the newer NSAIDs is illustrated by the benoxaprofen story where certain less common side effects of a new NSAID were only recognized after the drug had been prescribed for 500 000 patients (Editorial, 1982).

7.12.3   Costs

It is clear that many NSAIDs have roughly similar efficacies and frequencies of side effects. In view of this considerations of cost become relevant. We have calculated the cost of one week's treatment with an average adult dose of each NSAID on the basis of prices negotiated by our hospital pharmacy using the cheapest generic equivalent of the drug where available (Table 7.2). These costs represent an approximate, comparative guide only. It can be seen that, not surprisingly, the longest established and best known NSAIDs (including soluble aspirin), ibuprofen and indomethacin, tend to be the cheapest.

7.13   REFERENCES

Adams, S. S. and Buckler, J. W. (1979) Ibuprofen and flurbiprofen. *Clinics Rheum. Dis.*, 5, 359–79.

Andrade, L. and Fernandez, A. (1978) Sulindac in the treatment of osteoarthritis: a double-blind 8-week study comparing sulindac with ibuprofen and 96 weeks of long term therapy. *Eur. J. Rheumatol. Inflammation*, 1, 36–40.

Andreasen, P. B., Simonsen, K., Brooks, R., Dimo, B. and Bouchelouche, P. (1981) Hypoglycaemia induced by azapropazone – tolbutamide interaction. *Br. J. Clin. Pharmacol.*, 12, 581–3.

Antilla, M., Haataja, M. and Kasanen, A. (1980) Pharmacokinetics of naproxen in subjects with normal and impaired renal function. *Eur. J. Clin. Pharmacol.*, 18, 263–8.

Bach-Andersen, R., Lund, B., Grae, A. and Sonne, I. (1982) (Abstract) A 12 months' study of the effects of fenclofenac and gold in the treatment of patients with rheumatoid arthritis. *Scand. J. Rheumatol.*, Suppl. 45, 43.

Baker, N., Sibeon, R., Laws, E., Halliday, L., Orme, M. and Little, T. (1980). Indomethacin in rheumatoid arthritis: comparison of oral and rectal dosing. *Br. J. Clin. Pharmacol.*, 10, 387–92.

Balogh, Z., Papazoglou, S. N., MacLeod, M. and Buchanan, W. W. (1979) A crossover clinical trial of piroxicam, indomethacin and ibuprofen in rheumatoid arthritis. *Curr. Med. Res. Opinion*, 6, 148–53.

Bartter, F. C., Pronove, P., Gill, J. R. *et al.* (1962) Hyperplasia of the juxtaglomerular complex with hyperaldosteronism and hypokalemic alkalosis. *Am. J. Med.*, 33, 811–28.

Bartter, F. C. and Schwartz, W. B. (1967) The syndrome of inappropriate secretion of antidiuretic hormone. *Am. J. Med.*, **42**, 780–806.

Berry, H., Ford-Hutchinson, A. W., Camp, A. V., Heywood, D., Molloy, M. G., James, D. W. and Hamilton, E. B. D. (1980) Antirheumatic activity of fenclofenac. *Ann. Rheum. Dis.*, **39**, 473–5.

Blackman, W. J. and Leckner, B. (1979) Clinical comparative evaluation of choline magnesium trisalicylate and acetylsalicylic acid in rheumatoid arthritis. *Rheumatol. Rehabil.*, **18**, 119–24.

Boardman, P. L. and Hart, F. D. (1967) Clinical measurement of the anti-inflammatory effects of salicylates in rheumatoid arthritis. *Br. Med. J.*, **4**, 264–8.

Bowden, R. E., Gill, J. R., Radfar, N., Taylor, A. A. and Keiser, H. R. (1978) Prostaglandin synthetase inhibitors in Bartter's syndrome. Effect on immunoreactive prostaglandin E excretion. *J. Am. Med. Assoc.*, **239**, 117–21.

Brewis, I. D. P. (1977) Ibuprofen and indomethacin in the treatment of rheumatoid arthritis. *Curr. Med. Res. Opinion*, **5**, 48–52.

Brezin, J. H., Katz, S. M., Schwartz, A. B. and Chinitz, H. L. (1979) Reversible renal failure and nephrotic syndrome associated with non-steroidal, anti-inflammatory drugs. *N. Engl. J. Med.*, **301**, 1271–3.

Brogden, R. N., Pinder, R. M., Speight, T. M. and Avery, G. S. (1977) Fenoprofen: a review of its pharmacological properties and therapeutic efficacy in rheumatic diseases. *Clinics Rheum. Dis.*, **13**, 241–65.

Brogden, R. N., Heil, R. C., Speight, T. M. and Avery, G. S. (1978) Tolmetin: A review of its pharmacological properties and therapeutic efficacy in rheumatic diseases. *Drugs*, **15**, 429–50.

Brogden, R. N., Heil, R. C., Speight, T. M. and Avery, G. S. (1979) Flurbiprofen: a review of its pharmacological properties and therapeutic use in rheumatic diseases. *Drugs*, **18**, 417–38.

Brogden, G. E., Speight, T. M., Pakes, G. E. and Avery, G. S. (1980) Diflunisal: a review of its pharmacological properties and therapeutic use in musculoskeletal strains and sprains and pains in osteoarthritis. *Drugs*, **19**, 84–106.

Brooks, P. M., Bell, M. A., Lee, P., Rooney, P. J. and Dick, W. C. (1974a) The effect of frusemide on indomethacin plasma levels. *Br. J. Clin. Pharmacol.*, **1**, 485–9.

Brooks, P. M., Bell, M. A., Sturrock, R. D., Famaey, J. P. and Dick, W. C. (1974b) The clinical significance of indomethacin–probenecid interaction. *Br. J. Clin. Pharmacol.*, **1**, 287–90.

Brooks, P. M. and Buchanan, W. W. (1976a) Azapropazone – its place in the management of rheumatoid conditions. *Curr. Med. Res. Opinion*, **4**, 94–100.

Brooks, P. M. and Buchanan, W. W. (1976) Current management of rheumatoid arthritis in *Recent Advances in Rheumatology* (ed. W. W. Buchanan and W. C. Dick), No. 1, Churchill Livingstone, Edinburgh, pp. 33–87.

Brooks, P. M., Mason, D. I. R., McNeil, R., Anderson, J. A. and Buchanan, W. W. (1976a) An assessment of the therapeutic potential of azapropazone in rheumatoid arthritis. *Curr. Med. Res. Opinion*, **4**, 50–6.

Brooks, P. M., Walker, J. T., Dick, W. C., Anderson, J. A. and Fowler, P. D. (1975) Phenylbutazone: a clinico-pharmacological study in rheumatoid arthritis. *Br. J. Clin. Pharmacol.*, **2**, 437–42.

Buchanan, W. W., Rooney, P. J. and Rennie, J. A. N. (1979) Aspirin and the salicylates. *Clin. Rheum. Dis.*, **5**, 499–539.

Buxton, R., Grennan, D. M. and Palmer, D. G. (1978) Fenbufen compared with indomethacin in osteoarthritis. *Curr. Med. Res. Opinion*, **5**, 682–7.

Calabro, J. J. (1978) Sulindac in the treatment of gout: multicase studies. *Eur. J. Rheumatol. Inflammation*, **1**, 21–33.

Cartwright, K. C., Trotter, T. L. and Cohen, M. C. (1979) Naproxen nephrotoxicity. *Arizona Med.*, 36, 124–6.

Ceuppens, J. L., Rodriguez, M. A. and Goodwin, G. S. (1982) Non-steroidal anti-inflammatory agents inhibit the synthesis of IgM rheumatoid factor *in vitro*. *Lancet*, i, 528–30.

Cohen, A. (1979) Fecal blood loss and plasma salicylate study of salicylsalicylic acid and aspirin. *J. Clin. Pharmacol.*, 19, 242–7.

Co-operating Clinics Committee of the American Rheumatism Association (1967) A three month trial of indomethacin in rheumatoid arthritis, with special reference to analysis and influence. *Clin. Pharmacol. Ther.*, 8, 11–37.

Cuthbert, M. F. (1974) Adverse reactions to non-steroidal anti-rheumatic drugs. *Curr. Med. Res. Opinion*, 2, 600–10.

Davies, J., Dixon, A. St. J. and Ring, E. F. J. (1981) A double-blind cross-over comparison of piroxicam and indomethacin in the treatment of rheumatoid arthritis. *Eur. J. Rheumatol. Inflammation*, 4, 314–17.

Davison, C. (1971) Salicylate metabolism in man. *Ann. N. Y. Acad. Sci.*, 179, 249–68.

Daymond, T. J., Thompson, M., Abbar, F. A. and Chertney, V. (1979) A controlled trial of tiaprofenic acid versus ibuprofen in rheumatoid arthritis. *Rheumatol. Rehabil.*, 18, 257–60.

Deodhar, S. D., McLeod, M. M., Dick, W. C. and Buchanan, W. W. (1977) A short term comparative trial of salsalate and indomethacin in rheumatoid arthritis. *Curr. Med. Res. Opinion*, 5, 185–8.

Donnelly, P., Lloyd, F. and Campbell, H. (1967) Indomethacin in rheumatoid arthritis: an evaluation of its anti-inflammatory and side effects. *Br. Med. J.*, 1, 69–75.

Doyle, D. (1981) An articular index for the assessment of osteoarthritis. *Ann. Rheum. Dis.*, 40, 75–8.

Dieppe, P. A., Doherty, M., Whicker, J. T. and Walter, G. (1981) The treatment of gout with azapropazone: clinical and experimental studies. *Eur. J. Rheumatol. Inflammation*, 4, 392–400.

Douthwaite, A. H. and Lintott, G. A. M. (1938) Gastroscopic observation of the effect of aspirin and certain other substances on the stomach. *Lancet*, ii, 1222–5.

Editorial (1979) Anti-inflammatory drugs and tumour growth. *Lancet*, i, 420–1.

Editorial (1980) Prostaglandin synthetase inhibition in obstetrics and after. *Lancet*, i, 185–90.

Editorial (1982) Benoxaprofen. *Br. Med. J.*, 285, 459–60.

Ehrlich, G. E. (1979) Tometin sodium: meeting the clinical challenge. *Clinics Rheum. Dis.*, 5, 481–97.

Ehrlich, G. E., Muller, S. B. and Seider, R. S. (1980) Choline magnesium trisalicylate versus ibuprofen in rheumatoid arthritis. *Rheumatol. Rehabil.*, 19, 30–41.

Emori, H. W., Paulus, H., Bluestone, R., Champion, G. D. and Pearson, C. (1976) Indomethacin serum concentrations in man. Effects of dosage, food and antacids. *Ann. Rheum. Dis.*, 35, 333–8.

Fields, W. S., Lemak, N. A., Frankouski, R. F., Hardy, R. J. and Bigelow, R. H. (1980) Implications of aspirin trials in transient ischaemic attacks and strokes. *Aspirin Symposium*. Academic Press, London, pp. 33–42.

Flower, R., Gryglewski, R., Harbaczyuska-Cectro, H. and Vane, J. R. (1972) Effects of anti-inflammatory drugs on prostaglandin biosynthesis. *Nature, New Biol.*, 238, 104–6.

Fowler, P. D. (1979) Voltarol: diclofenac sodium. *Clinics Rheum. Dis.*, 5, 427–64.

Geaney, P. D., Carver, J. G., Aronson, J. R. and Warlow, C. P. (1982) Interaction of azapropazone with phenytoin. *Br. Med. J.*, 284, 1372.

Godfrey, R. G. and De La Cruz, S. (1975) Effect of ibuprofen dosage on patient response in rheumatoid arthritis. *Arthr. Rheum.*, 18, 135–7.

Goldberg, A. A. J. and Godfrey, R. E. (1980) Fenclofenac. *Clinics Rheum. Dis.*, 6, 647–74.

Good, A. and Mena, H. (1977) Treatment of ankylosing spondylitis with flurbiprofen and indomethacin. *Curr. Med. Res. Opinion*, 5, 117–21.

Grennan, D. M., Aarons, L., Siddiqui, M., Richards, M., Thompson, R. and Higham, C. (1983) Dose–response study with ibuprofen in rheumatoid arthritis: clinical and pharmacokinetic findings. *Br. J. Clin. Pharmacol.*, 15, 311–16.

Grennan, D. M., Ferry, D. G., Ashworth, M. E., Kenney, R. E. and MacKinnon, M. (1979) The aspirin–ibuprofen interaction in rheumatoid arthritis. *Br. J. Clin. Pharmacol.*, 8, 497–503.

Grennan, D. M., Jolly, J., Holloway, C. J. and Palmer, D. G. (1979) Vasculitis in a patient receiving naproxen. *N. Z. Med. J.*, 89, 48–9.

Grennan, D. M., McLeod, M., Watkins, C. and Dick, W. C. (1976) Clinical assessment of azapropazone in rheumatoid arthritis. *Curr. Med. Res. Opinion*, 4, 44–9.

Hart, F. D. and Boardman, P. L. (1975) Ibuprofen (4-isobutylphenyl acetic acid). *Ann. Rheum. Dis.*, 24, 61.

Helberg, L. (1981) Clinical pharmacokinetics of indomethacin. *Clin. Pharmacokinet.*, 6, 245–58.

Henry, D. A. and Langman, M. J. S. (1981) Drugs as gastric irritants, in *Gastrointestinal Haemorrhage* (eds P. W. Dykes and M. R. B. Keighley), Wright, Bristol, pp. 49–59.

Herrich, W. L. (1983) Nephrotoxicity of non-steroidal anti-inflammatory agents. *Am. J. Kidney Dis.*, 2, 478–88.

Higgs, G. A. and Vane, J. R. (1983) Inhibition of cyclo-oxygenase and lipoxygenase. *Br. Med. Bull.*, 39, 265–70.

Higham, C., Aarons, L., Holt, P. J. L., Lynch, M. and Rowland, M. (1981) A chronic dose-ranging study of the pharmacokinetics of phenylbutazone in rheumatoid arthritic patients. *Br. J. Clin. Pharmacol.*, 12, 123–9.

Hurst, A. and Lintott, G. A. M. (1939) Aspirin as a cause of haematemesis. *Guy's Hosp. Rep.*, 89, 173–6.

Huskisson, E. C. (1978) Sulindac. *Eur. J. Rheumatol. Inflammation*, 1, 3–6.

Huskisson, E. C., Woolf, D. L. Baum, H. W., Scott, J. and Franklyn, S. (1979) Four new anti-inflammatory drugs: responses and variations. *Eur. J. Rheumatol.*, 2, 29–32.

Inman, W. H. W. (1977) Study of fatal bone marrow depression with reference to phenylbutazone and oxyphenbutazone. *Br. Med. J.*, 1, 1500–5.

Jones, C. J. (1976) The pharmacology and pharmacokinetics of azapropazone – a review. *Curr. Med. Res. Opinion*, 4, 3–16.

Kakkar, V. V. (1980) Aspirin – the prevention of venous thrombosis. *Aspirin Symposium 1980*. Academic Press, London, pp. 63–8.

Kent, T. H., Cordell, R. M. and Stamler, F. W. (1969) Small intestinal ulcers and intestinal flora in rats given indomethacin. *Am. J. Pathol.*, 54, 237–45.

Lasagna, L. (1961) Analgesic drugs. *Am. J. Med. Sci.*, 242, 620–7.

Lassus, A. (1976) A comparative study of azapropazone and indomethacin in the treatment of psoriatic arthritis and Reiter's disease. *Curr. Med. Res. Opinion*, 4, 65–9.

Levy, M. (1974) Aspirin use in patients with major upper gastro-intestinal bleeding and peptic-ulcer disease. *N. Engl. J. Med.*, 290, 1158–62.

Lewis, G. P. (1983) Immunoregulatory activity of metabolites of arachidonic acid and their role in inflammation. *Br. Med. Bull.*, 39, 243–8.

McGiff, J. C. (1977) Bartter's syndrome results from an imbalance of vasoactive hormones. *Ann. Intern. Med.*, 87, 369–72.

McLean, W. (1983) Personal communication. DHSS Statistics and Research Division.

Marbet, G. A., Auckert, F., Walter, M., Six, P. and Airenne, H. (1977) Interaction study between phenprocoumon and flurbiprofen. *Curr. Med. Res. Opinion*, 5, 16–31.

Mavrikakis, M. E., MacLeod, M., Buchanan, W. W., Hernandez, L. A. and Rennie, J. A. N. (1977) Mefenamic acid: an under-rated antirheumatic? *Curr. Med. Res. Opinion*, 4, 535–9.

Mawdsley, P. (1979) Fenbufen. *Clinics Rheum. Dis.*, 6, 615–32.

Mielants, H., Veys, E. M., Verbrugen, G. and Schielstraeti, H. (1979) Salicylate-induced gastrointestinal bleeding. *J. Rheumatol.*, 6, 210–8.

Mintz, G. and Fraga, A. (1976) Gastro-intestinal bleeding in patients with rheumatoid arthritis: the effects of azapropazone treatment. *Curr. Med. Res. Opinion*, 4, 89–93.

Mitchell, W. S., Scott, P., Kennedy, A. C., Brooks, P. M., Templeton, R. and Jeffries, M. G. (1975) Clinicopharmacological studies in ketoprofen (Orudis). *Curr. Med. Res. Opinion*, 3, 423–30.

Mowat, A. G., Ansell, B. M., Gumpel, F. M., Hill, A. E. H., Hill, A. G. S. and Stoppard, M. (1979) Naproxen in rheumatoid arthritis. Extended trial: further report. *Eur. J. Rheumatol. Inflammation*, 2, 19–24.

Muir, A. (1963) Salicylates, dyspepsia and peptic ulceration in *Salicylates, an International Symposium* (ed. A. St. J. Dixon, M. J. H. Smith, B. K. Martin and P. N. H. Wood), Churchill, London, p. 231.

New Zealand Rheumatism Association (1974) Aspirin and the kidney. *Br. Med. J.*, 1, 593–6.

Norby, L., Flamenbaum, W., Leutz, R. *et al.* (1976) Prostaglandins and aspirin therapy in Bartter's syndrome. *Lancet*, ii, 604–6.

O'Grady, J. and Moncada, S. (1978) Aspirin: a paradoxical effect on bleeding time. Lancet, ii, 780.

Palmer, D. G., Barbezat, G. O., Gibbons, B. L., Grennan, D. M., Lunn, J., Myers, D. B. and Wilson, K. (1981) A single-blind trial of the anti-inflammatory drug sodium meclofenamate, including an evaluation of the dynamics of grip and of lymphocyte responsiveness. *Curr. Med. Res. Opinion*, 7, 359–69.

Palmer, D. G., Ferry, D. G. and Gibbons, D. C. (1981) Ibuprofen and diflusinal in rheumatoid arthritis – a double-blind trial. *N. Z. Med. J.*, 94, 45–7.

Paulus, H. E. and Furst, D. E. (1979) Aspirin and non-steroidal anti-inflammatory drugs. in *Arthritis and Allied Conditions* (ed. J. McCarty), Lea and Febiger, Philadelphia, pp. 331–54.

Petersen, P. B., Husted, S., Mortensen, A. and Andreasen, F. (1979) The effect of daily administration of naproxen in the antithrombin complex activity in patients under long-term therapy with phenprocoxen. *Scand. J. Rheumatol.*, 8, 54–6.

Pottier, J., Berlin, D. and Raynaud, J. P. (1977) Pharmacokinetics of the anti-inflammatory tiaprofenic acid in humans, mice, rats, rabbits and dogs. *J. Pharmacol. Sci.*, 66, 1030–6.

Ranlov, P. J., Nielsen, S. P. and Barenholdt, D. (1983) Faecal blood loss during administration of acetylsalicylic acid, ketoprofen and two new ketoprofen sustained release compounds. *Scand. J. Rheumatol.*, 12, 280–4.

Rees, W. D. W. and Turnberg, L. A. (1980) Reappraisal of the effects of aspirin on the stomach. *Lancet*, ii, 410–12.

Rennie, J. A. W., MacLeod, M. M., Reynolds, R. G. and El-Ghobarvey, A. F. (1977) Comparison of sodium meclofenamate and indomethacin in rheumatoid arthritis. *Curr. Med. Res. Opinion*, 4, 580–3.

Rhymer, A. R. (1979) Sulindac. *Clinics Rheum. Dis.*, 5, 553–68.

Rhymer, A. R. and Gengos, D. C. (1979) Indomethacin. *Clinics Rheum. Dis.*, 5, 541–52.

Ridolfo, A. S., Nichander, R. and Mikulasckek, W. M. (1979) Fenoprofen and benoxaprofen. *Clinics Rheum. Dis.*, 5, 393–410.

Ritch, A. E. S., Perera, W. N. R. and Jones, C. J. (1982) Pharmacokinetics of azapropazone in the elderly. *Br. J. Clin. Pharmacol.*, 14, 116–19.

Rogers, H. J., Spector, R. G., Morrison, P. J. and Bradbrook, I. D. (1981) Comparative steady state pharmacokinetic study of piroxicam and flurbiprofen in normal subjects. *Eur. J. Rheumatol. Rehabil.*, 4, 303–8.

Ruest, O., Biland, L., Thilo, D., Nyman, D. and Duckert, F. (1975) Testing of the antirheumatic drug tolmetin for interaction with oral anticoagulants. *Schewize Med. Wochenschr.*, 105, 752–3.

Sasisekhar, P. R., Penn, R. G., Haslock, I. and Wright, V. (1973) A comparison of benorylate and aspirin in the treatment of rheumatoid arthritis. *Rheumatol. Rehabil.* (Suppl.), 31–8.

Seaman, W. E., Ishak, K. G. and Plotz, P. H. (1974) Aspirin-induced hepatotoxicity in patients with systemic lupus erythematous. *Ann. Int. Med.*, 80, 1–8.

Segre, E. S. (1979) Naproxen. *Clinics Rheum. Dis.*, 5, 411–26.

Sheldrake, F. E., Webber, J. M. and Marsh, B. P. (1977) A long-term assessment of flurbiprofen. *Curr. Med. Res. Opinion*, 5, 106–16.

Sydnes, O. A. (1969) A controlled trial of flufenamic acid in rheumatoid arthritis. *Ann. Phys. Med.*, Suppl. 93–8.

Sydnes, O. A. (1981) Comparison of piroxicam with naproxen in rheumatoid arthritis: a double-blind, cross-over multicentre study. *Eur. J. Rheumatol. Inflammation*, 4, 318–22.

Tamisier, J. N. (1979) Ketoprofen. *Clinics Rheum. Dis.*, 5, 381–91.

Templeton, J. S. (1981) Azapropazone – Twice or four times daily? *Eur. J. Rheumatol. Inflammation*, 4, 401–7.

Tudhope, G. R. (1967) Comparison of flufenamic acid with aspirin and paracetamol in terms of gastrointestinal blood loss. *Ann. Phys. Med.*, Suppl., 58–61.

Vaisrub, S. (1978) Bartter's syndrome – limelight on prostaglandins. *J. Am. Med. Assoc.*, 239, 137–8.

Vakil, B. J., Kulkami, R. D., Kulkanja, V. N., Mehta, D. J., Granpure, M. B. and Pisfati, P. K. (1977) Estimation of gastro-intestinal blood loss in volunteers treated with non-steroidal anti-inflammatory agents. *Curr. Med. Res. Opinion*, 5, 32–7.

Vergara-Castro, J. M., Avias, L. F. and Greenberg, B. P. (1976) A comparative clinical trial of fenbrufen and indomethacin in patients with rheumatoid arthritis. *J. Int. Med. Res.*, 4, 418–26.

Watkins, J., Abbot, E. C., Hensby, C. N., Webster, J. and Dollery, C. T. (1980) Attenuation of hypotensive effect of propranolol and thiazide diuretics by indomethacin. *Br. Med. J.*, 281, 702–5.

Wax, J., Clinger, W. A., Varner, P. *et al.* (1970) Relationship of the enterohepatic cycle to ulcerogenesis in the rat small bowel with flufenamic acid. *Gastroenterology*, 58, 772–80.

Widmark, P. (1978) Safety and efficacy of piroxicam in the treatment of acute gout. *Eur. J. Rheumatol. Inflammation*, 1, 346–8.

Winder, C. V., Kaump, D. J., Glazko, A. J. and Holmes, E. L. (1967) Pharmacology of the fenemates. Experimental observations on flufenamic mefenamic and meclofenamic acids. *Ann. Phys. Med.*, Suppl. 7–49.

Wiseman, E. H. and Boyle, J. A. (1980) Piroxicam (Feldene). *Clinics Rheum. Dis.*, 6, 585–613.

Wojtulewski, J., Walter, J. and Thornton, E. J. (1981) Tiaprofenic acid (Surgam) in the treatment of osteoarthritis of the knee and hip. *Rheumatol. Rehabil.*, 20, 177–80.

CHAPTER 8

Corticosteroids in

rheumatic diseases

Vera C. M. Neumann

8.1 INTRODUCTION

The view popularly held by rheumatologists in the UK today is that there is little or no justification for the use of systemic corticosteroids (steroids) in rheumatoid arthritis (RA). Yet, in a recent survey of our own rheumatology clinic we have found that 30% of patients were currently taking systemic steroids, and a further 6% had previously been on steroids (Wright *et al.*, unpublished observations). We believe our clinic is not unusual in this respect. Whatever the reasons for this discrepancy between what we preach and what we practise, it is clear that the role of steroids in RA urgently needs reappraisal. The aim of this chapter is to weigh up the benefits and risks of steroids in rheumatoid arthritis and some other rheumatic disorders.

8.2 SYSTEMIC THERAPY IN RHEUMATOID ARTHRITIS

The benefits are both obvious and predictable; immediate relief of pain and stiffness in the joints, associated with a reduction in the clinical signs of inflammation. These effects are often accompanied by a general sense of well-being. Also in the short term, there are few overt adverse effects. Patients may notice fluid retention or dyspepsia, but generally in the short term they tolerate all steroids well, and therefore compliance is good.

This must be weighed against the disadvantages of systemic steroids, the most important of which is the vast array of side effects. The major problem with the side effects listed above is that they are not only dose related but also detectable at daily doses of corticosteroids that are insufficient to control the inflammation of RA. Interference with the hypothalamo-pituitary-adrenal (HPA) axis has been detected with doses as low as 3 g nocte for two years (Chamberlain and Keenan, 1976). In this study significant clinical improvement after two years was only seen in patients taking 5 mg nocte. Furthermore, with larger doses of prednisolone (40–100 mg m^{-2}) adrenal suppression is detectable by an impaired response to synacthen after only seven days' treatment (Spiegel *et al.*, 1979). This problem of suppression of the HPA axis varies from one corticosteroid to another and is not directly related to the ability to reduce inflammation. Thus, 1 mg of betamethasone is equivalent to a maximum of 8 mg prednisolone in terms of ability to reduce inflammation. However, at these doses betamethasone produces significantly more suppression of endogenous cortisol production than prednisolone (Downie *et al.*, 1978). Table 8.1 shows doses of steroids producing equivalent suppression of inflammation.

TABLE 8.1
Steroid doses producing equivalent anti-inflammatory effects

	mg
Prednisolone or prednisone	5
Cortisone	25
Hydrocortisone (cortisol)	20
Methylprednisolone or triamcinolone	4
Paramethasone	2
Dexa- or betamethasone	0.7

Another worrying aspect of the use of corticosteroids is their ability to produce osteoporosis. The problem is complex in RA, for it has been known for over 100 years that RA itself can produce osteoporosis. Though this is most pronounced in bone next to affected joints, cortical thinning and increased bone resorption have been observed in rib biopsies from patients who have not received steroids, implying a generalized effect of the disease (Duncan *et al.*, 1965). This observation of a generalized reduction in bone density has been confirmed by different workers using various methods. With the exception of a study by Oka *et al.* (1975) it is generally agreed that osteoporosis is related to disease duration and severity (McConkey *et al.*, 1965; Kennedy *et al.*, 1974). However, there is little doubt that corticosteroids can produce osteoporosis over and above that due to the disease itself. In a recent survey by Reid *et al.* (1982), patients with RA on less than 10 mg per day of prednisolone had a significant reduction of total body calcium (measured by neutron activation analysis) when compared with RA patients treated without steroids. In this study, as in the earlier work by Kennedy et al. (1974), postmenopausal women fared worst when treated with steroids. However, the longer disease duration and greater steroid dosage used in the patients in Reid's study make the findings difficult to interpret.

One point to note is that osteoporosis alone is not a problem unless it is severe enough to lead to fractures. Whilst vertebral crush fractures or wedging were often reported in the early days of steroid use, with the advent of a more cautious use of steroids in lower doses in RA such complications are probably less common. The true frequency is not known. The more sensitive methods now available for estimating bone mass, such as neutron activation analysis, may be detecting a laboratory abnormality too small to be of clinical relevance (Reid's paper makes no mention of the frequency of fractures or other complications of osteoporosis in his patients).

Several disease factors as well as steroid therapy may interact in the development of osteoporosis in RA. Immobilization has long been recognized as a cause of bone loss both in man and experimental animals (Hulley et al., 1971; Mattson, 1972). Bone mass is initially lost at a rate of 4% per month. Thus, diffuse osteoporosis in RA could be a consequence of the disease process itself or due to immobilization by bed rest and splintage. Since immobilization was a popular form of therapy at a time when steroids were in vogue for RA, the problem of osteoporosis would have been aggravated. Since small doses of steroids can provide pain relief they could potentially allow a patient greater mobility, and, paradoxically, increase bone mass. There is already some evidence that modest physical exercise can increase lumbar vertebral density in postmenopausal women (Krolner et al., 1983). No such work has been done in patients with RA.

Linked with the problem of osteoporosis is that of ligamentous or tendon damage in RA. Once again the disease process itself can lead to injury of these structures. Nevertheless, the study by Rasker and Cosh (1978) clearly showed an association between steroids on cervical subluxation and arthritis mutilans in RA over and above that due to the disease itself. Recently, Rudge and Lloyd-Jones (1980) have demonstrated that patients who have never had a rheumatic disorder involving the neck can develop cervical subluxation if treated with chronic steroids for other disorders such as chronic chest diseases. Achilles tendon rupture has also been reported in patients taking systemic steroids for conditions other than RA (Haines, 1983).

Avascular necrosis of bone, particularly of the femoral head, is another of the steroid side effects that deserves special mention here. Once again, it is not confined to patients receiving steroids for rheumatic disorders, but has been reported in patients with such diverse disorders as glomerulonephritis and Addison's disease (Williams and Corbett, 1983). Its aetiology is unknown. The most likely hypothesis so far proposed is that steroids cause hyperlipidaemia;

fat emboli may then lodge in the vasculature supplying areas such as the femoral head (Cruess *et al.*, 1975).

So far this review has discussed insidious side effects of steroids. Other more dramatic adverse effects were well recognized in the original MRC trial (Joint Committee, 1959) of prednisolone versus aspirin in RA. Out of eight patients on 20 mg prednisolone daily for three months, four developed bleeding or perforation of peptic ulcers and a further patient developed psychosis. The paper concludes that this frequency of life-threatening side effects is 'clearly unacceptable'. Two questions then arise; can steroids be given in other ways to minimize their adverse effects, and do other methods of steroid administration affect their efficacy?

Although the prevailing view is that steroids do not modify the course of RA (Dick, 1978), the first reports of the combined MRC and Nuffield Foundation Studies showed that patients on cortisone had marginally less radiological progression of their RA than patients treated with aspirin alone (Joint Committee, 1957). This finding was confirmed when the Joint Committee reported again in 1959. An improvement in functional capacity of the prednisolone treated patients was also seen. However, since these large studies were performed the efficacy of daily oral prednisolone has not been closely examined. A recent study of 97 elderly patients (greater than 65 years old) with RA, treated with an average daily dose of 5–7.5 mg prednisolone, showed clinical improvement in all but three patients. Seventy-three patients showed a persistent fall in ESR. This study was retrospective and uncontrolled, and can tell us little about radiological progression. However, it does show that prednisolone is well tolerated in the elderly. Only three patients stopped this drug, one because of an osteoporotic fracture, one because of gastrointestinal problems, and one because she 'felt better' (Lockie *et al.*, 1983).

Another approach to the problem of trying to achieve clinical improvement with the minimum of side effects has been to use intermittent dosage. One of the earliest methods was to give oral prednisolone on alternate days. This was advocated by Harter *et al.* (1963). This produces less adrenal suppression than daily steroid regimes, and more recently has been shown to produce significantly less growth retardation in children given steroids for juvenile chronic arthritis (Byron *et al.*, 1983).

Where a daily dose of prednisolone is used, it is better to opt for a single morning dose, since this produces less adrenal suppression than divided doses (Myles *et al.*, 1971). This may be the best alternative for patients already established on steroids. Such patients often find symptomatic relief inadequate with the alternate day regimes. In a recent study of 24 such patients who had been on oral prednisolone for a mean of 8.5 years, only 10 were able to change to alternate day dosage (Fitzcharles *et al.*, 1982). Interestingly, two-thirds of the patients who found conversion to alternate day treatment impossible in this study were poor responders in a short synacthen test. Possibly, patients with adrenal insufficiency are unable to use endogenous steroid production to compensate for variation in steroid levels produced by an alternate day regime. Thus, initiating steroids on alternate days only may achieve a more satisfactory response than later conversion to alternate day treatment.

8.3   STEROIDS FOR THE SYSTEMIC COMPLICATIONS OF RHEUMATOID ARTHRITIS

The value of systemic steroids in patients with the more serious complications of RA, such as systemic vasculitis, pulmonary involvement, or pericardial involvement, is widely accepted. In fact, few controlled trials have been carried out on the use of steroids for these complications; such trials would be difficult because of the relative rarity of the complications. Also, as the patients are often severely ill, there is a tendency to try all possible therapies. Our own policy is to try pulsed methylprednisolone, either alone or combined with cytotoxic therapy such as cyclophosphamide or chlorambucil.

8.4   STEROIDS IN SYSTEMIC LUPUS ERYTHEMATOSUS

Whereas in RA many rheumatologists condemn the use of systemic steriods at any time, a viewpoint which the author regards as extreme, in systemic lupus erythematosus (SLE) the reverse is true. Steroids, often in high doses, are prescribed for most patients despite a paucity of supporting evidence and plenty of evidence showing that high dose steroids can lead to increased morbidity. For example, the frequency of aseptic hip necrosis in patients with SLE shows an almost linear relationship with the magnitude and duration of corticosteroid dosage (Dimant, 1978). Steroids are also likely to be the most important factor leading to the increased frequency of infection in SLE (Quismorio and Dubois, 1975). SLE usually runs a benign course. In a prospective study of 50 patients, Grigor *et al.* (1978) showed that the disease has a 98% 5-year survival rate. Most SLE patients in the study were managed on 7.5–15 mg of prednisolone on alternate days; at these doses, the frequency of infection was low and no new cases of aseptic bone necrosis occurred. Conventional textbook teaching is that steroids are required for active disease involving the central nervous system (CNS), kidneys or lungs, or causing a haemolytic anaemia (Hughes, 1977). There is tendency to give steroids in very high doses, often as intravenous pulsed therapy, to treat these complications. The rationale for the use of pulsed steroids for renal involvement is that the morphological lesions in renal biopsies obtained from patients with lupus nephritis are similar to those obtained from patients with renal transplants during rejection episodes. In the 1970s it became fashionable to manage acute rejection episodes with pulsed methylprednisolone. This fashion was then transferred to the treatment of lupus nephritis with encouraging results. However, since recent evidence has suggested that low dose oral prednisolone is as effective in the treatment of renal transplant rejection episodes, the treatment of lupus nephritis needs to be reviewed (Adu and Cameron, 1982; Orta-Sibu *et al.*, 1982). Furthermore, in a survey of 107 patients with lupus nephritis, 7 out of 28 patients treated with prednisolone developed end-stage renal failure, whereas only 4 out of 38 patients treated with oral or intravenous tri-monthly cyclophosphamide developed renal failure. Thus, the treatment choice for SLE with renal involvement should be cyclophosphamide in combination with steroids rather than steroids alone.

Intravenous cyclophosphamide has also been found effective in agranulocytosis in SLE previously unresponsive to steroids. Full CNS involvement in SLE is usually treated with high-dose steroids. The value of this therapy must again be questioned. There is little doubt that high-dose steroids can cause as well as cure CNS problems. Ayoub (1983) described three cases of SLE with no previous CNS problems who developed severe neurological abnormalities shortly after receiving three 1 g pulses of methylprednisolone. However, all three patients were also on oral steroids in doses of up to 80 mg daily. Another argument against the use of aggressive steroid therapy for CNS involvement is that milder disease, particularly neuro-psychiatric problems, are far commoner and more benign than originally thought. There is evidence suggesting that this manifestation of SLE waxes and wanes independently of steroid dosage (Grigor *et al.*, 1978). For severe CNS involvement steroids remain the best available therapy and can sometimes produce dramatic and clinical improvement. We have recently observed a patient with chorea in whom the disease had been present for nearly a month and disappeared within 24 hours of a 1 g pulse of methylprednisolone (McKenna *et al.*, 1986).

Pulmonary involvement in SLE is varied in its manifestation and in its response to steroids. Thus, pleural effusions usually resolve whereas pneumonitis responds less well and carries a more serious prognosis. As with CNS or renal involvement, there is good reason for cautious use of steroids since the frequency of lung infections in SLE is high (Turner-Stokes and Turner-Warwick, 1982).

Conclusions: Steroids are not required routinely in SLE. They are often helpful in the more severe manifestations of the disease but controversy surrounds the necessary dose for each complication. Other therapies may be more effective and supersede steroids. These include cyclophosphamide which is already gaining importance in the treatment of lupus nephritis. The value of other alternative therapies, such as antimalarials, has probably been underestimated. These may prove a useful adjunct, even in patients with the more severe manifestations of SLE (Lanham and Hughes, 1982). Regarding steroids in dermatomyositis, as with SLE, conventional teaching is that large doses are required. However, a survey by Miller *et al.* (1958) showed that small doses

(1 mg/kg) were successful in severe juvenile dermatomyositis. These doses were not associated with severe complications.

8.5   STEROIDS IN POLYARTERITIS NODOSA AND WEGENER'S GRANULOMATOSIS

These diseases appear to be partially responsive to steroids. Thus an early report by the MRC Collagen Diseases Panel (1960) found that 5-year survival of patients with polyarteritis nodosa (PAN) improved from 13 to 43% with steroid treatment. Pulsed methylprednisolone has also been found successful in two cases of PAN with glomerular nephritis and pulmonary involvement that were previously unresponsive to oral steroids. However, in Wegener's granulomatosis, a combination of steroids plus cyclophosphamide is more effective than steroids alone, the former giving a mean remission time of four years, whereas the latter only gave a mean survival time of 12.5 months (Fauci, 1982).

8.6   STEROIDS IN POLYMYALGIA RHEUMATICA AND GIANT CELL ARTERITIS

These disorders are characterized by their dramatic response to steroids and are the most clear-cut indication for their use in rheumatology. Steroids are obligatory in giant cell arteritis (GCA) where they can prevent blindness, and almost always necessary in polymyalgia rheumatica (PMR).

PMR is an insidious disorder in which the virtual absence of physical signs can make diagnosis difficult. The response to steroids can be used as a diagnostic test. The patient is given one week's treatment with placebo (usually a vitamin tablet), followed by one week's oral prednisolone, followed by one week's placebo; the patient should respond only in the middle week. The main debate about steroids in PMR and GCA is how much prednisolone to use and for how long. This question has recently been tackled by Behn *et al.* (1983) in a prospective study of 176 patients, 114 of whom had PMR and 62 of whom had GCA. In patients with PMR, 10 mg of prednisolone was sufficient as an initial dose, and for most patients with GCA 20 mg of prednisolone per day was adequate. In this study, once an ESR of less than 30 had been achieved, daily prednisolone was reduced by 1 mg per month. For those receiving 10 mg per day, the dosage reduction was slightly quicker with patients on higher doses. Seventy-two patients were able to stop treatment after a mean of 31 months, but 30 of these subsequently relapsed and had to re-start steroids. The main lessons we can learn from this study are that the very high initial steroid doses formally used in GCA are seldom required and that the diseases are so variable in duration that rigid treatment regimes are inappropriate. The authors also recommend monitoring patients for at least two years after stopping steroids.

Patients with PMR on steroids are said to be less prone to side effects than patients with other rheumatic disorders. However, this view is based on anecdotal evidence. Pharmacokinetic data indicate that the drug is metabolized equally well in PMR and RA (Taggart, unpublished observations). Therefore, a sensible policy is to use the minimum effective dose of steroids, preferably as a single morning dose as divided doses are likely to produce more adrenal suppression. About two-thirds of patients can be converted from daily to alternate-day prednisolone once their disease is under control (Bengtsson and Malmvall, 1981). Once again this would reduce the tendency to develop side effects.

Azathioprine has been tried as a steroid sparing agent, but with limited success. The mean daily steroid dose could only be reduced by less than 3 mg (De Silva and Hazleman, 1983). Two-thirds of the patients in this study 'dropped out' before completion so no definite conclusions can be reached.

8.7   STEROIDS IN ANKYLOSING SPONDYLITIS

There is no place for continuous systemic steroids in ankylosing spondylitis (AS). This chronic disorder is usually adequately managed with anti-inflammatory drugs and physiotherapy alone. There may, however, be a place for short courses of steroids to alleviate pain and stiffness and thus facilitate physiotherapy in those few patients who are otherwise unable to tolerate conventional physiotherapy. Good results have also been reported using pulsed methylprednisolone in five patients with severe AS previously unresponsive to treatment (Mintz *et al.*, 1981). Prolonged or delayed effects on immune function have been reported after this therapy (Richter *et al.*, 1983). However, the clinical relevance of these effects is doubtful since in this study maximum clinical improvement was seen at one week and deterioration had occurred at 4 weeks, whilst disturbance of some immune functions only appeared after 8 weeks. Both the above studies were uncontrolled. We are currently evaluating pulsed methylprednisolone in combination with physiotherapy in patients with severe ankylosing spondylitis in a double-blind controlled study.

Local steroids may be required occasionally for peripheral joint involvement and local or systemic steroids are used for treatment of iritis occurring in association with AS, although their role may be superseded by chlorambucil or cyclosporin A.

8.8   STEROIDS IN OSTEOARTHROSIS

The hazards of administering systemic steroids to the older population affected by osteoarthrosis (OA) are considerable. This population already has an increased frequency of osteoporosis and is thus more likely to develop complications if steroids worsen the osteoporosis. Peptic ulceration is potentially more dangerous in the elderly. Moreover, there is no evidence that systemic steroids improve osteoarthrosis. The risks of intra-articular steroids are the same as in rheumatoid arthritis but the efficacy of steroids given this way is not established. Early studies by Wright *et al.* (1960) and Miller *et al.* (1958) failed to show that hydrocortisone was superior to placebo. As discussed later, triamcinolone is likely to be superior to hydrocortisone and needs a fuller evaluation in OA. Radio-isotope synovectomy has also been recommended, both in OA and pyrophosphate arthropathy. In the latter disorder, clinical improvement with yttrium 90 plus triamcinolone was superior to triamcinolone alone, but radiological progression was unaffected by both treatments (Doherty and Dieppe, 1981).

Very little work has been done on the use of chemical agents or synovectomy in OA.

8.9　LOCAL STEROIDS AND OTHER LOCAL THERAPIES

8.9.1　Local steroids

In contrast to systemic steroids this form of steroid administration is widely accepted as safe and useful for RA and for certain other non-infective inflammatory arthropathies (e.g. those of the spondarthritis group). Though most often used for intra-articular injections, steroids can also be useful for soft tissue lesions associated with RA. The carpal tunnel syndrome can be controlled by between one and three injections of triamcinolone avoiding the need for surgical decompression in over 80% of patients. This is particularly useful when the syndrome occurs during pregnancy. 'Trigger' fingers can also be helped by a local injection into the synovial sheath, though the risk of tendon rupture must be remembered.

Intra-articular steroids are most useful in RA when one or a few joints are causing particular problems, and should be regarded as an adjunct but not a substitute for systemic therapy. Their effect is transient, its duration depending on which steroid preparation is used; hydrocortisone acetate has effects lasting two weeks, methylprednisolone acetate three to four weeks, and triamcinolone hexacetonide six weeks. Giving steroids intra-articularly does not completely avoid the risk of systemic side effects. Adrenal suppression occurs after repeated intra-articular injections of triamcinolone (Esselinckx *et al.*, 1982), methylprednisolone or prednisolone (Bird *et al.*, 1979). The effect is transient and less profound than after oral steroids. Other problems associated with intra-articular injections are an acute inflammatory synovitis occurring within a few hours of the injection. This is thought to be due to irritation produced by crystals within the joint and occurs in 2% of injections. This seems to be linked to the use of steroids with particular characteristics; poor water solubility, crystal size of 0.5–20 μm. Hydrocortisone acetate, which is particularly liable to cause these 'flares' of synovitis, has these characteristics (McCarty and Hogan, 1964). Infection is another potential hazard after intra-articular injection, which fortunately occurs very rarely. In Hollander's (1972) large series of 250 000 injections, only 18 cases of infection were reported. This hazard is minimized by careful skin cleansing and the use of a 'no-touch' technique with a sterile syringe and needle. Full operation cleansing procedures are unnecessary. A wise precaution is to aspirate fluid from a joint before injection. This ensures that steroid injections are not placed into infected joints. It also reduces the likelihood of injecting steroid into the soft tissues outside the joint. Steroids injected into the skin can cause local atrophy. The final hazard associated with intra-articular steroids is that the steroid may cause fissuring and cystic lesions in articular cartilage (Salter *et al.*, 1967). It may also lead to decreased cartilage and matrix synthesis (Mankin and Conger, 1966) and increased proteoglycan loss from cartilage suggesting cartilage degradation (Sedgwick *et al.*, 1983). However, this evidence is all derived from animal work. The only evidence of joint damage occurring in man as a result of intra-articular steroids is from patients in whom repeated injections were given over prolonged periods. Chandler *et al.* (1959) reported the case of a doctor's wife who presented with mild osteoarthrosis of the hip and later developed a Charcot-like derangement of the joint. A review of this patient's history showed that she had had a total of 900 mg of hydrocortisone injected into her hip. Alarcon-Segovia and Ward (1966) reported a similar problem in a woman who had had over 3000 mg of intra-articular steroid injections for osteoarthrosis in the hands and had developed gross derangement of several joints. However, used sparingly (two to three times a year) this complication does not present a problem and most patients treated with intra-articular steroids do well (Balch *et al.*, 1977).

8.9.2   Liposomes

These are microscopic spheres varying in diameter between 25 nm and several microns, composed of one or more concentric phospholipid bi-layers. They are formed simultaneously by contact of dry phospholipids with excess water and can trap solids in the process. By varying lipid composition and size, an almost infinite number of liposome versions can be produced. The relevance of liposomes here is that they have been used as vehicles for the injection of steroids into joints. Their advocates have claimed that liposomes prolong retention of steroids within joints (De Silva *et al.*, 1979). However, the pattern of thermographic improvement in joints reported by this group resembles that of short-acting rather than long-acting steroids, and their superiority over conventional intra-articular steroid injections is disputed (Bird *et al.*, 1979).

The liposomes described above were synthesized with cortisol palmitate. Recently more stable liposomes, where the steroid is chemically linked to the phospholipids, have been synthesized and may yield more promising results.

8.9.3 Other local therapies in rheumatoid arthritis

Apart from steroids, a number of other substances have been injected intra-articularly in order to achieve a remission of synovitis. These fall into two broad categories: (a) beta emitting radio-isotopes and (b) chemical agents.

(a) Radio-isotopes

These were introduced many years ago and have been found useful in the treatment of malignant effusions in serous cavities. Ansell *et al.* (1963) had the good idea of applying this kind of treatment to chronic effusions of the knee. Their first results using 10 mCi of radioactive gold were encouraging, but the colloid was not particularly effective when the knee effusion was associated with marked soft tissue swelling. Ansell suggested that yttrium 90 was more suitable for treating thick synovitis in the knee. The choice of isotopes for use in a particular joint should depend on a number of factors: the isotope should be reasonably easy to obtain, it should be non-toxic and chemically pure. Tissue destruction should be effected by a beta emission of sufficient energy to penetrate the synovium. To minimize radiation damage to tissues outside the joint there should be little or no associated gamma emission, as its energy is released not only in the joint but also far away from it. Whole body irradiation due to leakage of isotope from a joint can also be much reduced by using a short half-life isotope. Colloids are used instead of soluble isotopes, since the latter would rapidly diffuse out of the joint injected. Very large colloid particles might lead to an uneven radiation, and a particle size of about 100 nm is usually chosen. Whereas yttrium is suitable for knee synovectomy, there is too much penetration of radiation for safe use of this isotope in smaller joints. Rhenium 186 is suitable for medium-sized joints and erbium 169 for small joints such as digital joints. The joint should also be immobilized for three days after injection. This has been shown to restrict the spread of isotopes and to decrease the frequency of chromosomal damage in peripheral blood lymphocytes (Chapelle *et al.*, 1972; Lloyd and Reeder, 1978).

Despite the fact that yttrium synovectomies of the knee compare well with surgical synovectomy and are preferred by patients (Gumpel and Roles, 1975), the technique of radiation synovectomy has never gained widespread popularity. There are several reasons for this. Intra-articular steroids are more freely available than isotopes, and the longer-acting steroids such as triamcinolone can give comparable results. Clinicians administering isotopes are required to attend a period of instruction in the handling of isotopes. The possibility of teratogenesis precludes the use of radioactive material in patients of child-bearing age. Finally, the need to immobilize injected joints has until recently required hospital admission and bed rest, though Williams *et al.* (1981) have shown that for knee injection, allowing patients to mobilize with a plaster of Paris cylinder around the injected joint is satisfactory.

(b) *Chemical synovectomy*

A large number of chemicals have been tried and include lactic acid, aspirin, methotrexate, nitrogen mustard, thiotepa, rifamycin SV, orgotein, and osmic acid. Aspirin was found to be no better than saline alone (Rylance *et al.*, 1980), though this controlled study was too small for firm conclusions to be made. Methotrexate has been tried by several groups (Marks *et al.*, 1976; Bird *et al.*, 1977; Wigginton *et al.*, 1980) and has been found to be less effective than intra-articular steroids. Nitrogen mustard failed to produce a lasting remission and has the potential hazards of severe leukopenia and thrombocytopenia, as well as producing nausea from systemic spread of the drug (Vainio and Julkunen, 1960). In an uncontrolled study of thiotepa, only seven out of 30 patients did well, 50% showed increasing deformity or X-ray progression, a response rate that does not justify the use of this therapy (Ellison and Flatt, 1971). Intra-articular orgotein – a metallo-protein with superoxide dismutase activity – has been reported to be effective in both RA and OA (Huskisson and Scott, 1979; Goebel *et al.*, 1981) though this substance was ineffective in experimental osteoarthrosis in rabbits (Rosner *et al.*, 1980) and induced synovitis in most patients. Rifamycin SV has been tried in RA and provided substantially more clinical improvement than joint aspiration alone, but has not been shown to influence radiological progression of RA (Caruso *et al.*, 1982).

Osmic acid is the most widely used agent for chemical synovectomy, particularly in France. Intra-articular injection of this substance was introduced in 1951 by the Scandinavians Von Reis and Swensson (1951) for the treatment of persistent knee synovitis in RA or osteoarthrosis. Local reactions were common and osmic acid is now given as a 'cocktail', together with lignocaine and hydrocortisone. Using this 'cocktail' in a series of 447 knee injections, 46% were improved one year after injection (Kajander and Ruotsi, 1967). Osmic acid has been compared directly with yttrium 90 (Sheppeard *et al.*, 1981) and with triamcinolone (Anttinen and Oka, 1975) for the treatment of RA knee synovitis and produces comparable or even slightly better results.

8.9.4 Chemical and radiation synovectomy versus intra-articular steroids

Chemical and radiation synovectomy are unlikely to displace steroids from their present major role in intra-articular injections due to the relative ease and safety with which the latter can be given. However, newer methods to improve the safety and efficacy of isotopes are being developed. One of these is to chelate the radio-isotope with another agent and then administer this compound as a liposome. So far this technique has only been applied to experimental animals but has obvious potential in man (Bard *et al.*, 1983). Of the various agents for chemical synovectomy, only osmic acid has been well tried and tested. There is some experimental animal work indicating that it produces growth retardation in young but not adult rabbit cartilage (Menkes *et al.*, 1972). However, in man the agent appears safe. A reasonable policy is therefore to try local steroids, but if these fail proceed to chemical or radiation synovectomy before considering surgical synovectomy. The latter is not only more expensive and time-consuming, but also carries the risk of limiting the range of movement in the joint as well as general risks associated with any anaesthetic or operation.

8.10 APPROACHES TO REDUCE SIDE EFFECTS

8.10.1 Enteric-coated prednisolone

Enteric coating of steroid preparations has been advocated as a method to reduce the gastrointestinal complications of oral steroids. Unfortunately, these enteric-coated drugs may reduce, but do not eliminate, the risk of mucosal damage since the latter results partly from a systemic effect of steroids. Furthermore, enteric-coated prednisolone is absorbed erratically, making it an unpredictable form of therapy in RA (Hayes *et al.*, 1983).

8.10.2 Pulsed systemic steroids

One further approach to the problem of achieving efficacy with the minimum of side effects has been the use of pulsed intravenous steroids (usually methylprednisolone) at infrequent intervals. This form of therapy was introduced for the treatment of lupus nephritis and for renal allograft rejection episodes, and was then tried in RA by Liebling *et al.* (1981). Liebling reported dramatic clinical benefit with few adverse effects in the original double-blind crossover study. His results are open to criticism since patients were allowed varying doses of gold, penicillamine and oral prednisolone during the trial, as well as intra-articular steroids. However, encouraging clinical results were also achieved with methylprednisolone infusions 1 g monthly in a better controlled study by Williams *et al.* (1982). Our own findings in an open study of three consecutive pulses given on alternate days to a group of patients with severe rheumatoid arthritis showed biochemical as well as clinical improvement. Significant falls in ESR and CRP were shown and persisted for about seven weeks (Forster *et al.*, 1982). We have recently investigated the efficacy of pulsed methylprednisolone given as three 1 g pulses on alternate days, either alone or at the start of therapy with second-line agents such as penicillamine. Our results show that solumedrone given alone provides an improvement that is too short-lived to be of practical value in RA (Neumann *et al.*, 1985). Combining methylprednisolone pulses with other long-term agents does not appear to modify the final outcome, but provides immediate improvement. This would be helpful to patients with severe pain where three months' wait for other therapy to work can seem interminable.

It was hoped that pulsed methylprednisolone would be free of the side effects associated with more long-term prednisolone treatment. However, adrenal suppression, albeit minor and transient, has been shown after single 1 g intravenous pulses (Novak *et al.*, 1970). Cardiac arrests immediately after infusions have occurred (Bocanegra *et al.*, 1981; Barrett, 1983). These have occurred in association with diuretic therapy or impaired renal function. Severe infections have occasionally followed methylprednisolone infusions, but in our own experience are rare (Forster *et al.*, 1982). Avascular necrosis of the femoral heads has also been reported. A recent editorial in the *Lancet* (Anon, 1983) discussed the question of whether steroids in collagen diseases should be given in grams or milligrams and points out that 'if a drug is given in very high doses this ought to be because smaller doses are known to be less effective. If a drug is given intravenously this ought to be because oral treatment is contraindicated by poor or variable absorption and unpredictable first-pass metabolism or side effects avoidable by the intravenous route'. In our own experience pulsed methylprednisolone has been a safe therapy. However, direct comparisons must be made between pulsed methylprednisolone and oral prednisolone given in short courses, before the much greater cost and inconvenience of the intravenous therapy can be justified. Pulsed methylprednisolone has been a popular form of therapy for the treatment of renal allograft rejection episodes. However, when high dose methylprednisolone (600 mg m^{-2}) was compared with lower dose oral prednisolone (3 mg kg^{-1}) for the treatment of such rejection episodes in children, both therapies were equally effective and equally well tolerated (Orta-Sibu *et al.*, 1982).

8.10.3 Targeting steroid therapy

This is an interesting and novel approach to the problem of steroid side effects. Mizushima *et al.* (1982) have developed a lipid emulsion into which dexamethasone can be incorporated. This liposteroid, when injected intravenously into rats, is selectively trapped in the reticulo-endothelial system and inflamed tissue. Its effects persist for nine days. A similar dose of dexamethasone, given intramuscularly in saline, is concentrated in muscle and its effects last only six days. This technique will have tremendous potential if it can be used in humans.

8.11 GENERAL CONCLUSIONS

Over the last two decades the popularity of steroids for use in rheumatic diseases has waxed and waned. They are at present out of favour for RA. In many collagen disorders, notably RA and SLE, high-dose intravenous pulses of prednisolone are fashionable, yet evidence that this is preferable to a short course of high- or even low-dose steroids is lacking. Antagonism to all steroids dates from the 1960s when the long-term complications of this therapy were first recognized. However, we now know safer methods of administering steroids – notably alternate day dosage and intermittent short courses. Steroids will never supplant long-term agents as systemic therapy in rheumatoid arthritis, particularly now that safer long-term agents such as sulphasalazine are emerging. However, as an adjunct to other therapy, for example, to tide a patient over an exacerbation, their value has been underestimated. Local steroids are also valuable, and there is little evidence that they do any harm in RA, provided they are used in moderation.

In the other collagen disorders, and in PMR and GCA, the tendency has been to use too large a dose of steroids too frequently. Here again, moderation is the key to safe and successful treatment.

8.12 REFERENCES

Adu, D. and Cameron, J. S. (1982) Lupus nephritis. *Clinics Rheum. Dis.*, 8, 153–82.

Alarcon-Segovia, D. and Ward, L. E. (1966) Osteoarthritic finger joints after intra-articular injection of corticosteroids. *Arthr. Rheum.*, 9, 443–63.

Anon (1983) Prednisolone pulses in collagen disease: grammes or milligrammes. *Lancet*, i, 280–1.

Ansell, B. M., Crook, A., Mallard, J. R. and Bywaters, G. L. (1963) Evaluation of intra-articular colloidal gold, [198]Au, in the treatment of persistent knee effusions. *Ann. Rheum. Dis.*, 22, 435–9.

Antinen, J. and Oka, M. (1975) Intra-articular triamcinolone hexacetonide and osmic acid in persistent synovitis of the knee. *Scand. J. Rheumatol.*, 4, 125–8.

Ayoub, J. (1983) Central nervous system manifestations after pulse therapy for systemic lupus erythematosus. *Arthr. Rheum.*, 26, 809–10.

Balch, H. W., Gibson, J. M. C., El-Ghobarey, A. F., Bain, L. S. and Lynch, M. P. (1977) Repeated corticosteroid injections into knee joints. *Rheum. Rehabil.*, 16, 137–40.

Bard, D. R., Knight, C. G. and Page-Thomas, D. P. (1983) Treatment of a rabbit experimental arthritis with ^{177}Lu in chelator liposomes. *Heberden Soc. Abstracts* Nov. 1983, No. 16, p. 40.

Barrett, D. F. (1983) Pulsed methylprednisolone therapy. *Lancet*, ii, 800.

Behn, A. R., Perera, T. and Myles, A. B. (1983) Polymyalgia rheumatica and corticosteroids: how much and for how long? *Ann. Rheum. Dis.*, 42, 374–8.

Bengtsson, B. A. and Malmvall, B. E. (1981) Prognosis of giant cell arteritis including temporal arteritis and polymyalgia rheumatica; a follow-up study on 90 patients treated with corticosteroids. *Acta Med. Scand.*, 209, 337–45.

Bird, H. A., Ring, E. F. J. and Bacon, P. A. (1979) A thermographic and clinical comparison of three intra-articular steroid preparations in RA. *Ann. Rheum. Dis.*, 38, 36–9.

Bird, H. A., Ring., E. F. J., Daniel, R. and Bacon, P. A. (1977) Comparison of intra-articular methotrexate with intra-articular triamcinolone hexacetonide by thermography. *Curr. Med. Res. Opinion*, 5, 141–6.

Bocanegra, T. S., Castaneda, M. O., Espinoza, L. R., Vasey, F. B. and Germain, B. F. (1981) Sudden death after methylprednisolone pulse therapy. *Ann. Int. Med.*, 95, 122.

Byron, M. A., Jackson, J. and Ansell, B. M. (1983) Effect of different corticosteroid regimens on hypothalamic-pituitary-adrenal axis and growth in J.C.A. *J. Roy. Soc. Med.*, 76, 452–7.

Caruso, I., Montrone, F., Fumagalli, M., Patrono, C., Santandrea, S. and Gandini, M. C. (1982) Rheumatoid knee synovitis successfully treated in intra-articular rifamycin S.V. *Ann. Rheum. Dis.*, 41, 232–6.

Chamberlain, M. A. and Keenan, J. (1976) The effect of low doses of prednisolone compared with placebo on function and on the hypothalamic pituitary adrenal axis in patients with RA. *Rheum. Rehabil.*, 15, 17–24.

Chandler, G. N., Jones, D. T., Wright, V. and Hartfall, S. J. (1959) Charcot's arthropathy following intra-articular hydrocortisone. *Br. Med. J.*, 1, 952–3.

Chapelle, A. de la, Oka, M., Rekonen, A. and Ruotsi, A. (1972) Chromosome damage after intra-articular injections of radioactive yttrium. Effect of immobilisation on the biological dose. *Ann. Rheum. Dis.*, 31, 508–12.

Cruess, R. L., Ross, D. and Crawshaw, E. (1975) The aetiology of steroid-induced avascular necrosis of bone. A laboratory and clinical study. *Clin. Orthop.*, 113, 178–83.

De Silva, M. and Hazleman, B. L. (1983) Azathioprine in polymyalgia rheumatica – giant cell arteritis. A double-blind study. *Heb. Soc.*, Leeds, Abstr. 16.

De Silva, M., Hazleman, B. L. and Page-Thomas, D. P. (1979) Liposomes in arthritis: a new approach. *Lancet*, i, 1320–2.

Dick, W. C. (1978) Drug treatment of R.A. in *Copeman's Textbook of the Rheumatic Diseases* (ed. J. T. Scott), 5th edn, Churchill Livingstone, Edinburgh, p. 405.

Dimant, J. (1978) Computer analysis of factors influencing the appearance of aseptic necrosis in patients with systemic lupus erythematosus. *J. Rheumatol.*, 5, 136–41.

Doherty, M. and Dieppe, P. A. (1981) Effects of intra-articular ^{90}Y on chronic pyrophosphate arthropathy of the knee. *Heb. Soc. Abstracts*, September, No. 32.

Doherty, M., Dieppe, P. and Watt, I. (1982) The influence of primary osteoarthrosis on the development of secondary osteoarthrosis. *Ann. Rheum. Dis.*, 41, 642.

Downie, W. W., Dixon, J. S., Lowe, J. R., Rhind, V. M., Leatham, P. A. and Pickup, M. E. (1978) Adrenocortical suppression by synthetic corticosteroid drugs: a comparative study of prednisolone and betamethasone. *Br. J. Clin. Pharmacol.*, 6, 397–9.

Duncan, H., Frost, H. M., Villanueva, A. R. and Sigler, J. W. (1965) The osteoporosis of rheumatoid arthritis. *Arthr. Rheum.*, 8, 943–54.

Ellison, M. R., Flatt, A. E. (1971) Intra-articular thirotepa in rheumatoid disease. A clinical analysis of 123 injected MCP and PIP joints. *Arthr. Rheum.*, 14, 212–22.

Esselinckx, W., Kolanowski, J. and Nagant de Deuxchaisnes, C. (1982) Adrenocortical function and responsiveness to tetracosactrin infusions after intra-articular treatment with triamcinolone hexacetonide and hydrocortisone acetate. *Clin. Rheumatol.*, 1, 176–84.

Fauci, A. S. (1982) Wegener's granulomatosis: prospective clinical experience with 85 patients for 21 years. *Ann. Intern. Med.*, 98, 76–85.

Fitzcharles, M. A., Halsey, J. and Currey, H. L. F. (1982) Conversion from daily to alternate day corticosteroids in rheumatoid arthritis. *Ann. Rheum. Dis.*, 41, 66–8.

Forster, P. J. G., Grindulis, K., Neumann, V., Hubball, S. and McConkey, B. (1982) High-dose intravenous methylprednisolone in rheumatoid arthritis. *Ann. Rheum. Dis.*, 41, 444–6.

Goebel, K. M., Storck, U. and Neurath, F. (1981) Intrasynovial orgotein therapy in RA. *Lancet*, i, 1015–7.

Grigor, R., Edmunds, J., Lewkonia, R., Bresnihan, B. and Hughes, G. R. V. (1978) Systemic lupus erythematosus. A prospective analysis. *Ann. Rheum. Dis.*, 37, 121–8.

Gumpel, J. M. and Roles, N. C. (1975) A controlled trial of intra-articular radiocolloid versus surgical synovectomy in persistent synovitis. *Lancet*, i, 488–9.

Haines, J. F. (1983) Bilateral rupture of the Achilles tendon in patients on steroid therapy. *Ann. Rheum. Dis.*, 42, 652–4.

Harter, J. G., Reddy, W. J. and Thorn, G. W. (1963) Studies on an intermittent corticosteroid dosage regime. *N. Engl. J. Med.*, 269, 591–6.

Hayes, M., Alam, A. F. M. S., Bruckner, F. E., Doherty, S. M., Myles, A., English, J., Marks, V. and Chakraborty, J. (1983) Plasma prednisolone studies in rheumatic patients. *Ann. Rheum. Dis.*, 42, 151–4.

Hollander, J. L. (1972) in *Arthritis and Allied Conditions* (eds J. L. Hollander and D. J. McCarty), 8th edn, Lea and Febiger, Philadelphia, p. 520.

Hughes, G. R. V. (1977) *The Connective Tissue Disorders*. Blackwell Scientific, London.

Hulley, S. B., Vogel, J. M., Donaldson, C. L., Bayers, J. H., Friedman, R. J. and Rosen, S. N. (1971) The effect of supplemented oral phosphate on the bone mineral changes during prolonged bed rest. *J. Clin. Invest.*, 50, 2506.

Huskisson, E. C. and Scott, J. (1979) Orgotein in OA of the knee joint. Presented at Orgotein Workshop, Aachen.

Joint Committee of the M.R.C. and Nuffield Foundation (1957) Clinical trials of cortisone, ACTH and other measures in chronic rheumatic diseases; long term results in early cases of RA treated with either cortisone or aspirin. *Br. Med. J.*, 1, 847–50.

Joint Committee of the M.R.C. and the Nuffield Foundation (1959) A comparison of prednisolone with aspirin or other analgesics in the treatment of RA. *Ann. Rheum. Dis.*, 18, 173–86.

Kajander, A. and Ruotsi, A. (1967) The effects of intra-articular osmic acid on rheumatoid joint affections. *Ann. Med. Int. Fenn.*, 57, 87–91.

Kennedy, A. C., Smith, D. A., Buchanan, W. W., Anderson, J. B., Samuels, B. B. and Jasani, M. K. (1974) Osteoporosis in RA; its natural history and statistical reduction. *Rheumatology*, 4, 23–35.

Krolner, B., Toft, B., Nielsen, S. P. and Tondevold, E. (1983) Physical exercise as prophylaxis against involutional vertebral bone loss; a controlled trial. *Clin. Sci.*, 64, 541–6.

Lanham, J. G. and Hughes, G. R. V. (1982) Anti-malarial therapy in systemic lupus erythematosus. *Clinics Rheum. Dis.*, 8, 279–98.

Liebling, M. R., Lieb, E., McLaughlin, K., Blocka, K., Furst, D., Nyman, K. and Paulus, H. (1981) Pulsed methylprednisolone in rheumatoid arthritis. *Ann. Int. Med.*, 94, 21–6.

Lloyd, D. C. and Reeder, E. J. (1978) Chromosome aberration and intra-articular yttrium-90. *Lancet*, i, 617.

Lockie, L. M., Gomez, E. and Smith, D. M. (1983) Low dose adrenocorticosteroids in the management of elderly patients with RA: selected examples and summary of efficacy in the long-term treatment of 97 patients. *Semin. Arthr. Rheum.*, 12, 373–81.

Mankin, H. J. and Conger, K. A. (1966) The acute effects of intra-articular hydrocortisone on articular cartilage in rabbits. *J. Bone Jt. Surg.*, 48-A, 1383–8.

Marks, J. S., Stewart, I. M. and Hunter, J. A. A. (1976) Intra-articular methotrexate in RA. *Lancet*, ii, 857–8.

Mattson, S. (1972) The reversibility of disease osteoporosis – experimental studies in the adult rat. *Acta Orthopaed. Scand.* (Suppl.) 144, 1.

McCarty, D. J. and Hogan, J. M. (1964) Inflammatory reaction after intrasynovial injection of microcystalline adrenocorticosteroid esters. *Arthr. Rheum.*, 7, 359–67.

McConkey, B., Frazer, G. and Bligh, A. (1965) Transparent skin and osteoporosis – a study in patients with rheumatoid disease. *Ann. Rheum. Dis.*, 24, 219–23.

McKenna, F., Eccles, J., Newmann, V. (1986) *Br. J. Rheum.* (in press).

Menkes, C. J., Piatier-Piketty, D., Zucman, J. and Delbarre, F. (1972) Effets des injections articulaires d'acide osmique chez le lapin. Repercussion sur la croissance osseuse. *Rev. Rheum.*, 39, 513–21.

Miller, J. H., White, J. and Norton, T. H. (1958) The value of intra-articular injections in OA of the knee. *J. Bone Jt. Surg.*, 40-B, 636.

Mintz, G., Enriquez, R. D., Mercado, U., Robles, E. J., Jimenez, F. J. and Gutierrez, G. (1981) Intravenous methylprednisolone pulse therapy in severe ankylosing spondylitis. *Arthr. Rheum.*, 24, 734–6.

Mizushima, Y., Hamano, T. and Yokoyama, K. (1982) Tissue distribution and anti-inflammatory activity of corticosteroids incorporated in lipid emulsion. *Ann. Rheum. Dis.*, 41, 263–7.

MRC Collagen Diseases Panel (1960) Treatment of polyarteritis nodosa with cortisone. *Br. Med. J.*, 1, 1399–400.

Myles, A. B., Bacon, P. A. and Daly, J. R. (1971) Single daily dose corticosteroid treatment. *Ann. Rheum. Dis.*, 30, 149–53.

Neumann, V. C., Hopkins, R., Bird, H. A. and Wright, V. (1985) Pulsed methylprednisolone in rheumatoid arthritis – alone or in combination. *Annals Rheum. Dis.*, 44, 747–51.

Novak, E., Stubbs, S. S., Seckman, C. E. and Hearron, M. S. (1970) Effects of a single large IV dose of methylprednisolone sodium succinate. *Clin. Pharm. Ther.*, 11, 711–17.

Oka, M., Rokonen, A., Kuikka, J. and Anttinen, J. (1975) Bone mineral density in RA measured by the gamma transmission method. *Scand. J. Rheumatol.*, 4, 28–32.

Orta-Sibu, N., Chantler, C., Bewick, M. and Haycock, G. (1982) Comparison of high dose IV methylprednisolone with low dose oral prednisolone in acute renal allograft rejection in children. *Br. Med. J.*, 285, 258–60.

Quismorio, F. P. and Dubois, E. L. (1975) Septic arthritis in systemic lupus erythematosus. *J. Rheumatol.*, 2, 73–82.

Rasker, J. and Cosh, J. A. (1978) Radiological study of cervical spine and hand in patients with RA of 15 years' duration: an assessment of the effects of corticosteroid treatment. *Ann. Rheum. Dis.*, 37, 529–35.

Reid, D. M., Kennedy, N. S. J., Smith, M. A., Tothill, P. and Nuki, G. (1982) Total body calcium in RA: effects of disease activity and corticosteroid treatment. *Br. Med. J.*, 285, 330–2.

Richter, M. B., Woo, P., Panayi, G. S., Yrull, A., Unger, A. and Shepherd, P. (1983) The effect of intravenous pulse methylprednisolone on immunological and inflammatory processes in A.S. *Clin. Exp. Immunol.*, 53, 51–9.

Rosner, I. A., Goldberg, V. M., Getzy, L. and Moskovitz, R. W. (1980) A trial of intra-articular orgotein, a superoxide dismutase, in experimentally-induced OA. *J. Rheumatol.*, 7, 24–9.

Rudge, S. R. and Lloyd-Jones, K. (1980) Cervical subluxation and long term corticosteroids in non-rheumatoid patients. *Heb. Soc. Abstr.*, Sept., No. 22, p. 32.

Rylance, H. J., Chalmers, T. M. and Elton, R. A. (1980) Clinical trials of intra-articular aspirin in RA. *Lancet*, ii, 1099–102.

Salter, R. B., Gross, A. and Hall, J. H. (1967) Hydrocortisone arthropathy – an experimental investigation. *Can. Med. Assoc. J.*, 97, 274.

Sedgwick, A. D., Sin, M. Y., Moore, A. R., Edwards, J. C. W. and Willoughby, D. A. (1983) The effect of local corticosteroid on cartilage degredation in vivo. *Heb. Soc. Abstr.* Nov., No. 3.

Sheppeard, H., Aldin, A. and Ward, D. J. (1981) Osmic acid versus yttrium-90 in rheumatoid synovitis of the knee. *Scand. J. Rheumatol.*, 10, 234–6.

Spiegel, R. J., Vigersky, R. A., Oliff, A., Echelberger, C. K., Bruton, J. and Poplack, D. G. (1979) Adrenal suppression after short term corticosteroid therapy. *Lancet*, i, 630–3.

Turner-Stokes, L. and Turner-Warwick, M. (1982) Intra-thoracic manifestations of SLE. *Clinics Rheum. Dis.*, 8, 229–42.

Vainio, K. and Julkunen, H. (1960) Intra-articular nitrogen mustard treatment of rheumatoid arthritis. *Acta Rheumatol. Scand.*, 6, 25–30.

Von Reis, G. and Swensson, A. (1951) Intra-articular injections of osmic acid in painful joint affections. *Acta Med. Scand. (Suppl. 259)*, 140, 27–32.

Wigginton, S. M., Chu, B. C. F., Weisman, M. H. and Howell, S. B. (1980) Methotrexate pharmacokinetics after intra-articular injection in patients with RA. *Arthr. Rheum.*, 23, 119–22.

Williams, I. A., Baylis, E. M. and Shipley, M. E. (1982) A double blind placebo-controlled trial of methylprednisolone pulse therapy in active rheumatoid disease. *Lancet*, ii, 237–40.

Williams, P. L. and Corbett, M. (1983) Avascular necrosis of bone complicating corticosteroid replacement therapy. *Ann. Rheum. Dis.*, 42, 276–9.

Williams, P. L., Crawley, J. C. W., Freedman, A. M., Lloyd, D. C. and Gumpel, J. M. (1981) Feasibility of outpatient management after intra-articular yttrium-90: comparison of two regimens. *Br. Med. J.*, 282, 13–14.

Wright, V., Chandler, G. N., Morison, R. A. H. and Hartfall, S. J. (1960) Intra-articular therapy in OA. Comparison of hydrocortisone acetate and hydrocortisone tertiary butylacetate. *Ann. Rheum. Dis.*, 19, 257–61.

CHAPTER 9

Slow-acting antirheumatoid drugs

H. Berry

9.1 GENERAL

In order to ascertain which drugs are slow-acting antirheumatoid drugs (see Section 2 onwards), it is essential that we define what we mean by slow-acting antirheumatoid. Traditionally, slow-acting antirheumatoid drugs are those that induce either disease remission, or perhaps to be more precise, disease modification. Some would refer to these drugs as disease modifying antirheumatic drugs. Disease modification can be defined by clinical, laboratory or radiological means.

9.1.1 Clinical measurement (Table 9.1)

Clinical measurements used in investigating all drugs in this area are the same. These include: (a) morning stiffness, (b) articular index, (c) ring size, (d) grip strength, (e) PIP joint size, and (f) pain using 4 point and visual analogue scales. These clinical measurements are carried out over a long time, probably over the space of at least six months in order to assess the slow-acting nature of a drug. Unfortunately, all these measurements will respond to NSAIDs as well

TABLE 9.1
Clinical measurement

Morning stiffness
Articular index
Ring size
Grip strength
PIP joint size
Pain (4 point or VAS)

as disease modifying antirheumatoid drugs. It is likely that the only one of these that is slow to change is the ring size, and this is a reflection of the ability of the joints to show a pure anti-inflammatory response. Also, the disease process itself can cause changes in these measurements: if rheumatoid arthritis gets better, being a disease of exacerbations and remissions, then this will be mirrored by improvement in these measurements. It is therefore arguable how useful these measures are in the assessment of the disease modifying anti-rheumatoid drug.

9.1.2 Laboratory measurements (Table 9.2)

Many different tests can be carried out in the laboratory. These vary from rheumatoid factor and anti-nuclear factor, often found in rheumatoid arthritis, to the immune complex levels. This may be assessed by measuring either complement (C3 or C4), or complement degradation products (C3d or C4d). One can also measure lymphocytes (T and B cell populations). There is a lot of conflict in the reports over T and B cell numbers in the peripheral blood in rheumatoid arthritis. Most suggest that T and B cell proportions in patients with rheumatoid arthritis are the same as in control populations (Williams *et al.*, 1953; Mellbye *et al.*, 1972; Williams and Messner, 1975). Two studies have shown an increase in B cells (PapaMichail *et al.*, 1971; Vernon Roberts *et al.*, 1974), as assessed by Sig staining in this disease. This probably reflects absorbed immunoglobulin rather than a true change in B cell proportions. T cell subset studies show a normal percentage of Tg and Tm in the blood of rheumatoid arthritis patients, but in synovial fluid Tg cells are reduced, Tm cells are normal. The ratio between the OKT4+ and OKT8+ cells, which has been used as an index of help compared with suppression, is high in the peripheral blood of patients with active rheumatoid arthritis (Bach and Bach, 1981; Raeman *et al.*, 1981).

TABLE 9.2
Laboratory measurement

Rheumatoid factor
Antinuclear factor
Immune complex levels
C3, C4
C3d, C4d
Lymphocyte function
T cell and B cell numbers
Skin testing
Lymphocyte response to PHA and Con A
Acute phase reacting proteins
ESR, C reactive protein
Measurement of sulphydryl radicals
Haemoglobin improvement

The usefulness of the T4:T8 ratio in clinical trials is yet to be validated, although Veys (1984) has looked at it in a clinical trial context. The use of skin testing to reveal long-acting activity by drugs is relatively controversial, as it is open to question on ethical grounds.

However, rheumatoid patients do show positive skin testing with a battery of common antigens in practice. Treatment with these remission-inducing agents may cause conversion to response from non-response. The lymphocyte response to PHA and con A appear fairly consistently depressed in patients with rheumatoid arthritis (Lockshin *et al.*, 1975; Silverman *et al.*, 1976; Percy *et al.*, 1978). Pokeweed mitogen has been reported as being normal (Silverman *et al.*, 1976), reduced (Lockshin *et al.*, 1975), or enhanced (Percy *et al.*, 1978). There is a suggestion that myocrisin *in vitro*, perhaps via an effect on macrophages, inhibits mitogen-triggered human lymphocyte DNA synthesis (Lipsky and Ziff, 1977; Highton *et al.*, 1981). Penicillamine, if combined with copper, produces a similar result. This would support the view that decreases in activity of the disease itself cause improvement in the lymphocyte response.

Measurement of rheumatoid factor is often used for recording response to disease modifying drugs. One particular problem in multicentre trials is the need to collect sera from patients at regular intervals and to deep freeze these because all measurements should be carried out in the same laboratory at the same time. Quantitation of complement protein, whilst of interest and of considerable value diagnostically in SLE or in vasculitis, is of little help in the monitoring of patients with rheumatoid arthritis and in assessing their changing state in clinical trials.

Acute phase proteins have been largely studied in the context of clinical trials, among these are caeruloplasmin, alpha $[\alpha_1]$ acid glycoprotein, $[\alpha_1]$ antitrypsin, $[\alpha_1]$ antichymotrypsin, haptoglobin, fibrinogen, CRP and SAA. The ESR is a useful, non-specific test. However, there are patients with rheumatoid arthritis in whom the ESR may be normal but the disease highly active. C-reactive protein has been used extensively as an estimate of disease activity as the concentrations can rise rapidly from normal levels. CRP levels change much more rapidly than ESR levels and therefore it may well be a much more acute index of change. This has been shown in juvenile chronic arthritis, where a pauci-articular or quiescent disease can be differentiated from polyarticular or systemic disease, by the finding of increased levels of CRP in active disease (Pepys, 1981). Other laboratory tests have included analysis of sulphydryl radicals (Hall *et al.*, 1981).

In summary, a large number of laboratory tests have become available for the assessment of the patient with rheumatoid disease, but the specificity of these tests is limited. Whether it is a drug-related effect or whether it is a consequence of change of disease is open to argument. Whether any tests give more information than the C-reactive protein and the ESR is open to discussion. Perhaps haemoglobin improvement appears to be a more reliable means than any of the others in assessing whether the drug is capable of inducing remission. The NSAIDs will lead to no change or a fall in the haemoglobin level whereas improvement in the disease for any reason will lead to a rise.

9.1.3   Radiological changes (Table 9.3)

Radiographic assessment of clinical trials is difficult and hazardous. The pathological lesion of rheumatoid arthritis is the erosion. Other factors are joint space narrowing and osteoporosis. An attempt to improve magnification has been carried out by Gelman (1981), whose technique has been to evaluate ten joints of the hand, six joints of feet, and the radiocarpal compartment of the wrist. He counted joint space narrowing and bone erosion by grading the narrowing on a scale from 0 to 4, and in addition, evaluates bone erosion on the same scale, i.e. 1 = questionable, 2 = minimal, 3 = moderate, and 4 = severe.

TABLE 9.3
Radiological changes

Measurement of erosions
Measurement of joint space narrowing
Measurement of osteoporosis

Osteoporosis is analyzed by measuring the total bone width and the medullary canal of the mid-portion of the second metacarpal using a measuring magnifier. The difference between the total bone width and the medullary canal width equals the width of the cortex. Magnification may lead to demonstration of earlier erosive changes but is cumbersome and expensive. Larsen (1981) has also looked into the effect of drugs on radiological change in some detail. He has used standard radiographs and compared changes to the standards. The question of what actually to measure on X-rays is somewhat difficult as Larsen's technique is still in the experimental phase.

TABLE 9.4
ARA definition of remission

Absence of pain
Absence of swelling
Absence of fatigue
Drop in morning stiffness to below 15 minutes
Fall in ESR to below 20 in males or 30 in females

In summary, the best measurement of remission is a composite. The council of perfection is as described by Decker for the ARA (1981) (Table 9.4). This is absence of pain, swelling, fatigue, and a drop in morning stiffness to 15 minutes or below together with a fall in ESR to the normal level, i.e. below 20 in males or below 30 in females. Our view is that disease remission or modification should include a rise in haemoglobin, a fall in ESR, a *status quo* in radiological changes, and an improvement in the clinical measure elucidated. Only on this basis over a period of time can one really talk about disease remission. The question is how long should this time interval be, a six month trial is but a drop in the ocean to the rheumatoid arthritis sufferer. What is really required for true disease remission is to measure for at least two if not five years before being convinced.

9.2 CHLOROQUINE

Chloroquine is a synthetic antimalarial drug introduced in 1943 at the same time as hydroxychloroquine. The earliest work using it in medicine suggested that it was beneficial for the treatment of systemic lupus erythematosus and discoid lupus erythematosus.

First reports of successful treatment in rheumatoid arthritis were published in 1951 at a dose level 20 times that which was used to treat malaria. Unfortunately, it became all too apparent early on that the dosages being employed were toxic to the retina.

9.2.1 Pharmacology

Few data are available in terms of absorption, distribution, metabolism or excretion of this drug and there have been very few dose–response studies. It would appear to be absorbed from the upper intestinal tract rapidly and almost completely. It is then localized in the liver, spleen and heart, has an affinity for melanin, and high concentrations are subsequently found in the iris, the choroid and the skin. Urinary excretion is slow and discontinuous. When the drug is withdrawn the output falls by 50% per week over a four-week period, then the excretion rate becomes stable at around 7.5 µg per 24 hours, remaining at this level for months. It continues to be excreted for a long time, even years after discontinuing therapy. Metabolic breakdown in man proceeds by the formation of a secondary amine, the primary amine, the 4-aldehyde and the 4-carboxy derivative.

9.2.2 In the clinic

In 1953 Haydu described 28 patients who had active rheumatoid arthritis in whom he studied the drug at dosages of 900 mg per week for six months.

A further open study by Bagnell in 1957 on 108 patients treated for more than eight months showed that 70% had a complete remission after one year of therapy, with parallel improvement in haemoglobin levels and fall in ESR levels. Part of this study was double blind, 12 of 19 patients showed improvement with none of 12 showing improvement in the control group.

Young (1959) showed that a variable dose gave better results. The highest dose utilized was up to 1800 mg weekly. Freedman and Steinberg (1960) conducted a double-blind study of 53 patients who received chloroquine and 54 placebo. Patients were also allowed to continue with aspirin and physiotherapy. In 40 control patients and 42 in the chloroquine group, one year's treatment was completed. Of the chloroquine-treated patients 80% improved compared with 30% of the control patients, 300 mg a day being the dose used in this study.

In 1965, Lansbury had stated that chloroquine is less harmful in its side effects than corticosteroids, phenylbutazone or gold salts for the treatment of rheumatoid arthritis. He used chloroquine for ten years in a dosage between 125 and 250 mg daily and considered it safe. Chloroquine has been extensively used in discoid lupus and has even been tried in such unrelated conditions as basal cell epithelioma and squamous cell carcinoma of the skin, resistant asthma, rosacea, scleroderma, polyarteritis nodosa, granuloma annulare, dermatitis herpetiformis, and chronic acrodermatitis atrophicans.

9.2.3   Therapeutic usage

It is unclear whether it is wiser to use a dose of 300 mg of chloroquine or 400 mg of hydroxychloroquine as a starting dose and then reducing to half that dose at the end of three months, or starting initially at the lower dose. Like all long acting antirheumatoid drugs it does not have an immediate effect, taking up to three months before having its main therapeutic effect. It should probably be given in combination with NSAIDs until remission is achieved. It should be reserved for those patients who are seropositive and/or erosive early in the course of the disease, or those where NSAIDs are ineffective.

9.2.4   Side effects

(a) *Rash*

This occurs in 1% of patients and subsides on stopping the drug.

(b) *Digestive tract*

Increased flatus, bloating, and audible peristalsis is heard in many patients on this drug, and the irritable bowel syndrome may occur.

(c) *Pigment change*

Reversible greying or bleaching of the hair often occurs in patients who receive excess dosage of the drug.

(d) *The eye*

This fear has led to chloroquine being somewhat unpopular. There is little doubt that the original dosages did lead to eye damage, probably because they were too high. There is a modern school of thought that believes that lower doses are associated with an almost negligible number of ophthalmological complications. Bernstein (1967) indicated that a dose of 250 mg was associated with a frequency of retinopathy of under 1%, and he studied 1906 patients. At 500 mg per day the frequency rises to between 3 and 6%, this in a study of 515 patients. At 750 mg a day the frequency is greater than 15% in 596 patients. Retinal effects include premaculopathy, which is defined as a reversible change without permanent anatomical or functional injury (reversible scotoma to red characterizes this phase and correlates with exceeding the toxic threshold of dosage).

A maculopathy is the next lesion showing a bull's-eye pattern of pigment. Both the scotoma and reduced vision are reversible. Finally, a fully fledged retinopathy causing permanent functional injury to vision can occur with a visible anatomical counterpart in the form of a bull's-eye pigment ring. In this condition there is both a scotoma and diminished visual activity. This is a preventable tragedy occurring sooner at high dosage than at lower dosages. The question is how to prevent this tragedy occurring. One test recommended by Percival and Behrman (1969) was to check visual field defects to red targets. This had been successfully used as a way of detecting premaculopathy, but other authorities have challenged this work. In the light of observations by Marks and Power (1979), the argument against using chloroquine on the grounds of retinopathy and production of corneal opacities has probably been over stated, and at lower dosages the patient is probably safe. It is, however, advisable to continue examining by means of three-monthly slit lamp examinations, including a preliminary base line examination. The usefulness of available tests that pick out premaculopathy is controversial. Marks and Power (1979) recommend the use of recording visual activity, slit lamp corneal microscopy and fundal examination under mydriasis. Further tests include visual field testing to red target, fluorescein fundal angiography, colour vision, and electroretinopathy.

9.2.5 Summary

The favourable benefit-to-risk ratio when giving antimalarial drugs has been reconfirmed in every clinical study of the last decade. The efficacy is less than that of gold, penicillamine or azathioprine, but the only major toxic manifestation is retinopathy which would appear to be a preventable lesion at the correct dose. Therefore careful monitoring of patients with regular periodic ophthalmalogical examination will rid the patient of the risk of early lesions that can be detected, and, by stopping the drug, be reversed. As this drug would appear to have less risk it would seem reasonable to start the use of hydroxychloroquine or chloroquine before other more hazardous remission-inducing drugs.

9.3   GOLD

9.3.1   Introduction

Gold was first introduced into rheumatology by Forestier in 1929 on an empirical basis because the drug seemed to have an effect on tuberculosis, which was then considered to be a possible aetiological factor in the production of rheumatoid arthritis. The history of gold since that time has been one of waxing and waning. It was really the Empire Rheumatism Council report in 1961 that finally established the clinical benefit of gold beyond all reasonable doubt in a long-term controlled trial. It is the last heavy metal in common practice, although knowledge on how it works has not progressed in the 50 years that it has been available. If gold is used early in the course of disease, remissions appear to occur early, and in these circumstances frequency of injections may be reduced at the time of clinical remission.

9.3.2   Gold formulation

Until recently the only formulation of gold which has been available commercially has been injectable. The two commonest have been sodium aurothiomalate in a 5% solution (Myocrisin) and 5% aurothioglucose (Solganal). Sodium aurothiomalate is in an aqueous solution and aurothioglucose is in an oily suspension. This means that aurothiomalate is quickly absorbed, whereas the latter is more slowly absorbed. More recently an alternative means to administer gold has been through an oral preparation, auranofin.

9.3.3   Pharmacokinetics

Much work exists on the pharmacokinetics of gold in blood and urine, and it has been compared during intramuscular and oral treatment. Gold levels are three to ten times higher with injectable thioglucose and thiomalate than with auranofin, but serum half-life of the injectable compound is significantly shorter – 5.5 days compared with the oral agents in which it is 14–21 days with a mean of 19 days. Gold content of the urine is ten times higher with intramuscular than with the oral compound. Excretory pathway and tissue distribution of gold during conventional intramuscular therapy suggests that 40% of the 50 mg injectable thiomalate is excreted in 7 days, of which 70% is recovered in the urine. The highest gold concentrations are found in the reticulo-endothelial system, adrenal glands and kidneys, whilst the bone marrow, liver, skin and bone contain the greatest quantities of gold. Using slowly increasing injectable gold, levels rise to around 3 µg ml^{-1} after four weeks. Elimination occurs with a half-life of three to five days. During maintenance treatment using 50 mg monthly serum gold concentration is held at around 1 µg ml^{-1}, the maximum values being around 6 µg ml^{-1}, with an elimination half-life of eleven days. Fifty per cent of the blood gold content is found associated with cellular components.

9.3.4 Monitoring faeces and urine

Gottleib (1979) showed 95% of auranofin gold was recovered in the faeces and 5% in the urine. This contrasts with thiomalate where 70% of an injectable dose is recovered in the urine. Comparing 20 weeks with auranofin 6 mg daily with 20 weeks of Myocrisin 50 mg weekly, 66 mg of gold was retained in the auranofin group, compared with 300 mg from the Myocrisin group, less tissue gold than with parenteral therapy.

9.3.5 Gold and the immune response

The effects of administering gold is often followed by a fall in serum immunoglobulin levels and rheumatoid factor titres in rheumatoid arthritis.

Gold inhibits stimulation of immunoglobulin cells. It also inhibits activation of complement pathways either mediated through the classical or alternative pathways. The inhibition may be due to the effects of gold on macrophages (which act as helper cells in these reactions). Both auranofin and Myocrisin seem to be effective in this way.

9.3.6 Who should receive gold?

Because the side effects are so hazardous it would be convenient to be able to predict who is likely to respond. Studies have been made of responders and non-responders and it has been shown that gold concentrations are similar, in blood, urine and faeces, skin, hair and nails in both these groups. Concentrations are also similar in patients with or without toxicity. There is, however, a suggestion that gold toxicity relates to dosage schedules; higher than conventional doses increase prevalence and severity of adverse responses. There is some suggestion that certain of the commoner side effects of Myocrisin, such as dermatitis, stomatitis and proteinuria, may be fewer with the oral preparations, although diarrhoea may be commoner (Gottleib, 1979).

9.3.7 Dosage regimes

The first properly designed controlled clinical trial showing Myocrisin to be active was the Empire Rheumatism Council trial in which 50 mg weekly was compared with 0.05 mg weekly. The response to the higher dose was significantly superior in all measurements. Later studies have set out to assess whether such doses are necessary or whether higher doses should be employed. Furst et al. (1977) compared 50 mg weekly with 150 mg weekly. Conventional doses were found to be as efficacious as high dosage with respect to rapidity and degree of response, but side effects were much more frequent and much more severe in the high dose group. Sharp et al. (1977) compared one group treated with 25 mg weekly up to 30 weeks and then biweekly or monthly for up to 2 years of treatment with another group who received double the dose at the same intervals. No difference was observed in therapeutic response in the two groups and the conclusion was that 25 mg or less a week may be the correct dose. Again, in both these studies there appeared to be little correlation between either plasma levels or the rate at which gold disappeared from serum and therapeutic response. McKenzie (1981) compared a lower dose still of 10 mg weekly with 50 mg weekly. Her results showed no difference in terms either of efficacy of toxicity between these two groups in up to five years.

Cats (1976) evaluated the effect of different initial doses followed by maintenance dosage in the treatment of rheumatoid arthritis. A high dose of gold compound offered no advantage over a lower dose. After a high dose, a significantly higher number of side effects occurred, but the development of toxicity did not influence the ultimate results. A second course of gold hardly appeared to have any beneficial effect. Prolonged administration of gold is usually well tolerated, although whether it has any substantial therapeutic effect is dubious. Progression of radiological abnormality can be observed at the same time as other signs and symptoms of the disease show improvement.

9.3.8   Recommendations

(a) *Myocrisin*

The main aim of crysotherapy is to induce a remission. A dose of 50 mg weekly until remission is obtained appears still to be a reasonable therapeutic approach. After this maintenance therapy 50 mg monthly or six-weekly according to patient requirement would appear to be a reasonable continued approach. Regular monitoring 2–4 weekly for unwanted effects remains essential, especially a full blood count, differential white count, platelet count, urine analysis, and checks of the skin for rash.

(b) *Auranofin*

This relatively new agent has been submitted to various exhaustive clinical trials, 9 mg has been compared with 1 mg, and 6 mg to 9 mg daily dosage. It would appear that 6 mg would be the recommended starting dose for most patients. It may be necessary for patients to continue this oral medication indefinitely. A long-term study suggests that this may be the main problem – that patient compliance, whilst it can be regularized by injections, may be more difficult to achieve when patients are having to swallow daily tablets once the disease remits. Meyers (1982) suggests that breakthrough of activity occurring after three to four years of therapy occurs because of poor compliance rather than efficacy. Again, haematological, dermatological and urinary monitoring remain essential.

9.3.9 Side effects

Side effects from gold have been well documented over the 50 years that the drug has been available. Most important of these are renal lesions, particularly proteinuria, rashes and bone marrow problems, particularly pancytopenia.

(a) *Renal lesions*

The predominant renal complication is a minimal-change lesion leading to persistent proteinuria or nephrotic syndrome. Skrifvars *et al.* (1979) described patients with microhaematuria which appears rarely to lead to progressive renal failure. In these patients renal biopsy has disclosed granulomatous glomerulonephritis. Rovenska *et al.* (1979) described a similar case using gold in juvenile chronic polyarthritis when membranous glomerulonephritis was seen and immunofluorescent examination revealed that the deposits contained IgG suggestive of an immune complex mechanism. Nelson and Birchmore (1979) described renal vein thrombosis associated with nephrotic syndrome and gold therapy.

(b) *Dermatological effects*

The rash consists of an exanthematous lesion often in the form of round plaques which can occur over any part of the body, particularly over the trunk. If gold therapy is continued the rash can become confluent and ultimately can exfoliate. A maculopapular rash occurs which also becomes confluent. It is often difficult to decide whether a rash appearing during gold treatment is due to the drug or to some unrelated coincidental cause. In all probability a large number of patients have had their gold therapy terminated as a result of a rash that may well not have been gold induced.

(c) *Bone marrow suppression*

The commonest form of bone marrow suppression is pancytopenia, but neutropenia is also a frequent finding. For these reasons it is recommended that patients have weekly full blood counts, including differential white counts and platelet counts, for the first eight weeks of starting therapy, followed by two-weekly blood counts up to the 1 g dosage, followed by four-weekly counts thereafter.

(d) Other side effects

Gold lung has been described. Mouth ulceration is fairly common and can be difficult to overcome. Hydrocortisone sodium succinate pellets (Corlan) are useful for alleviating this. Griffin (1979) described cholestatic hepatitis.

(e) Analysis of the frequency of side effects

An elegant study from Cape Town (Majoos *et al.*, 1981) over an eight-year period from 1971 to 1979 studied 114 patients with rheumatoid arthritis who had been treated with Myocrisin. Seventy of 104 patients benefited from the drug with 40 going into complete remission. Therapy was discontinued in 58 patients, side effects accounting for this in 33 patients. Adverse reactions included rashes in 41 patients (39%), renal complications in 16 patients (14%) and 7 (6%) developed haematological complications leading to death in two patients. Tissue typing in 37 patients with side effects showed no increase in frequency of HLA DW2 or 3 antigen. There was, however, a significant increase in HLA DW4 antigen in both whites and blacks. Other studies have suggested that the dropout rate on gold is anywhere between 50 and 75% by the end of eight months' treatment.

(f) Side effects on auranofin

Side effects on auranofin appear to be fewer and less severe. Side effects appear to be more predominantly diarrhoea, and this appears to be dose related – the dose of 6 mg being associated with a lower frequency of diarrhoea than a 9 mg dose. Other side effects such as rash, thrombocytopenia and proteinuria do occur but appear to be much less common. However, further reports are necessary before drawing any firm conclusions about the toxicity of this compound.

(g) Are there more side effects on D-penicillamine after gold therapy?

This therapeutic problem does arise and has now been extensively studied. In a study of 151 patients submitted to D-penicillamine, 125 took only D-penicillamine and 45 developed side effects from the drug, whereas of the 27 patients with a history of gold toxicity, 18 also reacted adversely to penicillamine. All patients who took penicillamine within 6 months after an adverse reaction developed side effects. Fourteen patients developed similar reactions to D-penicillamine and gold. The interval between treatments in this group was significantly shorter than in those who developed either differing adverse reactions to both drugs, or no reaction to D-penicillamine after treatment with gold. It would seem that if a gap of 6 months is left between two treatments this would reduce the risk of adverse reactions to D-penicillamine.

Webley and Coombs (1979) considered 114 patients with rheumatoid arthritis who received treatment with penicillamine, having previously received gold. The side effects occurred in 50 patients, 60 were considered to have improved with the drug. Low and high maintenance regimes were compared and there was no significant difference in side effects or clinical improvement. Previous gold therapy did not influence therapeutic response or total frequency of side effects observed with penicillamine. Rashes were perhaps more common in patients who received gold.

(h) *Tissue antigens and side effects*

Wooley *et al.* (1980) attempted to relate HLA antigens and toxicity. A total of 91 patients were studied, 71 had toxic reactions to either penicillamine or gold or to both drugs. Of 24 patients in whom proteinuria developed 19 were positive for HLA B8 and DRW3. Fourteen out of 15 episodes of aurothiomalate-induced proteinuria and 9 out of 13 episodes of penicillamine-induced proteinuria occurred in patients with these antigens. All 13 episodes of proteinuria in which urinary protein exceeded 2 g in 24 hours occurred in patients who were DRW3 positive. No significant association was found between any HLA antigen in the development of rashes or haematological complications.

Latts *et al.* (1980) studied 32 patients receiving gold. Adverse reactions appeared to be found in increased frequency in patients who were B12 antigen positive.

9.4 PENICILLAMINE

9.4.1 Introduction

Penicillamine was discovered by Abraham *et al.* in 1943 when they found that acid hydrolysates of penicillin gave a strong blue–violet colouration with the ninhydrin agent. It was also found that 59% of total nitrogen of the pure penicillin preparation could be estimated as amino nitrogen after one hour's hydrolysis with 0.1N sulphuric acid using the Van Slyke method. This observation showed that the substance responsible for the results of these reactions was an integral part of the penicillin molecule, and they were able to report its isolation as a crystalline hydrochloride. To this amino acid degradation product of penicillin they gave the name penicillamine. The chemical structure was determined later by Sir Ernst Chain in 1949. Subsequent experiments showed that the L enantiomorph is the more toxic isomer and therefore only D-penicillamine is now used therapeutically in man, either as the hydrochloride or free amino acid.

9.4.2   Animal toxicity

Experiments carried out under the auspices of Dr Hugh Lyle at the Dista Laboratories found that D-penicillamine is not lethal to most rats, although some died following a dose of 10 000 mg kg^{-1} body weight. The drug appears to exhibit anti-pyridoxine activity in rats which is correctable with vitamin B$_6$. It also appears to have lathyrogenic effects in the same animal.

9.4.3   General clinical applications

Walshe (1953) identified penicillamine in the urine of patients with advanced liver disease receiving parenteral penicillin therapy. As the compound is excreted in the reduced-SH state he deduced that the thiol group might prove active in the chelation of copper. Further investigations confirm that penicillamine prompted the urinary excretion of copper both in healthy people and patients with Wilson's disease. Penicillamine forms chelates with other cations such as lead.

Disulphide exchange with cysteine

Tabachnick et al. (1954) showed that penicillamine reacted readily with cysteine with the formation of a mixed disulphide. It was not until ten years later that this observation was used in the treatment of patients with cystinuria. The excessive urinary excretion of cysteine was shown to be reduced or abolished according to the dose of penicillamine administered. Penicillamine is capable of producing dissolution of cysteine calculi in patients with cystinuria when added to other conventional techniques of treatment.

9.4.4   Pharmacological applications

All administered D-penicillamine is largely resorbed from the gastrointestinal tract, but half the effective dose is rapidly excreted in the urine, mostly as a mixed D-penicillamine cysteine disulphide leading to cysteine depletion. Only a relatively small porportion of D-penicillamine taken up by the body is turned into S-methyl-D-penicillamine. It is partly excreted and partly catabolized by way of D-amino acid oxidase in the liver. Roughly 20% of the administered dose is stored in the tissue, from which the serum pool is slowly refilled. This results in a steady rise in serum penicillamine level during continuous treatment and leads to an increase in storage of penicillamine in the tissues. These

observations are based on work by Perret (1981) who himself swallowed
[14]C-labelled D-penicillamine. He recovered 35% of the radioactivity in the
faeces indicating incomplete resorption from the intestines, or metabolic
breakdown in the liver followed by biliary excretion. He recovered almost
50% of the administered dose from the urine. Other results came from
intravenous studies. One subject took a single intravenous dose of 50 mg of
D-penicillamine and results were compared with the effect of an oral dose of
1000 mg. In both instances a serum peak level of 8 mg per mole was reached.
However, after intravenous administration, 75% of the dose administered was
recovered from the urine, but from the oral dose only 28% was recovered.

In summary, it appears that from an oral dose administered, two thirds are
resorbed from the gut, and one third or more is circulating as free D-penicillamine in the body and is partly excreted as disulphide with itself or with cysteine
and as a copper complex. Part of the free D-penicillamine becomes tissue bound
from which the serum pool is constantly refilled, presenting as a slow pool. The
remainder, about 20%, is converted into S-methyl-D-penicillamine which is
partly oxidized in the liver, followed by a further breakdown, whilst another
part of the S-methyl-D-penicillamine is excreted in the urine.

9.4.5 Effects in rheumatoid disease

Jaffe (1962) demonstrated the dissociation of rheumatoid factor in synovial
fluid when penicillamine was injected into the knee joint of a patient with
rheumatoid arthritis. Later, he proved that oral administration in such a
patient produced a consistent reduction of circulating rheumatoid factor
accompanied by clinical improvement, but only after a latent period of a
month or so on this treatment. He also reported a beneficial response in a
patient with rheumatoid arthritis and a return to normal values of laboratory
measurements of disease activity. Jaffe observed a drug-induced fall in IgG and
IgM. Other workers have subsequently confirmed the drug's ability to lower
all major immunoglobulin classes to normal. This does not necessarily correlate with clinical improvement. Jaffe also showed that penicillamine was
capable of causing the level of immune complexes to decline on treatment.

9.4.6 Effects on lymphocyte function

There is a dose-related inhibition of lymphocyte transformation in the presence
of D- and L-penicillamine. Schumacher (1975) has shown that pre-exposure of
male spleen T cells to D-penicillamine *in vitro* results in striking inhibition of
cellular immune responses measured by the sheep erythrocyte rosette technique. This phytohaemagglutinin-induced lymphocyte transformation inhibition has since been confirmed by Maini and Roff (1977) but only after using
high D-penicillamine concentrations. This leads to the speculation that the

therapeutic action of the drug might be through modulation of T cell function *in vivo*. Kendell and Hutchins (1978), experimenting on mouse spleen cells stimulated in culture by concavalin A, observed that the true effect of penicillamine is enhancement of lymphocyte transformation. This was observed when it was in the medium long enough to deplete cysteine supply, the rate of the depletion being dependent on penicillamine concentration. These apparently conflicting views are compatible in a truly biological system, when enhancement and suppression both present evidence of effectiveness.

9.4.7   Specific clinical applications

(a) *Progressive systemic sclerosis (PSS)*

Penicillamine seems to be of use for patients with morphoea particularly in children (Moynahan, 1973). However, its use in PSS is somewhat more controversial. Jayson *et al.* (1977) have concluded that it was of limited value for the cutaneous features of PSS and of no value for the vascular or visceral manifestations of the disease.

(b) *Liver disease*

There have been three trials in the use of penicillamine in primary biliary cirrhosis. The most significant finding appears to be a reduction in serum aspartate transaminase after three months which is maintained for at least to nine months. Liver copper concentrations fell in the penicillamine-treated patients (Jain *et al.*, 1977). In chronic active hepatitis D-penicillamine therapy appears to be a useful alternative therapy to corticosteroids in some patients (Stern *et al.*, 1977).

(c) *Rheumatoid arthritis*

(i) Dosage

First studies in rheumatoid arthritis were originally carried out at 1500 mg of penicillamine a day. The Multicentre Study Group (1973) first confirmed efficacy in a placebo controlled double-blind study. Dixon *et al.* (1975) reported that 600 mg a day was as effective as 1200 mg a day, with a significant reduction in withdrawal for adverse effects. Response has been observed in some patients with as low a dose as 125 mg although the response is slow. The probability is that the right dose to start with is 250 mg daily. If there is improvement in six weeks to two months, this may well be sufficient. Some patients will, however, need 500 or 750 mg daily. However, the tendency now is to increase the dose slowly, possibly allowing a further two or three months to elapse before the final increase to 750 mg. Only on very rare occasions will it be necessary to use a dose of 1 g daily.

(ii) Evidence for disease modifying effect

There are now a large number of papers showing that D-penicillamine is capable of improving all clinical measurements, inducing remission in some patients, certainly inducing disease modification in others, and causing some reversion towards normal disease-related immunological changes (Jaffe, 1965). Comparative trials against azathioprine (Berry *et al.*, 1980), gold (Huskisson *et al.*, 1974), pyrithioxine (Camus *et al.*, personal communication), fenclofenac (Berry *et al.*, 1981) and levamisole (Mowat and Mowat, 1981) have all confirmed the ability of penicillamine to induce remission in rheumatoid arthritis.

(iii) Unwanted effects

Unfortunately, penicillamine leads to a Pandora's Box of unwanted drug-related effects.

Haematological. Neutropenia, thrombocytopenia, pancytopenia and anaemia have all been described (Multicentre Study Group, 1973).

Renal. Proteinuria (early and often transient) or later, especially at nine months, leading to nephrotic syndrome often occur (10% of patients) (Dische *et al.*, 1976). A rare renal complication is seen in some patients who develop frank haematuria and renal failure from an associated Goodpasture's syndrome (Gibson *et al.*, 1976).

Skin complications. Classically an early rash occurs which may well go away even if the treatment is continued. Certainly on stopping treatment the rash will disappear and on re-introducing treatment it will not necessarily reappear. A later and more troublesome complication is that of pemphigus or pemphigoid-like rashes. These all have the bullous appearance on the mucous membranes and on the skin around the mucous membranes and this needs treatment with corticosteroids.

Alimentary tract. Taste loss is described in early treatment with at least 10% of patients afflicted. It may last for up to two years, but all cases so far described are reversible (Jaffe, 1965). Nausea is sometimes encountered, leading to up to 10% of patients being withdrawn from the drug. A thorough search has failed to confirm peptic ulceration as being caused by penicillamine therapy. In patients in whom this does occur, it would seem more likely to be due to the NSAID that the patient is taking in addition to the penicillamine. Diarrhoea and constipation appear to be described in equal numbers in most trials, and in all probability the drug is not the cause either.

Muscular. There have been case reports of polymyositis which appears to be drug related (Fernandes *et al.*, 1977).

Lung complications. An obliterative bronchiolitis and pulmonary fibrosis have been described as being possibly drug induced. It is hard to be sure that these are drug induced as both these complications can occur as a complication of the disease itself rather than the drug (Turner-Warwick, 1981).

Immunological disease. Myasthenia gravis with anti-acetylcholine and anti-motor end plate antibodies is now well substantiated as being caused by penicillamine (Bucknall *et al.*, 1975). Lupus-like reactions with antinuclear antibodies are also well described (Camus *et al.*, 1977a; Walshe, 1981; Chalmers *et al.*, 1982). If the drug is stopped soon after onset of symptoms, they will disappear. On the other hand, there are case reports of patients in whom the drug has been continued and in whom the disease has become fixed.

(iv) Effects in pregnancy

Penicillamine can be given during pregnancy, as it is for Wilson's disease, but the ideal would be to avoid the drug in pregnancy if possible. However, the only death described in an infant was not related to the drug, the child dying of small bowel atresia. On the other hand the skin of the infant did exhibit features of the Ehlers–Danlos syndrome. Subsequently, in a series described by Lyle (1973), 27 patients taking penicillamine at some stage in pregnancy delivered children and all were normal except for one with a ventral septal defect. Although it is still wise to withhold administration of the drug during pregnancy, it is no longer deemed a necessary indication for termination of that pregnancy.

(v) Continuation of therapy

Penicillamine, like all disease remittive agents takes three to six months before showing its maxima effect. At the end of that period it seems reasonable to reduce the dose to the lowest at which the patient still obtains clinical remission. There is some evidence suggesting that lower doses produce fewer side effects, although this is by no means universally agreed. It may well be necessary to continue the medication together with NSAIDs. There are now many patients who have been treated successfully with penicillamine for at least ten years. There seems no particular reason for stopping the drug if it is keeping the patient in clinical remission. It is, however, important to emphasize that continuing vigilance should be exercised by carrying out monthly full blood and platelet counts, checking also the urine and skin. Side effects can occur at any point during the therapeutic use of the drug and patients have been known to develop proteinuria or neutropenia as late as 8 years after starting treatment.

9.5 CYTOTOXIC DRUGS

The use of cytotoxic drugs in rheumatoid arthritis comes from the concept of immuno-dysfunction in this disease. Jimenez Diaz (1951) first used a nitrogen mustard. There are still questions as to their mode of action. Do they act through a real immunodepressor process, or simply through a generalized anti-proliferative effect on cells, or is it by combination of the two?

9.5.1 Chlorambucil

This alkylating agent which acts directly on DNA synthesis has an action on cells in tissue culture that depends exponentially on dosage. Its effect is particularly evident during the phase of DNA synthesis and the post-mitotic phase.

(a) *Metabolism*

Little is known of its metabolism in man. In animals, studies have been carried out using ^{14}C-labelled chlorambucil. In the rat absorption is very rapid, the molecule is split into two fragments and the butyric radical undergoes β-oxidation which renders active the alkylating group of chlorambucil. It is excreted in the urine and bowel. In the rat chlorambucil is fixed in the thymus and bone marrow.

(b) *Pharmacology*

(i) Anti-inflammatory effect

This was demonstrated by Currey (1971) in a dose–effect study on rat paw swelling after an injection of irritant. The drug was active but only at high dose. Other studies in carrageenan-induced oedema showed similar dose-related effects (Brouilhet *et al.*, 1971). Similar studies on phagocytosis and bacterial action by Kahan and Amor (1971) confirmed this cytotoxic effect. Chlorambucil significantly inhibits development of polyarthritis induced by Freund's adjuvant, and it also significantly reinforces arthritis induced by complete *Mycoplasma arthritidis* (as does anti-lymphocyte serum). If one compares the effects of chlorambucil, 5-fluorouracil, azathioprine, cyclophosphamide and methotrexate in the same pharmacological test, both Brouilhet *et al.* (1971) and Currey (1971) have been able to demonstrate some notable differences. 5-Fluorouracil and azathioprine seem to be immunosuppressors, the action of methotrexate, cyclophosphamide and chlorambucil being anti-proliferative, anti-inflammatory and immunosuppressive.

(ii) Clinical work

The effect of the cytotoxic drugs in rheumatoid arthritis has been demonstrated by several controlled trials carried out notably by the American Medical Association using cyclophosphamide (Co-operating Clinic's Committee of the American Rheumatism Association, 1970) and Mason *et al.* (1969) using azathioprine. The only controlled trial with chlorambucil was made in 1972 (Hatchuel, 1972). In this study a double-blind comparison of 25 patients receiving chlorambucil and 23 receiving placebo over a three-month period was studied. The initial dose of chlorambucil was 0.2 mg kg^{-1} per day which was eventually reduced with the appearance of leucopenia. The total active dose received by patients during the three month controlled trial was 920 mg. From the results of this study the drug is capable of decreasing the Rose Waaler test in some 50% of the patients studied, causing the ESR to fall in the same 50% of patients to at least half of the initial level. It also gave an overall clinical improvement on the basis of a four category scale that took into account pain, morning stiffness, number of joints affected and functional ability in 72% of the patients studied as compared with 27% of the patients receiving placebo.

Further open data from Kahan and Amor (1971) studying 528 patients show that around 50% responded favourably in terms of clinical or biological measures involving inflammation, particularly the sedimentation rate. A decrease in the rheumatoid factor appears to be real, although less spectacular than with penicillamine. The remission induced by the drug, whilst it may start in as little as two months, may take up to nine months before it begins to work. On stopping therapy the remission may be maintained often for more than a year.

(iii) Therapeutic control

Again, it is very important that full blood counts and platelet counts are studied at least monthly on this therapy, and it is advisable to suggest a two-month run-in period where patients receive their blood tests two weekly.

(c) *Side effects*

(i) Infections

Viral infections include those of Herpes zoster: whilst most are innocuous, occasionally they can be fatal. This particular side effect can appear some time after treatment has been halted.

Mycotic infections have consisted essentially of moniliasis, particularly of the digestive tract.

Bacterial infections. These are primarily urinary or bronchopulmonary, but other types also noted include cholecystitis, septic arthritis, and subcutaneous or muscular abscess. These can lead to septicaemia, and rarely death. Common predisposing factors to septicaemia include leucopenia and patients who have had corticosteroids for a considerable time.

(ii) Endocrine effects

Amenorrhoea and azoospermia have been described.

(iii) Cutaneous effects

Alopecia is rare. Rashes are occasionally seen.

(iv) Digestive effects

Digestive problems are usually minor and only occasionally lead to withdrawal of treatment.

(v) Haematological effects

Leucopenia is common but rarely fatal, providing it is investigated and managed adequately. Thrombocytopenia, anaemia and pancytopenia are also encountered. Reviewing a controlled study comparing chlorambucil with placebo, it seems that Herpes zoster, amenorrhoea, digestive disorders and blood disorders are certainly drug related, but the bacterial infections seem to appear equally in patients with placebo as to those on chlorambucil and could be unrelated to the drug.

(d) *Mortality*

There is an increase in certain malignant disorders in patients treated with chlorambucil. The Oxford study (Kinlen *et al.*, 1979) on 3823 patients who had received renal transplants, and 1349 other patients including cases of rheumatoid arthritis receiving cytotoxic drugs, particularly azathioprine, showed that the risk of malignant disorders was tripled particularly for non-Hodgkin lymphomas and squamous cell skin cancer. Kahn *et al.* (1979), using results from the collective retrospective study, calculated the frequency of acute leukaemia during and after cytotoxic treatment of rheumatic disorders. Results of this survey, which included 2006 patients, showed an increased frequency of leukaemia. Delay between the beginning of treatment and the appearance of the disease appears to be 5.7 ± 2.9 years (Menkes *et al.*, 1975; Kahn *et al.*,

1979). No leukaemia has been observed in patients who have received less than 1 g and for whom the duration of treatment was less than six months.

(e) Conclusion

Chlorambucil appears to be active for the treatment of rheumatoid arthritis. The best results appear to be in those patients who are not receiving corticosteroids, and therefore there might be an argument for giving chlorambucil early in the course of the disease. However, this positive advantage has to an extent to be weighed by the risks of possible infection or the development of cancer. This moderates the enthusiasm for the drug and makes one reserve it for patients with arthritis in whom other treatments have failed and where the severe nature of the disease justifies the risks. This effectively stops the drug being suitable for children.

9.5.2 Azathioprine

This antimetabolic drug has been studied in the hope that it would be able to suppress the immune alteration seen in patients with rheumatoid arthritis. Azathioprine has been the subject of many clinical trials. The first was carried out by Galens *et al.* (1964) where two patients, treated from 4 to 9.5 months, both improved. A further small study of 11 patients treated by Meons and Blocteur (1965) from 1 to 5 months showed improvement in four patients. Mason *et al.* (1969) carried out another open clinical study of 9 cases in which 8 improved, although the duration of treatment and total dose was not clear from the paper. Further studies also showed an improvement in patients. However, a more formal study carried out by Mason *et al.* (1969) in 25 patients at 2.5 mg per day from 3 to 18 months' duration of treatment was double blind with 24 matched controls, and showed a steroid dose reduction of 36%. Criticism of this trial was that showing steroid sparing was not necessarily an index of disease-modifying antirheumatic activity. Nevertheless, further studies (Woodland *et al.*, 1974) showed that azathioprine is comparable with, if inferior to, cyclophosphamide, but comparable with gold. Berry *et al.* (1976) have shown that penicillamine is slightly more effective than azathioprine.

(a) Toxic effects

The same problems with azathioprine exist as have been described with cyclophosphamide. The risk of malignancy is still an unanswered question, despite prolonged attempts to discover whether or not the drug is or is not mutagenic. This is certainly of sufficient worry to preclude the use of azathioprine in pregnancy.

(b) *Haematological problems*

Bone marrow suppression is a major problem with this drug, as with all drugs in this group. A more acute explosive type of bone marrow depression early in the course of treatment has also been described and has been seen by this author, with death within two weeks of the start of treatment despite careful monitoring.

(c) *Gastrointestinal effects*

Sickness and nausea appear to be a considerable problem with this drug; and certainly in our hands this has precluded its use in half the patients treated (Berry *et al.*, 1976).

(d) *Summary*

This drug appears to have a role in the treatment of rheumatoid arthritis when penicillamine, gold and chloroquine have been tried first. Otherwise, the risk-to-benefit ratio appears to be too great. The possibility of malignancy, the risk of severe nausea, and the bone marrow depression being of sufficient concern to make it not the first choice of drug in this group.

9.5.3 Levamisole

Levamisole is an established anti-worming agent that has been used for many years and has been given safely to pregnant women (Mowat and Vischer, 1979). The observation that the drug exerted an effect on the immune system led to its use where the fault was primary or secondary immune deficiency, particularly in malignancy or lymphoma. The early results of these studies showed that the drug was able to improve the immunological status of such patients, although the way in which the drug works remains unknown. There is no certainty that this is an effect on lymphocytes, but the drug may exert its effect by interference with phagocytic cell function. In rheumatoid arthritis the earliest reports consisted of uncontrolled data from Lewis and Symoens (1978). These suggest an antirheumatic effect in patients with rheumatoid arthritis and the ability of the drug to reduce rheumatoid factor titres. Side effects that have been seen include rashes and dyspepsia. There have also been reports of leucopenia. The dosage used varies widely, there are data at 150 mg daily on a continuous basis, but other studies have looked at once-weekly and twice-weekly administration (Mielants and Veys, 1978; Mowat and Mowat, 1981). It is absorbed when administered orally and has a short half-life of 1–2 hours. There is no evidence that the drug is accumulated in any organ. Control trial data (Multicentre Study Group, 1981) suggest that the drug is an alternative, but that it is highly toxic. More studies are necessary to establish whether the toxicity may be modified by dose reduction, and it remains to be seen if the drug will still be active at lower dosage.

9.5.4 Cyclophosphamide

This drug selectively depletes lymphocyte sub-populations (Hurd and Ziff, 1968). It is the only drug that materially alters a continued secondary cellular or antibody mediated immune response (Berenbaum and Brown, 1964; Levy *et al.*, 1970; Arinoviche and Loewi, 1970). Unfortunately, side effects are more frequent and severe with cyclophosphamide than with other cytotoxic drugs. Metabolism is very complex and several of the many metabolities possess biological activity that may lead to mediation either of clinical effects or side effects. The liver biotransforms the drug, and the effects of the drug may be influenced by drugs that affect hepatic microsomal enzymes (Struck and Hill, 1972). The best-controlled clinical trials that have been carried out on this drug include a comparison between azathioprine, cyclophosphamide and gold (Woodland *et al.*, 1974), as well as the six-year data from Fosdick *et al.* (1968). In these studies cyclophosphamide was seen to be an effective drug but the toxicity, including haemorrhagic cystitis, alopecia, azoospermia and severe nausea, together with neutropenia and thrombocytopenia, as well as the potential risk of increased tumour frequency, were common enough to reduce the use of the drug for rare cases where a remission cannot be induced by any others means. Unfortunately, this is the only drug that has been shown actually to influence the erosive pattern of the disease. This is based on the Multicentre Americal Trial organized by the Co-operating Clinics (1970). In this there was definite slowing down of erosions.

9.6   THIOL DERIVATIVE DRUGS

Penicillamine has been shown to be a useful and effective drug for the treatment of rheumatoid arthritis. Unfortunately, it would appear that patients who experienced a major side effect on gold appear to be more likely to develop a serious side effect with penicillamine. Therefore, if there were other compounds with a similar remission-inducing property, the physician may well have larger numbers of drugs from which to choose. Since penicillamine is a thiol compound, further studies of this class have been undertaken in an effort to identify similar SH compounds with penicillamine-like activity. The first of these is 5-thiopyridoxine (5-TP). It is a sulphydryl compound structurally dissimilar to penicillamine because it is a ring compound rather than a straight-chain amino acid. It was first used in an attempt to produce intervascular dissociation of cold agglutinin macroglobulin antibodies by the SH–SS inter-change *in vivo* (Ritzmann and Leven, 1961). 5-TP was effective in that disorder. The study showed that the reduction in cold agglutinin titres persisted long after the treatment was continued – a similar response to that which is seen with penicillamine in rheumatoid factor titre in rheumatoid arthritis. Therefore a pilot study in which 5-TP was compared with penicillamine was carried out by Jaffe in 1963, and showed similar results. Similar side effects appeared, including loss of taste. Other studies showed an improvement in clinical state accompanied by a reduction in ESR and rheumatoid factor titre, and there was an improvement in haemoglobin levels comparable with that produced on penicillamine. It also appeared to work slowly, possibly even more slowly than penicillamine, taking up to six months to produce its maxima effect.

Similar side effects to D-penicillamine were encountered, including loss of taste, rash, pemphigus and proteinuria, and immune complex deposition appeared responsible for some of these immunological toxic problems. It was noteworthy that individual patients receiving 5-TP did not necessarily develop the same adverse effect on that drug as had been responsible for their withdrawal from penicillamine. This supports the concept that although the spectrum of side effects among these agents may be similar, a particular patient is not necessarily liable to the development of the identical toxicity of each member of this class compound.

9.6.1 Pyrithioxine

Pyrithioxine is the disulphide of 5-thiopyridoxine. Unlike penicillamine disulphide, it is readily absorbed from the gastrointestinal tract and is much more freely dissociable. It is presumed to exist *in vivo* in equilibrium with the sulphydryl form (5-TP), and the pattern of urinary metabolites is similar with the two compounds. It is sold in some countries as a central nervous system energizer for the treatment of senile and depressive states. The studies have therefore been carried out in countries where it is freely available such as France, and Camus *et al.* (1977b) have shown it to be an effective agent. When 150 patients with rheumatoid arthritis given 600 mg daily were studied for one year or longer, the effects of morning stiffness, articular index, ESR and rheumatoid factor were evaluated. A total of 47% were good responders, 30% non-responders, 10% had late relapses, and 13% were withdrawn for side effects, mainly cutaneous and mucocutaneous. Camus' conclusions were that the drug is somewhat less effective but better tolerated than either penicillamine or gold.

A study in Warsaw, involving 23 rheumatoid arthritis patients in whom both gold and penicillamine had to be withdrawn because of side effects or lack of activity, has been carried out. In 12 of these patients after six months of therapy there was marked improvement in 7, associated with a fall in ESR of at least 50%, and a significant drop in the rheumatoid factor titre (Bruhl *et al.*, 1979).

The results of these trials support the concept that 5-TP and pyrithioxine do have penicillamine-like activity in rheumatoid arthritis, although they appear to be less effective in the degree of disease suppression achieved, and take a longer period to reach their maxima effectiveness. They also appear to be less likely to give rise to the more serious side effects of penicillamine therapy, such as acute haematological toxicity. It is of interest that immune-complex nephropathy has been encountered with 5-TP and pyrithioxine. Another patient treated with pyrithioxine developed myasthenia gravis, with development of antibodies for the acetylcholine receptor (Camus and Darkins, personal communication).

9.6.2 Thiopronine

Thiopronine was studied by Jaffe (1983) for its effectiveness on circulating rheumatoid factor in a limited number of rheumatoid arthritics. It appeared to have no activity in this regard. However, a further open study from the University of Pisa showed a good to excellent clinical response from four to eighteen months (Pasero and Ciompi, 1979). There were no serological data in their report. The side effects, however, bore a remarkable similarity to those encountered with penicillamine, including loss of taste, stomatitis, rash, and nephrotic syndrome in two patients. There was no haemotological toxicity in their small series. Amor et al. (1979) showed in an open study of 23 patients improvement in morning stiffness, articular index, grip strength, sedimentation rate, and joint swelling. Again, similar side effects to penicillamine were encountered.

9.6.3 Summary

It would appear therefore that these three drugs are capable of offering an alternative to penicillamine. Penicillamine may well be the parent compound of a group of compounds, and further developments may occur in this area.

9.7   FENCLOFENAC

This drug was introduced as a conventional NSAID. However, it is not conventional in its effect on certain of the animal models, particularly adjuvant arthritis, and its effect on the ability to ulcerate the rat gastric mucosa is minimal. It was this that led to investigation of its likely role as a long-term agent.

In a comparative trial of fenclofenac against penicillamine the drug was found to be useful in some patients, and it appeared to exert a disease-modifying antirheumatic role. This was accompanied by a fall in ESR but not an improvement in haemoglobin. It was also accompanied by a fall in C-reactive protein, a fall in immunoglobulins, and a reversion to normal in some patients with raised rheumatoid factor titres. The side effects from this drug are those of a NSAID, namely gastrointestinal intolerance in some patients (Berry *et al.*, 1980). Other workers have subsequently confirmed these observations. Cox *et al.* (1981) compared fenclofenac with gold. Their one-year data would certainly support the concept of an equal effect of fenclofenac and gold in patients with rheumatoid arthritis. Bach-Anderson *et al.* (1981) have confirmed these findings in their comparative study of fenclofenac against gold.

9.7.1 Conclusions

The importance of these observations is that this might be a suitable drug to be used in early disease. This needs to be confirmed on the basis of other controlled clinical trials. However, it appears likely that this drug is capable in some patients of inducing and holding patients in remission.

Whether it is indeed capable of interfering with the erosive changes seen on X-rays is much more controversial and again is the subject of other controlled clinical trials.

9.8 SULPHASALAZINE

Sulphasalazine is in fact an 'old' therapy in which there has been a resurgence of interest. Introduced by Svartz in 1942 for the treatment of rheumatoid arthritis (its use for inflammatory bowel disease came later), it quickly fell into disfavour after an unenthusiastic British report (Sinclair and Duthie, 1948). However, recently encouraging reports of its efficacy as a long-term agent in rheumatoid arthritis have been published (McConkey *et al.*, 1978, 1980), although this enthusiasm has not been universal (Currey and Chaput de Saintonge, 1980; James and Reebach, 1980). Nevertheless, fresh interest in the drug is being maintained (Bird *et al.*, 1982), and recent trials (Farr *et al.*, 1984; Bax and Amos, 1985) have shown the drug to be a safe and effective drug for prolonged control of rheumatoid arthritis.

9.9 THE FUTURE

Whereas gold and penicillamine seem to be active in interfering with some elements of the disease they are not good at interfering with radiological change, the most accurate way of demonstrating effectiveness or otherwise of drugs in this group. At best, these drugs are capable of 'buying time', although everybody will quote patients who have been 'cured' by these agents. There is still the risk of recurrence of arthritis later on. There is also the risk that, despite the absence of physical signs, the disease grumbles on and that repeat X-rays, even in patients who appear to be normal, show continuation of the disease changes. Cyclophosphamide appears to be the one drug capable of having a profound effect even on erosive changes, but it would appear to be too toxic for routine use. Azathioprine and other immunodepressive drugs appear to work, but are probably less effective than gold or penicillamine. The group of thiol derivative drugs which resemble penicillamine also appear to resemble this drug in their side effects and in their pattern of efficacy.

There is clearly a need in this area for new drugs capable of offering better efficacy with lower toxic manifestations. It is of note that a large number of pharmaceutical companies are investigating these agents and have instituted long-term disease-modifying drug programmes. Unfortunately, recent events with benoxaprofen have caused a cut back in this area as drug companies wonder whether the cost-to-risk benefit is viable. These drugs also need meticulous monitoring, and toxic manifestations must be carefully researched before the drugs are tried in man. However, only this sort of research programme will be helpful to patients. There is a strong feeling that we should stop producing yet more NSAIDs, which, however safe they may be to the patients, and however financially useful to the drug companies, are not in fact providing anything new to the rheumatoid patient. However, the real solution to rheumatoid arthritis will not be forthcoming until such time that we know more about what produces the disease and what keeps it going.

9.10   REFERENCES

Abraham, E. P., Chain, E., Baker, W. and Robinson, R. (1943) Penicillamine: a characteristic degradation product of penicillin. *Nature*, 151, 107.

Amor, B., Mery, C. and de Gery, A. (1979) Thioprine a new long acting drug in R.A. *Communication, IXth Congress of Rheumatology*, Wiesbaden, West Germany, Abstract 170.

Arinoviche, R. and Loewi, G. (1970) Comparison of the effects of two cytotoxic drugs and of anti-lymphocytic serum on immune and non-immune inflammation in experimental animals. *Ann. Rheum. Dis.*, 29, 32–9.

Bach, M. A. and Bach, F. J. (1981) The use of monoclonal anti-T cell antibodies to study T cell imbalance in human diseases. *Clin. Exp. Immunol.*, 45, 449–56.

Bach-Anderson, R., Lund, B. and Graae, A. (1981) A 12-month comparison of the effects of fenclofenac and gold in patients with rheumatoid arthritis. *Communication, XVth International Congress of Rheumatology*, Paris.

Bagnell, A. W. (1957) The value of chloroquine in rheumatoid disease. *Can. Med. Assoc. J.*, 77, 182–94.

Bax, D. E. and Amos, R. S. (1985) Sulphasalazine; a safe, effective agent for prolonged control of rheumatoid arthritis. A comparison with sodium aurothiomalate. *Ann. Rheum. Dis.*, 44, 194–8.

Berenbaum, M. D. and Brown, I. N. (1964) Dose response relationships for agents inhibiting the immune response. *Immunology*, 7, 65–74.

Bernstein, H. N. (1967) Chloroquine ocular toxicity. *Survey Ophthalmol.*, 12, 415–47.

Berry, H., Camp, A. V., Molloy, M. G., Heywood, D., James, D. W., Bloom, B. and Hamilton, E. B. D. (1981) Anti-rheumatic properties of fenclofenac in comparison with D-penicillamine and placebo. *Communication, XVth International Congress of Rheumatology,* Paris.

Berry, H., Camp, A. V., Molloy, M., Heywood, D., James, D. W., Bloom, B. and Hamilton, E. B. D. (1981) Anti-rheumatic properties of fenclofenac in comparison with D-penicillamine and placebo. in *Modulation of Autoimmunity and Disease* (eds R. N. Maini and H. Berry), Praeger Scientific, Eastbourne and New York, pp. 249–52.

Berry, H., Ford-Hutchinson, A. W., Camp, A. V., Heywood, D., Molloy, M. G., James, D. W. and Hamilton, E. B. D. (1980) Anti-rheumatic activity of fenclofenac. *Ann. Rheum. Dis.,* 39, 473–5.

Berry, H. and Huskisson, E. C. (1974) Experience with penicillamine and azathioprine in rheumatoid arthritis. *Postgrad. Med. J.,* 50, 61–2.

Berry, H., Liyanage, S. P., Durance, R. A., Barnes, C. G., Berger, L. and Evans, S. (1976) Azathioprine and penicillamine in the treatment of rheumatoid arthritis: a controlled trial. *Br. Med. J.,* 1, 1052–4.

Bird, H. A., Dixon, J. S., Pickup, M. E., Rhind, U. M., Lowe, J. R., Lee, M. R. and Wright, V. (1982) Chemical assessment of sulphasalazine in rheumatoid arthritis. *J. Rheum.,* 9, 36–45.

Brouilhet, H., Kahan, A. and Jouanneau, M. (1971) Etudes cytostatiques et du sérum anti-lymphocytaire sur les differents aspects de l'immunité chez l'animal. in *Colloque Immunodepression, Bases Expérimentales – Résultates Thérapeutiques,* Paris, Inserm. pp. 69.

Bruhl, W., Swierczymska, Z. and Cygler, B. (1979) Clinical and immunological effects of pyrithioxine in RA patients. *Communication, IXth European Congress of Rheumatology,* Wiesbaden, West Germany, Abstract 243).

Bucknall, R. C., Dixon, A. St. J., Glick, E. N., Woodland, J. and Zutshi, D. W. (1975) Myasthenia gravis associated with penicillamine treatment for rheumatoid arthritis. *Br. Med. J.,* 1, 600–2.

Camus, J. P., Crouzet, J., Homberg, J. C. and Bach, J. F. (1977a) *Penicillamine Research in Rheumatoid Disease.* Fabritus and Sonner, Oslo, pp. 125–9.

Camus, J. P., Jaffe, I. A., Crouzet, J., Prier, A. and Lavent, C. (1977b) La pyrithioxine, nouveau traitment de fond de la polyarthrite rhumatoide. *Ann. Med. Interne,* 128, 907–91.

Camus, J. P., Jaffe, I. A., Crouzet, J., Prier, A., Mercier, A. and Dubois, A. (1978) La pyrithioxine nouveau traitment de fond de la polyarthrite rhumatoide. *Rev. rhum.,* 45, 95–100.

Cats, A. (1976) *Agents Actions,* 6, 355–63.

Chalmers, A., Thompson, D., Stein, H. E., Reid, G. and Patterson, A. C. (1982) Systemic lupus erythematosus during penicillamine therapy for rheumatoid arthritis. *Ann. Intern. Med.,* 97, 659–63.

Co-operating Clinics Committee of the American Rheumatism Association (1970) A controlled trial of cyclophosphamide in rheumatoid arthritis. *N. Engl. J. Med.,* 283, 883.

Cox, N. L. and Goodall, W. (1981) A long-term comparative study of fenclofenac and gold in patients with rheumatoid arthritis. *Communication, IXth International Congress of Rheumatology,* Paris, Abstract 167.

Currey, H. L. F. (1971) A comparison of immunosuppressive and anti-inflammatory agents in the rat, in *Colloque Immunodepression, Bases Expérimentales – Résul-* measurement in patients with rheumatoid arthritis treated with D-penicillamine, in

Currey, H. L. F. and Chaput de Saintonge, D. M. (1980) Sulphasalazine in rheumatoid arthritis. *Br. Med. J.,* 280, 861.

Dische, F. E., Swinson, D. R., Hamilton, E. B. D. and Parsons, V. (1976) Immunopathology of penicillamine-induced glomerular disease. *J. Rheumatol.*, 3, 145–54.

Dixon, A. St. J., Davis, J., Dormandy, T. L., Hamilton, E. B. D., Holt, P. J. L., Mason, R. M., Thompson, M., Weber, J. C. P. and Zutshi, D. W. (1975) Synthetic D-penicillamine in rheumatoid arthritis. Double blind controlled study of a high and low dosage regime. *Ann. Rheum. Dis.*, 34, 416–21.

Dodd, M. J., Griffith, I. D. and Thompson, M. (1980) Adverse reactions to D-penicillamine after gold toxicity. *Br. Med. J.*, 280, 1498–500.

Empire Rheumatism Council (1961) Gold therapy in rheumatoid arthritis. Final report of a multicentre controlled trial. *Ann. Rheum. Dis.*, 23, 315–54.

Farr, M., Tunn, E., Crockson, A. P. and Bacon, P. A. (1984) The long term effects of sulphasalazine in the treatment of rheumatoid arthritis and a comparative study with penicillamine. *Clin. Rheumatol.*, 3, 473–82.

Fernandes, L., Swinson, D. R. and Hamilton, E. B. D. (1977) Dermatomyositis complicating penicillamine treatment. *Ann. Rheum. Dis.*, 36, 94–5.

Forestier, J. M. (1929) L'aurothérapie dans les rhumatismes chroniques. *Bull. mem. Soc. Med. Hopitaux de Paris*, 53, 323–27.

Fosdick, W. M., Parsons, J. L. and Hill, D. F. (1968) Long-term cyclophosphamide therapy in rheumatoid arthritis. *Arthr. Rheum.*, 11, 151–61.

Freedman, A. and Steinberg, V. L. (1960) Chloroquine in rheumatoid arthritis: a double blindfold trial of treatment for 1 year. *Ann. Rheum. Dis.*, 19, 243–50.

Furst, D. E., Levine, S., Srinivasen, R., Metzger, A. L., Bangst, R. and Paulus, H. E. (1977) A double-blind trial of high versus conventional dosages of gold salts for rheumatoid arthritis. *Arthr. Rheum.*, 20, 1473–80.

Galens, G. J., Bull, F. E. and Bartholomew, L. E. (1964) The treatment of rheumatoid arthritis with 6-mercaptopurine and azathioprine. *Arthr. Rheum.*, 7, 735.

Gelman, M. (1981) *Symp. Med. Hoechst*, 18, 315–23.

Gibson, T., Burry, H. C. and Ogg, C. (1976) Goodpasture's syndrome and D-penicillamine. *Ann. Intern. Med.*, 84, 100.

Gottlieb, N. L. (1979) Gold excretion and retention during auranofin treatment: a preliminary report. *J. Rheumatol.*, 6, 61–7.

Griffin, A. J. (1979) Cholestatic hepatitis induced by gold. *Rheumatol. Rehabil.*, 18, 174–6.

Hall, N. D., Blake, D. R. and Bacon, P. A. (1981) The significance of serum sulphydryl measurement in patients with rheumatoid arthritis treated with D-penicillamine. in *Modulation of Autoimmunity and Disease* (eds R. N. Maini and H. Berry), Praeger Scientific, Eastbourne and New York, pp. 143–50.

Hatchuel, R. (1972) Efficacité et mode d'action du chlorambucil dans la polyarthrite rhumatoide. Etude contrôlée en double insu. A propos de 47 observations. Mémoire pour l'obtention du Certificate d'Etudes Spéciales en Rhumatologie. Paris.

Haydu, G. G. (1953) Rheumatoid arthritis therapy: rationale and the use of chloroquine diphosphate. *Am. J. Med. Sci.*, 225, 71–5.

Highton, J., Panayi, G. S., Shepherd, P., Griffin, J. and Gibson, T. (1981) Changes in immune function in patients with rheumatoid arthritis following treatment with sodium aurothiomalate. *Ann. Rheum. Dis.*, 40, 254–62.

Hurd, E. R. and Ziff, M. (1968) Studies on the anti-inflammatory action of 6-mercaptopurine. *J. Exp. Med.*, 128, 785–800.

Huskisson, E. C., Gibson, T. J., Balme, H. W., Burry, H. C., Grahame, R., Hart, F. D., Henderson, D. R. F. and Whatulewski, J. A. (1974) Trial comparing D-penicillamine and gold in rheumatoid arthritis: preliminary report. *Ann. Rheum. Dis.*, 33, 532–5.

Huskisson, E. C., Jaffe, I. A., Scott, J. and Dieppe, P. A. (1980) 5-thiopyridoxine in rheumatoid arthritis: clinical and experimental studies. *Arthr. Rheum.*, 23, 106–10.

Jaffe, I. A. (1962) Intra-articular dissociation of the rheumatoid factor. *J. Lab. Clin. Med.*, 60, 409–21.

Jaffe, I. (1963) Thiol compounds with penicillamine like activity and possible mode of action in rheumatoid arthritis. In *Antirheumatic Drugs* (ed. E. C. Huskisson). Praeger, Eastbourne and New York.

Jaffe, I. A. (1965) The effect of penicillamine on the laboratory parameters in rheumatoid arthritis. *Arthr. Rheum.*, 8, 1064–79.

Jaffe, I. A. (1983) Thiol compounds with penicillamine-like activity and possible mode of action in rheumatoid arthritis, in *Anti-rheumatic Drugs* (ed. E. C. Huskisson), Praeger Scientific, Eastbourne and New York.

Jain, S., Scheuer, P. J., Samourian, S., McGee, J. O. D. and Sherlock, S. (1977) A controlled trial of D-penicillamine therapy in primary biliary cirrhosis. *Lancet*, i, 831–4.

James, D. and Reebach, J. (1980) Sulphasalazine in rheumatoid arthritis. *Br. Med. J.*, 280, 861–2.

Jayson, M. I. V., Lovell, C., Black, C. M. and Wilson, R. S. E. (1977) Penicillamine therapy in systemic sclerosis. *Proc. R. Soc. Med.*, 70, 82.

Jimenez Diaz, C. (1951) Treatment of dysreaction diseases with nitrogen mustard. *Ann. Rheum. Dis.*, 2, 144.

Kahan, A. and Amor, B. (1971) Phagocytose et immunodépression. in *Colloque Immunodepression, Bases Expérimentales – Résultates Thérapeutiques*, Paris, Inserm. p. 23.

Kahn, M. F., Bedoiseau, M., Six, B., Le Goff, P. and De Seze, S. (1971) Le chlorambucil dans la polyarthrite rhumatoide. *Rev. Rhum. malades osteoarticulaire*, 38, 741.

Kahn, M. F., Arlet, J., Blockmichael, A., Caroit, Y. and Renier, J. C. (1979) 19 leucoses äigue apres traitment de rhumatisme inflammatoire chronique et de connectivites par les agents cytolytiques à visée immunodépressive résultates é une enquête rétrospective portant 2006 cas. *Rhum. malades osteoarticulaire*, 49, 163.

Kendell, P. A. and Hutchins, D. (1978) The effect of thiol compounds on lymphocytes stimulated in culture. *Immunology*, 35, 189–201.

Kinlen, W., Sheil, A. G. R., Peto, J. and Doll, R. (1979) Collaborative United Kingdom-Australian study of cancer in patients treated with immunosuppressive drugs. *Br. Med. J.*, 2, 1461.

Lansbury, J. (1965) Chloroquine in rheumatoid arthritis. *Ann. Intern. Med.*, 62, 1065.

Larsen, A. (1981) *Symp. Med. Hoechst*, 18, 323–30.

Latts, J. R., Antel, J. P., Levinson, D. J., Amason, B. G. and Medef, M. E. (1980) Histocompatibility antigens and gold toxicity: a preliminary report. *J. Clin. Pharmacol.*, 20, 206–9.

Levy, J., Barrett, E. V., MacDonald, N. S. and Klineberg, J. R. (1970) Altered immunoglobulin metabolism in systemic lupus erythematosus and rheumatoid arthritis. *J. Clin. Invest.*, 49, 708–15.

Lewis, P. J. and Symoens, J. (1978) Levamisole in rheumatoid arthritis – a multivariate analysis of a multicentric study. *J. Rheumatol.*, 5, 17–25.

Lipsky, P. E. and Ziff, M. (1977) Inhibition of antigen and mitogen induced human lymphocyte proliferation by gold compounds. *J. Clin. Invest.*, 59, 455–66.

Lockshin, M. D., Eisenhauer, A. C., Kohn, R., Weksler, M., Block, F. and Mushlin, S. B. (1975) Cell mediated immunity in rheumatic diseases. II. Mitogen response in RA, SLE and other illnesses: correlation with T and B lymphocyte populations. *Arthr. Rheum.*, 18, 245–9.

Lorber, A., Wilcox, S. A., Viebert, G. J. and Simon, T. M. (1979) Carbon rod atomisation analysis: application to *in vivo* lymphocyte gold quantitation. *J. Rheumatol.*, 6, 31–9.

Lyle, W. H. (1973) Penicillamine in pregnancy. *Lancet*, i, 606–7.

McConkey, B., Amos, R. S., Butler, E. P., Crockson, R. A., Crockson, A. P. and Walsh, L. (1978) Salazopyrin in rheumatoid arthritis. *Agents Actions*, 8, 438–41.

McConkey, B., Amos, R. S., Durham, S., Forster, P. J. G., Hubbal, S. and Walsh, L. (1980) Sulphasalazine in rheumatoid arthritis. *Br. Med. J.*, 280, 442–4.

McKenzie, J. M. (1981) Report on a double-blind trial comparing small and large doses of gold in the treatment of rheumatoid disease. *Rheumatol. Rehabil.*, 20, 198–202.

Maini, R. N. and Roff, I. (1977) *Penicillamine Research in Rheumatoid Disease*, Fabritus and Sonner, Oslo, pp. 172.

Majoos, F. L., Klemp, P., Meyers, O. L. and Briggs, B. (1981) Gold therapy in rheumatoid arthritis. *S. Afr. Med. J.*, 59, 971–4.

Marks, J. S. and Power, B. J. (1979) Is chloroquine obsolete in treatment of rheumatic disease? *Lancet*, i, 371–3.

Mason, M., Currey, H. L. F., Barnes, C. G., Dunne, J. F., Hazleman, B. L. and Strickland, I. D. (1969) Azathioprine in rheumatoid arthritis. *Br. Med. J.*, 1, 420.

Meilants, H. and Veys, E. M. (1978) A study of the haematological side-effects of levamisole in rheumatoid arthritis, with recommendations. *J. Rheumatol.*, 5, 77–83.

Mellbye, O. J., Messner, R. P., De Board, J. R. and Williams, R. C. (1972) Immunoglobulins and receptors for C3 on lymphocytes from patients with rheumatoid arthritis. *Arthr. Rheum.*, 15, 371–80.

Menkes, C. J., Levy, J. P., Wells, B., Deirieu, F., Mathiot, C. and Delbarre, F. (1975) Leucémie äigue à mégacaryoblastes servenue apres traitment amino de proceur d'une polyarthrite rhumatoide. *Nouvell Presse Med.*, 4, 2869.

Meons, C. and Blocteur, J. (1965) *Acta Rheumatol. Scand.*, 11, 212.

Mowat, A. G. and Vischer, T. L. (1979) Levamisole. *EULAR Monograph No. 5*.

Moynahan, E. J. (1973) D-penicillamine in morphoea (localised scleroderma). *Lancet*, i, 428–9.

Multicentre Study Group (1973) Controlled trial of D-penicillamine in severe rheumatoid arthritis. *Lancet*, i, 275–8.

Multicentre Study Group (1982) Levamisole in rheumatoid arthritis. Final report on a randomised double-blind study comparing a single weekly dose of levamisole with placebo. *Ann. Rheum. Dis.*, 41, 159–63.

Nelson, D. C. and Birchmore, D. A. (1979) Renal vein thrombosis associated with nephrotic syndrome and gold therapy in rheumatoid arthritis. *S. Med. J.*, 72, 1616–8.

Papamichail, M., Brown, J. C. and Holborow, E. J. (1971) Immunoglobulins on the surface of human lymphocytes. *Lancet*, ii, 850–2.

Pasero, G. and Ciompi, M. L. (1979) Thiopronine therapy in rheumatoid arthritis. *Arthr. Rheum.*, 22, 803–4.

Pepys, M. B. (1981) Serum C-reactive protein (CRP), serum amyloid P component (SAP) and serum amyloid A protein (SAA) in autoimmune disease, in *Clinics in Immunology and Allergy*, vol. 1 (ed. E. J. Holborow), W. B. Saunders, Eastbourne.

Percival, S. P. B. and Behrman, J. (1969) Ophthalmological safety of chloroquine. *Br. J. Ophthalmol.*, 53, 101–9.

Percy, J. S., Davis, P., Russell, A. S. and Brisson, E. (1978) A longitudinal study of *in vitro* tests for lymphocyte function in rheumatoid arthritis. *Ann. Rheum. Dis.*, 37, 416–20.

Perrett, D. (1981) The metabolism and pharmacology of D-penicillamine in man. *J. Rheumatol.*, 7, 41–50.

Pinals, R. S., Masi, A. T. and Larsen, R. A. (1981) Preliminary criteria for clinical remission in rheumatoid arthritis. The Sub-committee for criteria of remission in rheumatoid arthritis of the American Rheumatism Association. Diagnostic and therapeutic criteria Committee. *Arthr. Rheum.*, 24, 1308–15.

Raeman, F., Decock, W., Debeukelaar, T., Decree, J. and Verhaegen, H. (1981) Enumeration of T lymphocytes and T lymphocyte sub-sets in autoimmune disease using monoclonal antibodies. *Clin. Exp. Immunol.*, 45, 475–9.

Ritzmann, S. E. and Levin, W. C. (1961) Effect of mercaptans in cold agglutinin disease. *J. Lab. Clin. Med.*, 57, 718–32.

Rovenska, E., Kappeller, K. and Rossman, P. (1979) *Czech. Med.*, 2, 125–33.

Schumacher, K., Maerker-Alzer, G. and Preuss, R. (1975) Effect of D-penicillamine on lymphocyte function. *Drug Res.*, 23, 603–9.

Sharp, J. T., Lidsky, M. D., Duffy, J., Thomson, H. K., Person, B. D., Fattah, A. and Andrianokos, A. A. (1977) Comparison of two dosage schedules of gold salts in the treatment of rheumatoid arthritis: relationship with serum gold levels to therapeutic response. *Arthr. Rheum.*, 20, 1179–87.

Silverman, A. H., Johnson, J. S., Vaughan, J. H. and McGlomary, J. C. (1976) Altered lymphocyte reactivity in rheumatoid arthritis. *Arthr. Rheum.*, 19, 509–15.

Sinclair, R. J. G. and Duthie, J. J. R. (1948) Salazopyrin in the treatment of rheumatoid arthritis. *Ann. Rheum. Dis.*, 8, 226–31.

Skrifvars, B. (1979) Hypothesis for the pathogenesis of sodium aurothiomalate (Myocrisin) induced immune complex nephritis. *Scand. J. Rheumatol.*, 8, 113–8.

Stern, R. B., Wilkinson, S. P., Howarth, P. J. N. and Williams, R. (1977) Controlled trial of synthetic D-penicillamine and prednisone in maintenance therapy for active chronic hepatitis. *Gut*, 18, 19–22.

Struck, R. F. and Hill, D. L. (1972) Investigation of the synthesis of aldophosphamide (AP), a toxic metabolite of cyclophosphamide (CTX). *Proc. Am. Assoc. Cancer Res.*, 13, 50, Abstract 199.

Svartz, N. (1942) A. Therapeutic results in rheumatic polyarthritis. B. Therapeutic results in ulcerative colitis. C. Toxic manifestations in treatment with sulfanilamide preparations. *Acta Med. Scand.*, 110, 577–98.

Symeons, J. and Schuermans, Y. (1979) Levamisole. *Clinics Rheum. Dis.*, 5, 603–30.

Tabachnick, M., Eisen, H. N. and Levine, B. (1954) New mixed disulphides; penicillamine-cysteine. *Nature*, 174, 701–2.

Talal, N. (1981) Congress Report. *Rheumatol. Int.*, 1, 150.

Turner-Warwick, M. (1981) Adverse reactions affecting the lung: possible association with D-penicillamine. *J. Rheumatol.*, 8, 166–8.

Van der Korst, J. K., Van de Stadt, R. J., Miujsers, A. O., Ament, H. J. W. and Henrichs, A. M. A. (1982) Pharmacokinetics of D-penicillamine in rheumatoid arthritis, in *Modulation of autoimmunity and disease* (eds R. N. Maini and H. Berry), Praeger Scientific, Eastbourne and New York, pp. 165–71.

Vernon-Roberts, B., Currey, H. L. F. and Perrin, J. (1974) T and B cells in the blood and synovial fluid of rheumatoid patients. *Ann. Rheum. Dis.*, 33, 430–3.

Veys, E. M. and Mielant, S. H. (1978) Experience and recommendations for treatment schedule of levamisole in rheumatoid arthritis. *J. Rheumatol.*, 5, 31–41.

Walshe, J. M. (1953) Disturbances of amino acid metabolism following liver injury. *Q. J. Med.*, 22, 483–505.

Walshe, J. M. (1981) Penicillamine and the SLE syndrome. *J. Rheumatol.*, 8, 155–61.

Webley, M. and Coombs, E. N. (1979) An assessment of penicillamine therapy in rheumatoid arthritis and the influence of previous gold therapy. *J. Rheumatol.*, 6, 20–4.

Williams, R. C., De Board, J. R., Mellbye, O. J., Messner, R. P. and Lindström, F. D. (1953) Studies of T and B lymphocytes in patients with connective tissue diseases. *J. Clin. Invest.*, 52, 283–95.

Williams, R. C. and Messner, R. P. (1975) Alterations in T and B cells in human disease states. *Ann. Rev. Med.*, 26, 181–92.

Woodland, J., Mason, R. M., Harris, J., Dixon, A. St. J., Currey, H. L. F., Brownjohn, A. M. M., Davis, J. and Owen-Smith, B. D. (1974) Trial of azathioprine, cyclophosphamide and gold in rheumatoid arthritis. *Ann. Rheum. Dis.*, 33, 399–401.

Wooley, P. H., Griffin, A. J., Panayi, G. S., Batchelor, S. R., Walshe, K. I. and Gibson, T. J. (1980) HLA-DR antigens and toxic reactions to sodium aurothiomalate and D-penicillamine in patients with rheumatoid arthritis. *N. Engl. J. Med.*, 303, 300–2.

Young, J. P. (1959) Chloroquine phosphate (Aralen) in the long-term treatment of rheumatoid arthritis. *Ann. Intern. Med.*, 51, 1159–78.

CHAPTER 10

New drugs and

experimental progress

V. Wright

There is a wide divergence between the prevalence of rheumatic diseases seen in hospital practice and those for which antirheumatic medication is prescribed in the community (Fig. 10.1). In a rheumatism clinic inflammatory joint disease predominates. In general practice degenerative conditions are far commoner. In a recent analysis of side effects of indoprofen in general practice I surveyed the types of arthritis for which it was prescribed in Leeds. Of 427 patients only 10% had inflammatory arthritis.

Moreover, despite a deprecation of polypharmacy, an analysis of our outpatients showed 35% were receiving more than one analgesic and/or NSAID, suggesting that complete efficacy of these preparations is far from being achieved. Medical and financial considerations, therefore, justify a continued search for more pain-relieving drugs, whilst at the same time seeking compounds that affect the rheumatic disorders fundamentally.

10.1 ANALGESICS AND NSAIDs

Despite the plethora of NSAIDs available, little that is truly novel has emerged in recent years.

10.1.1 Analgesics

That there is a demand for a new analgesic was shown by the popularity of zomepirac before it was withdrawn from the market. Other drugs marketed predominantly as analgesics, such as diflunisal and flufenamic acid, might

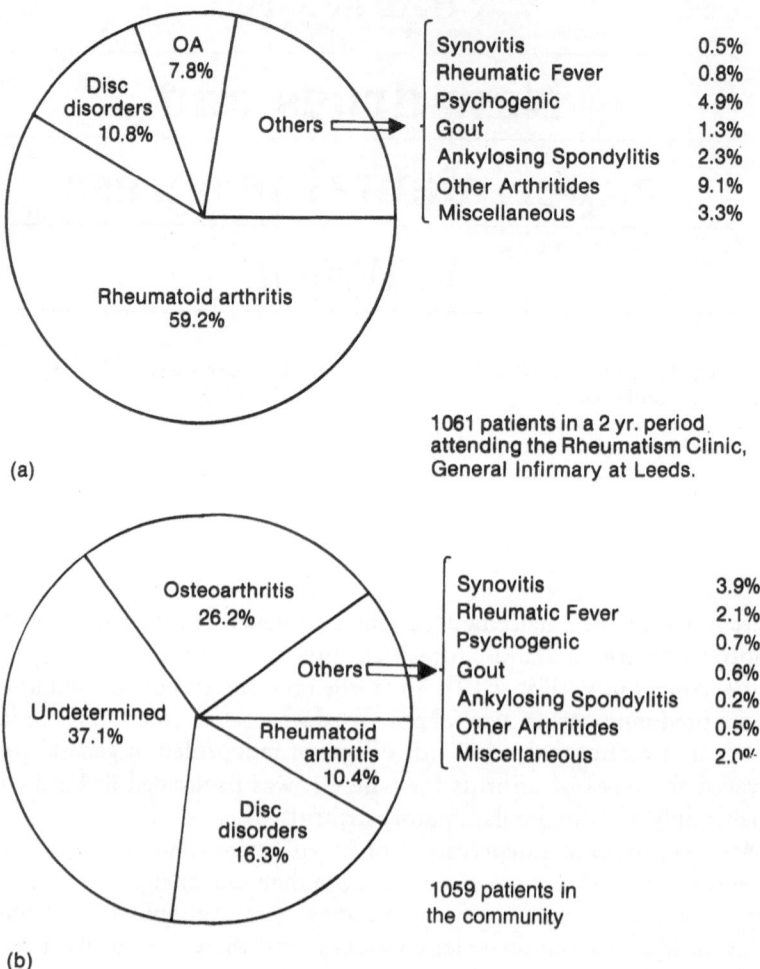

Synovitis	0.5%
Rheumatic Fever	0.8%
Psychogenic	4.9%
Gout	1.3%
Ankylosing Spondylitis	2.3%
Other Arthritides	9.1%
Miscellaneous	3.3%

1061 patients in a 2 yr. period attending the Rheumatism Clinic, General Infirmary at Leeds.

(a)

Synovitis	3.9%
Rheumatic Fever	2.1%
Psychogenic	0.7%
Gout	0.6%
Ankylosing Spondylitis	0.2%
Other Arthritides	0.5%
Miscellaneous	2.0%

1059 patients in the community

(b)

Figure 10.1 Diagnoses in patients with rheumatic complaints: (a) in a hospital clinic; (b) within the community.

more properly be considered as anti-inflammatory agents in that they have an inhibitory effect on prostaglandin synthetase.

The methods to measure pain relief in animals are standard, using tests such as acetylcholine-induced writhing in mice, the rat foot carageenin test, and the mouse hot plate test (examples of pain elicited by chemical, mechanical, and thermal stimulation respectively). Some tests use combinations of these methods (Randall and Selitto, (1957). In man the methods used remain subjective, with visual analogue pain rating scales being the most popular (Huskisson, 1974; Downie *et al.*, 1978). Sources of error in these scales have been increasingly recognized. It is fallacious to believe that all divisions on the scale have equal importance in the eyes of the patient (Lasagna, 1960). Errors occur if the scale is not directly beneath the patient's eye. Similar errors occur when photocopying the scale lengthens the line by up to 5%, a clear source of error since scores are usually measured to 1 mm (Greenfield and Hawks, 1981). Our own work has also shown that the reproducibility varies along the length of a 10 cm scale, presented either vertically or horizontally (Dixon and Bird, 1981). For these and other reasons the use of visual analogue scales has been termed a pseudo-science (Dixon *et al.*, 1981).

In an attempt to estimate analgesia objectively, we have begun work on the assessment of sleep disturbance. A review of 200 outpatients and 255 inpatients with rheumatic diseases showed that 68% and 65% respectively claimed that their sleep was disturbed by pain. Interestingly, the frequency of sleep disturbance was equal among patients with rheumatoid arthritis and with osteoarthrosis. We have constructed a Sleep Laboratory and analysed EEG and EMG traces from rheumatic patients receiving different drug regimes. It has been suggested that such polysomnographic data are of diagnostic value (Moldofsky *et al.*, 1983). Recordings from patients with fibrositis are similar to those found in normal subjects with deliberate sleep deprivation (Moldofsky and Scarisbrick, 1976). Our preliminary experience suggests that there are considerable inter- and intra-patient variations that make analysis difficult. Nor is it yet clear how the electrical patterns correlate with 'perceived sleep', nor which is the more relevant clinically. We are comparing these studies with both the Middlesex and the Leeds sleep questionnaires (Parrott and Hindmarch, 1980; Ellis *et al.*, 1981). Our Bioengineering Group has also devised means of telemeterizing EEG and EMG signals, obviating the need for trailing wires, and this may improve variability. At the same time transducers incorporated into the bed legs will quantitate the amount of movement during the night using different regimes.

Future trends in pain research will doubtless endeavour to exploit the finding of natural opiate-like alkaloids present in the brain (Henry, 1976; Levine *et al.*, 1978). A non-narcotic inhibitor of P-substance release would be a most useful drug, particularly if it is confirmed that opioids such as pethidine act pre-synaptically to inhibit substance-P release and the onward transmission of pain (Hughes, 1975; Hughes *et al.*, 1975; Cox *et al.*, 1976; Jessel and Iversen, 1977). Agonists are always associated with receptors, and the current evidence favours at least three such receptors at which naturally occurring compounds might act. Morphine appears to interact with both μ receptors and δ receptors, whilst other narcotics appear to interact with a third receptor, the $\varkappa$ receptor. Interaction of morphine at the δ receptor is much less readily reversed by antagonists with interaction at the new receptor – at least in the mouse vas deferens, though this role appears to be reversed in the guinea-pig ileum (Kosterlitz *et al.*, 1980). There is much activity in trying to produce synthetic polypeptide morphine analogues that react at one or the other receptors in the hope of separating the toxic and therapeutic actions of opiates.

The relevance of these types of studies to a particular rheumatic disease is exemplified by our experience with a patient having severe psoriatic arthropathy who was also a drug addict. He was insistent that heroin and amphetamine relieved his pain, whilst morphine and barbiturates did not (Bird and Wright, 1982).

10.1.2   NSAIDs

Our study of desiderata for anti-rheumatic preparations by doctors and by patients puts absence of toxicity at the top of the list, followed by efficacy (Wright and Hopkins, 1983). Less frequent administration figures high on the list also. Drugs with long half-lives have been, and are being, developed to enable once or twice daily administration, thus facilitating less frequent administration. Isoxicam and tenoxicam are the two newest preparations of this type. Other drugs have been put in a sustained-release formulation to achieve the same end.

In the realm of formulation there have been interesting new developments. Many factors influence the rate and extent of drug absorption. Drug bioavailability can vary as a function of the physical characteristics of specific formulations, such as the amount of compression, size of drug crystals, and hardness of coating. Rate of absorption depends not only on the disintegration of the drug, but also on the rapidity with which it goes into solution. The role of ionization is of particular importance. Most drugs are either weak acids or weak bases, which exist in an equilibrium of ionized and non-ionized states that vary with the pH of the biological fluid tissue. Small fluctuations of intercellular or plasma pH can produce significant shifts in the proportion of polar (ionized) or non-polar (non-ionized) drug. In rheumatology many of the drugs employed are acidic and have similar, and often competing, actions (Robinson, 1981). This contributes to their potential for initial absorption in the stomach, where the pH is low.

Use of liposomes represents a new way of attempting to localize the response (Gregoriadis, 1980). For drugs taken orally a formulation which permits slow and constant release throughout the length of the gastrointestinal tract has obvious attractions when applied to drugs that have a short half-life. It would make absorption kinetics the over-riding factor instead of elimination kinetics in governing plasma and tissue levels of the drug. The problems are that the rate and extent of drug dissolution depend on factors such as the contents of the stomach, intestinal motility, gastrointestinal pH, and temperature. Enteric coating is often useful in this respect, but the dissolution of the coat can be erratic, and can even occur in the stomach when emptying is delayed. More complex formulations include a polymeric condensation with aluminium oxide (aloxiprin) and a microgranular sustained release preparation (safapryn). Sustained release formulations rely on an outer shell or capsule with a variable release of drug from within. Drug release from these systems is a function of diffusion through a membrane or erosion of form. A recent innovation has deposited ketoprofen on to a small but inert central core of starch and sucrose, and then coated the pellets with a dialysing membrane. After ingestion, the capsule shell dissolves completely, individual pellets are released and scatter in the stomach, passing slowly into the intestine. Water diffuses into the pellet under an osmotic gradient, the ketoprofen dissolves to form a saturated solution, and the drug diffuses out. The pellets are so designed that ketoprofen diffusion through the membrane increases in alkaline conditions. Faecal blood was less than that following aspirin and generic ketoprofen, and a new ketoprofen sustained-release compound, although this may have little relevance to clinical practice (Ranlov *et al.*, 1983). Another novel system of drug delivery was that used for osmosin (Jaffe, 1983). Unfortunately, because of gastrointestinal side effects, including gut perforation, the drug has been withdrawn. Nevertheless, the delivery system was of great interest. A core of drug is surrounded by a semi-permeable membrane, punctured by a single laser-drilled hole. The system functions by imbibing water at a controlled rate through the membrane as a result of an osmotic gradient. The rate of absorption is controlled by the properties of the delivery orifice, the membrane, and the core formulation. The device pumps a volume of saturated solution of drug equal to the volume of water uptake at any given period, and continues at a constant rate as long as there is solid drug in the core (Heilman, 1978; Theuwes, 1981). The attraction of the system is that the drug itself functions as the osmotic agent, therefore allowing the elimination of any drug bag which had previously been present in 'mini-osmotic pumps' (Theuwes and Yum, 1976).

There may be unforseen effects as with those that caused the withdrawal of osmosin. Some patients with diverticulosis sequestered the capsule in a diverticulum. The continued release of the drug at this localized site produced perforation. The high frequency of other gastrointestinal side effects was probably due to the failure of many doctors to realize that it was only the formulation that was new and not the drug. It is likely that patients who had previously experienced gastrointestinal side effects from indomethacin were exposed once more to the drug.

Increasing interest has been devoted to drug metabolism in the elderly. Poor compliance amongst this group of patients is notorious (Smith and Rawlins, 1973). It should, however, be recognized that there are three distinct groups of elderly people. One group is in hospital, a second is in residential Part 3 accommodation, and the third is at home. The common practice of considering the hospitalized group to be representative of all geriatric patients is erroneous. For reliable information, investigations need to be done on each group. Poor compliance in the elderly may be due to physical impairment (poor eyesight, disabled hands), mental deterioration with forgetfulness compounded by frequency of dosage, polypharmacy, hoarding of tablets, and lack of understanding of the nature of the treatment. Effective compliance on occasions is a self-protective mechanism for patients, so this is an added reason for seeking the highest therapeutic ratio where efficacy far outweighs toxicity.

The major side effect of this group of drugs continues to be dyspepsia, although to prove the association is not easy. The Boston Collaborative Drug Surveillance Program studied over 16000 admissions to prove an association between aspirin and various gastrointestinal pathologies (Levy, 1974; Jick and Porter, 1978; Jick, 1981). Enteric coating, as with diclofenac, reduces the frequency of dyspepsia, although it does not obviate it entirely, because of the systemic circulation of the drug and subsequent excretion in the stomach. Pro-drugs, such as benorylate and fenbufen, have similar advantages and problems.

The attempts to develop new preparations will be determined by one's view of the important features of inflammation. This aspect has been reviewed recently by Bird and Wright (1982). Pharmacologists tend to concentrate on prostaglandins, biochemists on free oxygen and hydroxyl radicals, cell biologists on lysosomal enzymes and cells such as macrophages, and immunologists on lymphocytes and their activation products. It is interesting to ask why NSAIDs do not completely alleviate pain produced by inflammation. It may be that the concentration of the drug at the site of inflammation is insufficient. It may be because only part of the arachidonic acid cascade is inhibited. On the other hand it may be that other mechanisms of pain are equally important. The question must be raised as to whether complete pain relief in these circumstances is desirable. The evidence from steroid arthropathy suggests that pain may be protective (Chandler and Wright, 1958). Prostaglandins tend to be highlighted, partly because of their link with salicylates, the yardstick against which new NSAIDs are usually compared, but peptides, enzymes, lymphokines, and complement may be equally important. A multiplicity of drugs may be necessary to combat arthritis in a given patient, a precise combination being determined by the particular inflammatory pathway involved at the time. The marked variability and unpredictability in patient responses cast doubt on the value of comparison trials of these preparations (Scott *et al.*, 1982).

Polypharmacy tends to be deprecated by all clinicians, but until a definitive cure is available, this may be a short-sighted policy. Little work has been done on the possible potentiation of NSAIDs, either by analgesics or by other NSAIDs. In the few clinical trials done on more than one NSAID simultaneously, a mild degree of clinical potentiation has been observed at certain doses only (Grennan *et al.*, 1979). One might expect therapeutic potentiation from drugs of different families, and it would be interesting to see results of trials of these combinations. Another interesting therapeutic concept has been the concomitant administration of blockers of both cyclo-oxygenase and lipoxygenase. The simultaneous prescription of H1 and H2 anti-histamine blockers could also be of interest.

10.2   CORTICOSTEROIDS

The dramatic and immediate effects of high-dose corticosteroids have been more than offset by undesirable side effects. Although rheumatologists (our group included) speak disparagingly of these drugs for the treatment of rheumatoid arthritis, in an analysis of our outpatients a third were receiving prednisolone or betamethasone. The basic tenets that led Hench to use cortisone in the treatment of rheumatoid arthritis remain unchallenged, namely that rheumatoid arthritis commonly goes into remission in pregnancy and during liver disease. It may still be worth trying to develop compounds which separate side effects from efficacy. It may be possible to separate the beneficial effects of steroids from the toxic side effects by more judicious prescribing. Regimens clearly requiring evaluation in the treatment of rheumatoid arthritis include high-dose pulse steroid therapy with methylprednisolone and its combination with a second-line agent. Treatment of ulcerative colitis provides a model for this, where remission by steroids is maintained by subsequent use of a long-term agent such as sulphasalazine (see Chapter 9).

In conditions where steroids are mandatory, studies are still required to determine when and how they should be withdrawn. From this point of view we have investigated acute phase reactants in patients with polymyalgia rheumatica. The ESR was the most useful variable, a rise antedating symptomatic relapse when patients were progressively weaned from steroids. C-reactive protein behaved oddly; it is quick to respond if present but sometimes is not raised. It may be that plasma viscosity and ESR are complementary and should both be considered in steroid withdrawal.

10.3 SECOND-LINE DRUGS

It is difficult to develop and to evaluate second-line drugs for the treatment of rheumatoid arthritis in the absence of an animal model. The models commonly

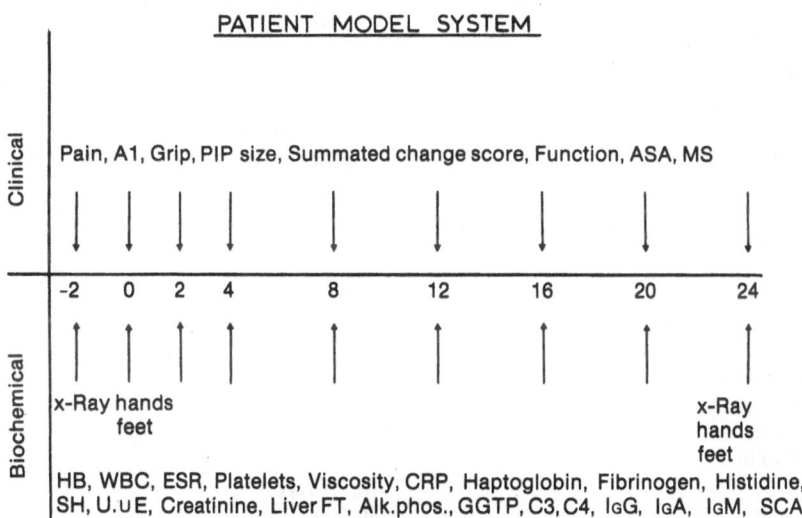

Figure 10.2 Patient model system.

used more closely resemble Reiter's disease than rheumatoid arthritis. For this reason in the Clinical Pharmacology Unit in Harrogate we have developed a patient model system (Dixon et al., 1982). This is shown diagrammatically in Fig. 10.2. Groups of 15 patients with definite rheumatoid arthritis for at least six months' duration are allocated for the first time to a second-line drug. The disease is sufficiently active to fulfil three of the following five criteria:

1. Tenderness of more than 6 joints.
2. Swelling of more than 3 joints.
3. Early morning stiffness of more than 45 minutes.
4. A Ritchie articular index of more than 20.
5. ESR of more than 28 mm in the first hour.

After a two week run-in period on enteric-coated aspirin alone, in a dose of up to 3.6 g daily, patients are allocated to the test drug in therapeutic dose for a 24-week period. During this period only aspirin is allowed as back-up therapy; all other NSAIDs are excluded. Patients attend a special clinic on two occasions before, and over the treatment period at 2, 4, 8, 12, 16, 20, and 24 weeks. On each occasion eight clinical assessments and 26 biochemical or immunological assessments are performed (Table 10.1). Since the hallmark of an anti-rheumatoid preparation is that biochemical change occurs simulta-

TABLE 10.1
Eight clinical variables and 25 laboratory variables used in the construction of correlation matrices

CLINICAL VARIABLES:

Articular index (AI)	Early morning stiffness (EMS)
Summated change score (SCS)	Pain score (PS)
Joint circumference (JC)	Grip strength (GS)
Aspirin dose (AD)	Functional grade (FG)

LABORATORY VARIABLES:

Haemoglobin	ESR
White count	Plasma viscosity
Platelets	Haptoglobin
	Fibrinogen
Urea	
Creatinine	RA latex titre
Bilirubin	IgM
SGOT	IgA
Alkaline phosphatase	IgG
Gamma glutamyl transpeptidase (GGTP)	
Total proteins	C3
Albumin	C4
Globulin	
	Sulphydryl
Salicylate	Histidine

neously with clinical improvement, correlation matrices are plotted between the clinical and biochemical variables for each group. If a drug has second-line activity, simultaneous clinical and biochemical improvement will occur, and this will show by significant correlations. Two specimen matrices are shown for response to penicillamine and aspirin (Table 10.2a and b). The value of this system is that it can be used to screen a wide variety of compounds that might have anti-rheumatoid activity. Compounds that show promise can then be submitted to formal clinical trial. It may well be that with adequate refinement the system could circumvent the need for formal and expensive clinical trials. In developing the system we have devised a mini-matrix including plasma viscosity, C-reactive protein, IgM, sulphydryl, histidine, and the haemoglobin.

TABLE 10.2
Correlation matrices between clinical and biochemical variables in groups of 15 patients treated for the first time on antirheumatoid drug. The correlation coefficient is calculated between each biochemical and clinical variable for mean patient data at each of 8 clinic visits. For clarity the r values are converted to p values, those reaching statistical significance being depicted in the matrices. Where correlation did not reach statistical significance, it is omitted from the matrix. Abbreviations: AI, articular index; SCS, summated change score; JC, joint circumference; AD, aspirin dose; EMS, early morning stiffness; PS, pain score; GS, grip strength; FG, functional grade.

(a) D-*penicillamine*

Laboratory variables	Clinical variables							
	AI	SCS	JC	AD	EMS	PS	GS	FG
SH	0.001	0.001	0.001	0.001	0.01	0.01	0.01	—
PV	0.001	0.001	0.001	0.01	0.01	0.01	—	—
C3	0.01	0.001	0.01	—	—	—	0.01	—
Platelets	0.001	0.001	0.001	0.01	0.01	—	—	—
Bilirubin	0.001	0.01	0.01	0.01	0.01	—	0.01	—
CRP	0.001	0.01	0.01	—	0.001	—	—	—
IgM	0.01	0.01	—	0.001	—	0.01	—	—
ESR	0.001	0.01	0.01	0.01	0.01	—	—	—
Hb	—	0.01	—	0.01	—	—	0.01	0.01
Albumin	0.01	—	0.01	—	0.01	—	—	—
Haptoglobin	—	—	—	—	0.01	—	—	—
GGTP	0.01	—	—	—	—	—	—	—
Alk.phos.	—	—	—	—	—	—	—	—
Fibrinogen	—	—	—	—	—	—	—	—
Creatinine	—	—	—	—	—	—	—	—
C4	—	—	—	—	—	—	—	—
Protein	—	—	—	—	—	—	—	—
Histidine	—	—	—	—	—	—	—	—
WBC	—	—	—	—	—	—	—	—
SGOT	—	—	—	—	—	—	—	—
IgG	—	—	—	—	—	—	—	—
IgA	—	—	—	—	—	—	—	—
Globulin	—	—	—	—	—	—	—	—

(b) Aspirin

Laboratory variables	Clinical variables						
	PS	AI	GS	FG	AD	JC	EMS
Haptoglobin	—	—	0.01	—	—	—	—
PV	0.001	0.01	—	—	—	—	—
Platelets	—	—	0.01	—	—	—	—
ESR	0.01	—	—	—	—	—	—
Albumin	0.01	0.001	—	—	—	—	—
IgA	0.01	0.001	—	—	—	—	—
CRP	—	—	—	—	—	—	—
GGTP	—	—	—	0.01	—	—	—
Alk.phos.	—	—	—	—	—	—	—
WBC	0.001	—	—	0.01	—	—	—
Globulin	—	—	—	—	—	—	—
Protein	—	—	—	—	—	—	—
Fibrinogen	—	—	—	—	—	—	0.01
C3	—	—	—	—	—	—	—
IgM	—	—	—	—	—	—	—
Hb	—	—	—	—	—	—	—
SH	—	—	—	—	—	—	—
Histidine	—	—	—	—	—	—	—
C4	—	—	—	—	—	—	—
Bilirubin	—	—	—	—	—	—	—
SGOT	—	—	—	—	—	—	—
IgG	—	—	—	—	—	—	—
Creatinine	—		—	—	—	—	—

The only biochemical variable we might wish to see replaced is IgM, which could be replaced by a measure of rheumatoid factor. Recent analysis of our considerable file of data has suggested on the clinical side that the measurement of one inflamed joint may be more appropriate in the assessment of joint size than the time-consuming measurement of the mean circumference of 10 proximal interphalangeal joints. Another difficult clinical variable is the salicylate dosage used as back-up therapy. Almost invariably up to 20% of patients cannot tolerate high-dose aspirin, giving incomplete data in the final tables with the statistical problems this poses. Similarly, some patients entering a study may have been on one or other NSAID, and when transferred to aspirin show some deterioration. This could, therefore, bias results. It may well be that we can cope with this situation by allowing the patient to remain on an NSAID of their choice. The summated change score, which has been developed in the Unit (Rhind *et al.*, 1980) has proved useful despite the inherent errors involved in its use. A numerical global symptom scale is an alternative possibility. The scale of +2, +1, 0, −1, −2 for grip strength may be preferable to readings based on sphygmomanometer cuffs. We find that functional grade lacks sensitivity. The Ritchie articular index is one of the most successful measurements. It is important that the same assessor carries out the assessment on a given patient throughout the period of study as the inter-observer error is considerable, although the intra-observer error is acceptable. For pain score the patient should be asked to fill out diary cards on a daily basis so that he gets into the habit of doing it.

We have used the patient model system to look at a number of compounds. Drugs worth considering are listed in Table 10.3. In view of the proven efficacy of gold, analogues are worth considering. Gold thioglucose is an alternative formulation, but appears to be little different from aurothiomalate. The oral compound, auranofin, in our experience has an efficacy comparable with hydroxychloroquine, but its side effects are fewer than the intra-muscular preparation. Diarrhoea in the form of soft motions (sufficient to cause the patient discomfort) may occur.

Similarly analogues of penicillamine are worth investigating. One useful analogue is 5-thiopyridoxine (Huskisson *et al.*, 1980). It appears rather slower acting than penicillamine, but pemphigus, which is seen only occasionally with penicillamine, appears to be a particular characteristic of this drug. The disulphate of 5-thiopyridoxine is pyrithioxine, which is marketed in Europe as a stimulant. In open studies it has appeared active (Camus *et al.*, 1978), and it has been advocated for use in patients who develop side effects on D-penicillamine (Bruhl *et al.*, 1979). Another analogue, thiopronine, in an open study appeared to have an antirheumatoid effect (Pasero and Ciompi, 1979).

TABLE 10.3
Drugs or methods of treatment with proved or possible antirheumatoid activity

DRUGS OF PROVEN ANTIRHEUMATOID ACTIVITY:

Hydroxychloroquine	Sulphasalazine
Sodium aurothiomalate	Clozic
D-penicillamine	Captopril

DRUGS WITH LESS CERTAIN ANTIRHEUMATOID ACTIVITY OR UNPROVEN ANTIRHEUMATOID ACTIVITY:

Gold thioglucose	Fenclofenac
Auranofin	Benoxaprofen
5-thiopyridoxine	Sodium cromoglycate
Pyrithioxine	Metronidazole
Thiopronine	
Dapsone	
Retinoic acid derivatives	

IMMUNOACTIVE DRUGS OR MECHANICAL METHODS WITH PROVEN OR SUSPECTED ANTIRHEUMATOID ACTIVITY:

Azathioprine	Thymopoetin
Methotrexate	Anti-lymphocyte serum
Chlorambucil	Thoracic duct drainage
Cyclophosphamide	Total body irradiation
Thiotepa	Plasmapheresis and lymphopheresis
Levamisole	

The side effects are essentially those of penicillamine. We have looked at compounds to see whether the thiol group or the chelating properties of pencillamine are important factors in its efficacy in patients with rheumatoid disease. We have studied trien hydrochloride, which is sometimes used in the treatment of Wilson's disease when patients are unable to tolerate penicillamine. It is a chelater of copper, but lacks an SH group. It did not prove effective in rheumatoid arthritis (Bird *et al.*, 1982b). We have also looked at methylcysteine, which is structurally similar to D-penicillamine, and is used for the treatment of bronchitis as a mucolytic agent. A number of general practitioners in our area have seen patients with chronic bronchitis whose rheumatoid disease appeared to improve on this drug. However, in our system we were not able to confirm this efficacy (McKenna *et al.*, 1983). Steven *et al.* (1982) studied the effect of gold, penicillamine, and levamisole in a prospective trial, and concluded that an adverse reaction to one of these should not prejudice the selection of another.

We have also studied the effect of captopril which is used as a hypotensive agent. It is a thiol-containing molecule, with a spectrum of side effects similar to penicillamine. We have found it to be effective in treating rheumatoid arthritis (Martin *et al.*, 1983). It would be of interest to test other angiotensin-converting enzyme inhibitors without a thiol group.

Dapsone has a beneficial effect in rheumatoid arthritis compared with placebo, but its tendency to cause haemolysis is its main limiting factor (Swinson *et al.*, 1981). Clozic was undoubtedly active also, although animal toxicology and the occurrence of some cases of Stevens–Johnson syndrome stopped its general release (Bird *et al.*, 1983). It was sufficiently promising, however, to merit the development of analogues in the hope that the toxicity

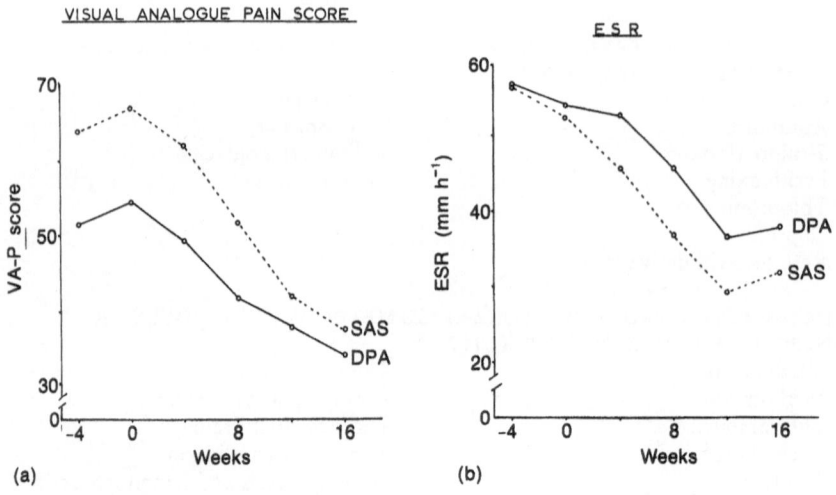

Figure 10.3 Effect of sulphasalazine on patients with rheumatoid arthritis: (a) on pain (Visual Analogue Pain Score); (b) on ESR.

would be eliminated. A study of thymopoietin pentapeptide showed the preparation to be active intravenously but not intramuscularly (Veys *et al.*, 1982). Although attractive on theoretical grounds, there is little to encourage one in these results.

Sulphasalazine, originally developed by Dr Nanna Svartz (1942, 1948), has proved active in the treatment of rheumatoid arthritis in our patient model system (Bird *et al.*, 1982a). Two controlled trials have subsequently confirmed this efficacy (Neumann *et al.*, 1983; Pullar *et al.*, 1983). A comparison of its effects on pain and ESR with that of penicillamine is shown in Fig. 10.3. The main drawback of the drug is upper gastrointestinal intolerance, which is only partly overcome by enteric coating. The amazing thing is that Dr Svartz had her patients taking 4–5 g uncoated tablets daily, whereas few of ours can tolerate more than 2 g. It is little wonder that the Edinburgh group could not confirm the usefulness of the preparation over the short period for which they used it (Sinclair and Duthie, 1948).

Recent work by Amos and Bax (personal communication) has shown that over a two-year period the success rate with sulphasalazine is comparable with that for gold. However, with sulphasalazine, failure was largely due to inefficacy, whereas with gold it was due to toxicity (mainly rashes).

Sulphasalazine is split in the colon by bacterial action to sulphapyridine and 5-aminosalicylic acid. Sulphapyridine is mainly absorbed while 5-aminosalicylic acid either remains largely in the bowel or undergoes enterohepatic circulation. Sulphapyridine is acetylated in the liver to acetylsulphapyridine, and this is excreted more rapidly by the kidney than the unacetylated form. Higher plasma concentrations of sulphapyridine, therefore, occur with slow acetylators (Khan *et al.*, 1980). The Glasgow study suggested that gastrointestinal intolerance occurred more commonly in slow acetylators, whereas lack of effect occurred in fast acetylators (Pullar *et al.*, 1983). It may be possible to manipulate the dose in the light of the acetylator status of individual patients. Both the Glasgow group and our own have shown that sulphapyridine is the active moiety rather than 5-aminosalicylic acid (Paller *et al.*, 1985; Neumann *et al.*, 1986). A study of a sulphonamide not absorbed from the bowel would be of particular interest, therefore.

Combination treatment with two or more second-line agents is a logical development by analogy with the cancer field. McCarty and Carrera (1982) have reported treatment with combined cyclophosphamide, azathioprine and hydroxychloroquine in 17 rheumatoid patients. We have used our patient model to explore this approach further (Martin *et al.*, 1982b). Hydroxychloroquine and penicillamine appear to be a useful combination, but gold and penicillamine do not (McKenna *et al.*, 1975).

Although mildly encouraging results of plasmapheresis and of total lymphoid irradiation have been reported in rheumatoid arthritis, they remain expensive unproved methods of treatment (Dequeker *et al.*, 1981; Kotzin, 1981; Jones *et al.*, 1981; Leading Article, 1982), and are unlikely to take over the role of drug therapy.

10.4   SERONEGATIVE SPONDARTHRITIDES

10.4.1   Ankylosing spondylitis

Although 85% of patients with ankylosing spondylitis never lose a day from work, continued treatment is important, and the other 15% must not be neglected. Systemic complications may occasionally be severe e.g. blindness from iritis, amyloidosis, or aortitis. Problems of evaluation of response are considerable. Some of the NSAIDs are highly effective in relieving pain and stiffness, allowing the all-important exercises. Our own experience suggests that statement of patient drug preferences at the end of a cross-over double-blind comparison is as useful as any measure (Bird *et al.*, 1980). For longer-acting drugs radiological changes are slow and serial changes at the sacro-iliac joints hard to quantify. It is doubtful whether isotope studies will be of value in drug evaluation. Serum IgA rises with increased clinical activity, and in conjunction with the ESR (or plasma viscosity), these may be the most useful variables to measure (Calin *et al.*, 1981; Calguneri *et al.*, 1981). Since IgA is a useful mark of disease activity, it may be that cytotoxic drugs could be a useful alternative therapy, but there have been few trials of these. We have looked at clozic as a non-specific antagonist of certain plasma proteins, but detected no beneficial effect (Hopkins *et al.*, 1984).

10.4.2   Psoriatic arthritis

This has received considerable attention in terms of clinical description, but less in terms of therapeutic response. There is little evidence that improvement of the skin affects the joints, except for PUVA therapy – long-wave ultra-violet radiation combined with topical psoralens (Purlman *et al.*, 1979). The most recent systemic drugs to be considered are oral retinoic acid derivatives (Bitter *et al.*, 1981). These vitamin A derivatives often have side effects on the skin and mucous membranes with cheilosis, and, like vitamin A, may be teratogenic. Our own experience in a controlled trial of cis-retinoic acid compound with ibuprofen showed that articular index improved with tigason, although other clinical variables did not. Biochemically there were more improvements in the cis-retinoic acid than in the ibuprofen group. This lends encouragement to the development of less toxic analogues for the treatment of psoriatic arthritis (Hopkins *et al.*, 1983).

Of the drugs with known antirheumatoid activity, aurothiomalate, azathioprine and D-penicillamine have all been tried (Leading Article, 1978). There is evidence that aurothiomalate benefits the condition, and has no adverse effect on the skin lesions (Bird and Wright, 1982).

It would be worth evaluating the new oral gold preparation, auranofin, in this connection.

10.4.3 Reiter's syndrome

The non-specific urethritis is commonly treated with 1.5 g tetracycline daily for 10 days, but this does not affect the arthritis. It could be useful to study the use of the antibiotic prophylactically before sexual exposure to determine its effect on the joint disease. The paucity of suitable patients, the tendency of the condition to spontaneous remission, and the poor compliance amongst this group of patients, make detailed trials difficult.

10.5 OSTEOARTHROSIS

The two major therapeutic approaches of the future would be firstly to halt or prevent the degeneration of the joints, and secondly to alleviate the pain (which is the main symptom) by reducing the inflammatory component. The difficulties of the first approach have been discussed by Bird and Wright (1982). One possibility is a specific inhibition of enzyme degradation, although some would see this as closing the stable door after the horse has bolted. If crystal deposition is shown to be of aetiological importance, and the evidence for that is tenuous, an attempt to prevent their formation or to stabilize them would be worthwhile. The crystals may well be contributory to the inflammatory phase, and modification of their deposition should be considered. Chelating high local excesses of calcium ions has only provoked attacks of acute inflammation (Bennett *et al.*, 1976). The use of local inhibitors such as 9-furyladenine to block adenylcyclase is unlikely to be acceptable and systemic blockade of adenylcyclase is likely to be dangerous, since the enzyme plays an important role in many biological systems. If a reliable animal model of osteoarthrosis, in which raised pyrophosphate levels in the synovial fluid and cartilage played an integral part, could be developed, then work on inhibiting pyrophosphate production could be pursued more easily.

Animal experience with diphosphonates shows that some will strongly inhibit apatite deposition and slow the natural resorption of the apatite plaque, but the clinical significance of this is unproven.

There has been a good deal of interest in orgotein, a generic name for a drug version of Cu-Zn superoxide dismutase, on the basis of arresting local damage by superoxide radicals (Dieppe, 1977). In 24 double-blind, placebo controlled trials of a week's duration in patients with osteoarthrosis of the knee, by 12 intra-articular injections at bi-weekly intervals, both the physician and the patients reported significant advantages of orgotein over placebo (Lund-Olesen and Menander-Huber, 1983). There has also been interest in the intra-articular use of glycosaminoglycan polysulphate to inhibit enzymatic degradation. One further promising approach may be the suppression of anti-collagen antibody formation. This does, of course, presuppose an immunological component to the development of the disease.

Intra-articular synthetic lubricants have long been an attractive proposition and their desiderata have been well defined (Cooke and Gvozdanovic, 1981). They should have acceptable frictional characteristics and a structure similar to that of mucin, resistance to degradation, tolerance within the joint space, retention within the synovial cavity, cheapness and ease of production, compatibility with synovial fluid in respect to rheology and surface properties, and no interference with the nutrient supplied to chrondrocytes. A group of such lubricants has been elaborated, but the major problem is that of retaining them within the joint space. The feasibility of an encapsulated lubricant should be considered. It may well be possible with endoprostheses, but it is difficult to see how it could be used in natural joints.

10.6 VASCULITIS

Over the past few years the introduction of new therapeutic agents that have their action at a cellular level has highlighted the need to study the microcirculation in more detail. Several methods are available for evaluating blood supply to an extremity, but few of them are able to distinguish between thermoregulatory flow via shunt vessels, and nutritional flow directed through the capillary circulation (Fagrell, 1977). The method of laser light scattering depends on analysis of the frequency spectrum of laser light scattering by moving red cells in the skin (Nilsson et al., 1980). However, this method probably records blood flow at a depth below the superficial capillaries and will, therefore, include both plexus and anastomotic vessels (Tooke et al., 1984). The technique that indisputably records capillary events is dynamic capillaroscopy (Fagrell et al., 1977), and this method has been developed to the extent that quantified measurements can now be made directly on the capillary circulation (Martin and Tooke, 1982).

Microvascular changes are a recognized feature of most connective tissue diseases. Rheumatoid vasculitis is characterized by changes that vary from a mild obliterative endarteritis to a severe necrotizing arteritis depending on the size of vessels involved. Similar changes are seen in SLE, and in both these diseases an immune complex mediated tissue injury has been demonstrated (Gilliam and Smiley, 1976).

In systemic sclerosis vascular obstruction and ischaemic atrophy are frequently seen. The most common subjective clinical feature is Raynaud's phenomenon. The vascular changes in the microvessels range from an altered vascular endothelium to a marked intimal proliferation that results in lumen obliteration (Campbell and Leroy, 1975).

The pathological mechanisms associated with many of these vascular changes remain obscure. Whenever possible treatment should be aimed at fundamental disease processes, but as most are poorly, if at all, understood, therapy is directed at preventing vessel damage, at improving vascular flow both thermoregulatory and nutritional, and by altering local factors that may contribute to the clinical picture.

For the treatment of severe disseminated necrotizing arteritis, cytotoxic agents, in particular cyclophosphamide, with or without corticosteroid therapy, have been recommended, as well as for vasculitic conditions where other treatments have failed (Fauci *et al.*, 1978). Some benefits have also been reported after the use of repeated plasma exchange. The mechanism by which these effects occur are poorly understood, but may involve alterations in platelet function, blood rheology and circulating immune complexes (Scott *et al.*, 1983). Plasma exchange has also been successfully used in the treatment of severe Raynaud's phenomenon, producing prolonged clinical benefit with healing of digital ulceration (O'Reilly *et al.*, 1979). The administration of stanazolol, an anabolic steroid which enhances fibrinolysis and lowers fibrinogen levels, has also been reported to improve symptoms of Raynaud's phenomenon (Jarrett *et al.*, 1978). Further studies of this drug are underway to determine whether it acts as a modulator of the immune system, but until results are available this form of treatment is reserved for severely affected males and post-menopausal women who have normal liver function.

Recent pilot studies of other therapeutic approaches have shown some interesting results. Topical application of glyceryl trinitrite has been reported to be beneficial in Raynaud's phenomenon (Franks, 1982), as has oral nifedipine, a slow calcium channel antagonist, which is the first of a new class of agents which blocks cellular uptake of calcium. It has emerged as a potent vasodilator which affects both the coronary and peripheral arterial beds. Nifedipine was effective in reducing the frequency and severity of Raynaud's phenomenon but was not shown to influence skin temperature recovery times (Smith and McKendry, 1982). Ketanserin, a selective 5-hydroxytryptamine receptor blocking agent, has been shown to increase finger blood flow and skin temperature measurements after intravenous administration (Stranden *et al.*, 1982). This drug antagonizes both the vasoconstricting and platelet aggregatory effect of serotonin, and an oral preparation of this drug may offer a new approach in the treatment of vascular disease.

Prostaglandins E_1, E_2 and prostacyclin (PGI_2) are known potent vasodilators and inhibitors of platelet aggregation, and are important in the maintenance of normal vascular function. In the connective tissue diseases, where vessel abnormalities are associated with pathophysiological abnormalities, each of these substances has been evaluated. In a single blind, cross-over study comparing intravenous PGE_1 with placebo 0.15 m saline, patients with systemic sclerosis reported an improvement in symptoms of Raynaud's phenomenon with PGE_1 lasting up to 6 weeks, but no change was seen in the placebo group or in the response to cold challenge (Martin *et al.*, 1981). However, further work by Kyle *et al.* (1982) has demonstrated improved skin temperature recovery times following PGE_1 treatment. Similar vascular changes have been reported following intravenous prostacyclin (Dowd *et al.*, 1982), with improved Raynaud's symptoms and response to cold challenge (Pardy et al., 1980). Each of these compounds requires intravenous administration and the associated side effects have reduced their use to conditions in which vascular changes are severe or life threatening. Topically administered prostaglandin E_2 is being evaluated as an acceptable alternative, and this novel method of administration overcomes the known gastrointestinal side effects associated with these compounds.

Although short intravenous prostaglandin infusions are potent vasodilators and anti-platelet agents, both these effects are short lived and do not explain the long duration of response recorded following infusion. PGE_1 is known to alter lymphocyte aggregation (Dunn et al., 1976) as well as modulate immune function (Stobo et al., 1979), and PGI_2 inhibits leucocyte adherence to endothelial cells in vitro (Boxer et al., 1980). It is possible that these components can alter the immunological mechanisms associated with vasculitis and with Raynaud's phenomenon. This approach is being evaluated in the treatment of rheumatoid vasculitis.

An alternative approach for treating vascular disease has been to use oral treatment with dazoxiben, a thromboxane synthetase inhibitor (Menys and Davies, 1983), that blocks the production of thromboxane A_2 by platelets and thus prevents the potent vasoconstrictor effect of this substance in plasma. The selective inhibition of thromboxane A_2 synthesis might, therefore, enhance the local production of PGI_2 by the vessel wall, but long-term treatment with oral dazoxiben resulted in no significant changes in finger skin temperature or in capillary red cell velocity (Tindall et al., 1984).

For the future the research that offers the greatest interest in treating vascular disease with or without immunological phenomena is the use of oral prostaglandin analogues. Not only do these compounds increase peripheral blood flow, thereby increasing hand temperature (Clifford et al., 1980), but this simultaneous increase in capillary pressure and red cell velocity (Martin and Tooke, 1982) has led to marked healing of ischaemic ulcers as a direct result of both improved thermoregulatory and nutritional blood flow.

10.7 REFERENCES

Bennett, R. M., Lehr, J. R. and McCarty, D. J. (1976) Crystal shedding and acute pseudogout. Arthr. Rheum., 19, 93–7.

Bird, H. A., Dixon, J. S., Finney, B. L., Leatham, P. A., Lowe, J. R., Pickup, M. E., Rhind, V. M., Rushton, A., Sitton, N. G. and Wright, V. (1983) A clinical and biochemical evaluation of Clozic, a novel disease modifying drug in rheumatoid arthritis. Clin. Exp. Rheumatol., 1, 93–100.

Bird, H. A., Dixon, J. S., Pickup, M. E., Rhind, V. M., Lowe, J. R., Lee, M. R. and Wright, V. (1982a) A biochemical assessment of sulphasalazine in rheumatoid arthritis. J. Rheumatol., 9, 36–45.

Bird, H. A., Leatham, P. A., Dixon, J. S., Sitton, M. G. and Wright, V. (1982b) Failure of trien to improve rheumatoid arthritis. Ann. Rheum. Dis., 41, 314–15.

Bird, H. A., Rhind, V. M., Pickup, M. E. and Wright, V. (1980) A comparative study of benoxoprofen and indomethacin in ankylosing spondylitis. *J. Rheumatol.*, 7 (Suppl. 6), 139–42.

Bird, H. A. and Wright, V. (1982) *Applied Drug Therapy of Rheumatic Diseases*, Wright, Bristol.

Bitter, T., Bahous, I. and Rosenthal, M. (1981) All-trans retinoic acid (R): a remission aim in the treatment of psoriatic arthritis. *Ann. Rheum. Dis.*, 40, 209.

Boxer, L. A., Allen, J. M., Schmidt, M., Tocler, M. and Badiner, R. L. (1980) Inhibition of polymorphonuclear-leucocyte adherence by prostacyclin. *J. Lab. Clin. Med.*, 95, 672–5.

Bruhl, W., Swierczynska, Z. and Cygler, B. (1979) Clinical and immunological effects of pyrithioxine treatment in RA patients. *9th Eur. Congr. Rheumatol.*, Wiesbaden, West Germany, Abstract 243.

Calguneri, M., Swinburn, L., Cooke, E. M. and Wright, V. (1981) Secretory IgA immune defence pattern in ankylosing spondylitis and Klebsiella. *Ann. Rheum. Dis.*, 40, 600–4.

Calin, P., Ebringer, R. and Ebringer, A. (1981) Association of inflammation with elevated serum IgA in ankylosing spondylitis. *Ann. Rheum. Dis.*, 39, 545–9.

Campbell, P. M., and Leroy, E. C. (1975) Pathogenesis of systemic sclerosis: a vascular hypothesis. *Seminars Arthr. Rheum.*, 4, 351–68.

Camus, A., Jaffe, I. A. and Grouzet, J. (1978) La pyrithioxine: nouveau traitement de fond de la polyarthrite rhumatoide. *Rev. Rhum.*, 45, 95–100.

Chandler, G. N. and Wright, V. (1958) Deleterious effect of intra-articular hydrocortisone. *Lancet*, ii, 661–3.

Clifford, P. C., Martin, M. F. R., Sheddon, E. J., Kirby, J. D., Baird, R. N. and Dieppe, P. A. (1980) Treatment of vasospastic disease with prostaglandin E$_1$. *Br. Med. J.*, 281, 1031–4.

Cooke, A. F. and Gvozdanovic, D. D. (1981) Synthetic lubricants of synovial joints. In (eds D. Dowson and V. Wright), *Introduction to the Biomechanics of Joints and Joint Replacements* Mechanical Engineering Publications, London, pp. 139–43.

Cox, B. M., Goldstein, A. and Li, C. H. (1976) Opioid activity of a peptide, β lipotropin-(61–91), derived from β-lipotropin. *Proc. Nat. Acad. Sci.*, USA, 73, 1821–3.

Dequeker, J., Naesens, M. and Martens, J. (1981) The effect of plasma exchange on synovitis in rheumatoid arthritis. *Scand. J. Rheumatol.*, 10, 273–90.

Dieppe, P. A. (1977) Crystal-induced inflammation and osteoarthritis, in *Perspectives in Inflammation: Future Trends and Developments* (eds D. A. Willoughby, J. P. Giraud and G. P. Vely), MTP Press, Lancaster, pp. 225–37.

Dixon, J. S. and Bird, H. A. (1981) Reproducibility along a 10 cm vertical visual analogue scale. *Ann. Rheum. Dis.*, 40, 87–9.

Dixon, J. S., Bird, H. A., Pickup, M. E. and Wright, V. (1982) A human model screening system for the detection of specific anti-rheumatic activity. *Seminars Arthr. Rheum.*, 12, 185–90.

Dixon, J. S., Bird, H. A. and Wright, V. (1981) The pseudo-science of visual analogue scales. *15th Int. Congr. Rheumatol.*, Paris. Abstract 1388. Revue Rheumatologie. Special Issue.

Dowd, P. M., Martin, M. F. R., Cooke, E. D., Bowcock, S. A., Jones, R., Dieppe, P. A. and Kirby, J. D. T. (1982) Treatment of Raynaud's phenomenon by intravenous infusion of prostacyclin (PGI$_2$). *Br. J. Dermatol.*, 106, 81–9.

Downie, W. W., Leatham, P. A., Rhind, V. M., Wright, V., Branter, J. A. and Anderson, J. A. (1978) Studies with pain rating scales. *Ann. Rheum. Dis.*, 37, 378–81.

Dunn, C. J., Willoughby, D. A., Giroud, J. P. and Yamamoto, S. (1976) An appraisal of the interrelationships between prostaglandins and cyclic nucleotides in inflammation. *Biomedicine*, **24**, 214–20.

Ellis, B. W., Johns, M. W., Lancaster, R., Raptopoulos, P., Angelopoulos, N. and Priest, R. G. (1981) The St. Mary's Hospital sleep questionnaire: a study of reliability. *Sleep*, **41**, 93–7.

Fagrell, B. (1977) The skin microcirculation and the pathogenesis of ischaemic necrosis and gangrene. *Scand. J. Clin. Lab. Invest.*, **37**, 473–6.

Fagrell, B., Fronek, A. and Intaglietta, M. (1977) A microscope-television system for studying flow velocity in human skin capillaries. *Am. J. Physiol.*, **233**, 318–21.

Fauci, A. S., Haynes, B. F. and Katz, P. (1978) The spectrum of vasculitis. *Ann. Intern. Med.*, **89**, 660–6.

Franks, A. G. (1982) Topical glyceryl trinitrate as adjunctive treatment in Raynaud's disease. *Lancet*, i, 76–7.

Gilliam, J. N. and Smiley, J. D. (1976) Cutaneous necrotising vasculitis and related disorders. *Ann. Allergy*, **37**, 328–39.

Greenfield, S. S. and Hawks, G. W. (1981) Visual analogue scale. *Br. J. Clin. Pharmacol.*, **11**, 98.

Gregoriadis, G. (1980) Tailoring liposome structure. *Nature*, **283**, 814–15.

Grennan, D. M., Ferry, D. G. and Ashworth, M. E. (1979) The aspirin–ibuprofen interaction in rheumatoid arthritis. *Br. J. Clin. Pharmacol.*, **8**, 497–504.

Heilman, K. (1978) Therapeutic systems. *Patterns Specific Drug Delivery: Concepts and Development*, Georg Thieme, Stuttgard.

Henry, J. L. (1976) Effect of substance P on functionally identified units in cats' spinal cord. *Brain Res.*, **114**, 439–52.

Hopkins, R., Bird, H. A., Hill, J., Surrall, K., Miller, A. and Wright, V. (1983) A double-blind controlled trial of tigason (etretinate) in psoriatic arthritis. *Communication, Xth Eur. Congr. Rheumatol.*, Moscow, USSR.

Hopkins, R. and Bird, H. A. Personal communication.

Hughes, J. (1975) Isolation of an endogenous compound from the brain with pharmacological properties similar to morphine. *Brain Res.*, **88**, 295–308.

Hughes, J., Smith, D. W. and Kosterlitz, H. (1975) Identification of two related pentapeptides from the brain with potent opiate agonist activity. *Nature*, **285**, 577–9.

Huskisson, E. C. (1974) Measurement of pain. *Lancet*, ii, 1127–31.

Huskisson, E. C., Jaffe, I. A. and Scott, J. (1980) 5-thiopyridoxine in RA: clinical and experimental studies. *Arthr. Rheum.*, **23**, 106–10.

Jaffe, M. E. (1983) Osmosin. A new continuously acting anti-arthritic. *Curr. Med. Res. Opinion*, Suppl. 2.

Jarrett, P. E. M., Morland, M. and Browse, N. L. (1978) Treatment of Raynaud's phenomenon by fibrinolytic enhancement. *Br. Med. J.*, ii, 523–5.

Jessel, T. M. and Iversen, L. L. (1977) Opiate analgesic inhibits substance P-release from rat trigeminal nucleus. *Nature*, **268**, 549–51.

Jick, H. (1981) Effects of aspirin and acetaminophen in gastrointestinal haemorrhage. *Arch. Intern. Med.*, **141**, 316.

Jick, H. and Porter, J. (1978) Drug-induced gastrointestinal bleeding. *Lancet*, ii, 87.

Jones, J. V., Clough, J. D., Klinberg, J. R. and Davis, P. (1981) The role of therapeutic plasmapheresis in the rheumatic diseases. *J. Lab. Clin. Med.*, **97/5**, 589–98.

Khan, K. A., Howes, D. T., Piris, J. and Truelove, S. C. (1980) Optimum dose of sulphasalazine for maintenance treatment in ulcerative colitis. *Gut*, **21**, 232–40.

Kondo, H., Rabin, B. S. and Rodnan, G. P. (1976) Cutaneous-antigen-stimulating lymphokine production by lymphocytes of patients with progressive systemic sclerosis (scleroderma). *J. Clin. Invest.*, **58**, 1388–94.

Kosterlitz, H. N., Lord, J. A. H. and Patterson, S. J. (1980) Effects of changes in structure of enkephalins and narcotic analgesic drugs on their interactions with receptors and receptors. *Br. J. Pharmacol.*, 68, 333–42.

Kotzin, B. L. (1981) Treatment of intractable rheumatoid arthritis with total lymphoid irradiation. *N. Engl. J. Med.*, 17, 969–76.

Kyle, M. V., Parr, G., Salisbury, R., Page Thomas, P. and Hazleman, B. L. (1982) PGE₁ vasospastic disease and thermography. *Ann. Rheum. Dis.* 41, 310.

Lasagna, L. (1960) The clinical measurement of pain. *Ann. N. Y. Acad. Sci.*, 86, 28–37.

Leading article (1978) Treatment of arthritis associated with psoriasis. *Br. Med. J.*, 1, 262–3.

Leading article (1982) Total lymphoid irradiation in rheumatoid arthritis. *Lancet*, i, 25–7.

Levine, J. G., Gordon, N. C. and Fields, H. L. (1978) The mechanism of placebo analgesia. *Lancet*, ii, 654–6.

Levy, M. (1974) Aspirin use in patients with major upper gastrointestinal bleeding and peptic ulcer disease. *N. Engl. J. Med.*, 290, 1158.

Lund-Olesen, K. and Menander-Huber, K. B. (1983) Intra-articular orgotein therapy in osteoarthritis of the knee. A double-blind, placebo-controlled trial. *Arzneimittelforschung*, 33, 1199–203.

McCarty, D. J. and Carrera, G. F. (1982) Intractable rheumatoid arthritis: treatment with combined cyclophosphamide, azathioprine and hydroxychloroquine. *J. Am. Med. Assoc.*, 248, 1718–23.

McKenna, F., Hickling, P., Martin, M. F. R., Sitton, N., Dixon, J. S. and Wright, V. (1983) Why is methylcysteine not an anti-rheumatoid drug? *Heberden Soc.*, Leeds.

McKenna, F., Hopkins, R., Hinchcliffe, M. P., Bird, H. A. and Wright, V. (1985) Gold and penicillamine, alone and in combination, in active rheumatoid arthritis. Abstract D158, p. 221. XVIth International Congress of Rheumatology, Sydney.

Martin, M. F. R., Dowd, P. M., Ring, E. F. J., Cooke, E. D., Dieppe, P. A. and Kirby, J. D. T. (1981) Prostaglandin E₁ infusions for vascular insufficiency in progressive systemic sclerosis. *Ann. Rheum. Dis.*, 40, 350–4.

Martin, M. F. R., Dixon, J., Hickling, P., Bird, H., Golding, J. and Wright, V. (1982) A combination of D-penicillamine and hydroxychloroquine for the treatment of rheumatoid arthritis. *Ann. Rheum. Dis.*, 41, 208.

Martin, M. F. R., Surrall, K., McKenna, F., Dixon, J. S., Bird, H. A. and Wright, V. (1983) Captopril: a new long-term agent for treating rheumatoid arthritis. *Ann. Rheum. Dis.*, 42, 231.

Martin, M. F. R. and Tooke, J. E. (1982) Effect of prostaglandin E₁ on microvascular haemodynamics in progressive systemic sclerosis. *Br. Med. J.*, 285, 1688–90.

Menys, V. C. and Davies, J. A. (1983) Selective inhibition of thromboxane synthetase with dazoxiben-basis of its inhibitory effect in platelet adhesion. *Thrombosis Haemostasis*, 49, 96–101.

Moldofsky, H., Lue, F. A. and Smythe, H. A. (1983) Alpha EEG sleep and morning symptoms in rheumatoid arthritis. *J. Rheumatol.*, 10, 373–9.

Moldofsky, H. and Scarisbrick, P. (1976) Induction of neurasthenic musculo-skeletal pain syndrome by selected sleep deprivation. *Psychosom. Med.*, 38, 35–44.

Neumann, V. C., Grindulis, K. A., Hubball, S., McConkey, B. and Wright, V. (1983) Comparison between penicillamine and sulphasalazine in rheumatoid arthritis. Leeds-Birmingham trial. *Br. Med. J.*, 287, 1099–102.

Neumann, V. C., Taggart, A. J., Legauer, P., Astbury, C., Hill, J. and Bird, H. A. (1986) A study to determine the active moiety of sulphasalazine in rheumatoid arthritis. *J. Rheum.* (In press)

Nilsson, G. E., Tenland, T. and Oberg, P. A. (1980) Evaluation of a laser doppler flowmeter for measurement of tissue blood flow. *IEEE Trans. Biomed. Engng*, **27**, 597–604.

O'Reilly, M. J. G., Talpos, G., Roberts, V. C., White, J. M. and Cotton, L. T. (1979) Controlled trial of plasma exchange in treatment of Raynaud's syndrome. *Br. Med. J.*, i, 113–15.

Pardy, B. J., Lewis, J. D. and Eastcott, H. H. G. (1980) Preliminary experience with prostaglandins E_1 and I_2 in peripheral vascular disease. *Surgery*, **88**, 826–32.

Parrott, A. C. and Hindmarch, I. (1980) The Leeds sleep evaluation questionnaire in psychopharmacological investigations – a review. *Psychopharmacology*, **71**, 173–9.

Pasero, G. and Ciompi, M. L. (1979) Thiopronine therapy in rheumatoid arthritis. *Arthr. Rheum.*, **32**, 882–4.

Pullar, R., Hunter, J. A. and Capell, H. A. (1983) Sulphasalazine in rheumatoid arthritis: a double-blind comparison of sulphasalazine with placebo and sodium aurothiomalate. *Br. Med. J.*, **287**, 1102–4.

Pullar, T., Hunter, J. A., Capell, H. A. (1985) Which component of sulphasalazine is active in rheumatoid arthritis. *Br. Med. J.*, **290**, 1535–8.

Purlman, S. G., Gerber, L. H. and Roberts, M. (1979) Photochemotherapy and psoriatic arthritis: a prospective study. *Ann. Intern. Med.*, **91**, 717–22.

Randall, W. and Selitto, J. F. (1957) A method for measurement of analgesic activity on inflamed tissue. *Arch. Int. Pharmacodynam. Ther.*, **111**, 409–19.

Ranlov, P. J., Nielsen, S. P. and Barenholdt, O. (1983) Faecal blood loss during culmination of acetylsalicylic acid, ketoprofen and a new ketoprofen sustained-release compound. *Scand. J. Rheumatol.*, (In press).

Rhind, V. M., Bird, H. A. and Wright, V. (1980) A comparison of clinical assessments of disease activity in rheumatoid arthritis. *Ann. Rheum. Dis.*, **39**, 135–7.

Robinson, D. (1981) Principles of pharmcodynamics. in *Textbook of Rheumatology* (eds W. N. Kelly, E. Harris, S. Ruddy and C. Sledge), Saunders, Philadelphia, pp. 721–7.

Scott, D. G. I., Bacon, P. A., Bothamley, J., Allen, C., Elson, C. J. and Wallington, T. (1986) Plasma exchange in rheumatoid arthritis. (in preparation)

Scott, D. L., Roden, S., Marshall, T. and Kendall, M. J. (1982) Variations in responses to non-steroidal anti-inflammatory drugs. *Br. J. Pharmacol.*, **14**, 691–4.

Sinclair, R. J. G. and Duthie, J. J. R. (1948) Salazopyrin in the treatment of rheumatoid arthritis. *Ann. Rheum. Dis.*, **8**, 226–31.

Smith, C. D. and McKendry, R. J. R. (1982) Controlled trial of nifedipine in the treatment of Raynaud's phenomenon. *Lancet*, ii, 1299–301.

Smith, S. E. and Rawlins, M. D. (1973) *Variability in Human Drug Response*, Butterworths, London.

Stranden, E., Roald, O. K. and Krohg, R. (1982) Treatment of Raynaud's phenomenon with the $5\text{-}HT_2$-receptor antagonist ketanserin. *Br. Med. J.*, **285**, 1069–71.

Steven, M. M., Hunter, J. A., Murdock, R. M. and Capell, H. A. (1982) Does the order of second-line treatment in rheumatoid arthritis matter? *Br. Med. J.*, **284**, 79–80.

Stobo, J. D., Kennedy, M. S. and Goldyne, M. E. (1979) Prostaglandin E modulation of the mitogenic response of human T cells. *J. Clin. Invest.*, **64**, 1188–95.

Stone, P. H., Antman, E. M., Muller, J. E. and Braunwald, E. (1980) Calcium channel blocking agents in the treatment of cardiovascular disorders. Part II: Haemodynamic effects and clinical applications. *Ann. Intern. Med.*, **93**, 886–904.

Svartz, N. (1942) Salazopyrin, a new sulfanilamide preparation. *Acta Med. Scand.* **110**, 577–98.

Svartz, N. (1948) The treatment of rheumatic polyarthritis with acid azo compounds, in *Rheumatism*, **4**, pp. 56–60.

Swinson, D. R., Zlosnick, J. and Jackson, L. (1981) Double-blind trial of dapsone against placebo in the treatment of rheumatoid arthritis. *Ann. Rheum. Dis.*, 40, 235–9.

Theuwes, F. (1981) Drug delivery systems. *Pharmacol. Ther.*, 13, 149–191.

Theuwes, F. and Yum, S. I. (1976) Principles of the design and operation of generic osmotic pumps for the delivery of semisolid or liquid drug formatulations. *Ann. Biomed. Engng*, 4, 343–53.

Tindall, H., Tooke, J. E., Menys, V. C., Martin, M. F. R. and Davies, J. A. (1985) Effect of dazoxiben, a thromboxane synthetase inhibitor, on skin-blood flow following cold challenge in patients with Raynaud's phenomenon. *Eur. J. Clin. Invest.*, 15(1), 20–30.

Tooke, J. E., Ostergren, J. and Fagrell, B. (1986) Synchronous assessment of human skin microcirculation by laser doppler flowmetry and dynamic capillaroscopy. (in preparation)

Veys, E. M., Huskisson, E. C., Rosenthal, M., Vischer, T. L., Mielants, H., Thrower, P. A., Scott, J., Ott, H., Scheijgrond, H. and Symoens, J. (1982) Clinical response to therapy with thymopoietin pentapeptide (TP-5) in rheumatoid arthritis. *Ann. Rheum. Dis.*, 41, 441–3.

Wright, V. and Hopkins, R. (1983) Administration of anti-rheumatic drugs. *Ann. Rheum. Dis.*, 35, 229–31.

Clinical applications and implications

INTRODUCTION

J. M. H. Moll

The previous sections have dealt with the general principles underlying rheumatological therapeutics (Part one) and details of drugs comprising the 'rheumatological pharmacopoeia' (Part two).

This section is intended to outline how this knowledge is applied to the specific management of individual rheumatic entities.

It is a curious fact that whatever speciality is considered, the advice authors give in their writing bears relatively little relationship to what they do in practice! 'Classical' guidelines tend to be perpetuated, perhaps because of an intrinsic fear of breaking from 'conservatism'. However, it is clear from professional discussions between practising clinicians that the 'craft' of medical therapeutics, not least rheumatological therapeutics, differs significantly from textbook pronouncements.

Therefore, one of the main remits of this section, carefully specified to contributors at the planning stage of the book, was to encourage 'not so much what you preach, but what you actually do'.

In requesting this from the authors, certain areas of rheumatological therapeutics were especially highlighted for particular consideration. These areas included the following:

1. What drugs do you use in particular circumstances?
2. What is your policy regarding the titration of dosage according to symptomatology?
3. How do you manage toxic effects?

It was hoped that this approach would create a realistic picture of rheumatological *management*, as opposed to *treatment*, using the latter term in its more pragmatic and confined sense.

In order to further the management (L. manus = hand; It. maneggiare = to handle) approach, that is an approach in which the general handling of the patient is important, authors were also encouraged to add a note on non-drug aspects of therapy. Although this book is largely concerned with antirheumatic drugs, it was felt that this more generous compass would help to provide the necessary dimension to enable a realistic overview. Thus, wherever possible, brief comments have been included on elements comprising 'general management' such as patient education, rest, and the control of anaemia. The place of physiotherapy and occupational therapy has also been commented on where applicable.

The division of this section provided some problems in that it seemed necessary to avoid two extremes. One extreme concerned the dangers of collective handling of unrelated rheumatic diseases; the other being the hazards of the 'catalogue approach', in which the therapies of disorders might be handled in an encyclopaedic fashion. A compromise seemed to be a construct in which relatively few chapters were chosen, each encompassing disorders that fell as comfortably as possible into natural therapeutic groupings.

It has, of course, been necessary to vary this approach a little between chapters, perforce the individual characteristics of the rheumatic problems under review. However, it is hoped the general message of 'management', as opposed to explicit categorization of treatments, will be apparent throughout.

CHAPTER 11

Rheumatoid arthritis

L. P. J. Holt

11.1 INTRODUCTION

Patients with rheumatic diseases often experience a fluctuant chronic illness characterized by periods of exacerbation and remission. Simple measures other than drugs may serve to reduce the symptoms of an exacerbation; drug therapy is less likely to be needed when the patient is undergoing lengthy periods of remission. *Patient education* plays an important role in the management of disease, and the supervising physician should ensure that either a physician or adequately trained paramedical colleagues are providing adequate education in the hope of preventing joint damage and subsequent deformity. Occupational therapists and physiotherapists should be asked to advise on splinting and the appropriate type of rest required for the patient's condition. Patients should be instructed in the *exercises* they should perform at home. Attention given to providing adequate *footwear*, for example, might relieve the strain on joints higher up the lower limbs, in turn reducing the need for analgesics and anti-inflammatory agents to control the patient's symptoms. Immobilization of a joint by *splinting* may also reduce the patient's consumption of analgesics or anti-inflammatory agents. (Conversely, the active physiotherapy that will be provided for a patient with ankylosing spondylitis may require the addition of extra analgesics in order to allow the physiotherapist to mobilize the joints through their full range of movements.) Close collaboration between the *prescribing physician and the paramedical attendant* is essential. Neither should physicians forget the value of *rest* in certain inflammatory polyarthritides before embarking upon drug therapy. Physical rest may be indicated when rheumatoid arthritis is in exacerbation (though may be contraindicated for the chronic phase of ankylosing spondylitis). However, there is support for the philosophy of physical exercise even when active inflammation is present. This has been mainly advocated in Scandinavian countries. Relief of mental anxiety is also important. On the one hand, this may require adequate *career guidance*, social worker support and information on the management of finances as a wage earner in the family finds his career is to be limited by arthritis. Drug therapy including the use of *anxiolytic agents* and appropriate hypnotics may also be required to promote rest. A recent survey in Leeds suggested that a large proportion of patients with arthritis experience *sleep disturbance*; this is often forgotten as prescribers plunge into the one track tunnel of anti-inflammatory agents as a universal panacea for arthritis complaints.

Patients with arthritis may become *anaemic*. Patients on anti-inflammatory agents develop a hypochromic microcytic iron deficiency anaemia that responds to iron therapy. Patients with rheumatoid arthritis (and even the systemic seronegative spondarthritides) may develop a normochromic normocytic anaemia of prolonged disease activity. Management of the former is likely to be with investigation, adjustment in drug therapy to minimize dyspepsia and gastrointestinal bleeding, and oral iron supplements. (Management of the latter is likely to be unresponsive to oral iron supplements and intramuscular iron injections may be needed.) A serum ferritin level less than 60 µ/L indicates true iron deficiency (Rajapakse, Holt and Perera, 1980).

Drug therapy forms only part of the overall management of a patient with rheumatoid arthritis and should be approached in this context. It may be the most effective; it may also be the most disastrous. Not only are many of these drugs potentially toxic, their use may prevent other simple and less dangerous procedures being employed. Thus it is essential to view the rheumatoid patient in total context, including in this the family, occupation and pastimes. In determining goals, there are three groups of people to consider, all with slightly different points of view:

(1) The patient. Young children have not formed their views on the future, nor usually realistically evaluated their place in society. They will usually want to join their friends in play and not be separated from their home by in-patient care. It is only later that the worries of examinations and work appear. Adults will usually worry about independence and supporting their families.

(2) The parents, spouse or relatives. Parents obviously worry about the suffering of their children and foresee problems with the future for which they may make long-term plans. Their views are often influenced by how other patients they see are managing, in which case it is usually only those who are badly affected that are obvious, and thus their outlook is coloured by this.

(3) The doctor. The doctor has objectively to weigh up the various possibilities open to him; particularly in children, admission to hospital or home care? In adults similar problems may arise. Will a spell in hospital jeopar-

dize career prospects? Is it better to go for certain benefit with corticosteroid rather than wait for benefit from antirheumatic treatment that may not materialize? (See Paulus, 1982.)

The cause of the patient's problems should be as clearly defined as possible, and this definition reassessed often for it usually changes. The patient's view of his problem may be radically different from that of the physician and, in particular, the feasibility of treating different problems may be out of keeping with the disability they cause. Similar disabilities may have completely different causes. Thus, the treatment of mechanical pain may be quite different from that of inflammatory pain; one needing analgesic to allow exercise and other physical activities, and the other anti-inflammatory therapy to reduce inflammation (and pain) and joint destruction, and to allow exercise. Further, the timing of therapy may also be quite different; the inflammatory pain often being worse before exercise, i.e. in the morning, and the mechanical pain, after exercise, in the evening. In both types of pain treatment needs to be given well before intended exercise, i.e. the night before in patients with morning symptoms. Inflammatory pain usually takes longer to settle than mechanical pain.

The initial assessment is that of *pain tolerance* (i.e. the amount of pain the patient can stand) and *pain threshold* (the level at which pain is appreciated). If either of these is low it is necessary to enquire why. Depression, in any of its forms, is a frequent cause of low pain tolerance (Von Knorring *et al.*, 1983), and treatment of depression may relieve the pain (Ward *et al.*, 1982). This may be linked with altered sleep patterns, a suggested cause of the 'fibrositis' syndrome (Smythe, 1981).

Another frequent cause of enhanced pain is 'selective attention', i.e. where the patient selectively focuses on the pain signals ignoring the many other competing sensory inputs. By reducing the psychological import of these selected inputs by full explanation and discussion, their importance and effect can often be lessened, thus reducing pain and the need for analgesia. It should be noted that the drugs given may depress the patient; e.g. sedatives and NSAIDs (aspirin in children has seemed to be a particular offender). Acupuncture, transcutaneous electrical nerve stimulation (TENS), hypnosis, and biofeedback may all be adjuvants to a reduction in drug therapy.

The second assessment is of *prognosis*. In determining the type of treatment to employ an assessment of progress is helpful. Four factors are important — chronicity, disability, compliance, and potential toxicity.

Generally, if arthritis has persisted for four months it is unlikely to subside spontaneously. However, patients with disease of explosive acute onset often have a better outlook (Duthie *et al.*, 1964). Disease complications such as Felty's syndrome, vasculitis, and pulmonary involvement all carry a worse prognosis. Serum markers, such as the presence of rheumatoid factor, reinforce this. Raised acute phase reactants, immunoglobulins, and rheumatoid factors, especially IgG type, suggest that there will be more damage and that extra-articular complications may occur. Recently, interest has centred on the genetic make-up of the patient and an association with DR4/DW4 and DR4/DR7 haplotypes with joint destruction shown (Young *et al.*, 1984). Often, by the time the patient is seen, the pattern of damage will already be in train and the problems of disability obvious.

A third assessment to make is that of probable *compliance* and access to therapy and monitoring facilities.

Fourthly, an estimate of *toxic reaction* due to treatment may be possible by genetic markers (see later). Also, the susceptibility to peptic ulceration after NSAID therapy is increased in blood group O patients (Semble *et al.*, 1982).

Increasing knowledge of these associations will allow a prognostic profile to be built up for each patient. This can then be compared with the risk of treatment.

11.2 ANTIRHEUMATIC THERAPY

In general 'antirheumatic' therapy takes five forms: (a) analgesic; (b) anti-inflammatory; (c) antirheumatic; (d) anti-depressant and (e) hypnotic.

In addition, other drugs such as antacids and H_2 antagonists are given to overcome gastrointestinal side effects. It is possible that these added drugs may also have an effect on the rheumatic process or the metabolism of anti-rheumatic drugs. The H_2 antagonists may have considerable effects on the inflammatory and immune system. Interaction between administered drugs and variation in drug metabolism could occur at several levels – intestinal absorption, plasma protein binding, hepatic function – particularly enzyme induction – and renal excretion (Salem *et al.*, 1978; Kampmann and Molholm Hansen, 1979; Olason, 1983; Bird *et al.*, 1981). The rate of hepatic metabolism has the greatest influence on the efficacy of these drugs. The most important effect of the NSAIDs on each other is their relative degree of protein binding. These interactions have been discussed in Chapter 3 and elsewhere (Bird and Wright, 1982). The NSAIDs may influence the effectiveness of other drugs used in the treatment of rheumatic patients, such as diuretics (decreased), sulphonylurea (increased with aspirin, causing hypoglycaemia), and anticoagulants (increased bleeding tendency).

The antirheumatic drugs can be divided into several groups according to their efficacy and safety. The basis for this grouping will be discussed later.

Probable antirheumatic activity
    4-aminoquinolones
    Chloroquine/hydroxychloroquine
    Sodium aurothiomalate/aurothioglucose
    D-penicillamine
Drugs with uncertain antirheumatic activity
    Auranofin
    5-thiopyridoxine
    Sulphasalazine

Dapzone
Clozic (Discontinued)
Cytostatic drugs
Azathioprine
Methotrexate
Cyclophosphamide
Chlorambucil
Immunoregulating drugs
Levamizole
Thymopoetin
Antilymphocyte globulin
Immunoregulating techniques
Thoracic duct drainage
Total body irradiation
Local irradiation (e.g. yttrium 90)
Aphoresis

This list is by no means exhaustive, and indeed a fuller list would reflect the marked differences in prescribing possibilities and habits between countries. The evaluation of these drugs varies greatly, and, since no clinician can have useful experience of more than a few, comparisons are difficult. If the practising clinician can master the use of a few he will be better placed than many to treat his patients well. Too often a form of treatment has been followed without thought to the alternatives.

It has been fashionable to consider the use of drugs in stages, i.e. 'first-line' used for early or less severe disease, 'second-line' if these fail or in more severe disease, and 'third-line' if second-line drugs do not control symptoms. This simple approach is useful as a convenient classification implying both increasing efficacy and frequency of side effects; but in clinical practice stages may be bypassed.

| FIRST-LINE DRUGS | Essentially the NSAIDS. | These have few side effects, some of which may be individual. The evidence that they prevent joint destruction is poor. Little toxicity monitoring necessary. Analgesic and anti-inflammatory. |
| SECOND-LINE DRUGS (Remission inducing) | Chloroquine, gold, penicillamine. | These drugs have potentially serious side effects and need careful monitoring. Delayed onset of benefit, but more evidence of prevention of joint destruction. Anti-inflammatory. |

| THIRD-LINE DRUGS | Corticosteroid and cytotoxic drugs. | Almost inevitable that sooner or later greater or lesser side effects will occur. May be very effective in symptomatic relief. May protect the joints at expense of side effects. Cytotoxic drugs need monitoring. Anti-inflammatory. |

11.3   ANALGESICS AND ANTI-INFLAMMATORY DRUGS

11.3.1   General

The relief of pain is in most cases the main desire of patients. Many patients attend with what may be termed 'pain syndromes' rather than rheumatic problems. Although an NSAID is often given and is sometimes effective, the more logical approach, where there is no inflammation, is often with an analgesic (Kantor, 1982). This reduces the risk of side effects. The mode of action of analgesics is poorly understood but is thought to be both peripherally on the peptide substance-P in the spinal tracts and centrally on the endorphins and enkephalins. It is probable that analgesics act *via* a competitive action for receptors for these substances on cells. It follows that in competing for cerebral cell receptors the chances of producing other cerebral effects, such as drowsiness, will be high. Thus the use of peripherally acting analgesics, although often less effective, is preferable.

The NSAIDs have many actions; in addition to the anti-inflammatory function they have analgesic and antipyretic activity. They also affect other metabolic pathways both directly and *via* their antiprostaglandin and antileukotriene activities. The group characteristics are of being weakly acidic and highly protein bound. In spite of much research, there is at present no convincing evidence that any of the NSAIDs have an antirheumatic property, that is, prevent progressive joint destruction. There are suggestions, and counter suggestions, that newer examples may alter some of the indices of disease activity, most notably the acute phase reactants. This lack of antirheumatic effect is the more disappointing, but illuminating, since it would obviously be a valuable propaganda feature for the relevant pharmaceutical firm.

Several general comments about antirheumatic therapy with NSAIDs may be made.

In general, the patient is the best guide to the drug required, and dosage should be adjusted according to response (Gumpel, 1978). Often, larger doses than those suggested by the manufacturers, especially when a drug is first introduced to clinical practice, are necessary. However, excessive doses should not be given in an attempt to remove the last remaining symptom, since the dose required to remove these residual symptoms tends to rise rapidly. Perhaps more important is correct administration; thus, doses of NSAID on awakening, taking up to one and a half hours for adequate absorption, may be too late to alleviate morning pain and stiffness. A large dose last thing at night before going to sleep may avoid side effects and continue to work in the morning. There is some evidence to support the clinical feeling that a given dose of NSAID last thing at night has a more prolonged effect than a similar dose given during the day. An alternative stratagem is to leave out at the bedside the required dose of drug in a teacup or egg cup together with a glass of water, so that the patient can take it on waking up at night, as many do. The drug will then have time to work before the patient has to get up in the morning.

Rectal suppositories and enteric-coated tablets are alternative ways to avoid gastrointestinal side effects. However, uniform absorption cannot always be guaranteed. Where possible, tablets should be taken when sitting and with fluid. Otherwise, they may remain in the oesophagus leading to delayed absorption and mucosal irritation.

The NSAIDs are usually given systemically, and the possible disadvantages of flooding the body with these drugs to treat a local monoarthritis problem must be considered. In these circumstances it may be better to give a potentially more toxic drug (e.g. corticosteroid) locally in a smaller dose than that used systemically.

The interpretation of pharmacokinetics is often difficult since many of these drugs have short half-lives, and may be effective even when in very low levels in the serum. Indeed, we have seen children in whom it has been impossible to achieve normally accepted therapeutic levels of salicylate.

Regular therapy is usually better than intermittent therapy. If patients note no difference if they miss their NSAID, then its efficacy should be questioned. Normally the rebound symptoms of missing a dose of NSAID are greater than the relief obtained by a similar dose. The main causes of irregular therapy are lack of effectiveness of the drug, or a belief that habituation or lack of effectiveness will occur with continuous use. There is no evidence of either significant habituation or decreasing effectiveness with use.

Proprietary products are sometimes the combination of two drugs, often an analgesic and an anti-inflammatory drug. Although popular because of the facility of administration, they should be avoided. There is little evidence of synergism.

A persistent worry must be whether the continuing use of NSAID in a patient by producing complacency in doctor and patient may put off the use of more definitive treatment. NSAIDs may reduce pain in an inflamed joint without necessarily reducing the mediators of joint destruction within that joint. The theory of suppressing pain, without suppressing inflammation and progressive joint destruction, has been raised and is still unresolved. However, it would seem a bad policy to treat pain, and not inflammation, when the latter is the main problem. Some of the NSAIDs have acquired a reputation for efficacy in certain diseases; for instance, indomethacin in osteoarthrosis of the hip and ankylosing spondylitis and phenylbutazone in the treatment of ankylosing spondylitis. Except that they are effective drugs, there is little justification for these claims. The use of NSAIDs in primary psychogenic pain, depression, and 'fibrositic' syndromes is usually relatively ineffective and this poor response suggests the true diagnosis. Indeed, depressive symptoms may be worsened by NSAIDs.

The paucity of disease-modifying drugs and the consequent introduction of more NSAIDs has led to the inevitable increased occurrence of side effects, some fatal in this group. The phenylbutazone and oxyphenbutazone drugs have acquired a particularly bad reputation, principally for their ability to cause aplastic anaemia and agranulocytosis. This is rare, but these very effective drugs should only be used if others fail. Many patients have taken them for years and have found no other drugs help them.

11.3.2 Side effects

(a) *Cerebral*

Several of the NSAIDs have psychogenic effects. Thus indomethacin in large doses may cause severe depression and an unusual depersonalization syndrome. In this, patients feel that they are outside their body and able to view themselves as a separate person. Aspirin in the high doses used may make children very miserable; in the adult, aspirin sometimes has a euphoric effect, especially if taken with alcohol.

Unsteadiness may be a complaint. A degree of high-tone deafness is common with aspirin therapy in the elderly but is normally only detected by formal testing. High-tone hearing being essential for clear differentiation of the spoken word, its loss is an obvious disadvantage and leads to increasing isolation of the elderly.

(b) *Renal*

Fluid retention is usually mild and, in particular, some antagonism of diuretics occurs with most NSAIDs. This appears to be due to reduced prostaglandin production and reduced renal blood flow.

(c) *Gastrointestinal*

The main problem is gastric ulceration and occult blood loss. The first may warrant treatment with ranitidine or cimetidine. The mechanism (or mechanisms) of this toxicity are unknown but suggestions have been reviewed

(Duggan, 1981). Local mechanical damage and cytotoxicity occur. However, parenterally administered NSAIDs also cause gastric lesions, suggesting a systemic effect, and it may be that it is the reduction of vaso-active prostaglandins that leads to mucosal ischaemia and ulceration. Many of these gastric erosions are asymptomatic and are only discovered on routine endoscopy (Caruso and Biachi Porro, 1982). They are more frequent when multiple drugs are given. The more recent theories depend on an effect on cyclo-oxygenase, and thus would be operative whether the drug was given orally or parenterally. If this were so, their effect might be lessened if the tissue cyclo-oxygenase inhibiting effect of drugs could be relatively increased and the effect on gastric cyclo-oxygenase decreased.

(d) Drug interactions

Mainly due to competitive binding for carrier protein, the effects of coumarin anticoagulants, oral hypoglycaemic agents, oral contraceptives, anticonvulsants, and thyroid hormones, may all be disturbed (see Chapter 3 for further details).

(e) Hypersensitivity

A wide range of minor rashes and pruritus may occur. More serious, but very rare, is acute asthma, pulmonary oedema, and, in severe cases, anaphylactoid shock. This very rare syndrome may be fatal. Although classically associated with aspirin, the other NSAIDs are potentially capable of producing it.

11.3.3 Delivery systems

Pharmokinetic studies have shown the importance of controlling the uptake of drugs from the gastrointestinal tract. It is especially with the short-acting drugs that an even and sustained absorption is required to avoid fluctuations in serum levels. The evidence suggests that side effects such as nausea are related to some drug levels but that clinical efficacy may be less closely related. Packaging of orally administered drugs may have other benefits, for example, to disguise taste and odour and to prevent physical damage to the stomach mucosa (e.g. aspirin and indomethacin). Slow-release systems include:

1. Coatings that are pH dependent, i.e. insoluble in acid but soluble in alkali;
2. Semipermeable coatings of methyl cellulose, etc.;
3. Enzyme-dependent coatings, which are slowly removed in the small intestine;
4. Controlled release *via* measured capsular pores and osmosis;
5. Layered capsules that alternate between layered active drug and coating;
6. Conjugated drugs in which the conjugate has to be split to enable absorption, i.e. the so-called 'pro-drug' principle.

To ensure more even absorption, the preparation is often made up of multiple microspheres placed within a larger container. Alternatively, conjugates may be given that are non-irritant and absorbed intact, but depend on liver enzymes to be cleaved into the active constituents.

As an alternative to oral presentation, rectal suppositories are sometimes used, but are inconvenient and difficult for some patients. Some patients may not be able to retain them and may not know that they have been voided. This is particularly a problem in the elderly.

11.4   SLOW-ACTING ANTIRHEUMATIC DRUGS

The terms slow-acting antirheumatic drugs (SAARDs), disease-modifying antirheumatic drugs (DMARDs), penicillamine-like, or remission-inducing drugs have been used interchangeably for a group of drugs that have several features in common:

1. Delayed action usually taking at least six weeks and more, often 8–10 weeks, before benefit starts.
2. Reversal of most of the clinical symptoms of inflammation, i.e. stiffness, pain of non-mechanical origin, and reduction in ill health.
3. Reversal of most of the clinical signs of inflammation, i.e. effusion, thickening, tenderness, and warmth.
4. Restoration to normal of biochemical evidence of disease – ESR reduced to or toward normal ranges, and other acute phase reactants similarly affected. Elevated immunoglobulins, including antiglobulins, may be reduced.
5. A slow, progressive relapse of the disease after stopping treatment.
6. Little or no convincing evidence of radiological benefit.
7. Limited disease spectrum, i.e. primarily effective against rheumatoid arthritis and closely similar conditions, but only benefiting 70–80% of these patients.
8. A potential for serious side effects.
9. All were developed as antirheumatic drugs for the wrong reasons, i.e. either by serendipity or from false hypothesis.
10. In spite of long usage the *in vivo* mode of action can only be surmised.
11. None appears to be locally effective, i.e. by local injection. This may simply represent the long latent period of their mode of action.

The use of antirheumatic drugs depends on remembering the above points and explaining the position fully to the patient – 'a 70% chance of success, but not before three months at the earliest, with the possibility of side effects requiring continuous blood and urine testing (monitoring), the degree of benefit to be gained being governed mainly by the degree of joint disease (secondary degenerative) already present'.

The choice of drug and stage at which it is used must be personal.

Chloroquine is thought to be slightly less powerful and tends to be used first and in the milder cases. It has an additional benefit that it is effective in both rheumatoid disease and systemic lupus erythematosus – the differentiation between these disorders not always being easy in clinical practice. Monitoring is minimal and toxicity rare. It is probably underrated as a form of therapy and it is of interest that it has not attracted any recent clinical trials.

After chloroquine, by injection gold and penicillamine are felt to be about equally effective. Each has its advantages and disadvantages. Gold is initially a weekly injection, thus compliance and monitoring are more easily assessed. For those who find injections unbearable then penicillamine is the alternative. With a 'go slow go low' regime therapeutic benefit may be delayed, and thus the importance of preliminary discussion with the patient. Compliance cannot be assessed. To insert personal dogma, but based on 30 years of gold and 20 years of penicillamine therapy, my preference would be gold before penicillamine and, in aggressive rheumatoid disease, both before chloroquine.

11.4.1 Chloroquine

The aminoquinolines have a long ancestry going back to the use of quinine primarily in lupus erythematosus (Payne, 1894; Davidson and Birt, 1938; Page, 1951). Later pamoquine, quinocrine, chloroquine, and hydroxychloroquine evolved. In practice only the last two compounds are used today. Their use is probably becoming more widespread, although increasing familiarity with, and confidence in, gold and penicillamine therapy, which are felt to be more effective, may prevent their widespread use.

Chloroquine has no significant interactions with other drugs. It is strongly bound to melanin, and hence its deposition in retina and skin. It has been suggested that retention in pigmented tissue such as the retina produces a concentration a thousand times more than in the serum. Other tissues bind chloroquine slightly and tissue saturation is soon reached. Excretion is almost exclusively renal, and therefore adequate renal function is important; otherwise reduced doses of chloroquine must be used. The aminoquinolines pass the placenta (Dencker and Lindquist, 1975), however results from malarial countries where chloroquine is used prophylactically have not shown chloroquine in low doses to be retinotoxic to the fetus. The fetus may be protected (until delivery) by the absence of light which seems to be necessary for retinotoxicity (Legros *et al.*, 1973). However, it is best avoided in pregnancy. My normal practice is to recommend withdrawing chloroquine about three months before conception is hoped for. However, chloroquine with its long half-life will still be present in the serum.

The problem of fetal injury with the antirheumatic drugs is not that they are very likely to cause damage but rather that *if* the baby is born damaged, as may happen in any pregnancy, the parents will blame the drug. This may lead to persisting psychological problems.

Antimalarials are used in a reduced dosage schedule, i.e. 250 mg of chloroquine phosphate-base or 400 mg hydroxychloroquine sulphate daily for four months to ascertain if they are effective. Then the dose is halved either by giving chloroquine phosphate on alternate days (e.g. on the odd days of each month) or 200 mg hydroxychloroquine sulphate daily. At these levels most, but not all, responding patients will be controlled and the chance of eye complications is negligible. This statement cannot at present be backed by data since sufficient patients have not been treated in a formal trial.

The impression is usually given that chloroquine should be reserved for the milder cases of rheumatoid arthritis and systemic lupus erythematosus. The justification for this is not clear and certainly it has seemed that chloroquine, either on its own or in combination with other drugs, may be very useful in treating all stages of systemic lupus erythematosus. Other similar diseases – Sjögren's syndrome, mixed connective tissue disease, and some myositic diseases in which there is evidence of immune dysfunction – may be suitable for chloroquine therapy. It is not believed that psoriasis is a contra-indication to this form of therapy.

Several good controlled trials of these drugs have been undertaken, and it has been perhaps easier to get statistically significant results because of the lower drop-out rate and greater compliance with antimalarials than with gold and penicillamine. Although clinical and biochemical improvement has occurred in some 70% of patients in most trials, radiological improvement has not occurred (Hamilton and Scott, 1962; Popert *et al.*, 1961; Mackenzie and Scherbel, 1980).

The mode of action of chloroquine is unknown, and it is of some interest that although considered by many to be an effective drug, research into its mode of action has not been as actively pursued as with gold and penicillamine in the last decade. The prime interest has been in membrane stabilization, but other factors may be invoked. (See Mackenzie and Scherbel, 1980.)

In determining the frequency of side effects, the main one being a maculopathy (Marks and Power, 1979; Rynes *et al.*, 1979; Marks, 1982), it is probable that the daily dose of chloroquine is more important than the length of treatment or total dose given. The early retinal lesion is probably reversible, but later lesions are irreversible and may, in fact, be progressive after stopping treatment.

Apart from maculopathy, other side effects are not a major problem. Presbyopia may occur but the patient soon accommodates to this. Deposition of chloroquine in the subepithelial layer of the cornea may give rise to a halo effect. This is especially frequent in xerophthalmia. These deposits are reversible. The impact of these symptoms can be greatly lessened by discussing the current views of chloroquine toxicity with the patient. In particular there is no evidence of significant ocular toxicity in under 6 months of treatment with chloroquine phosphate 250 mg daily, nor is there evidence of toxicity on longer-term therapy with chloroquine phosphate 250 mg on alternate days.

The question of ocular monitoring is debatable. In children it may be impossible. In the adult it may be physically impracticable if there are many patients, and it is still unresolved whether all cases of early retinotoxicity can be detected. As a precaution it is sometimes recommended that patients wear sun glasses in strong sunlight.

Muscle disease, other than as a result of inflammatory disease, is a contra-indication to treatment with chloroquine as the drug reduces skeletal and muscle contractability (Argov and Mastaglia, 1979). This is often difficult to detect, but is reversible.

Excessive doses may result in a dirty grey pigmentation of exposed areas and greying or bleaching of the hair.

Acute, as distinct from chronic, toxicity is rapid in onset, occurring in hours, and irreversible.

In view of the above limited toxicity, chloroquine qualifies as a useful drug to use in a wide spectrum of diseases over a prolonged time, either alone or in combination.

11.4.2 Gold

The clinical impression remains that gold has a beneficial effect and this is heightened by the effects of withdrawing the drug. The increasing use of gold may yet represent a gross misplacement of confidence; it has, however, comforted clinicians and patients.

In view of the long history of gold therapy (chrysotherapy) (Forestier, 1935), it is surprising that there is not more evidence of efficacy. The placebo controlled trial of The Empire Rheumatism Council (1961), which was probably one of the first properly conducted trials of this nature, only showed a beneficial effect for 18 months. It was not continued longer than this and thus demonstrates the changing concepts to that of long-term therapy now held. This particular trial treated patients for 20 weeks only, and it is perhaps remarkable that it was possible to show improvement up to 72 weeks, i.e. one year after ceasing treatment. Subsequent, more prolonged, trials using clinical and biochemical data have not shown continued evidence of benefit, more pertinently, radiological progression has not been delayed (American Rheumatism Association, 1973; Sigler *et al.*, 1974; Luukainen *et al.*, 1977).

These trials have problems of different therapy protocols, lack of adequate placebo groups and, in particular, the small numbers employed. The last problem is accentuated by the number of drop outs occurring over a period of a year (more than is often realized), which leaves even fewer patients for statistical analysis.

Several different treatment regimes have been recommended, low dose 10 mg and 50 mg sodium aurothiomalate weekly being the most popular with little to choose between them (McKenzie, 1981; Griffin *et al.*, 1983). Higher doses, e.g. 150 mg weekly, have been tried, but the toxicity is much greater (Furst *et al.*, 1977). An alternative technique for giving high doses of gold has been suggested by Norton and Donnelly (1983) in which 200 mg of aurothioglucose was given at about monthly intervals. The gold salt was given in an oil base to blunt peak gold levels and nitroid reactions. My preference is for a 10 mg weekly regime continued over a prolonged period, during which many patients can be taught to give their own intramuscular injections. If not effective then larger doses – 20 mg weekly or 50 mg every 2–3 weeks (but never monthly which I believe to be too infrequent) – can be given.

It has long been considered that second courses of gold treatment are less successful than the first (Evers and Sundstrom, 1983) and that, in particular, if there was no benefit in the first course there will be none in the second.

Recently an oral form of gold, auranofin (see Chapter 9 for further details), has been introduced. Systemic absorption seems to be poor, most of the drug being excreted in the faeces. There appear to be subtle differences in immunological effects of this compound which still needs full evaluation. It must be given daily and is less strongly tissue bound, with relatively higher unbound serum levels (Lorber *et al.*, 1983b). After injection the gold thiomalate molecule rapidly splits into gold and thiomalate moieties. Forty per cent of the thiomalate is retained in the tissues and may be pharmacologically active (Jellum and Munthe, 1982). With this preparation unbound gold constitutes less than 2% of total serum gold. However, after oral gold there is a higher unbound/bound gold ratio which may explain differences in effect (Lorber *et al.*, 1983a, b). The clinical evaluation of auranofin continues, but it is probably less effective, but less toxic, than gold sodium aurothiomalate (Ward *et al.*, 1982).

Chrysotherapy, although usually employed for the treatment of arthritis, may be of value in other systemic manifestations of the disease, such as Felty's syndrome (Luthra *et al.*, 1981). However, where serious problems such as arteritis or neuropathy are present, the delay and uncertainty of benefit usually indicate that treatment be initiated with corticosteroids or immunosuppressive agents.

(a) *Side effects*

Eosinophilia has been related to the severity of the disease (Panush *et al.*, 1971). Others disagree (Sylvester and Pinals, 1970). During gold therapy eosinophilia has been related to adverse reactions, especially cutaneous (Davis and Hughes, 1974), yet others disagree (Jessop *et al.*, 1974).

Thrombocytopenia is the commonest severe blood dyscrasia, but usually readily recovers. Many alarms are caused by technical errors in estimating the platelet count, especially when using old samples.

Proteinuria is a frequent problem in the clinic, a false picture occurring either from vaginal secretions or old test sticks. The severity of proteinuria is often related to its duration (Newton *et al.*, 1983). After moderate proteinuria it may be possible to restart gold therapy. The proteinuria, which is usually unaccompanied by other evidence of renal disease, may take months to subside and residual mild proteinuria is common.

The mechanism (or mechanisms) of these side effects is unknown. The genetic factor has already been mentioned. Much more work probably needs doing in this area, but at present HLA DR3 (or HLA DRW3) seems to be the major association with toxicity (Panayi *et al.*, 1978; Gran *et al.*, 1983), however B8 and CW7 may also be important (Bardin *et al.*, 1982).

Serum gold estimations have little part to play in everyday practice – fluctuating markedly between gold injections and being influenced by, among other things, smoking (Graham *et al.*, 1982; James *et al.*, 1982), the erythrocyte gold concentration rising in smokers who may get toxicity earlier!

An interesting study (Sambrook *et al.*, 1982) has shown that 27% of patients terminate their treatment at six months, 48% at a year, and 84% at 4 years, usually due to mucocutaneous reactions. Since a prolonged course of treatment is presumably necessary, less than half will be able to tolerate gold long enough to obtain significant benefit.

11.4.3 Penicillamine

Even fewer controlled trials have been undertaken with penicillamine. Introduced in 1965 by Jaffe, the only double-blind, prospective placebo controlled trial was undertaken in 1973 (Multicentre Trial Group, 1973). This showed improvement up to one year, the length of the trial. However, a third of the patients were withdrawn, and some of the doses used would be unacceptable by many today. As in all trials the clinical benefit was more impressive than the radiological improvement.

There has been a marked change in the use of pencillamine. Originally used in doses of about 1 g per day and more, this being the type of dose used in treating Wilson's disease, there were many side effects. More recently the concept has been to start with a smaller dose and increase it with spaced increments.

With all the second-line disease remitting drugs some 2–3 months elapse before benefit is apparent, whatever the daily dose. Thus, it is debatable whether incremental increases in doses more rapidly than every two months are justified. If a more rapid system is used, unnecessarily high therapy levels will be reached since the full effect of each increased therapy dosage level will not have had time to take effect. At present the therapeutic range has been some 125–750 mg of penicillamine daily. Comparisons of 'low dose' (125–300 mg day) and 'high dose' (500–600 mg day) suggest that although the larger doses are slightly more effective they are also more toxic (Nissila *et al.*, 1982; Williams *et al.*, 1983). A summary of trials would suggest that lower doses, although apparently less effective, can be continued for longer because of less side effects, and thus in the long term they may be more effective.

The pharmacokinetics of penicillamine are important. Absorption after oral administration is markedly reduced by food taken at the same time (Kukovetl *et al*; 1983 Osman *et al.*, 1983; Schuna *et al.*, 1983). Iron, as given for the correction of iron deficiency, and antacids also markedly reduce absorption. Thus penicillamine should be given one hour before, or one and a half hours after, food, and, since it can be given as a single daily dose, at the opposite end of the day to oral iron therapy. Lack of awareness of these interactions may lead to problems with therapy such as overdosage and toxicity (Harkness and Blake, 1982).

In recent years interest has centred on the relationship of genetic factors to the toxicity of gold and penicillamine (Panayi *et al.*, 1978; Bardin *et al.*, 1982). However, as in most studies of this nature the question of the most appropriate therapeutic regime arises, i.e. it is still unresolved whether the frequency of side effects in those genetically susceptible is dose related. Thus, do those experiencing the side effects belong mainly to patients receiving the higher dose, e.g. 50 mg gold instead of 10 mg, or treated with the more rapid increments of penicillamine? In view of shared genetic markers for toxicity, it is not surprising that toxic reactions to penicillamine may be more in patients who have had toxic reactions to gold (Dodd *et al.*, 1980; Smith *et al.*, 1982). Not all agree (Kean *et al.*, 1982).

Developing eosinophilia has been noted during penicillamine treatment (Jaffe, 1965), but recent suggestions (Smith *et al.*, 1983) conclude that routine platelet counts are probably of little value, eosinophilia being just as frequent in NSAID-treated patients. We would also feel that eosinophilia seldom indicates a serious side effect, many factors affecting the peripheral blood eosinophilia count. It is perhaps worth remembering that the eosinophil is primarily an extra vascular cell, comparatively few being present in the circulation. Anaemia and thrombocytopenia, which may occur, usually resolve.

How this is related to deficient sulphoxidation status, which is found in many patients developing thrombocytopenia and proteinuria, as shown using penicillamine carbocysteine (a structurally similar compound) is unknown (Pananyi *et al.*, 1983).

Myasthenic syndromes have been known for a little while to complicate some patients on penicillamine treatment; but recent investigations have opened up many new fields. Thus the work of Delamere *et al.* (1983) suggests that these patients have a different genetic make-up from other rheumatoid patients, and not that associated with haematological or renal side effects, or with other forms of myasthenia. The prime related HLA antigen appeared to be DR1, and there is an absence of DR3, an antigen associated with serious toxicity to both gold and penicillamine (Panayi *et al.*, 1978; Bardin *et al.*, 1982). Penicillamine has been shown to bind to the acetylcholine receptor of electric fish, thus reducing the binding of acetylcholine, and thereby affecting neuromuscular transmission (Bevar *et al.*, 1982). Alternatively this binding may alter the antigenicity of the acetylcholine receptor, with loss of tolerance.

In the 18 patients described by Delamere *et al.* (1983) diplopia and/or ptosis occurred as the initial symptom in all. In the author's experience increasing weakness, often rapidly progressive, has brought the patient to notice, and the history of ptosis/diplopia was charted later. Where diagnosis, which is often difficult, was delayed then muscle weakness progressed. Withdrawal of penicillamine resulted in increasing muscle strength in all, but some ptosis/diplopia remained in 3, and took over one year to improve in other patients. Choline esterase receptor site antibody was present in all patients and is probably the most useful screening test.

These patients may develop other features of systemic auto-immunity, especially systemic lupus erythematosus and liver disease. Delamere *et al.* (1983) make the observation that these patients' arthritis had responded well to treatment, and this raises the question of whether these patients had been overtreated or whether successful treatment demands that treatment is pushed to its limit.

No evidence of penicillamine toxicity was found in patients sensitive to penicillin (Bell and Graziano, 1983).

11.4.4 Newer and still controversial drugs

(a) *Sulphasalazine*

In 1948 Svartz described the use of an azo compound, sulphasalazine, in rheumatoid arthritis. This being the combination of aspirin and an antibiotic, infective theory of causation being fashionable. Subsequent trials gave mixed results (Sinclair and Duthie, 1948; Kuzell and Gardner, 1950). Little further interest was shown until McConkey *et al.* (1980) in an open study showed sulphasalazine to be beneficial. More recently Pullar *et al.* (1983) in a double-blind comparison with gold and placebo showed both test drugs to be beneficial, though nausea and vomiting proved a problem with sulphasalazine. However, there was a high drop out rate of about 40% at the end of the six months' trial which in terms of the long natural history of this disease is disappointing. Major side effects were few. A wide variation of doses have been used but not more than 3 g day^{-1}.

(b) *Dapsone*

Dapsone has been used in the treatment of leprosy for a long time. There are immunological similarities to rheumatoid arthritis and McConkey *et al.* (1976, 1979) undertook trials of this drug in rheumatoid arthritis. These suggested benefit and more recently in a double-blind study Swinson *et al.* (1981) showed dapsone to be effective, approaching the effectiveness of penicillamine. Fowler *et al.* (1984) have suggested that, although effective, dapsone is not as useful as chloroquine. All studies agree that a mild haemolytic anaemia and agranulocytosis can occur. The usual dose would be 100 mg a day.

Thus at present both sulphasalazine and, especially in view of its side effects, dapsone are controversial treatments only to be considered if all conventional therapies are invalid.

(c) *Levamisole*

As described elsewhere, various terms such as immunosuppressive, immune stimulator, and immune regulators have been used for drugs thought to affect and in particular correct the immune aberration of rheumatoid disease. Since new concepts of the immune defects appear yearly, this aspect of the pharmaceutical industry has a continuing future.

Levamisole is one such contender. It is one of several antihelminthics that have been tried. It appears to aid the maturation of T lymphocytes and restores depressed T lymphocyte function. Thus some of its effects are thymomimetic.

Trials have suggested that it has a beneficial effect similar to penicillamine (Multicentre Study Group, 1978, 1982; Miller *et al.*, 1980). However, various adverse reactions have occurred causing its withdrawal in 40% of patients at six months, and this in the most recently adopted conservative regime of 150 mg once a week. There is evidence that the side effects are dose related, as is benefit to a lesser degree. Once again, the trials have been too brief to fit into the natural history of the disease. The side effects have been diverse and include agranulocytosis. More interestingly many of the side effects appear to be of an auto-immune nature, perhaps indicating too vigorous treatment.

At present one cannot recommend levamisole as a form of treatment. However, developments of this therapeutic theme are appearing and may be more successful.

11.4.5   Corticosteroids

(a) *Systemic corticosteroids*

Failure of the second-line programme leads to a consideration of third-line drugs, i.e. corticosteroids and cytotoxic drugs. Corticosteroids (basically prednisolone and prednisone), and less often corticotrophins, are almost invariably effective in reducing various rheumatic inflammations and in reducing ill health, often in low dosage (Medical Research Council, 1960; Harris *et al.*, 1983). Inevitably there will be side effects, the degree depending on the dose used, the duration of therapy, and probably the constitution and previous condition of the patient. Less joint erosions and more joint freedom are found.

The unresolved question is whether the increased physical activity and nutrition outweighs the catabolic effect of corticosteroid. The work of Million *et al.* (1979) goes some way to suggesting that long-term therapy with corticosteroid is not as dangerous as has been feared. In which type of case are systemic corticosteroids indicated?

1. Obviously in those patients failing second-line therapy and needing suppressive therapy.
2. Juvenile arthritic patients with severe systemic illness may need corticosteroids whilst the disease is settling.
3. In older patients or patients with a limited life span, e.g. with progressive cancer, where a rapid predictable response for a limited period with least inconvenience is required (Lockie *et al.*, 1983). Osteoporosis is not, in my view, a contraindication in these older patients.
4. Where another condition such as bronchospasm would also be benefited. Thus treatment of two conditions by one therapy simplifies management.
5. Certain complications of rheumatoid disease such as neuropathies may benefit from corticosteroids more rapidly and better than with gold or penicillamine. The response of leucopenia and thrombocytopenia in Felty's syndrome is less reliable.
6. A short course of corticosteroid may be indicated for a specific problem such as tenosynovitis of the hands or inflammatory muscle spasm around joints, where these are not amenable to local injection.
7. Certain rheumatic conditions require corticosteroids – polymyalgia rheumatica, systemic lupus erythematosus, eosinophilic fasciitis, and the polyarteritis nodosa/Wegener's syndrome type of patient.

The question of disease severity is important. The implication is often given that in the more aggressive cases of rheumatoid arthritis the underlying immune abnormality is greater, and hence that stronger drugs are needed to treat the patient. There is little support for this. There is evidence that in complicated rheumatoid arthritis, e.g. Felty's syndrome, additional pathogenic mechanisms are operative other than that causing the arthritis (e.g. splenic dysfunction, abnormal antibodies, serum inhibitors of granulopoiesis), some of which may be genetically determined. But is this necessarily an indication for the use of drugs that are thought to be stronger, but also acknowledged to have more side effects? Perhaps the implication should be that in these patients, since progressive disease is occurring, there is greater need to persevere with trials of further treatments if the initial ones fail; and, in particular, treatments designed to correct these additional pathological processes. In many patients with rheumatoid arthritis some of the disease features respond to treatment more easily than others, vasculitis being particularly hard to control.

(b) *Local injection of corticosteroid*

The use of local injections of corticosteroid have been employed to reduce the total dose of corticosteroid administered and to increase the local concentration of the drug obtained. Age is no contraindication to this form of therapy, other than the psychological shock to which such patients may be prone.

The techniques and choices are well described and easy (Dixon and Graham, 1981). A simple aseptic 'no touch' method is adequate and complications rare.

Administration is often with a local anaesthetic to identify that the corticosteroid has reached the inflamed site. The choice of hydrocortisone salt or depot forms will have to be made but will not be discussed here. In general local corticosteroids are given either into a cavity (e.g. the synovial space) around which they circulate during joint movement, or into solid tissues where they only diffuse locally and thus have to be deposited at multiple sites over the inflamed area.

The main concern about local steroid injections is their effect. It is accepted that steroids will reduce inflammation, although how is less certain, i.e. as cellular regulators or cytotoxic agents. It is the question of cytotoxicity that is worrying. There are sufficient examples of tissue destruction either of skin or more particularly of tendons to suggest caution. Some of these problems may be due to direct injury from the injecting needle. Another problem is that of minor crystalline deposits provoking local inflammation similar to that of urate crystals. As with all antirheumatic treatment, the worry exists that loss of pain does not mean that the joint is protected. The processes of cartilage destruction and pain production are separate, and failure to curb both together could increase rather than reduce joint destruction. The cellular depressant, as distinct from the cytotoxic, effect of local corticosteroid must be recognized; thus reduction of cartilage anabolic activity may be marked (Mankin and Conger, 1966). The projected result of repeated injections is the production of cartilage destruction and secondary osteoarthrosis. Examples of this have been quoted (McCarty and Hogan, 1964) and found in animal models. However, if spaced injections, i.e. greater than six weeks, are used this probably does not occur. Similar problems may occur if corticosteroid is injected near a nerve or intracutaneously when skin atrophy may result; this effect is probably worse if depot forms are used.

Intra-articular corticosteroid has two distinct sites of action – synovial membrane and cartilage. The first is the preferred site and is in a sense protected by its blood supply which will remove corticosteroid. The chondrocytes will, however, remain exposed to relatively high concentrations of corticosteroid for a long time. It is this latter aspect that is of concern since corticosteroid at the level used may well be cytocidal. The prime aim is to reduce inflammation, and thus the main indication for their use is inflammation, especially that occurring in conditions less amenable to systemic noncorticosteroidal treatment (e.g. psoriatic or Reiter's arthropathy). The use of intra-articular corticosteroids in 'non-inflammatory' conditions such as osteoarthrosis is more controversial. The rate of passage into the systemic circulation is rapid, i.e. within minutes; this seems to depend in part on the size of the joint and its vascularity. Thus, there is a systemic effect from intra-articular corticosteroids, and this needs to be recognized in assessing their efficacy. Since the desired effect is within the joint, attempts have been made to localize the corticosteroid preparation either by producing insoluble compounds or by the use of liposomes. Although drug metabolism has been investigated in tissue culture, there is little evidence as to how this compares with *in vivo* conditions.

An alternative method to produce localized cytotoxicity is by the use of radioactive substances localized to the synovial cavity by size of carrier particle (Gumpel, 1973). Several isotopes have been described, originally colloidal ^{198}gold in 1959. But the most popular at present are ^{90}yttrium and ^{169}erbium. The latter has a weaker energy and can be used in the small joints of the hand. The rationale is to irradiate the synovial lining of the joint without involving the bone. The substance used should have a short half-life and should be attached to non-toxic carriers. It is important to avoid leakage along the needle track which may lead to a fistula track. Similarly, to reduce the risk of radioactive leakage the joint is usually immobilized for 24 hours. It will be obvious that to ensure accurate injection the joint must be predictably entered, and for this reason these compounds are usually used for large superficial joints, typically the knee.

Other intra-articular agents that have been tried include osmium tetroxide which is popular in Scandinavia and France (Nissila, 1979). In spite of enthusiastic reports from Europe, it has not been generally accepted in the UK or the USA. This chemical (which is used as a fixative for microbiological histology) causes death and necrosis of the tissues it reaches, irrespective of their nature. The concern here is in its effect on cartilage. However, effusions seem to decrease after treatment. It has been used in children but may increase the X-ray changes.

Various cytotoxic agents, especially methotrexate and nitrogen mustard compounds, have been injected in an attempt to localize their toxicity. The results are equivocal.

Not surprisingly, NSAIDs have been injected into the joint but there is no evidence of any clinical benefit.

Both radioactive drugs and cytotoxic agents are most effective against dividing cells (Gumpel, 1973). Yet they are usually used in patients whose disease is partially suppressed. The dramatic relapse in symptoms and signs that follows within 24 hours of withdrawing NSAIDs suggests perhaps that before using these forms of injection therapy NSAIDs should be temporarily stopped so that the synovial cells are 'unsuppressed' when radioactivity is administered.

All attempts to treat synovitis by local therapy may be flawed since the evidence suggests that the perpetuating influence comes from blood borne cells, particularly lymphocytes (Paulus *et al.*, 1977). Thus local measures aimed at the synovitis may have very temporary effects and should be considered an adjuvant to systemic therapy.

In spite of their widespread usage and numerous trials, there is little conclusive evidence of efficacy for intra-articular therapy, other than with corticosteroid and, in particular, none of long-term joint protection.

Intra-articular injection is an attempt to localize the therapeutic agent. However, as mentioned above, extrasynovial sites may be equally important in maintaining the disease. Unfortunately at present we have few markers for these sites (cells). But after the work in anti-tumour therapy – where metastases as well as primary tumours have to be sought out – monoclonal antibodies, to which are attached lethal chemicals such as protein A or ricin, may become available. There are many similarities in aetiopathogenesis and treatment between neoplastic diseases and autoimmune diseases.

11.4.6 Cytotoxic therapy

The aetiopathogenesis of these diseases being poorly understood, it is reasonable to try to reduce the activity of both the immune and inflammatory systems, which seem to be overactive. To this end cytotoxic therapy has been used. Other terminologies such as 'immunosuppressive' or 'immunoregulatory' are hopeful to say the least, particularly at the doses usually employed, which are much less than those used in cancer therapy or transplantation management.

Of the drugs presently used – azathioprine, cyclophosphamide, methotrexate, and chlorambucil – the first trials were done over a decade ago. The initial aim was to see if they would be steroid sparing and effective in patients unresponsive to gold and penicillamine.

With the correct dose schedule, clinical effect is more rapid than gold or penicillamine – about 4–6 weeks.

(a) *Azathioprine*

This drug succeeded 6-mercaptopurine (into which it is converted *in vivo*). It is an antimetabolite affecting purine synthesis, and it was to potentiate this approach to cancer chemotherapy that allopurinol was evolved before its usefulness in gout became apparent. Hence, if allopurinol is being used, e.g. as a gout prophylactic during lymphoma treatment, the dose of azathioprine must be reduced.

Azathioprine seems to have a strong anti-inflammatory effect as well as affecting the immune system. It is the least unpleasant to take and the most easily controlled of the cytotoxic agents. It has been used in various doses (reviewed by Whisnant and Pelkey, 1982). My own schedule is perhaps conservative, starting with 50 mg day^{-1} (i.e. 0.75–1 mg kg^{-1} body weight) and increasing to 100 mg after 1 month if necessary, and then to 150 mg. Rarely is it necessary to use 2.5 mg kg^{-1} body weight. In a trial comparing azathioprine, cyclophosphamide and gold, azathioprine appeared the most useful (Currey *et al.*, 1973). Once started, azathioprine needs to be continued apparently indefinitely (De Silva and Hazleman, 1981), which is worrying.

(b) *Methotrexate*

This antimetabolic interferes with folic acid metabolism and thus DNA synthesis in cells. It is therefore most effective where cellular division is most marked, e.g. in inflammatory states. Antimetabolites of this nature are probably the least likely of the cytotoxic agents to cause neoplasia. The original work was mainly in psoriasis and later psoriatic arthropathy. Comparatively little work has been done in rheumatoid disease (Michaels *et al.*, 1982; Steinsson *et al.*, 1982). Various schedules have been proposed, perhaps the easiest is 7.5–25 mg as a single oral dose once a week or in divided doses at the weekend. Intramuscular and intravenous schedules have been described (Michaels *et al.*, 1982). Initially gastric intolerance may be found. Other side effects are mucosal changes, megaloblastic anaemia, infertility, and 'mucosis' – a condition of capillary fragility and separation of skin most easily seen over prominences. The question of hepatic fibrosis is debatable, however, liver function tests should be regularly performed, and some authorities would suggest regular liver biopsies at yearly intervals.

(c) *Cyclophosphamide*

This alkylating agent has been more extensively tried in rheumatoid arthritis, systemic lupus erythematosus, and a variety of inflammatory granulomatous and other connective tissue diseases. In all of these diseases it appears to be effective. Most trials suggest that cyclophosphamide is effective in rheumatoid disease (Co-operating Clinics Committee, 1970, 1972; Townes *et al.*, 1976). Its main drawback is its toxicity which is wide ranging. Gastrointestinal disturbance, infections particularly with viruses, azoospermia and amenorrhoea, and bone marrow depression all occur. More typically alopecia and cystitis (the latter may be severe and haemorrhagic) are found. The cystitis may lead to bladder fibrosis and contracture and possibly malignant change.

As with many cytotoxic agents, there is the long-term anxiety concerning drug-induced malignant change. Sustained effects on the bone marrow have been demonstrated a decade after treatment (Thomas *et al.*, 1983). Their significance is unclear but malignancies, especially of lymphoreticular type, seem to be increased up to fourfold (Baltus *et al.*, 1983).

The various trials suggest that 150 mg day^{-1} is usually necessary to get benefit, and that there is little evidence of a graded effect to different dose levels. In order to increase the benefit/toxicity ratio, various techniques for giving cyclophosphamide have been tried (Hall *et al.*, 1979). Intravenous and alternate-day therapy schedules seem to have little to offer. The combination with prednisolone has been suggested to reduce both the dose of prednisolone necessary and the severity of acute side effects to cyclophosphamide. In one's own experience this type of combination has led to severe viral infections, especially of the herpes zoster type.

(d) *Chlorambucil*

The alkylating agent is a popular treatment for chronic lymphatic leukaemia. The hypothesis that abnormal lymphocyte function is important in rheumatic diseases led to its use in these diseases. Unfortunately there is little published evidence for its benefit (see Amor and Mery, 1980). It has been suggested as a possible form of treatment for amyloidosis complicating juvenile arthritis (Schnitzer and Ansell, 1977).

Taken orally, the main problem has been the rapid changes in blood count that can occur, fortunately usually reversible if detected early, but needing rather frequent blood tests.

Newer cytotoxic or 'immune-regulatory' drugs are becoming available. Cyclosporin A is a good example in which extensive experience is available in the short term, mainly from transplantation work.

Since there is a lack of specificity in their effect, these drugs can be used in all types of chronic non-infective inflammatory synovitis and in the systemic complications that may occur.

The late side effects of these drugs have still to be evaluated. They are limited in value by the length of time that they can be administered in what is usually a chronic disease.

11.5   EXPERIMENTAL FORMS OF THERAPY

The advent of machines capable of separating plasma or blood cells from the peripheral blood (apheresis) has led to this form of therapy in many diseases. There are many hypotheses as to why this form of treatment should work. Since none of them is really proven they will not be discussed further.

Initially this treatment was used for systemic lupus erythematosus (Jones *et al.*, 1979), the rationale being to remove immune complexes which seem to have a pathogenic role in that disease. In rheumatoid arthritis the rationale is less clear. However, the mechanisms involved in systemic lupus erythematosus and complicated rheumatoid disease may be quite different from that of uncomplicated rheumatoid disease. There seems to be considerable evidence that circulating lymphocytes are important in maintaining synovitis (Paulus *et al.*, 1977). Trials of both plasmapheresis and leucopheresis have given conflicting results. The best study showed no benefit (Dwosh *et al.*, 1983). In some of these trials, biochemical and immunological features may be improved, but these are not usually associated with clinical improvement. Recently 'on-line' cryofiltration of plasma has been used with benefit to reduce immune complexes (Krabauer *et al.*, 1983).

Leucopheresis was first tried in rheumatoid arthritis in 1977 (Paulus *et al.*, 1977). Clinical improvement was obtained but not maintained after treatment was discontinued, and side effects were frequent and sometimes serious. Further studies have suggested only modest and, most importantly, only temporary benefit. In view of these conflicting results, these forms of treatment, which are expensive, should be reserved at present for controlled trials to evaluate this form of therapy. It must be remembered that there is a very strong placebo effect in this therapy. At the present time only patients with vasculitis, hyperviscosity, or possibly those who have failed gold and penicillamine therapy should be considered.

An alternative method of inhibiting lymphocytes is by total body irradiation, again a technique taken from cancer therapy, which is apparently successful (Fuld *et al.*, 1983).

These forms of therapy have been used in a wide variety of other diseases – usually where there is a strong suspicion of autoimmunity.

11.6 PLACEBO

Does placebo therapy have any place in management today? The answer is probably yes. However, it must be clearly understood why it is being used, and only used when no other practical alternative exists. Many ethical problems are raised by its use, and it may lead to loss of confidence. It has been observed in many placebo controlled studies that the placebo group also improves, both clinically and biochemically, and this is usually put down to spontaneous remission. However, research in similar diseases, especially neoplasia, has shown that patients retaining an optimistic outlook have fared better than their more pessimistic controls. The reason for this is not clear but is presumably psychosomatic. A similar mechanism may underly placebo analgesia, which was thought to be similar to that of morphia, i.e. *via* opiate receptors (Levine *et al.*, 1978). However, more recent work suggests that placebos may have more diverse pathways of action. Although in formal trials many of the drugs that are prescribed are shown to be better than placebo, in any single patient it may be impossible to know if more than a placebo effect is being obtained unless a blank control is used. Thus, in everyday practice the use of what amounts to placebos is probably common. If one believes that the main benefit of alternative medicine, which is commonly sought, is a placebo effect then this too adds to the concept that many patients derive benefit, actual or perceived, from placebos. The main disadvantage of trials in this area is the short time the patients remain on the therapy – sometimes held to indicate how ineffective it is.

It is quite possible to get placebo responders who find that every drug apparently makes them *worse!*

11.7   COMBINATION THERAPY

The use of more than one antirheumatic drug is usually deplored unless there is a good reason, for example the addition of an analgesic such as paracetamol to remove pain. It is, of course, irrational to prescribe two prostaglandin inhibitor type drugs together, and some of the undesirable and unrecognized combinations occur in proprietary products. Ease of obtaining repeat prescriptions unmonitored may be all important. The usual debatable combination found in practice is of a corticosteroid and a disease-modifying drug. In theory, if either were adequately successful a combination would not be necessary, increasing as it does the variety of side effects. The question then arises whether both drugs – corticosteroid and disease modifying – given together perhaps in individually lower doses might result in a lower frequency of toxicity. If more than one inflammatory cascade were involved in a case of inflammatory arthritis it would be justifiable to use two or more drugs, one acting on each cascade. However, if a single drug acted on both cascades this must be preferable. Whereas clinical judgement suggests that a graded response in a patient may be obtained to corticosteroids, no similar evidence is available for chloroquine, penicillamine or gold, where the response seems to be much more of an all-or-nothing nature, i.e. unless given in adequate dose, benefit will not follow. However, because the modes of action of these disease-modifying drugs are probably different, there is reason to believe that they could have complementary therapeutic effects. The best combination is probably chloroquine and either gold or penicillamine since the potential side effects are different and could be correctly attributed if they occurred. Little work has been done on combined therapy. Bunch *et al.* (1980) found no benefit from the combination of penicillamine and chloroquine.

It was partly to improve compliance that compound medications were introduced.

11.8   PROBLEMS OF THERAPY IN CHILDREN

The management and treatment of juvenile arthritis (JA) demands at least as much expertise and paramedical support as that of the adult form; not least because poor management lays the foundation for future problems – both physical and psychological – to a greater extent. It is, therefore, perhaps fortunate that the prognosis for most cases is better. Time spent in full and frank discussion with the family is time well spent. Thus, these children should be seen at a more leisurely pace than is often possible in an adult clinic.

The importance of making an accurate diagnosis and evaluation of the prognosis is paramount. The different treatments necessary for juvenile arthritis which appears to be linked to the HLA B27 antigen (not responsive to chloroquine, gold or penicillamine) and those not so linked (who may fortuitiously have HLA B27 antigen and may be responsive to these drugs) is a simple example. Similarly, the different prognostic patterns, though less well documented, have value in influencing management decisions. A full discussion of this subject is impossible here and only a few considerations will be given.

Patterns of onset

Systemic	This often alarming and hectic onset will usually resolve to a milder form when an arthritic picture predominates. During the initial period, bed rest and corticosteroids may be necessary.
Pauci-articular	Often mild arthritis, often a single joint, and thus easy to dismiss. Very important because of symptomless iridocyclitis, especially if ANF positive. The eye problems are often the most important aspect.
Polyarticular	Articular prognosis often the worst, and aggressive treatment from onset may be justified.
Rheumatoid factor positive	As for adult rheumatoid arthritis.

The treatment must take account of age (1–16 years by definition). Physiotherapy can be undertaken in a play setting, especially if, as it should be, hydrotherapy is available. Splinting is usually not a problem.

For many children, and all the B27 antigen associated arthritics, NSAIDs are usually the only treatment necessary. Many of these drugs are not licensed for use in children, because they have not been through the required safety trials. They have seemed safe, often at higher dosage than that suggested by the manufacturer. There is little evidence of significant differences in drug handling in the young child from that in the adult. Many occur as syrups. It is preferable if the child can be encouraged to take tablets. Aspirin which is a traditional remedy may make the child very miserable and should be avoided. Side effects are rare.

If these are unsuccessful, progression to chloroquine, penicillamine or gold should be considered. All have their problems and there are few definitive therapeutic trials – very necessary when there is a high remission rate. In all cases therapy needs to be continued for at least 2 years.

Chloroquine is easy to give but has seemed relatively ineffective in childhood arthritis. Visual testing is more difficult in the young, and other toxicity monitoring is unnecessary. Acute toxicity may occur with small overdosage, e.g. 1 g.

Penicillamine is perhaps the most useful drug. On the stepwise schedule used in this department therapeutic levels may take a long time to be reached. Though the final doses reached tend to be lower (<10 mg kg^{-1} day^{-1}).

Gold is probably a little more effective than penicillamine but the injections are disliked by many patients. Corticosteroids in the early systemic illness may be essential treatment, and should be given at least twice daily, later graduating to morning and later alternate-morning therapy. In some cases of JA steroids may be necessary on a continuing basis to avoid crippledom. 'Immunosuppressive' therapy is controversial and will not be discussed.

Apart from adequate treatment the aim must be to interfere with the child's life as little as possible; thus schooling, and social contact including games should be encouraged. Throughout the treatment period the management is reassessed as the patient's requirements change, often imperceptibly. In practice it is too easy to regard a 13 or 15 year old boy as 9 years old and manage him as such, reduced physical stature being an important determinant of this attitude.

In terms of assessment of treatment, patient well being has seemed as useful as any. The presence of a typical rash indicates continuing disease activity. Biochemical measurements such as the ESR may remain fixedly elevated in inactive disease or may be normal in acute disease and are less reliable than in the adult. A depressed haemoglobin level rises with successful treatment.

Rising immunoglobulins, especially IgG, should be viewed with alarm. They may herald the onset of amyloidosis. However, there have been relatively few advances in our ability to diagnose patients with rheumatoid arthritis complicated by amyloidosis (Cathcart and Wohlgethan, 1981). Proteinuria continues to be the most helpful diagnostic clue, although nephrotoxic long-term agents (gold and D-penicillamine) may confuse the clinical picture. Measurement of specific serum amyloid proteins SAA and SAP (serum amyloid P component) have been of little diagnostic value, and the same can be said for enumeration of peripheral blood T and B cells (Scheinberg and Cathcart, 1976). The recent finding of a high frequency of HLA B27 and of the haplotype A2, B27 in patients with rheumatoid arthritis and secondary amyloidosis is of interest but these data are only preliminary (Pasternack and Tiilikainen, 1977).

11.9   PROBLEMS OF THERAPY IN THE ELDERLY

No significant differences in gastrointestinal absorption have been detected in the elderly. However, since the plasma albumin tends to fall in older people (normal as well as ill), there is less plasma binding, and a lower plasma drug level represents a relatively higher plasma/tissue gradient (Royal College of Physicians, 1984).

It is in the rate of hepatic metabolism that the greatest variability arises, for whereas there is a wide variability in the healthy young, in the elderly the rate of metabolism tends to fall. However, since this fall in hepatic metabolic rate is variable, some elderly patients will have metabolic rates in the normal range and others markedly below. Further, the degree of enzyme induction, i.e. the degree to which drugs oxidize liver enzymes, is reduced in the elderly (Salem *et al.*, 1978). Elimination of the drug by the kidney may be significantly impaired in the elderly. There is a decline in renal function; in particular the creatinine clearance, which may not be reflected by the serum creatinine levels since endogenous production of creatinine falls with age (Kampmann and Molholm Hansen, 1979).

The more subtle aspects of cell receptor sensitivity and density have not been adequately investigated for other than the hormonal receptors which seem to fall (Roth, 1979).

The problems of psychological depression, which is often a feature of chronic inflammatory disease, and dementia, which is more frequent in the elderly, may be worsened by NSAIDs. Indomethacin seems especially important in this context, although much of the data are from the early introduction period when much higher doses, 200–300 mg daily, were used. Ototoxicity, with reduction in high-tone reception, tinnitus, and even vertigo, may be important complications, especially the high-tone deafness which may not be appreciated by the patient yet impair his contact with his surroundings. Aspirin has usually been implicated, but other NSAIDs may have similar side effects.

The presence of cataracts may make the use of chloroquine difficult because of its reputation for retinotoxicity, but there is little evidence that it is more toxic in the elderly. Although gold has been shown to be effective in the elderly (Kean *et al.*, 1983), problems of mobility and occasionally lack of muscle bulk may make injections and routine blood tests difficult to undertake.

The difficulty of knowing exactly what medication the patient is taking is often compounded by the taking of additional 'over the counter' prescriptions and prescribing by both hospital and general practitioner without adequate communication.

These problems can be reduced by several methods:

1. Make sure patients understand their drug regime, written down if necessary.
2. Make sure a third party, family or friend, understands the regime.
3. Clearly mark all containers.
4. Keep the regime as simple as possible.
5. Unless necessary for safety reasons, use easily opened containers.
6. Use calendar dispensers.
7. Use injections of gold to ensure compliance and to aid toxicity monitoring.

11.10   MONITORING

How should treatment be monitored?

Safety monitoring should be fairly straightforward, and, apart from the obvious but often forgotten comment that all new drugs are potentially toxic and that they may show unsuspected side effects at any stage of use, will not be dealt with here. Most of the safety monitoring can be undertaken by general practitioners (Pullar *et al.*, 1982).

Efficacy monitoring is important not only to judge if the therapeutic regime is right but also to ensure that it is effective and thus indicated (Amos *et al.*, 1977). The extent of monitoring depends on how much time can be spent on this, and this will vary. Only variables potentially capable of changing are of value and these may never return to 'normal' in spite of the absence of inflammation, i.e. they remain fixed at a raised level (Holt, 1979; Dixon *et al.*, 1982; Grindulis and McConkey, 1982). In many cases it is impossible to know how reversible an abnormal result may be.

The duration (not severity) of morning stiffness, the degree and distribution of pain, and functional grade are rapid and subjective assessments. Grip strength, joint size and articular index take longer, but are less subjective. The biological tests take even longer, but are non-subjective. The erythrocyte sedimentation rate (ESR) has tended to be replaced by the C-reactive protein (CRP) estimation, but both have their independent value. Plasma viscosity, when available, is useful and can be performed on stored plasma. It is not altered by smoking, as the ESR may be (Larkin *et al.*, 1984). The haemoglobin is a useful indication of inflammation, but needs careful interpretation as it is influenced by factors such as iron deficiency. Serum sulphydryl (SH) levels and histidine measurement have yet to be fully evaluated and are not universally available. It will be noted that alterations in these tests (other than Hb) do not occur as a result of drug toxicity, and thus confusion will not arise.

Although improvement in subjective features and inflammatory signs is encouraging, most rheumatologists would prefer radiological evidence of improvement, mainly in the form of healing erosions and lessening osteoporosis. The evidence for this is poor (Iannuzzi *et al.*, 1983; Pullar *et al.*, 1984; Scott *et al.*, 1984).

11.11   REFERENCES

American Rheumatism Association (1973) A controlled trial of gold salt therapy in rheumatoid arthritis. *Arthr. Rheum.*, **16**, 353–8.

Amor, B. and Mery, C. (1980) Chlorambucil in rheumatoid arthritis, in *Anti Rheumatic Drugs II, Clinics in Rheumatic Diseases*, vol. 6, (ed. E. C. Huskisson). Saunders, London, p. 3.

Amos, R. S., Constable, T. J., Crockson, R. A., Crockson, A. P. and McConkey, B. (1977) Rheumatoid arthritis; relations of serum C-reactive protein and erythrocyte sedimentation rates to radiographic changes. *Br. J. Rheumatol.*, **1**, 195–7.

Argov, Z. and Mastaglia, F. L. (1979) Disorders of neuromuscular transmission caused by drugs. *N. Engl. J. Med.*, 301, 409–13.

Baltus, J. A. M., Boersma, J. W., Hartman, A. P. and Van den Broucke, J. P. (1983) The occurrence of malignancies in patients with rheumatoid arthritis treated with cyclophosphamide: a controlled retrospective follow up. *Ann. Rheum. Dis.*, 42, 368.

Bardin, T., Dryll, A., Deleyne, N. *et al.* (1982) HLA system and side effects of gold salts and D-penicillamine treatment of rheumatoid arthritis. *Ann. Rheum. Dis.*, 41, 598–601.

Bell, C. L. and Graziano, F. M. (1983) The safety of administration of penicillamine to penicillin sensitive individuals. *Arthr. Rheum.*, 26, 801–3.

Bevar, C. T., Hai Wang Chang, Penn, A. S., Jaffe, I. A. and Bock, E. (1982) Penicillamine induced myasthenia gravis: effects of penicillamine on acetylcholine receptor. *Neurology*, 32, 1077–82.

Bird, H., Rhind, V., Leatham, P. A. *et al.* (1981) Enteric coated aspirin in rheumatoid arthritis. *Rheum. Rehabil.*, 20, 116–21.

Bird, H. A. and Wright, V. (1982) *Applied Drug Therapy of the Rheumatic Diseases.* Wright, PSG, Bristol.

Bunch, T. W., O'Duffy, D. and Tomkins, R. B. (1980) Penicillamine and hydroxychloroquine singly and in combination in the treatment of rheumatoid arthritis. *Arthr. Rheum.*, 23, 659.

Caruso, I. and Biachi Porro, C. (1982) Gastroscopic evaluation of anti-inflammatory agents. *Br. Med. J.*, 280, 75–9.

Cathcart, E. S. and Wohlgethan, J. R. (1981) Amyloidosis, in *Scientific Basis of Rheumatology* (ed. G. S. Panayi), Churchill Livingstone, Edinburgh pp. 131–43.

Co-operating Clinics Committee of the American Rheumatism Association (1970) A controlled trial of cyclophosphamide. *N. Engl. J. Med.*, 283, 883–9.

Co-operating Clinics Committee of the American Rheumatism Association (1972) A controlled trial of high and low doses of cyclophosphamide in 82 patients with rheumatoid arthritis. *Arthr. Rheum.*, 15, 434.

Currey, H. L. F., Harris, J., Mason, R. M. *et al.* (1973) Comparison of azathioprine, cyclophosphamide and gold in treatment of rheumatoid arthritis. *Br. Med. J.*, 3, 763–6.

Davidson, A. M. and Birt, A. R. (1938) Quinine bisulphate as a desensitizing agent in treatment of lupus erythematosus. *Arch. Dermatol.*, 37, 247.

Davis, P. and Hughes, G. R. V. (1974) Significance of eosinophilia during gold therapy. *Arthr. Rheum.*, 17, 964–8.

Delamere, J. P., Jobson, S., Mackintosh, L. P., Well, L. and Walton, K. W. (1983) Penicillamine-induced myasthenia in rheumatoid arthritis: its clinical and genetic features. *Ann. Rheum. Dis.*, 42, 500–4.

Dencker, L. and Lindquist, N. C. (1975) Distribution of labelled chloroquine in the inner ear. *Arch. Otolaryngol.*, 101, 185–8.

De Silva, M. and Hazleman, B. L. (1981) Long term azathioprine in rheumatoid arthritis – a double blind study. *Ann. Rheum. Dis.*, 40, 560–3.

Dixon, A. St. J. and Graham, J. (1981) *Local Injection Therapy in Rheumatic Disease.* EULAR Publishers, Basle.

Dixon, J. S., Bird, H. A., Pickup, M. E. and Wright, V. (1982) A human model screening system for the detection of specific antirheumatic activity. *Seminars Arthr. Rheum.*, 12, 185–90.

Dodd, M. J., Griffiths, I. D. and Thompson, M. (1980) Adverse reactions to D-penicillamine after gold toxicity. *Br. Med. J.*, 199, 1498–504.

Duggan, J. M. (1981) The pathogenesis of the aspirin-related gastric lesion. *J. R. Coll. Physicians (Lond.)*, 15, 117–18.

Duthie, J. J. R., Brown, P. E., Truelove, L. H., Barago, E. and Lawrie, A. J. (1964) Course and prognosis in rheumatoid arthritis. A further report. *Ann. Rheum. Dis.*, 23, 193–204.

Dwosh, I. L., Giles, A. R., Ford, P. M., Pater, J. L. and Anastassiades, T. P. (1983) Plasmaphoresis therapy in rheumatoid arthritis: a controlled, double blind, cross-over trial. *N. Engl. J. Med.*, 308, 1124–9.

Empire Rhematism Council (1961) Gold therapy in rheumatoid arthritis. Final report of a multicentre controlled trial. *Ann. Rheum. Dis.*, 20, 315–33.

Evers, A. E. and Sundstrom, W. R. (1983) Second course gold therapy in the treatment of rheumatoid arthritis. *Arthr. Rheum.*, 26, 1071–5.

Forestier, J. (1935) Rheumatoid arthritis and its treatment by gold salts: results of 6 years' experiments. *J. Lab. Clin. Med.*, 20, 827–40.

Fowler, P. D., Shadforth, M. F., Crook, P. R. and Lawton, A. (1984) Report on chloroquine and dapsone in the treatment of rheumatoid arthritis: a 6-month comparative study. *Ann. Rheum. Dis.*, 43, 200–4.

Fuld, E. H., Strobar, S., Hoppe, R. T. *et al.* (1983) Sustained improvement of intractable rheumatoid arthritis after total lymphoid irradiation. *Arthr. Rheum.*, 26, 937–46.

Furst, D. E., Levine, S., Srinivasan, R. and Metizger, A. L. (1977) Double blind trial of high versus conventional dosages of gold salts for rheumatoid arthritis. *Arthr. Rheum.*, 20, 1473–80.

Goldberg, I. J. L., Lawton, K., Redding, J. R., Francois, P. E. and Phull, J. (1982) Influence of previous gold toxicity on subsequent development of penicillamine toxicity. *Br. Med. J.*, 285, 1659.

Graham, C. G., Haavisto, T. M., McNaught, P. J. *et al.* (1982a) The effect of smoking on the distribution of gold in blood. *J. Rheumatol.*, 9, 527–31.

Gran, J. T., Husky, G. and Thorsby, E. (1983) HLA DR antigens and gold toxicity. *Ann. Rheum. Dis.*, 42, 63–6.

Griffin, A. J., Gilson, T. and Huston, G. (1983) A comparison of conventional and low dose sodium aurothiomalate treatment in rheumatoid arthritis. *Br. J. Rheumatol.*, 22, 82–8.

Grindulis, K. A. and McConkey, B. (1982) Do drugs alter the course of rhematoid arthritis, in *Topical Reviews in Rheumatic Disorders*, Vol. II. (ed. V. Wright), Wright, Bristol, pp. 97–132.

Gumpel, J. M. (ed.) (1973) Symposium on radioactive colloids in the treatment of arthritis. *Ann. Rheum. Dis.*, Vol. 3, Suppl. 6.

Gumpel, J. M. (1978) Which anti-inflammatory drug in rheumatoid arthritis? *Br. Med. J.*, 2, 256.

Hall, N. D., Bird, H. A., Ring. E. F. J. *et al.* (1979) A combined clinical and immunological assessment of 4 cyclophosphamide regimes in rheumatoid arthritis. *Agents Actions*, 9, 97–102.

Hamilton, E. B. D. and Scott, J. T. (1962) Hydroxychloroquine sulphate (Plaquenil) in treatment of rheumatoid arthritis. *Arthr. Rheum.*, 5, 502–12.

Harkness, J. A. L. and Blake, D. R. (1982) Penicillamine nephropathy and iron. *Lancet*, ii, 1368–70.

Harris, E. D., Emkey, R. D., Nichols, J. E. and Newberg, A. (1983) Low dose prednisolone therapy in rheumatoid arthritis: a double blind study. *J. Rheumatol.*, 10, 713–21.

Holt, P. J. L. (1979) A critical comparison of the evaluation of anti-inflammatory therapy in animal models and man, in *Anti-Inflammatory Drugs*. (eds J. R. Vane and S. H. Ferreira), Springer-Verlag, Berlin.

Iannuzzi, L., Dawson, N., Zein, N. and Kushner, I. (1983) Does drug therapy slow radiological deterioration in rheumatoid arthritis? *N. Engl. J. Med.*, 309, 1023–8.

Jaffe, I. A. (1965) The effect of penicillamine on the laboratory parameters in rheumatoid arthritis. *Arthr. Rheum.*, 8, 1064–79.

James, D. W., Ludvigsen, N. W., Cleland, L. G. and Milazlo, S. E. (1982) The influence of cigarette smoking in blood gold distributions during chrysotherapy. *J. Rheumatol.*, 9, 522–35.

Jellum, E. and Munthe, E. (1982) Fate of the thiomalate part after intramuscular administration of aurothiomalate in rheumatoid arthritis. *Ann. Rheum. Dis.*, 41, 431–2.

Jessop, T. D., Dippy, J., Turnbull, A. and Bright, M. (1974) Eosinophilia during gold therapy. *Rheumatol. Rehabil.*, 13, 75–9.

Jones, J. V., Cumming, R. H., Bacon, P. A., Evers, J., Fraser, I. D., Bothamley, J., Tribe, C. R., Davies, P. G. and Hughes, G. R. V. (1979) Evidence for a therapeutic effect of plasmaphoresis in patients with systemic lupus erythematosus. *Q. J. Med.*, 448, 555–76.

Kampmann, J. P. and Molholm Hansen, J. D. (1979) Renal excretion of drugs, in *Drugs and the Elderly* (eds J. Crooks and I. H. Stevenson), University Park Press, Baltimore, pp. 77–87.

Kantor, T. G. (1982) Control of pain by non-steroidal anti-inflammatory drugs. *Med. Clinics N. Am.*, 66, 1053–9.

Kean, W. F., Bellamy, N. and Brookes, P. M. (1983) Gold therapy in the elderly rheumatoid arthritis patient. *Arthr. Rheum.*, 26, 705–11.

Kean, W. F., Lock, C. J. L., Howard-Lock, H. E. and Buchanan, W. W. (1982) Prior gold therapy does not influence the adverse effects of D-penicillamine in rheumatoid arthritis. *Arthr. Rheum.*, 25, 917–22.

Krabauer, R. S., Wysenbeck, A. J. and Wallace, D. J. (1983) Therapeutic trial of cryofiltration in patients with rheumatoid arthritis. *Am. J. Med.*, 74, 951–5.

Kukovetl, W. R., Beubler, E., Kreuzig, F., Moritz, A. J., Nirnberger, G. and Werner-Breitenecker, L. (1983) Bioavailability and pharmacokinetics of D-penicillamine. *J. Rheumatol.*, 10, 90–4.

Kuzell, W. C. and Gardner, G. M. (1950) Salisylazosulfapyridine in R. A. and experimental polyarthritis. *California Med.*, 73, 476–80.

Larkin, J. G., Lowe, G. D. O., Sturrock, R. D. and Forbes, C. D. (1984) The relationship of plasma and serum viscosity to disease activity and smoking habits in rheumatoid arthritis. *Br. J. Rheumatol.*, 23, 15–19.

Legros, J., Rosner, I. and Berger, C. (1973) Influence du niveau d'eclairment ambiant sur les modifications oculaires induites par l'hydroxychloroquine chez le rat. *Arch. Ophthalmol. (Paris)*, 33, 417–24.

Levine, J. D., Gordon, N. C. and Fields, H. L. (1978) The mechanism of placebo analgesia. *Lancet*, ii, 654–6.

Lisberg, R. B., Higham, C. and Jayson, M. I. V. (1983) Problems for rheumatic patients in opening dispensed drugs containers. *Br. J. Rheumatol.*, 22, 95–8.

Lockie, L. M., Gorney, E. and Smith, D. M. (1983) Low dose adrenocorticosteroids in the management of elderly patients with rheumatoid arthritis: selected examples and scanning of efficacy in long term treatment of 97 patients. *Seminar Arthr. Rheum.*, 8, 373–81.

Lorber, A., Vibert, G. J., Harralson, A. F. and Simon, T. M. (1983a) I. Unbound serum gold: procedure for quantitation. *J. Rheumatol.*, 10, 563–7.

Lorber, A., Kunishima, D. H., Harralson, A. F. and Simon, T. M. (1983b) II. Unbound versus total serum gold concentration: pharmacological action on cellular function. *J. Rheumatol.*, 10, 568–73.

Luthra, H. S., Conn, D. L. and Ferguson, R. H. (1981) Feltys syndrome: response to parenteral gold. *J. Rheumatol.*, 8/6, 902–9.

Luukainen, R., Kajander, A. and Isomaki, H. (1977) Effects of gold on progression of erosions in rheumatoid arthritis: better results with early treatment. *Scand. J. Rheumatol.*, 5, 481–7.

Mackenzie, A. H. and Scherbel, A. L. (1980) Chloroquine and hydroxychloroquine in rheumatological therapy. *Clinics Rheum. Dis.*, 6, 545–66.

McCarty, D. J. and Hogan, J. M. (1964) Inflammatory reaction after intra-synovial injection of microcrystalline adrenocorticosteroid esters. *Arthr. Rheum.*, 7, 359.

McConkey, B., Amos, R. D., Durham, S. *et al.* (1980) Sulphasalazine in rheumatoid arthritis. *Br. Med. J.*, 280, 442–4.

McConkey, B., Davies, P., Crockson, R. A. *et al.* (1976) Dapsone in rheumatoid arthritis. *Rheum. Rehabil.*, 15, 230–4.

McConkey, B., Davies, P., Crockson, R. A. *et al.* (1979) Effects of gold, dapsone, and prednisolone on serum C-reactive protein and haptoglobin and the erythrocyte sedimentation rate in rheumatoid arthritis. *Ann. Rheum. Dis.*, 38, 141–4.

McKenzie, J. M. M. (1981) Report on a double-blind trial comparing small and large doses of gold in the treatment of rheumatoid disease. *Rheumatol. Rehabil.*, 20, 198–202.

Mankin, H. J. and Conger, K. A. (1966) The acute effects of intra-articular hydrocortisone on articular cartilage in rabbits. *J. Bone Jt Surg.*, 48A, 1383–7.

Marks, J. S. and Power, B. J. (1979) Is chloroquine obsolete in treatment of rheumatic diseases? *Lancet*, i, 371–3.

Marks, J. S. (1982) Chloroquine retinopathy: is there a safe daily dose? *Ann. Rheum. Dis.*, 41, 52–8.

Medical Research Council (1960) A second report by the Joint Committee of the Medical Research Council and the Nuffield Foundation on clinical trials of cortisone, ACTH and other therapeutic measures in chronic rheumatic diseases. A comparison of prednisolone with aspirin or other analgesics in the treatment of rheumatoid arthritis. *Ann. Rheum. Dis.*, 19, 331–7.

Michaels, R. M., Nashel, D. J., Leonard, A., Sliwinski, A. J. and Derbes, S. J. (1982) Weekly intravenous methotrexate in the treatment of rheumatoid arthritis. *Arthr. Rheum.*, 25, 339–41.

Miller, B., De Merinex, P., Srinivasan, R. *et al.* (1980) Double blind placebo controlled cross-over evaluation of levamisole in rheumatoid arthritis. *Arthr. Rheum.*, 23, 172–82.

Million, R., Kellgren, J. H., Poole, P. H. *et al.* (1979) The long term management of early rheumatoid arthritis. *Ann. Rheum. Dis.*, 38, 573.

Multicentre Study Group (1978) Levamisole in rheumatoid arthritis. A randomised double blind study comparing two dosage regimes of levamisole with placebo. *Lancet*, ii, 1007–12.

Multicentre Study Group (1982) Levamisole in rheumatoid arthritis. *Ann. Rheum. Dis.*, 41, 159–63.

Multicentre Trial Group (1973) Controlled trial of D-penicillamine in severe rheumatoid arthritis. *Lancet*, i, 275–80.

Multicentre Trial Group (1974) Absence of toxic and therapeutic interaction between penicillamine and previously administered gold in a trial of penicillamine in rheumatoid disease. *Postgrad. Med. J.*, 50 (Suppl. 2), 77–8.

Neuman, V. C., Grindulis, K. A., Huball, S., McConkey, B. and Wright, V. (1983) Comparison between penicillamine and sulphasalazine in rheumatoid arthritis. Leeds–Birmingham trial. *Br. J. Med.*, 287, 1099–102.

Newton, P., Swinburn, W. R. and Swinsion, D. R. (1983) Proteinuria with gold therapy: when should gold be permanently stopped? *Br. J. Rheumatol.*, 22, 11–17.

Nissila, M. (1979) Role of osmic acid in the topical treatment of exudative synovitis of the knee joint. *Scand. J. Rheumatol.*, 8 (Suppl. 29), 6–44.

Nissila, M., Nuotio, P., Von Essen, R. and Makisara, P. (1982) Low dose penicillamine treatment of rheumatoid arthritis. Comparison of 600 mg and 300 mg regimes. *Scand. J. Rheumatol.*, 11, 161–4.

Norton, W. L. and Donnelly, R. J. (1983) High dose, low frequency parenteral gold administration. *J. Rheumatol.*, 10, 454–8.

Olason, B. (1983) Decreasing serum salicylate concentration during long-term administration of acetylsalicylic acid in healthy volunteers. Discussion of possible clinical implications. *Scand. J. Rheumatol.*, 12, 81–4.

Osman, M. A., Patel, R. B. and Schuna, A. (1983) Reduction in oral penicillamine absorption by food, antacid and ferrous sulphate. *Clin. Pharmacol. Ther.*, 33, 465–70.

Page, F. (1951) Treatment of lupus erythematosus with mepacrine. *Lancet*, ii, 755–8.

Panayi, G. S., Wooley, P. and Batchelor, J. R. (1978) Genetic basis of rheumatoid disease: HLA antigens, disease manifestations and toxic reactions to drugs. *Br. Med. J.*, 2, 1326–8.

Panayi, G. S., Huston, G., Shah, R. R. *et al.* (1983) Deficient sulphoidation studies and D-penicillamine toxicity. *Lancet*, i, 414.

Panush, R. S., Franco, A. E. and Schur, P. H. (1971) Rheumatoid arthritis associated with eosinophilia. *Ann. Intern. Med.*, 75, 199–205.

Pasternak, A. and Tiilikainen, A. (1977) HLA-B27 in rheumatoid arthritis and amyloidosis. *Tissue Antigens*, 9, 80–9.

Paulus, H. E., Machleder, H. I., Levine, S., Yu, D. T. Y. and MacDonald, N. S. (1977) Lymphocyte involvement in rheumatoid arthritis. Studies during thoracic duct drainage. *Arthr. Rheum.*, 20, 1249–62.

Paulus, H. (1982) An overview of benefit/risk of disease modifying treatment of rheumatoid arthritis as of today. *Ann. Rheum. Dis.*, 41 (Suppl. 1), 26–9.

Payne, J. F. (1984) A post-graduate lecture on lupus erythematosus. *Clin. J.*, IV, 223.

Popert, A. J., Meijers, K. A. E., Sharp, J. and Bier, F. (1961) Chloroquine diphosphate in rheumatoid arthritis, a controlled trial. *Ann. Rheum. Dis.*, 20, 18–35.

Pullar, T., Hunter, J. A. and Capell, H. A. (1982) Gold and penicillamine therapy: is shared care with general practitioners effective and safe? *Rheumatol. Rehabil.*, 21, 139–44.

Pullar, T., Hunter, J. A. and Capell, H. A. (1983) Sulphasalazine in rheumatoid arthritis: a double blind comparison of sulphasalazine with placebo and sodium aurothiomalate. *Br. Med. J.*, 287, 1102–5.

Pullar, T., Hunter, J. A. and Capell, H. A. (1984) Does second-line therapy affect the radiological progression of rheumatoid arthritis? *Ann. Rheum. Dis.*, 43, 18–23.

Rajapakse, C. N. A., Holt, P. J. L. and Perera, B. S. (1980) Diagnosis of true iron deficiency in rheumatoid arthritis. *Ann. Rheum. Dis.*, 39, 590.

Roth, G. S. (1979) Hormone receptor changes during adulthood and senescence: significance for ageing research. *Fed. Proc.*, 38, 1910–14.

Royal College of Physicians (1984) Medication for the Elderly. A report of the Royal College of Physicians. *J. R. Coll. Physicians London*, 18, 7–17.

Rynes, R. I., Krohel, G. and Falbo, A. (1979) Ophthalmological safety of long term hydroxychloroquine treatment. *Arthr. Rheum.*, 22, 832–6.

Salem, S. A. M., Rajjayabun, P., Shepherd, A. M. M. *et al.* (1978) Reduced induction of drug metabolism in the elderly. *Age Ageing*, 7, 68–78.

Sambrook, P. N., Browne, C. D., Champion, G. D. *et al.* (1982) Termination of treatment with gold sodium thiomalate in rheumatoid arthritis. *Aus. J. Rheumatol.*, 9, 932–4.

Scheinberg, M. A. and Cathcart, E. S. (1976) Casein-induced experimental amyloidosis. VI. A pathogenic role for B cells in the murine model. *Immunology*, 31, 443–53.

Schlumf, V., Meyer, M., Ulrick, J. and Friede, R. L. (1983) Neurologic complications induced by gold treatment. *Arthr. Rheum.*, 26, 825–31.

Schnitzer, J. T. and Ansell, B. M. (1977) Amyloidosis in juvenile chronic arthritis. *Arthr. Rheum.*, **20** (Suppl. 2), 245–52.

Schuna, A., Osman, M. A., Patel, R. B., Welling, P. G., Sunderstrom, W. R. and Middleton, W. S. (1983) Influence of food on the bioavailability of penicillamine. *J. Rheumatol.*, **10**, 95–7.

Scott, D. L., Grindulis, K. A., Struthers, G. R., Coulton, B. L., Popert, A. J. and Bacon, P. A. (1984) Progression of radiological changes in rheumatoid arthritis. *Ann. Rheum. Dis.*, **43**, 8–17.

Semble, E., Metcalf, D., Turner, R., Agudel, C. *et al.* (1982) Genetic prediction of patient response and side effects in the treatment of rheumatoid arthritis with a high dose nonsteroidal anti-inflammatory drug regime. *Arthr. Rheum.*, **25**, 370–4.

Sharp, J. T., Lidsley, M. D., Duffy, J., Thompson, M. K. *et al.* (1977) Comparison of two dosage schedules of gold salts in the treatment of rheumatoid arthritis: relationship of serum gold levels to therapeutic response. *Arthr. Rheum.*, **20**, 1179–87.

Sigler, J. W., Bluhm, G. B. and Duncan, H. (1974) Gold salts in the treatment of rheumatoid arthritis – a double-blind study. *Ann. Intern. Med.*, **80**, 21–6.

Sinclair, R. J. C. and Duthie, J. J. R. (1948) Salazopyrine in the treatment of rheumatoid arthritis. *Ann. Rheum. Dis.*, **8**, 226–31.

Smith, D. H., Scott, D. L. and Zaphiropoulos, G. C. (1983) Eosinophilia in D-penicillamine therapy. *Ann. Rheum. Dis.*, **43**, 408–10.

Smith, P. J., Swinburn, W. R., Swinson, D. R. and Stewart, I. M. (1982) Influence of previous gold toxicity on subsequent development of penicillamine toxicity. *Br. Med. J.*, **285**, 595–6.

Smythe, H. A. (1981) Fibrositis and other diffuse musculoskeletal syndromes, in *Textbook of Rheumatology* (eds W. N. Kelly, E. D. Harris, S. Ruddy and C. B. Sledge), W. B. Saunders, London, pp. 485–93.

Steinsson, K., Weinstein, A., Korn, J. and Abeles, M. (1982) Low dose methotrexate in rheumatoid arthritis. *J. Rheumatol.*, **9**, 860–6.

Svartz, N. (1948) The treatment of rheumatic polyarthritis with azo compounds. *Rheumatism*, **4**, 56–60.

Swinson, D. R., Zlosnick, J. and Jackson, L. (1981) Double-blind trial of dapsone against placebo in the treatment of rheumatoid arthritis. *Ann. Rheum. Dis.*, **40**, 235–9.

Sylvester, R. A. and Pinals, R. S. (1970) Eosinophilia in rheumatoid arthritis. *Ann. Allergy*, **28**, 565–8.

Thomas, A. R., Robinson, W. A., Boyle, D. J., Day, J. F., Entringer, M. A. and Steigerwald, J. F. (1983) Long term effects of cyclophosphamide on granulocyte colony formation in patients with rheumatoid arthritis. *J. Rheumatol.*, **10**, 778–83.

Townes, A. S., Sowa, J. M. and Shulman, L. E. (1976) Controlled trial of cyclophosphamide in rheumatoid arthritis. *Arthr. Rheum.*, **19**, 563–73.

Von Knorring, L., Perris, C., Eisemann, M., Eriksson, U. and Perris, H. (1983) Pain as a symptom in depressive disorders. 1. Relationship to diagnostic subgroup and depressive symptomatology. *Pain*, **15**, 19–26.

Ward, J. R., Williams, H. J., Eggar, M. J., Reading, J. C. *et al.* (1983) Comparison of auranofin, gold sodium thiomalate and placebo in the treatment of rheumatoid arthritis, a controlled clinical trial. *Arthr. Rheum.*, **26**, 1303–15.

Ward, N. C., Bloom, V. L., Dworkin, S., Fawcett, J., Narasimhacheri, N. and Friedel, R. D. (1982) Psychobiological markers in coexisting pain and depression: towards a unified theory. *J. Psychiat.*, **43**, 32–41.

Wernick, R., Merryman, P., Jaffe, I. and Ziff, M. (1983) IgG and IgM. Rheumatoid factors in rheumatoid arthritis. *Arthr. Rheum.*, **26**, 593–8.

Whisnant, J. K. and Pelkey, J. (1982) Rheumatoid arthritis: treatment with azathioprine Immuran. Clinical side effects and laboratory abnormalities. *Ann. Rheum.
Dis.*, 41 (Suppl. 1), 44–7.

Williams, H. J., Ward, J. R., Reading, J. C., Eggar, M. J. *et al.* (1983) Low dose
D-penicillamine therapy in rheumatoid arthritis, a controlled, double blind clinical
trial. *Arthr. Rheum.*, 26, 581–92.

Young, A., Jaraquemada, D., Awad, J., Festenstein, H., Corbett, M., Hay, F. C. and
Roitt, I. M. (1984) Association of HLA-DR4/DW4 and DR2/DW2 with radiologic
changes in a prospective study of patients with rheumatoid arthritis. *Arthr.
Rheum.*, 27, 20–5.

CHAPTER 12

The spondarthritides

Ian Haslock

The colligative concept of seronegative spondarthritis was introduced by Moll, Haslock, Macrae and Wright in 1974 (Table 12.1). At that time it was suggested that this concept would have aetiological, diagnostic and therapeutic importance, and each of these predictions has been born out in the subsequent decade.

Therapeutically, the central position of ankylosing spondylitis, with its considerable therapeutic dissimilarity to rheumatoid arthritis, has been dominant. In particular, there is a major place for non-drug treatment, especially exercise therapy, the importance of which cannot be overemphasized. In many instances there is also a need to integrate the treatment of the articular portions of the conditions with their non-articular parts, which themselves pose major therapeutic problems.

Although each of the diseases of the seronegative spondarthritis group will be considered separately here, there is considerable overlap amongst them. However, the concept of 'B27 disease' seems inappropriate, both from its

TABLE 12.1
The seronegative spondarthritides

Ankylosing spondylitis
Psoriatic arthritis
Arthritis associated with inflammatory bowel disease
  Ulcerative colitis
  Crohn's disease
Whipple's disease
Reactive arthritis
  Reiter's disease
  Sexually acquired reactive arthritis
  Enteropathic reactive arthritis

accent on a laboratory test rather than the essentially clinical threads that bind these diseases together, and also from the existence of numerous examples of each of the diseases under consideration where HLA-B27 is not present. 'B27 disease' is also likely to engender sufficient anxiety in normal B27-possessing individuals that a separate section on laboratory-based iatrogenic anxiety might well prove to be an integral part of such a concept.

12.1 ANKYLOSING SPONDYLITIS

Idiopathic ankylosing spondylitis (AS) used to be considered a rare disease with a prevalence of about 1 in 1000 men and a tenth of this in women. More recent studies have suggested a prevalence as high as 1% in either sex (Calin and Fries, 1975; Cohen *et al.*, 1976) and although this has been challenged (Christiansen *et al.*, 1979), there seems no doubt from the numbers of patients with AS seen in clinical practice that the frequency of AS has been considerably underestimated in the past, especially in females. It remains a disease where diagnosis is often delayed, with considerable disability resulting from this delay, as early treatment conveys the greatest benefit.

The essential treatment of AS is by exercises; deformities of former times resulted from immobilization in plaster shells. After initial physiotherapy to maximize mobility in the spine, the thoracic cage and the peripheral joints, especially the root joints, the patient is encouraged to undertake an exercise regime on a twice daily, lifelong basis. Without co-operation with this regime, drug treatment is of very limited effect, but it is important in relieving pain enough for the patient to do his regular exercises. Drugs also provide useful relief of morning stiffness, but there is no evidence that they affect the progression of the disease.

12.1.1 NSAIDs

These are the sole drug treatment used in over 90% of patients with AS. Phenylbutazone has traditionally been considered the most effective drug for this condition, with some clinicians using the patient's response to phenylbuta-zone as a diagnostic test for AS. However, the toxicity of phenylbutazone precludes its general use, and many clinicians restrict its use for intractable disease. Oxyphenbutazone has no advantages over phenylbutazone and is twice as dangerous (Cuthbert, 1974). It should not be used. The more modern pyrazole derivative Azapropazone has been shown to be better than placebo (Calcraft *et al.*, 1974) and comparable to indomethacin in AS.

Indomethacin has been shown to be effective in the management of ankylos-ing spondylitis (Shipley *et al.*, 1980), and the use of a large nightly dose is especially valuable in overcoming morning stiffness. It should be noted that the relief of morning stiffness by indomethacin suppositories is not a result of delayed absorption from the rectal mucosa but is dependent on the dose used, 100 mg by mouth being at least as effective (Huskisson *et al.*, 1970). Sustained-release preparations such as Indocid-R are valuable in providing equal symptomatic relief from a lower dose of indomethacin. Unfortunately, the efficacy of indomethacin is accompanied by a number of side effects, especially involving the central nervous system (headaches, dizziness, depression and depersonalization) and the gastrointestinal tract. These are rarely a problem in patients taking a night-time dose only, especially if it is taken with food. Side effects of more frequent dose regimes can be reduced by introducing the drug in a small dose and increasing it slowly. Many patients are able to tolerate daily doses of 250 mg indomethacin over long periods if this stepwise introductory period is used. The indomethacin derivative sulindac has proved less effective in the management of AS (Gibson and Laurent, 1980) and appears to have no fewer side effects.

Although aspirin has a venerable history in rheumatology, it has always been acknowledged that it is less effective in AS than in other arthritides. In contrast, the new non-steroidals, especially the propionic acid derivatives (which are now generally accepted as the first-line treatment of choice for most rheumatic diseases), are equally effective in this disease. Naproxen has been widely studied since the initial trial by Hill and Hill (1973) demonstrated its effectiveness. It has been shown to be equivalent to phenylbutazone (Van Gerwen *et al.*, 1978) although marginally less effective than enteric-coated phenylbutazone (Ansell *et al.*, 1978). It is equivalent to indomethacin in relieving sleep-disturbing pain in spondylitic patients (Peter and Veress, 1975). The long half-life of naproxen makes it a valuable drug for relief of morning stiffness using a night-time dose. Even when needed twice daily it is well tolerated, and many patients take doses of 1 g daily for many years. Higher doses have been used, and well tolerated, for shorter-term treatment of acute exacerbations of disease. Flurbiprofen has been shown to be equivalent to indomethacin in a study where back movement, measured by spondylometry, was improved by both active drugs when compared with placebo (Sturrock and Hart, 1974). Unfortunately, the efficacy of this drug is largely offset by its side effects, with dyspepsia being particularly troublesome. Ibuprofen (Nikolic and Lukacevic, 1975), fenoprofen (Godfrey *et al.*, 1977) and ketoprofen (Jessop, 1976) have all been used successfully in patients with AS, with some patients expressing strong preferences for each member of this apparently similar group. Individual patient preference is a greater factor than objective differences in efficacy when deciding which of these drugs to use. This was well demonstrated in rheumatoid arthritis by Huskisson *et al.* (1976) who showed that, although naproxen was more effective than ibuprofen when groups of patients were considered, some individuals showed a strong preference for the less potent agent. Similar strong individual preferences have also been found in AS (Wasner *et al.*, 1981). These individual differences apply equally to side effects, where patients may find almost all the available non-steroidals intolerable, but tolerate one or two quite easily. It is considerations such as these that make most practising rheumatologists welcome the introduction of new non-steroidals (Editorial, 1976) despite the disparaging comments made by some academic clinical pharmacologists about 'me too' drugs. Another welcome trend is the introduction of sustained-release forms of drugs with intrinsically short half-lives. Oruvail, the sustained-release version of ketoprofen, is a good example of this approach, and although no formal studies in AS exist, personal experience suggests it is reasonably effective in controlling morning stiffness with a reduced level of side effects compared with its parent preparation.

The fenamates, mefenamic acid and flufenamic acid, show activity more biased towards the analgesic rather than the anti-inflammatory end of the non-steroidial anti-inflammatory spectrum. They have been used in AS (Simpson *et al.*, 1966) and are reasonably well tolerated, although some patients develop diarrhoea.

The phenylacetic acid derivative diclofenac proved to be slightly better than sulindac in AS (Nahir and Sharf, 1980), and a multi-centre trial in Germany showed it to be as effective as indomethacin (Rheinberger, 1976). No formal studies have been published using the sustained-release preparation of diclofenac in AS, but its use in combating morning stiffness would be logical.

The oxicams are a recently introduced family of non-steroidals, of which piroxicam is the only one widely available so far. Comparative studies in AS have shown it to be comparable with phenylbutazone (McAdam *et al.*, 1981) and with 75 mg indomethacin (Sydnes, 1981). This last study epitomizes one of the major problems of evaluating clinical trials of non-steroidals in AS. The indomethacin dose was given as 25 mg t.d.s., which contrasts with the usual practice of giving a single, or augmented, night-time dose to overcome morning stiffness. The clinical trial evidence available almost universally uses established agents in this inappropriate fashion. Therefore, except in the case of newer agents such as piroxicam, with its intrinsically long half-life giving once daily dosage, the published work provides at best an inadequate guide to everyday practice. It is, however, clear from studying clinical trials that improvement is almost completely restricted to symptomatic benefit rather than increasing the patients' mobility. In general the only effect of NSAIDs on spinal movement is that produced by reduction in pain which allows patients to exercise more effectively. No drug should be considered as a substitute for exercise therapy – pain-free patients have just as great a capacity to fuse their spines as those with residual discomfort.

12.1.2 'Second-line' drugs

Terms such as 'disease modifying' are inappropriate in AS as no drug has been claimed to modify the course of the disease. In our experience to date gold has been found to be of no value in AS, although work elsewhere is underway to study this further. Although occasional patients have been reported in whom a response appears to have taken place to D-penicillamine (Golding, 1974), most experience has suggested that no such response occurs (Bird and Dixon, 1977) and the only controlled trial conducted so far showed no advantage of penicillamine over placebo (Stevens *et al.*, 1985). Systemic corticosteroids appear to have little place in AS, although the judicious use of pulsed methylprednisolone has yet to be evaluated. Intra-articular corticosteroids may be used for the treatment of peripheral synovitis involving the knees or, occasionally, the toes. Local steroid injections are also valuable in treating the enthesopathic lesions that occur so commonly in AS. Occasional patients appear to respond to methotrexate but this, too, is unevaluated.

12.1.3 Radiotherapy

Intra-articular ^{90}yttrium may be of value in peripheral synovitis involving the knee. It appears to be a reasonably safe form of treatment provided some form of immobilization of the injected joint is used during the 48 hours after injection. This minimizes isotope dissemination from the joint and hence irradiation of the groin lymph nodes. The usual dose is 5 MCi, although this might require repeating if the synovium is very thick, as the maximum penetration of the emitted β particles is 11 mm. Spinal radiotherapy had a considerable vogue in the 1940s and 1950s, but fell into disrepute when the association with an increased risk of leukaemia was described (Court Brown and Doll, 1965). This is reflected in a reduced survival rate in irradiated patients compared with those not treated by radiotherapy (Kapgrove *et al.*, 1980). Radiotherapy is now used only rarely, and it must be stressed that the relief of pain produced by radiotherapy does not imply a cure of the disease and that progressive painless stiffening may take place if the patients' regular exercise regime is neglected. Our own unit contains an unfortunate group of patients who have stiffened irrevocably during the pain-free period after radiotherapy, an outcome entirely due to neglect of their exercises during this period. Radiotherapy is now considered to be of more value in treating an isolated peripheral joint that is the site of disproportionate, uncontrolled synovitis. Stubborn enthesopathic lesions, such as those at the insertion of the spring ligament (syn. plantar calcaneonavicular ligament), may also respond to radiotherapy when local corticosteroid injections have failed. In these patients the risk of marrow irradiation is very small and this form of treatment appears to offer a reasonable risk:benefit ratio.

12.1.4 Management strategy

The initial drug treatment should be with a modern, safe non-steroidal. Naproxen has a high acceptability to AS patients (Wasner *et al.*, 1981) and some clinicians now regard this as the drug of first choice. During the initial phase after diagnosis, during which time the patient will be attending for regular, vigorous mobilizing physiotherapy, a regular dose of one 500 mg tablet twice daily should be used, increasing to 500 mg t.d.s. if necessary. If this fails to control the patient's symptoms, indomethacin is the suggested substitute. Side effects may be minimized by using a graduated dose regime, such as 25 mg t.d.s. and 50 mg nocte for the first two weeks, increasing the dose to 50 mg t.d.s. and 100 mg at night if necessary. Alternatively, a single night-time dose of one 75 mg Indocid-R capsule may be used, adding a morning dose if necessary. If this is unsuccessful, other non-steroidals should be tried in sequence until a suitable one is found. Some clinicians, however, still regard phenylbutazone as the drug of first choice, arguing that its impressive efficacy in spondylitis outweighs its acknowledged toxicity. Other clinicians reserve its use to patients in whom other non-steroidals have proved ineffective. Although combinations of non-steroidals are deplored by clinical pharmacologists they are often popular with patients, and several patients with more severe AS do well on 500 mg naproxen bd plus one 75 mg Indocid-R capsule at night. Persistent synovitis in a peripheral joint or painful enthesopathic lesions may be treated by local corticosteroid injection. Persisting knee synovitis can be treated at this time by injecting [90]yttrium provided the patient is over 45 years of age.

Most patients will respond to this regime and come under symptomatic control with a good posture and an adequate range of movement maintained by regular exercises. Drug treatment can then be reduced, usually to a single night-time dose of naproxen or indomethacin, and many patients require only intermittent medication at times of minor exacerbation. A few patients continue to have increasing pain and decreasing mobility requiring further intervention. At this time admission to hospital, predominantly for intensive physiotherapy with appropriate rest, including prone lying, may prove useful. Especially where there is significant peripheral synovitis it is worth considering the use of pulsed methylprednisolone. This approach is empirical and the success which we have had with it under these circumstances, while apparently dramatic, has not been proved in a double-blind fashion. Despite this we remain convinced of its utility. After successful treatment with pulsed methylprednisolone, usually after two or three 1 g pulses at 3-day intervals, methotrexate may be introduced in an attempt to maintain disease control. Our usual practice is to give single, weekly 10 mg intramuscular doses, with weekly blood counts to monitor the effect on white cells. It is not our custom to carry out routine liver biopsies in our patients, but liver function tests are repeated monthly, and we would be reluctant to introduce the drug in patients with significant abnormalities in liver function.

Although methotrexate has proved useful in some patients, most develop nausea which often precludes continuation of this drug. This has proved resistant to pharmacological attempts to control it (Mitchell and Schein,

1982), but is sometimes abolished by stopping concurrent NSAIDs. It is only in those few patients in whom this approach has failed that spinal radiotherapy is indicated, and the rarity of this need is indicated by the fact that only two patients under our care have required such treatment in the last 10 years. However, about twice this number of patients have been subjected to local radiotherapy to an isolated peripheral joint, usually the ankle, which has proved resistant to other measures.

While many consultations with the attending physician will concentrate on the effects, and side effects, of medication, every opportunity should be taken to reinforce the need for regular exercises. Clear and accurate patient education, especially self-help education is considered to be of general importance in most rheumatology departments (Lorig et al., 1985), but the benefits of this approach are most obvious in the management of patients with AS. This disease is also one in which there are great benefits in the formation of patient groups, with consequent increase in motivation for exercises and for an active lifestyle. The existence of these groups engenders an even greater than usual need for the physician to be clear in communicating to his patients the rationale of drug and non-drug treatments, the side effects of therapy and, especially in AS, the genetic implications of the disease.

12.2   PSORIATIC ARTHRITIS

Psoriatic arthritis exhibits three distinct patterns of peripheral arthritis – distal, deforming and identical. The distal form, sometimes erroneously thought to be the only pattern of psoriatic arthritis, involves the distal interphalangeal joints, often in association with psoriatic involvement of the associated nail – so-called 'topographical' psoriatic arthritis. The identical form is named after its similarity to rheumatoid arthritis, although it is in fact less symmetrical and usually involves fewer joints than that disease. In general, although the number of joints involved in psoriatic arthritis is less than that in RA the degree of destruction in each involved joint is often higher. This fact is epitomized by the destructive form of the disease, arthritis mutilans. Each pattern of psoriatic arthritis may be complicated by spondylitis, the treatment of which is predominantly by exercises, as in idiopathic AS.

12.2.1   Non-steroidal anti-inflammatories

These drugs will be the only ones used in most patients with psoriatic arthritis and are the agents of first choice in all. Fewer formal studies in psoriatic arthritis have been published, reflecting the lesser frequency of the disease and the continuing debate regarding its definition in some quarters. The patchy joint involvement also makes clinical assessment more problematical (Leatham et al., 1982), with greater emphasis on subjective variables such as pain and stiffness than in studies of some other diseases. Phenylbutazone has again been used extensively in this disease, but the availability of a wide range of alternatives decreases the need to use this relatively toxic drug. Indomethacin is usually used as the standard comparator, and drugs such as azapropazone (Lassus, 1976) and diclofenac (Leatham *et al.*, 1982) have been shown to have similar efficacy to that agent. Drugs with frequent skin side effects are probably best reserved as late choices in psoriatic arthritis. While there appears to be no increase in the frequency of side effects with most of them, patients with psoriasis are, understandably, unhappy at having an iatrogenic rash added to their natural one.

12.2.2 'Second-line' drugs

No drugs have been claimed to modify the progression of psoriatic arthritis. Most clinicians are agreed that antimalarials, such as chloroquine or hydroxychloroquine, should be avoided as they may cause exacerbations of psoriasis. Gold has been used for many years in the treatment of psoriatic arthritis, but controlled trials have not been undertaken until relatively recently. These confirm the clinical impression that this is a useful form of treatment and that side effects, especially rashes, are no more frequent than in rheumatoid arthritis (Dorwart *et al.*, 1978; Richter *et al.*, 1980). There are a few anecdotal reports of the use of penicillamine in psoriatic arthritis, but these are insufficient to give any impression that this drug has any value in this disease.

Systemic corticosteroids are required rarely in psoriatic arthritis, although quite high proportions of patients treated successfully with these drugs have been reported in some series (Roberts *et al.*, 1976). Attempted reduction of steroid dosage in patients with psoriatic arthritis may result in exacerbation of the skin disease thus increasing patient pressure to maintain higher dose therapy than might otherwise be thought desirable. This fact should be borne in mind when initiating oral corticosteroids. Local injections may prove useful both in controlling isolated synovitis in a joint or in the tendon sheath of a sausage digit. Psoriatic plaques may be quite heavily contaminated with bacteria, and injection through such lesions must be avoided. We have used pulsed methylprednisolone in patients with psoriatic arthritis, especially those with large-joint synovitis unresponsive to conventional therapy. Although this has appeared to be a valuable adjunct to treatment, this is an uncontrolled observation.

The major alternative to NSAIDs is methotrexate. Methotrexate has been used successfully to control the rash of psoriasis (Weinstein and Frost, 1971) and for treating psoriatic arthritis (Black *et al.*, 1964; Feldges and Barnes, 1974; Zachariae E. *et al.*, 1985). Dermatologists initially showed great concern regarding the development of hepatic fibrosis during methotrexate therapy, but experience in the treatment of rheumatic diseases suggests that the risks are small (Willkens *et al.*, 1985; Rubinstein *et al.*, 1985; Zachariae, H. *et al.*, 1985) and many people now undertake monitoring using liver function tests only without routine liver biopsies (Williams *et al.*, 1985). The dosage of the drug must be reduced in those with impaired renal function and care should be exercised in those who drink alcohol regularly.

The aromatic retinoid etretinate, which is effective in controlling the skin lesions of psoriasis, has also been used in psoriatic arthritis (Hopkins *et al.*, 1985). Significant clinical and laboratory improvement was seen, although side effects were common. This form of therapy deserves fuller evaluation.

12.2.3   Relationship between skin and joint disease

There is no clear pattern of relationship between psoriasis and psoriatic arthritis. Some patients find that the two components of the disease follow a synchronous course of exacerbation and remission. Other patients feel that their joints are at their best when their skin is at its worst and *vice versa*, while most can discern no co-ordination in the pattern of exacerbation and remission in the two components of their disease. With the exception of methotrexate, which benefits both skin and joints, other forms of treatment appear to affect only the tissue at which they are aimed, although systemic corticosteroids, if used, may also affect both tissues. Side effects of antirheumatic therapy may, however, involve the skin. The psychological, as well as physical, effects of such adverse reactions must not be ignored and treatment chosen with the greatest possible care in order to minimize this risk.

Both skin and joints may be subject to the Köebner phenomenon – that is exacerbation after trauma. Treatment of psoriatic patients under our care requiring surgery has been associated with exacerbated local psoriasis at the site of the incision. Therapists treating psoriatic patients must be reminded of their potential to exacerbate psoriasis by both mechanical and thermal trauma. Patients with psoriasis may require admission to dermatology wards in order to bring their skin disease under control. Advantage should always be taken of such admissions for the physiotherapists to review the patients' exercise needs, especially if they have spondylitis.

12.2.4   Management strategy

The essential first stage in management is a firm diagnosis. Thereafter, initial treatment is with NSAIDs, with naproxen giving a good balance between safety and efficacy. If this fails to control the patients' symptoms, indomethacin is the drug of second choice, with others being tried only if these two fail. Although the skin lesions require separate treatment they must not be ignored. Patients may be reluctant to participate in physiotherapy sessions because of embarrassment produced by their rash. Digital, and especially nail, psoriasis may be sufficiently painful to diminish hand function, and it is extremely important to distinguish the origin of the patients' symptoms if treatment is to be appropriate. This applies equally to the feet, where the psoriatic lesions themselves may be the source of the patients' discomfort.

If NSAIDs, supplemented by treatment of skin and nail lesions where appropriate, fail to control the disease, local injections into affected joints and tendon sheaths should be used. If the disease is still progressive, chrysotherapy is introduced. My own practice is to use myocrisin 10 mg intramuscularly in the first week, and 20 mg intramuscularly at fortnightly intervals thereafter. Full blood counts, including platelet and differential white counts, are carried out weekly for two months, fortnightly for four months, and monthly thereafter. Urine specimens are checked before each injection, but supervision of the skin is more problematic in these patients than in those with RA. For this reason we try whenever possible to arrange for our own specialist rheumatology nurses to give gold injections to psoriatic patients, and ask that we see patients personally before treatment is discontinued because of apparent dermal side effects. It is my policy, which I discuss with the patients before the initiation of therapy, to continue successful chrysotherapy on a lifelong basis, with the injection frequency being reduced to no less than fortnightly even when good control is established. It is also essential during this discussion to warn the patient about the delay in the effect of gold, and plan the treatment for the first, ineffective, three months. It might be that an admission to hospital for bed rest followed by intensive physiotherapy will be required to help the patient through this period. Admission may also be required during periods of disease progression later in the course of the disease. If adequate rest and local treatment, including local injection, fail to bring the disease under control, we have had short-term success using pulsed methylprednisolone, although the efficacy of this medication has not been subjected either to long-term appraisal or formal clinical trial.

If disease control with gold fails, or side effects necessitate its withdrawal, methotrexate is effective in controlling both the joint and skin disease. Once control is established it is our policy to reduce progressively the size of the weekly dose. In many patients control can be maintained for quite long periods with NSAIDs alone, giving 'courses' of the more toxic drug only intermittently.

12.3 ARTHRITIS ASSOCIATED WITH INFLAMMATORY BOWEL DISEASE

Both ulcerative colitis and Crohn's disease are associated with two types of arthritis. Enteropathic arthritis occurs in about 15% of patients with ulcerative colitis and 20% of those with Crohn's disease. Clinical ankylosing spondylitis or its *forme fruste*, sacroiliitis, occurs in about 15% of patients with either condition. Precise diagnosis of the type of arthritis is essential, as the treatment varies. Enteropathic arthritis is self-limiting, exacerbations of gut and joint disease occurring synchronously. The joints suffer no long-term damage irrespective of the number of episodes of synovitis and treatment may, therefore, simply be concerned with providing symptomatic relief. In contrast, AS associated with inflammatory bowel disease has the same long-term connotations as idiopathic AS and requires the same treatment strategy, modified by the presence of gut inflammation.

12.3.1 NSAIDs

These are effective in reducing inflammation, but considerable care is needed in the choice of drug that is to be introduced into the inflamed gut. My own policy is to use benorylate, which is a pro-drug, metabolized after absorption to aspirin and paracetamol, as the preparation of first choice. If this proves ineffective, fenbufen, which is also a pro-drug, may be used. Both these drugs appear to produce little gastrointestinal upset, even in patients with active intestinal inflammation. If these are ineffective, propionic acid derivatives should be tried, and only later the more toxic indomethacin. The use of sustained-release preparations, such as Oruvail or Indocid-R, might on theoretical grounds be considered to carry extra hazard as the drug is released in closer proximity to the inflamed area of gut. This has not been borne out by very limited experience, but the delivery system used in the now-withdrawn Osmosin proved capable of causing perforation in the normal small bowel (Day, 1983), and should not be used in inflammatory bowel disease. Similarly, suppository preparations of NSAIDs often produce local proctitis and are contraindicated in inflammatory bowel disease.

12.3.2 'Second-line' drugs

There is no need for 'second-line'-type medication in enteropathic arthritis as the disease is non-progressive. Spondylitis associated with inflammatory bowel disease is subject to the same reservations, with regard to the ability of pharmacological agents to modify disease progression, as idiopathic ankylosing spondylitis with which it is identical.

12.3.3 Relationship between gut and joint disease

Enteropathic arthritis is always associated with activity of the underlying gut disease. It follows that the ideal treatment is the cure or elimination of the inflammatory bowel disease. This is possible in ulcerative colitis by panproctocolectomy and ileostomy, but the presence of arthritis should not be considered as an indication for radical surgery as the articular disease is short-lived, non-deforming, and usually easily controlled. In Crohn's disease no such radical cure is available. In practice most patients with inflammatory bowel disease are now treated medically. The better the control of the underlying disease the less problematical enteropathic arthritis will be. There is little evidence that the drugs used to control inflammatory bowel disease have any direct effect on the joint disease, although some of them such as sulphasalazine azathioprine and corticosteroids are used in the treatment of other types of arthritis.

The progress and treatment of the underlying gut disease has no effect on associated ankylosing spondylitis.

12.3.4 Management strategy

Each episode of enteropathic synovitis is treated as a separate entity. Two forms of treatment are available. NSAIDs may be used, starting with benorylate either 5–10 ml or 1–2 sachets bd, substituting fenbufen 600 mg at night, increasing by a 300 mg morning dose if necessary. Thereafter other nonsteroidals, chosen with regard to safety, are tried sequentially. The alternative strategy, that may be used as the prime therapy for enteropathic arthritis, or at any stage at which non-steroidal therapy fails, is to inject the inflamed joint with local corticosteroid. This approach to treatment is particularly apposite because the synovitis is often monarticular and the treatment carries no extra hazard as far as the gut is concerned. It should not be used during bacteraemic or septicaemic episodes.

Ankylosing spondylitis complicating inflammatory bowel disease is treated in exactly the same fashion as idiopathic AS from which it cannot be distinguished either clinically or radiologically. Thus exercise therapy is the prime form of treatment, and it is extremely important to continue this throughout exacerbations of the bowel disease, otherwise serious immobility with consequent disability may result. This advice is very difficult to follow when a patient requires urgent surgery for life-threatening disease. However, even when the patient is too ill to co-operate with an active exercise regime, the attending nurses can assist by ensuring that the posture in bed is as good as possible. The physiotherapist can contribute too, at least by putting the peripheral joints through a full passive range on a regular basis. As with all rheumatic diseases, teamwork is intrinsic to success. Unfortunately we have under our care patients in whom the treatment of the inflammatory bowel disease was so urgent and complex that the needs of the stiffening locomotor system were ignored with crippling long-term consequences.

The choice of NSAID is tilted towards absence of side effects and despite its relative inefficiency in seronegative arthritis, aspirin in the form of benorylate sometimes proves useful because of its relative gastrointestinal safety. In these diseases the costive effect of aloxiprin may be used to advantage. This drug is also acceptable in view of its relative lack of other gastrointestinal side effects. The potential for the fenamates to produce diarrhoea makes them unsuitable for use in these patients. Fenbufen may also be tried because of its low gastrointestinal toxicity. Thereafter propionic acid derivatives are chosen with an eye to safety, with preparations such as naproxen or Oruvail usually proving to have the best tolerance. There is controversy as to the effect of NSAIDs on the underlying gut disorder. Rampton and Slader (1981) have implicated NSAIDs in producing relapses of ulcerative proctocolitis, suggesting that interference with protective prostaglandins by prostaglandin synthetase inhibition may be the mechanism of this effect. In contrast, others have suggested that the beneficial effect of sulphasalazine is mediated through the same mechanism (Sharon *et al.*, 1978). In practice this does not seem to have proved a serious problem, although there are no substantial studies of treatment of arthritis and inflammatory bowel disease to provide more than anecdotal experience.

12.3.5 Whipple's disease

Sixty per cent of patients with Whipple's disease present with arthritis of enteropathic pattern. Biopsy studies show the same PAS-positive particles in the synovium as in the gut. As might be expected, the arthritis responds to appropriate antibiotic therapy, usually with tetracycline, and no other treatment is required. If synovitis persists after apparently adequate antibiotic therapy, this must be taken as a sign of non-response of the disease in general, and an alternative antibiotic should be used.

There is dispute as to whether there is a real association between AS and Whipple's disease. This has been highlighted by a case report of a patient with apparently typical clinical AS associated with Whipple's disease which responded to antibiotic therapy (Bowman *et al.*, 1983). The authors used the term 'pseudospondylitis' in this patient. If a true association does exist, treatment is identical to that of idiopathic AS.

12.4 REITER'S DISEASE: REACTIVE ARTHRITIS

Classically, Reiter's disease has been defined as the occurrence of urethritis, conjunctivitis and arthritis after infectious diarrhoea or venereally acquired non-specific urethritis. In Britain and the USA venereally acquired disease predominates, whereas the literature from continental Europe shows a predominance of enteropathic disease. Incomplete forms of Reiter's disease have been recognized for many years, but recently an increased number of sporadic cases of predominantly large joint polyarthritis after a variety of gut infections has been recognized (Table 12.2). There now seems no need for the concept

TABLE 12.2
Organisms known to precipitate reactive arthritis

Brucella abortus
Brucella melitensis
Campylobacter spp.
Clostridium difficile
Salmonella enteritidis
Salmonella typhimurium
Salmonella schwarzengrund
Salmonella okatie
Shigella dystenteriae
Shigella flexneri
Strongyloides stercolonis
Yersinia enterocolitica
Yersinia pseudotuberculosis

'Reiter's disease' to be retained; the concepts of sexually acquired reactive arthritis (SARA) and enteropathic reactive arthritis (ERA) appear adequate to cover the diseases involved, and the arthritides of all forms of this syndrome are similar enough to enable all to be considered together.

The essential component which needs to be kept constantly in mind is the high risk of recurrence and chronicity in these patients. There appears to be an increased risk of development of reactive arthritis in patients carrying HLA-B27, and carriers also appear to have more severe chronic disease and a greater tendency to develop spinal disease similar to ankylosing spondylitis (Leirisalo *et al.*, 1982).

12.4.1 NSAIDs

As with other members of the seronegative spondarthritis group, these drugs are the cornerstone of treatment for reactive arthritis. There are few comparative studies as reference sources, but personal experience suggests that indomethacin is particularly effective in this disease, and it is our drug of first choice. There is limited supporting evidence for this view in the literature (Lassus, 1976). Other NSAIDs such as ketoprofen (Juvakoski and Lassus, 1982) may be tried sequentially if indomethacin fails.

12.4.2 Second-line drugs

Although reactive arthritis is now known to have a high rate of chronicity, long-term studies to identify disease-modifying drugs have not been done. There appear to be two reasons for this. The initial episodes are often managed by venereologists, when the disease is sexually acquired, or general physicians when enteropathic. In general, neither group has traditionally given the type of long-term care and study which is the hallmark of a rheumatologist, and many of these patients have, in consequence, been followed up sporadically, if at all. Secondly, the progression of reactive arthritis appears to be more by way of isolated recurrences rather than the steady flow of exacerbations and remissions that characterize most rheumatic diseases. These recurrent episodes often have periods of symptomatic normality between them; they may also affect different tissues at different times, with the significance of, say, a recurrent episode of conjunctivitis or iritis some years after an episode of SARA being overlooked. These patients, especially if B27 positive, do carry a high risk of developing spondylitis, and while exercises may be more important in the long-term than drugs, supervision is essential to prevent eventual disability.

For these reasons, experience of second-line drugs is confined to anecdotes regarding penicillamine, which appears to be ineffective, and methotrexate, corticosteroids, ACTH and pulsed methylprednisolone, all of which appear to convey short-term benefits to some patients, but have unquantified long-term effects.

Some patients with Reiter's disease have shown some apparent response to methotrexate (Mullins *et al.*, 1966; Owen and Cohen, 1979) and we have treated one patient with prolonged severe disease unresponsive to all other medication who was rendered asymptomatic by this drug. One open study of sulphasalazine in 15 patients with chronic enteropathic reactive arthritis showed 11 to go into prolonged remission and the others showed some improvement (Mielants and Veys, 1985). The relationship of these findings to the inflammatory changes found in these patients on colonoscopy requires further elucidation.

12.4.3 Relationship between other tissues and joint disease

The time course of typical reactive arthritis was characterized by Noer (1966) in the 'experimental' epidemic of Reiter's disease that he described. Diarrhoea lasted for about eight days and was followed by urethritis. This lasted from about the twentieth to the thirtieth day. Conjunctivitis occurred between days 22 and 26, the last element of the disease to appear being arthritis, starting on about day 23 and lasting a month or more. This temporal relationship between the predisposing infection and the joint symptoms needs to be considered when taking a history from a patient with a large-joint oligoarthritis. Similarly, it must be noted that the presence of urethritis does not necessarily denote a venereal precipitation of the disease.

Recurrences of elements of complete 'Reiter's syndrome' may occur together or separately. It has been suggested that recurrent arthritis may be precipitated by further episodes of sexually acquired NSU, and for this reason some authorities suggest that a patient with a history of reactive arthritis should minimize this risk by wearing condoms, especially if there should be any extramarital sexual contact. Certainly, recurrent arthritis may be precipitated by further enteric infections (Chalmers *et al.*, 1978) – the life of the ascetic celibate appears the only one conveying relative freedom from recurrent disease, especially in those with B27.

12.4.4 Management strategy

On diagnosing reactive arthritis, it seems logical to treat any residual infection rigorously with appropriate antibiotics, thus reducing the immediate antigen load as much as possible. In most patients, however, the infective precipitant has long passed. The synovitis of reactive arthritis is often sufficiently intense and painful to require admission to hospital for bed rest and splintage of the inflamed joints. The systemic upset, often characterized by deranged liver function tests (Dawes, unpublished observations) may produce admission under non-rheumatological care from which patients should be rescued as soon as possible. Medication with indomethacin is started, and tensely distended effusions may require urgent aspiration in order to control pain. We have found the synovitis of reactive arthritis stubborn to control despite various combinations of NSAIDs, rest and physical methods of treatment. We have therefore increasingly resorted to the use of pulsed methylprednisolone to cut short the acute attack, which otherwise appears to have a natural history of about six to eight months.

Although all patients with reactive arthritis have a tendency to relapses and chronicity, this appears to be particularly so in those who are B27 positive. I therefore tissue type these patients as a prognostic guide, and give particular emphasis to follow-up exercises in the B27-positive patients. Most patients require exercises, individual treatment for episodes of skin, eye and urethral disease, and individual management for each future episode of joint disease. Those with a spondylitic posture are treated identically to idiopathic AS. A few patients have a rapid aggressive course of peripheral synovitis and enthesopathy, as well as spinal disease. They may require local or more general radiotherapy. We have had success in such patients with methotrexate, but there are no controlled studies of this type of treatment.

12.5 CONCLUSIONS

As can be seen from the preceding descriptions, all the seronegative spondarthritides have strong similarities, not only in their clinical courses but also in the management strategies required by them. All are bedevilled by a paucity of good-quality scientific evaluation of the drugs used in their management, and especially by a complete absence of studies which tell us whether or not we can modify their courses. Fortunately, most patients with seronegative spondarthritides do well, but this overall impression conceals the fact that some do quite horrendously badly. Relentlessly progressive seronegative arthritis is rare, but when it occurs the poverty of our therapeutic armamentarium is tragically exposed.

Management of this group of diseases calls for the usual therapeutic team employed in all rheumatology units, including rheumatologists, surgeons, therapists and nurses as well as social workers, appliance makers and chiropodists. The patient inevitably is the key member of the team, both as an individual and as a member of a local therapeutic group, or of a national group such as the National Ankylosing Spondylitis Society. The treatment team is greatly extended in many of these conditions because of major disease occurring outside the locomotor system. Unfortunately this association with other disciplines is sometimes unhappy, with the fundamental tenets of good rheumatological practice and patient care being ignored to the patients' long-term detriment. The seronegative spondarthritides are a group of diseases in which education of patients by the therapeutic team assumes enormous importance. It is a sad reflection of the paucity of rheumatological training, especially in the medical and nursing professions, that an equal amount of educational effort appears to be required directed towards our colleagues in other disciplines who share the care of these patients with us.

12.6　REFERENCES

Ansell, B. M., Major, G., Lyanage, S. P., Gumpel, J. M., Seifert, M. H., Mathews, J. A. and Engler, C. (1978) A comparative study of Butacote and Naprosyn in ankylosing spondylitis. *Ann. Rheum. Dis.*, 37, 436–9.

Bird, H. A. and Dixon, A. St. J. (1977) Failure of D-penicillamine to affect peripheral joint involvement in ankylosing spondylitis or HLA B27-associated arthropathy. *Ann. Rheum. Dis.*, 36, 289.

Black, R. L., O'Brien, W. M., Van Scott, E. J. (1964) Methotrexate therapy in psoriatic arthritis – double-blind study on 21 patients. *J. Am. Med. Assoc.*, 189, 743–7.

Bowman, C., Dieppe, P. and Settas, L. (1983) Remission of pseudospondylitis with treatment of Whipple's disease. *Br. J. Rheumatol.*, 22, 181–2.

Calcraft, B., Tildesley, G., Evans, K. T., Gravelle, H., Hole, D. and Lloyd, K. N. (1974) Azapropazone in the treatment of ankylosing spondylitis: a controlled clinical trial. *Rheumatol. Rehabil.*, 13, 23–9.

Calin, A. and Fries, J. F. (1975) Striking prevalence of ankylosing spondylitis in 'healthy' W27 positive males and females. *N. Engl. J. Med.*, 293, 835–9.

Chalmers, A., Kapgrove, R. E., Reynolds, W. J. and Urowitz, M. B. (1978) Postdiarrhoeal arthropathy of *Yersinia pseudotuberculosis. Can. Med. Assoc. J.*, 118, 515–16.

Christiansen, F. T., Hawkins, B. R., Dawkins, R. L., Owen, E. T. and Potter, R. M. (1979) The prevalence of ankylosing spondylitis among B27 positive normal individuals – a reassessment. *J. Rheumatol.*, 6, 713–18.

Cohen, L. M., Mittal, K. K., Schmid, F. R., Rogers, L. F. and Cohen, K. L. (1976) Increased risk for spondylitis stigmata in apparently healthy HLA W27 men. *Ann. Intern. Med.*, 84, 1–4.

Court Brown, W. M. and Doll, R. (1965) Mortality from cancer and other causes after radiotherapy for ankylosing spondylitis. *Br. Med. J.*, 2, 1327.

Cuthbert, M. F. (1974) Adverse reactions to non-steroidal antirheumatic drugs. *Curr. Med. Res. Opinion*, 2, 600–10.

Day, T. K. (1983) Intestinal perforation associated with osmotic slow-release indomethacin capsules. *Br. Med. J.*, **287**, 1671–2.

Dorwart, B. B., Gall, E. P., Schumacher, H. R. and Krauser, R. E. (1978) Chrysotherapy in psoriatic arthritis. *Arthr. Rheum.*, **21**, 513–15.

Editorial (1976) Anti-rheumatic drugs; plenty is not enough. *Br. Med. J.*, **1**, 59–60.

Feldges, D. H. and Barnes, C. G. (1974) Treatment of psoriatic arthropathy with either azathioprine or methotrexate. *Rheumatol. Rehabil.*, **13**, 120–4.

Gibson, T. and Laurent, R. (1980) Sulindac and indomethacin in the treatment of ankylosing spondylitis: a double-blind cross-over study. *Rheumatol. Rehabil.*, **19**, 189–92.

Godfrey, R., Gum., O. B., and Maltz, B. A. (1977) Evaluation of fenoprofen calcium (Nalfon) in ankylosing spondylitis. *Abstr. XIV Int. Congr. Rheumatol, San Francisco*, 168.

Golding, D. N. (1974) D-penicillamine in ankylosing spondylitis and polymyositis. *Postgr. Med. J., Suppl.*, pp. 62–5.

Hill, H. F. H. and Hill, A. G. S. (1973) Naprosyn in ankylosing spondylitis. in *Naprosyn in the Treatment of Rheumatic Diseases* (ed. G. A. Christie), Syntex Pharmaceuticals, Maidenhead, pp. 42–6.

Hopkins, R., Bird, H. A., Jones, H., Hill, J., Surrall, K. E., Astbury, C., Miller, A. and Wright, V. (1985) A double-blind controlled trial of etretinate (Tigason) and ibuprofen in psoriatic arthritis. *Ann. Rheum. Dis.*, **44**, 189–93.

Huskisson, E. C., Taylor, R. T., Burston, D., Chuter, P. J. and Hart, F. D. (1970) Evening indomethacin in the treatment of rheumatoid arthritis. *Ann. Rheum. Dis.*, **29**, 393–6.

Huskisson, E. C., Woolf, D. L., Balme, H. W., Scott, J. and Franklyn, S. (1976) Four new anti-inflammatory drugs: responses and variations. *Br. Med. J.*, **1**, 1048–9.

Jessop, J. D. (1976) Double-blind study of ketoprofen and phenylbutazone in ankylosing spondylitis. *Rheumatol. Rehabil. Suppl.*, 37–42.

Juvakoski, T. and Lassus, A. (1982) A double-blind evaluation of ketoprofen and indomethacin in Reiter's disease. *Scand. J. Rheumatol.*, **11**, 106–8.

Kapgrove, R. E., Little, A. H., Graham, D. C. and Rosen, P. S. (1980) Ankylosing spondylitis: survival in men with and without radiotherapy. *Arthr. Rheum.*, **23**, 57–61.

Kersley, G. D. (1968) Amethopterin (methotrexate) in connective tissue disease – psoriasis and polyarthritis. *Ann. Rheum. Dis.*, **27**, 64–6.

Lassus, A. (1976) A comparative pilot study of azapropazone and indomethacin in the treatment of psoriatic arthritis and Reiter's disease. *Curr. Med. Res. Opinion*, **4**, 65–9.

Leatham, P. A., Bird, H. A., Wright, V. and Fowler, P. D. (1982) The run-in period in trial design: a comparison of two non-steroidal anti-inflammatory agents in psoriatic arthropathy. *Agents Actions*, **12**, 221–4.

Leirisalo, M., Skylv, G., Kousa, M., Voipio-Pulkki, L-M., Suoranta, H., Nissila, M., Hvidman, L., Nielsen, E. D., Svejgaard, A., Tillikainen, A. and Laitinen, O. (1982) Follow-up study on patients with Reiter's disease and reactive arthritis with special reference to HLA B27. *Arthr. Rheum.*, **25**, 249–59.

Lorig, K., Lubeck, D., Kraines, R. G., Seleznick, M. and Holman, H. R. (1985) Outcomes of self-help education for patients with arthritis. *Arthr. Rheum.*, **28**, 680–5.

McAdam, L. P., O'Hanlan, M. A. and Willkens, R. F. (1981) Piroxicam in ankylosing spondylitis: a 14-week controlled double-blind study comparing piroxicam to phenylbutazone, in *Proc. 15th Int. Congr. Rheumatol.*, Paris, France. Pub. Academy Professional Information Services, Maddison Avenue, New York, USA, pp. 87–94.

Mielants, H. and Veys, E. M. (1985) Sulphasalazine (Salazopyrin) in HLA–B27 related reactive arthritis. Abstracts of the XVIth International Congress of Rheumatology, Sydney, f. 107.

Mitchell, E. P. and Schein, P. S. (1982) Gastrointestinal toxicity of chemotherapeutic agents. *Seminars Oncol.*, 9, 52–64.

Moll, J. M. H., Haslock, I., Macrae, I. F. and Wright, V. (1974) Associations between ankylosing spondylitis, psoriatic arthritis, Reiter's disease, the intestinal arthropathies and Behçet's syndrome. *Medicine (Baltimore)*, 53, 343–64.

Mullins, J. F., Maberry, J. D. and Stone, O. J. (1966) Reiter's syndrome treated with folic acid antagonists. *Arch. Dermatol.*, 94, 335.

Nahir, A. M. and Scharf, Y. (1980) A comparative study of diclofenac and sulindac in ankylosing spondylitis. *Rheumatol. Rehabil.*, 19, 193–8.

Nikolic, J. and Lukacevic, D. (1975) Ibuprofen ('Brufen') in the treatment of ankylosing spondylitis. *Curr. Med. Res. Opinion*, 3, 573–5.

Noer, H. R. (1966) An 'experimental' epidemic of Reiter's syndrome. *J. Am. Med. Assoc.*, 197, 693–7.

Owen, E. T. and Cohen, M. L. (1979) Methotrexate in Reiter's disease. *Ann. Rheum. Dis.*, 38, 48–50.

Peter, E. and Veress, M. (1975) Comparison of the action of naproxen and indomethacin in the double-blind test on post-midnight pain in patients with ankylosing spondylitis. *Arzneimittelforsch*, 25, 324–5.

Rampton, D. S. and Slader, G. E. (1981) Relapse of ulcerative proctocolitis during treatment with non-steroidal anti-inflammatory drugs. *Postgrad. Med. J.*, 57, 297–9.

Rheinberger, K. (1976) Efficacy and tolerance of Voltaren and indomethacin in patients with ankylosing spondylitis. *Therapiewoche*, 26, 2916–19.

Richter, M. B., Kinsella, P. and Corbett, M. (1980) Gold in psoriatic arthropathy. *Ann. Rheum. Dis.*, 39, 279–80.

Roberts, M. E. T., Wright, V., Hill, A. G. S. and Mehra, A. C. (1976) Psoriatic arthritis: follow-up study. *Ann. Rheum. Dis.*, 35, 206–12.

Rubenstein, H., Klamut, M., Adams, E. and Sundstrom, W. (1985) Liver biopsy in patients with rheumatoid arthritis receiving methotrexate. Abstracts of the XVIth International Congress of Rheumatology, Sydney, p. 128.

Sharon, P., Ligumsky, M., Rachmilewitz, D. and Zor, U. (1978) Role of prostaglandins in ulcerative colitis: enhanced production during active disease and inhibition by sulphasalazine. *Gastroenterology*, 75, 638–40.

Shipley, M., Berry, H. and Bloom, B. (1980) A double-blind cross-over trial of indomethacin, fenoprofen and placebo in ankylosing spondylitis, with comments on patient assessment. *Rheumatol. Rehabil.*, 19, 122–5.

Simpson, M. R., Simpson, N. R. W., Scott, B. O. and Beatty, D. C. (1966) A controlled study of flufenamic acid in ankylosing spondylitis. *Ann. Phys. Med. (Suppl.)*, 126–8.

Stevens, M., Morrison, M. and Sturrock, R. D. (1985) Penicillamine in ankylosing spondylitis: a double-blind placebo-controlled trial. *J. Rheumatol.*, 12, 735–7.

Sturrock, R. D. and Hart, F. D. (1974) Double-blind cross-over comparison of indomethacin, flurbiprofen and placebo in ankylosing spondylitis. *Ann. Rheum. Dis.*, 33, 129–31.

Sydnes, O. A. (1981) Comparison of piroxicam and indomethacin in ankylosing spondylitis: a double-blind cross-over trial. *Br. J. Clin. Pract.*, 35, 40–4.

Van Gerwen, F., Van der Korst, J. K. and Gribnau, F. W. J. (1978) Double-blind trial of naproxen and phenylbutazone in ankylosing spondylitis. *Ann. Rheum. Dis.*, 37, 85–8.

Wasner, C., Britton, M. C., Kraines, G., Kaye, R. L., Bobrove, A. M. and Fries, J. F. (1981) Non-steroidal anti-inflammatory agents in rheumatoid arthritis and anky-losing spondylitis. *J. Am. Med. Assoc.*, **246**, 2168–72.

Weinstein, G. D. and Frost, P. (1971) Methotrexate for psoriasis. A new therapeutic schedule. *Arch. Dermatol.*, **103**, 33–8.

Williams, H. J., Willkens, R. F., Samuelson, C. O., Alarcón, G. S., Guttadavria, M., Yarboro, C., Polisson, R. P., Weiner, S. R., Luggen, M. E., Billingsley, L. M., Dahl, S. L., Egger, M. J., Reading, J. C. and Ward, J. R. (1985) Comparison of low-dose oral pulse methotrexate and placebo in the treatment of rheumatoid arthritis: a controlled clinical trial. *Arthr. Rheum.*, **28**, 721–30.

Willkens, Clegg, Ward, Marks, Greene, Tolan and Roth (1985) Liver biopsies in patients on low dose pulse methotrexate (MTX) for the treatment of R.A. Abstracts of the XVIth International Congress of Rheumatology, Sydney. f. 15. (NB: No initials quoted in abstract.)

Zachariae, E., Kragballe, K. and Zachariae, H. (1985) Methotrexate in psoriatic arthritis. Abstracts of the XVIth International Congress of Rheumatology, Sydney, p. 131.

Zachariae, H., Søgaard, H. and Zachariae, E. (1985) Methotrexate toxicity in psoriasis and psoriatic arthritis. Abstracts of the XVIth International Congress of Rheumatology, Sydney, p. 132.

CHAPTER 13

Osteoarthrosis, spinal degenerative disease and other back pain syndromes

Sunil P. Liyanage

13.1 Osteoarthrosis
13.2 Spinal degenerative disease

13.3 Other back pain syndromes
13.4 References

13.1 OSTEOARTHROSIS

13.1.1 Pathogenesis

This is perhaps the commonest form of joint disease. Its prevalence is difficult to estimate accurately, but it is generally believed that about five million people in the United Kingdom are affected, causing a loss of 4.7 million days from work per year (Wood, 1976). Even so, it was not recognized as a separate entity until the last century. The archaic name *arthritis deformans* gave way to *osteoarthritis*; but, as it is widely regarded as a degenerative disease, the term *osteoarthrosis* has been in vogue during the last two decades. However, the simplistic concept of 'wear and tear' occurring in those of advancing years is no longer tenable as new evidence sheds light on the likely series of pathogenetic changes that take place in the joint.

Chondrocyte injury is associated with the liberation of several enzymes (proteolytic and lysosomic), reducing the production of proteoglycans that mask and protect the collagen fibres. These in turn become rough and fissured, and cartilage is destroyed. Cartilage destruction is accompanied by synovial inflammation which potentiates cartilage breakdown, but whether synovial changes are the primary event is not known. Synovial inflammation is thought to be due to the presence of a free sulphated proteoglycan in the joint space

(Chrisman *et al.*, 1965). Bollet (1969) has shown that proteoglycan release is related to mechanical factors.

Subchondral bone is laid down, but this too becomes eroded. Synovitis, if present, is a secondary event, and is marked by lymphocytic infiltration. Crystals of hydroxyapatite and pyrophosphate have been found in the synovial fluid and soft tissues of patients with osteoarthrosis (Dieppe and Calvert, 1983). These crystals may serve a pathogenetic role by triggering chondrocytes after endocytosis.

These pathological changes lead to the typical radiographic appearances of localized loss of joint space, marginal sclerosis, osteophytes and subchondral cysts. Progressive changes are indicated by buttressing, bony collapse, loose bodies and malalignment (Moll, 1976).

13.1.2 Clinical features

The clinical picture of generalized osteoarthrosis with Heberden's nodes on the terminal interphalangeal joints is usually seen in middle-aged females. The first carpometacarpal, first metatarsophalangeal, knee and cervical apophyseal joints are often involved in this polyarticular form of degenerative disease (Kellgren, 1961). The genetic basis of this entity stems from a higher prevalence of multiple joint osteoarthrosis in relatives of both sexes, and also of Heberden's nodes in female relatives (Stecher, 1955). Multiple osteoarthrosis without Heberden's nodes is an entity usually observed in men, and mainly affects the hips and, less often, the first carpometacarpal joints. Relatives of these probands have an increased prevalence of polyarticular osteoarthrosis and of seronegative inflammatory polyarthritis. Monoarthrosis is usually related to obvious or non-recognized trauma where there may be occupational factors, repeated minor trauma in sports, or damage from other disease.

A form of osteoarthrosis ('erosive osteoarthritis') involving the interphalangeal joints of the fingers is characterized clinically by painful episodes of inflammatory swelling (Crain, 1961). Radiologically, the typical changes of osteophyte formation, joint narrowing and marginal sclerosis are seen, but there may be erosive changes particularly in the central parts of the joints (Fig. 13.1). The apophyseal joints of the cervical spine may be involved in this syndrome which has a genetic basis, and is commoner in women of middle age. There is a tendency to bony ankylosis. The histological appearances in the synovium are very similar to those of rheumatoid arthritis, but the changes in the cartilage resemble typical osteoarthrosis.

Kashin–Beck disease is of interest. In eastern Siberia, a form of arthritis has been seen in children, teenagers as well as adults. These patients have bilateral symmetrical degenerative disease of the wrists, fingers and some lower limb joints, leading to much functional disability. It has been found that the cereal grain in this area is contaminated with a fungus. With the removal of this grain from the market, the disease has virtually disappeared (Nesterov, 1964).

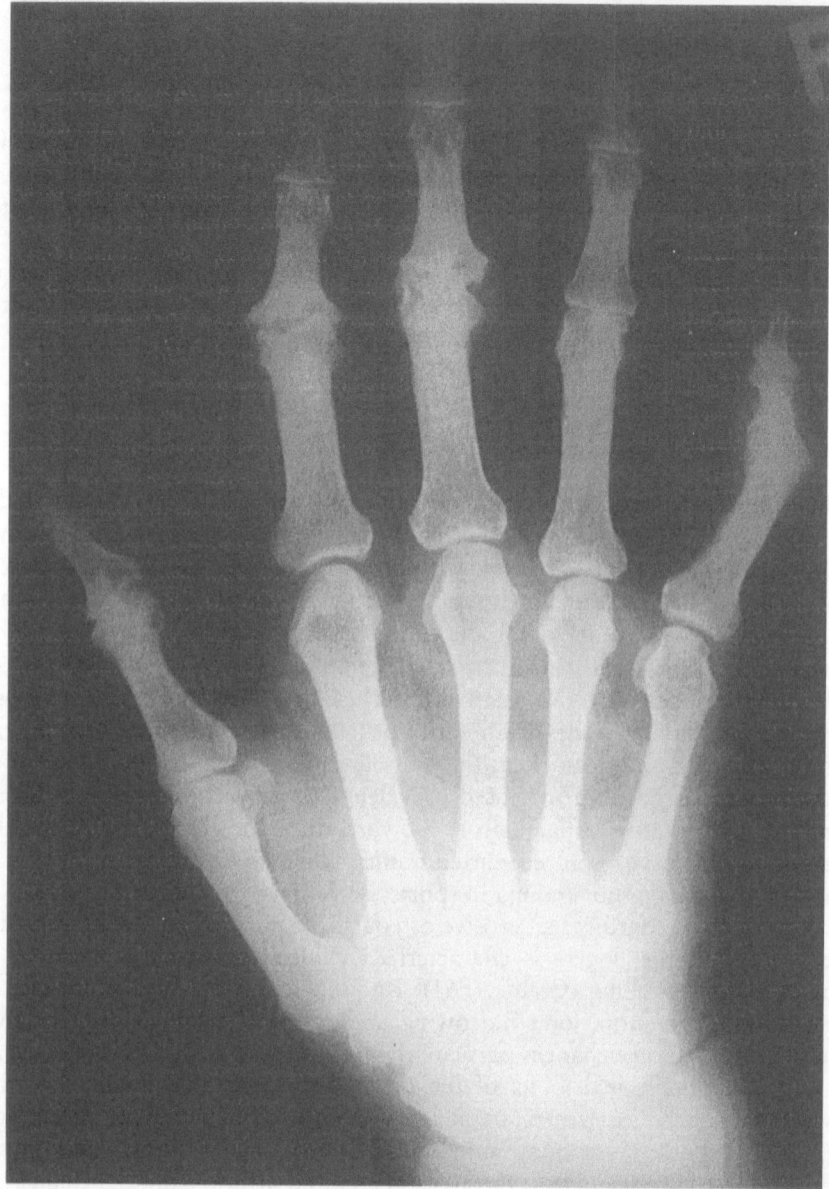

Figure 13.1 Erosive osteoarthritis, with predominant involvement of proximal inter-phalangeal joints. (The patient was a 67-year-old woman with no history of psoriasis, no Heberden's nodes, no morning stiffness, ESR 8, test for rheumatoid factor negative.)

13.1.3   Management

(a) *General*

Explanation of the nature of the condition, reassurance that it is not a systemic disease, that it will not usually lead to severe destructive changes, should be undertaken at the outset. Even though academics and research workers will continue to debate the role of inflammation in the causation of osteoarthrosis, it is probably best to stress to the patient the mechanical and local factors in terms of wear and tear. The degree of pain waxes and wanes spontaneously, but episodes may be triggered by trauma. With this explanation, it is helpful to issue a patients' handbook available free of charge from the Arthritis and Rheumatism Council. If the patient is already severely handicapped, information about Arthritis Care which is a voluntary organization with local branches may be welcome.

Patients may have to modify their habits to avoid remaining in one position for prolonged periods. They should be encouraged to remain active. Activities in daily living need to be assessed and the appropriate aids provided to help with dressing, cooking, bathing, showering and mobility. Dietary factors are probably of no relevance. Osteoarthrotic patients tend to be overweight, and it would seem reasonable to encourage them to lose weight, although this is a difficult task because of reduction in physical activity resulting from pain. However, there is no convincing evidence that weight reduction favourably influences the course of osteoarthrosis.

In the lower limbs it may be necessary to correct inequality of leg length, as osteoarthrosis occurs in the knee or hip joint of the longer leg. In the presence of valgus of varus deformity of the knee, a wedge correction is made either inside or outside the shoe.

(b) *Physiotherapy*

Physiotherapy, although not in any way curative, is helpful in relieving pain and stiffness in most patients (Robinson, 1981). Hot packs, infra-red heat, shortwave diathermy, wax, and ice packs can relieve pain, albeit temporarily. Whatever the mechanism of action, and whether it be placebo-mediated, the fact that pain can be relieved is relevant to the management of the problem, as it is reassuring. Exercises to strengthen muscles or increase the range of movement are more important in the longer term, and patients must follow a regular programme. In this regard, hydrotherapy is invaluable when dealing with the larger joints such as the hip or knee.

(c) *Drugs*

The aim of treatment is to relieve pain, thereby restoring function. At present, there are no drugs that modify the course of degenerative disease, and studies of experimental animals have been largely negative in this respect, with the exception of cartilage healing in salicylate-treated animals in one study (Simmons and Chrisman, 1965). Time spent in explaining the aims and limitations of treatment is time well spent, as co-operation and understanding will help acceptance. It may not be possible to abolish pain completely, but the patient may accept this as a very satisfactory outcome. On the other hand, the same degree of pain relief may continue to generate grumbles and dissatisfaction if the aims have not been adequately explained, or indeed if psychogenic factors predominate.

In most patients, and certainly in those with early osteoarthrosis, it would seem logical to use a simple analgesic such as paracetamol. This is effective in mild pain and produces very little gastric intolerance, but has no anti-inflammatory activity. Two tablets (1 g) may be taken on demand, and up to 8 tablets can be used in a day. Although safe in therapeutic doses, paracetamol is predictably associated with hepatic necrosis when taken in overdose, and the drug is becoming popular for suicidal purposes (Clark *et al.*, 1973) (mortality 2–3%); 15 g or more of the drug is invariably associated with hepatotoxicity, and in children the dose is proportionately smaller (Nogen and Bremner, 1978). Although the degree of liver damage is dose-related in animals (Mitchell *et al.*, 1973), in man the dose taken does not always correlate well with clinical outcome. Paracetamol should be used with caution in the presence of liver disease.

Dextropropoxyphene is an alternative preparation, but not often used on its own. It has a plasma half-life of 15 hours, and its active metabolite norpropoxyphene has a half-life of 23 hours. With regular dosage schedules there is accumulation over 4 days, producing blood levels five times as high as after initial dosage. The pharmacokinetics indicate that it is theoretically not a suitable drug for use as an 'on demand' analgesic. However, a combination tablet containing dextropropoxyphene and paracetamol (co-proxamol Distalgesic) is the most widely prescribed analgesic in general practice, and patient satisfaction is high. In the few controlled studies reported, this combination appears to be more effective than paracetamol alone in dealing with rheumatological pain. No more than 8 tablets of this combination should be given in a 24-hour period, and patients should be warned of interaction with alcohol. Self-poisoning with this drug has become frequent and has attained notoriety. The mortality rate is at least 15% (Carson and Carson, 1977). However, dextroproproxyphene is a useful drug when used as recommended.

In moderate pain, usually in the hip and knee joints, codeine phosphate 30 mg may be repeated up to four times a day. Constipation is a side effect, which unfortunately assumes greater significance because of old wives' tales linking constipation with the aetiology of most diseases, especially arthritic conditions! Dihydrocodeine is also effective in relieving such pain, and the use of one tablet (30 mg) rather than two, causes less problems without proportionate reduction in analgesic activity.

Buprenorphine is a newer drug with the novelty of sublingual administration. Pain relief is rapid in onset, and lasts several hours. Side effects such as nausea and light-headedness preclude its use more widely. Other narcotic analgesics, such as meptazinol and nefopam, may be used in more severe pain. Narcotics which may lead to dependence or addiction should be avoided in chronic joint disease. Most patients with osteoarthrosis do well with little drug medication, and this should not be forced on them if they do not require it. Indeed, some patients refuse medication on the grounds that taking it implies 'giving in' or that it may lead to 'addiction'.

In the more severe cases, and also with overt inflammation, one is more likely to succeed with the use of NSAIDs. This observation is in keeping with current concepts of the biochemical inflammatory changes that occur in osteoarthrotic joints (Lee *et al.*, 1974). Indeed, some clinicians always use this class of drugs rather than analgesic preparations. These drugs should be prescribed for regular use, rather than on demand. In the United States, aspirin is the favoured drug, but in the United Kingdom, where dozens of other NSAIDs are available and the State is expected to absorb drug costs, it is fashionable to start therapy with a non-aspirin drug. Only a specialist in the field could possibly know the full range of NSAIDs well. Others should familiarize themselves fully with a few of these agents, and use them with confidence and knowledge of adverse effects. Any drug used must be given an adequate trial, and if necessary the dose must be increased to the maximum recommended or to tolerable levels within the recommended range. On the other hand, if side effects occur with a useful drug, the dose may be lowered. It is usually possible to see a response within two weeks.

There is a marked individual variation in response, and it may be necessary to switch from one preparation to another, as it is difficult to predict response. No single drug has been shown to be superior to another. Thus, the initial choice of drug may depend on adverse effects, convenient dosage, familiarity, and other undefinable factors. Most of the drugs are associated with some degree of gastrointestinal intolerance, some produce rashes, and a few have side effects on the central nervous system. Drugs such as phenylbutazone, which was the only alternative to aspirin until about 20 years ago, cause marrow suppression and have no real place in the management of osteoarthrosis. Fortunately in the UK the prescription of this drug has recently been restricted to hospital use in ankylosing spondylitis only. One should be aware of drug interactions, especially with highly protein-bound preparations such as warfarin and anticonvulsants. Sulindac has little action on renal prostaglandins, and does not influence the hypotensive effect of diuretics. Benorylate suspension 10 ml b.d. delivers an anti-inflammatory dose of aspirin, but benorylate tablets 2 t.d.s. do not. Paracetamol is a constituent of benorylate and co-proxamol; hence these two drugs should not be prescribed together. Many of the patients will be elderly; the metabolism of drugs in this age group may be different from that in healthy volunteers and younger patients. A drug recommended once or twice a day is much more likely to result in good compliance than one which has to be taken several times a day. The question of avascular necrosis of the femoral head from the use of NSAIDs is an overstressed and doubtful concept, and is not an argument to deny a patient a potentially beneficial drug.

It is difficult to justify the use of one preparation and not another, but the popular choices are naproxen 500 mg b.d., ibuprofen 400 mg t.d.s., indomethacin 25 mg t.d.s., piroxicam 20 mg o.d, and fenbufen 600 mg nocte. In practice, a NSAID is given on a regular basis and this is supplemented with simple analgesics on demand.

Osteoarthrotic joints tend to stiffen after rest, and this immobility stiffness may be more troublesome than pain. Morning stiffness may be present, but is never as marked as in the inflammatory arthropathies. NSAIDs are indicated for the relief of stiffness in the joints. Morning stiffness may be relieved by the use of such an agent at bedtime. Indomethacin 75 mg orally or 100 mg as a suppository was one of the earliest regimens recommended, but many of the propionic acid derivatives or an oxicam may be used for this purpose.

The slow acting, disease-modifying drugs used in rheumatoid arthritis have not been considered to be indicated in osteoarthrosis. However, in view of the increasing knowledge of the inflammatory aspects, there is some interest in this field. Oral corticosteroids have no place in this disease.

For further details on NSAIDs see Chapter 7 and Huskisson (1978), Hart (1978, 1980), and Moll (1983).

(d) *Intra-articular injections*

Intra-articular therapy has less part to play in osteoarthrosis compared with rheumatoid arthritis, and Shah and Wright (1967) have shown normal saline to be as effective as corticosteroids in the treatment of osteoarthrosis of the knee. However, a single joint that remains troublesome, or shows signs of inflammation can be helped with an intra-articular corticosteroid injection. The first carpometacarpal and the knee joints are easily accessible, and respond well. Hydrocortisone acetate is the preparation used most, as it is cheap and effective. The longer-acting suspensions such as methylprednisolone and triamcinolone hexacetonide may be used if the effect of the standard injection is too short lived. A joint should not be injected if there is a suspicion of infection, or if there has been a recent fracture through the joint. An aseptic technique should be observed, but there is no need for operating-theatre sterility. With care, a joint may be injected just as safely in the patient's home or practitioner's surgery as in a hospital out-patient clinic. Unless the clinician is particularly skilled, it is kinder to use a local anaesthetic during this procedure. It is best to avoid repeated injections, and most rheumatologists would inject one joint only two or three times a year. In many discussions on this topic, reference is made to a report on joint damage after intra-articular steroid injections; this is a case report of one patient in whom one knee had been injected 32 times and the other knee 20 times within 14 months (Bentley and Goodfellow, 1969)! In a retrospective study of 65 knees injected, a minimum of 15 times in 4 years and up to a maximum of 167 in 12 years, the results did not support the contention that this led inevitably to rapid joint destruction (Balch *et al.*, 1977).

In painful osteoarthrosis of the knee, one may find that there is no effusion and that the tenderness is not over the joint line, but diffusely over the wide insertion of the medial collateral ligament into the tibia. This represents an enthesopathy, where there is inflammation of the soft tissue attachment to bone. Infiltration of the tender area with a mixture of local anaesthetic and hydrocortisone, a simple procedure, can result in surprisingly good relief of pain.

(e) *Surgery*

When pain is unrelieved by physical measures and drug therapy, and becomes intolerable, or restricts mobility or function, surgery should be considered. As synovitis, if present, is mild and probably 'secondary', synovectomy is very rarely recommended. If there is mechanical malalignment, this could be corrected with an osteotomy of one bone or both, sometimes incorporating a wedge resection. If the joint is stable and has a reasonable range of movement, this procedure is successful in relieving pain in about two-thirds of patients. In the presence of more severe damage, arthroplasy is necessary. This may comprise an excision of the joint or of a small bone. Replacement arthroplasty of the larger joints is carried out with a metal-on-polythene prosthesis; in the joints of the hand and big toe a silastic implant is used.

The results of hip arthroplasty are uniformly and predictably good whether the operation involves partial replacement (Apley *et al.*, 1969) or total replacement (McKee, 1971; Owens, 1971). Although total replacement has now largely superseded partial replacement, the latter is still useful in patients in whom the acetabulum is still intact, such as in avascular necrosis of the femoral head. Arthrodesis is rarely done, but offers good pain relief.

(f) *Acupuncture*

The resurgence of interest in acupuncture, even though this has been in use for over two thousand years, stems partly from the exchange of clinical expertise after the visit of former U.S. President Nixon to China.

Additional impetus has come in the last two decades from neurophysiological research (Wyke, 1976). According to the gate-control theory of pain, a gate-like mechanism may be opened or closed in varying degrees, such that signals from injured tissues may be blocked and fail to reach the brain (Melzack and Wall, 1965). Acupuncture stimulation activates a greater proportion of large fibres than small fibres, tending to close the gate and block pain signals. Acupuncture treatment after local anaesthetic blockade of skin and underlying muscle fails to increase the pain threshold in volunteers, whereas there was an increase in threshold when acupuncture was given without local anaesthetic or with blockage of skin only. A second modulating mechanism involves the powerful inhibitory influence of portions of the brainstem operating via descending fibres which act on the spinal gating system. Experimental electrical stimulation of the reticular formation of rats gives an analgesic effect which outlasts the period of stimulation. Pain perception may be modulated in yet another way involving descending fibres from the cortex. This is dependent on psychological processes such as anxiety, suggestion, and past memory, and may be associated with the placebo response.

The gate-control theory does not clarify how acupuncture needles may affect distant body areas. A breakthrough was the demonstration that a pain-relieving substance in the cerebrospinal fluid of an acupuncture-stimulated rabbit could be transmitted to another animal whose pain threshold rose immediately (Chang, 1978). These chemical substances are enkephalins and endorphins, and their effect could be blocked by naloxone.

Melzack (1978) has recently reviewed work on the mechanism of acupuncture pain relief, and 'hyperstimulation analgesia' is a term that provides a common thread through these studies. For example, dry needling or intense cold (Travell and Rinzler, 1952), injection of normal saline (Sola and Williams, 1956) and transcutaneous electrical stimulation (Melzack, 1978) relieve certain forms of myofascial or visceral pain, including low-back pain sometimes for days. Anderson *et al.* (1974) performed a controlled study and showed that intense stimulation of trigger points produces significantly greater pain relief than does placebo. Short-acting local anaesthetic blocks of trigger points will also give rise to prolonged and sometimes permanent pain relief (Livingstone, 1943; Travell and Rinzler, 1952; Bonica 1953).

How successful is acupuncture in clinical practice? The first point to be stressed is that the general evidence points to its success as an analgesic but not as a 'cure'. However, even claims regarding the former may not be as impressive as we have been led to believe from Chinese practitioners in the early 1970s. Indeed, in the field of surgical analgesia pooled impressions suggest that it is effective in only 10% of patients.

With regard to rheumatological applications of acupuncture, little is known about this from objective sources. However, the study of Godfrey and Morgan (1978) is worth noting. These authors showed that among 193 patients with painful conditions due to various rheumatic disorders (degenerative disc disease, osteoarthrosis, lumbosacral pain, cervical strain, tennis elbow, bursitis) reduced pain was achieved almost as effectively by inappropriate stimulation (56.5%) as by classical acupuncture (68.2%). Similar levels of success in locomotor disorders were achieved by Turban and Urlich (1978) using acupuncture but the 'success' rating was based entirely on patients' judgement.

In a study involving rheumatoid knees (Man and Baragar, 1974), one knee was injected with hydrocortisone and the other was treated on one occasion only with acupuncture needles placed either correctly or inappropriately. The steroid injection resulted in some local improvement and thus enabled comparison with the effects of acupuncture. All patients receiving correctly placed acupuncture obtained pain relief when assessed after 24 hours, and most had relief even after 3 months. There were no changes in the signs of local inflammation. In the control group, pain relief was transient and lasted less than a day.

Thus, acupuncture may have a role in offering pain relief in patients with degenerative joint disease. As a full knowledge of anatomy and sterilization techniques is essential, and diagnostic acumen is desirable, qualified medical practitioners would be in the best position to undertake acupuncture treatment.

It is concluded that further research is needed before acupuncture can enjoy a firmer grip on conventional medicine in the UK, and more particularly, in the field of rheumatology in which convincing objective evidence for its value is still sparse.

13.2   SPINAL DEGENERATIVE DISEASE

13.2.1   Types

This may involve the cartilaginous intervertebral discs, the synovial apophyseal joints, or the fibrous ligaments.

(a) *Disc degeneration*

Physiological changes within the discs occur with normal ageing. These include dehydration of the nucleus pulposus (Gower and Pedrini, 1969), decrease in the fixed charge density of the nucleus (Urban and Maroudas, 1979), and increase in its ratio of keratan to chondroitin (Adams and Muir, 1976). Clefts form and extend into the annulus fibrosus and the disc loses height. The outer fibres of the annulus bulge, the cartilaginous end plates undergo degeneration, and the adjacent bony trabeculae become thickened. Sometimes the protrusion may be into the body of the vertebra above or below. These changes result in the characteristic radiological appearances of loss of disc height, vacuum phenomenon, bony sclerosis and occasional Schmorl's nodes (Schmorl and Junghanns, 1971). The lower lumbar and cervical regions are commonly affected, and the process begins in the third or fourth decade. The usual posterolateral protrusion results in pressure on the corresponding nerve root.

(b) *Spondylosis*

The primary lesion is probably in the outer fibres of the annulus fibrosus. Their attachment to the vertebral rim is broken, and the disc material bulges forwards especially if the nucleus pulposus is still turgid and near normal. Osteophytes develop at the sites where the anterior longitudinal ligament is lifted off near the edge of the vertebrae. These bony outgrowths initially extend horizontally and later vertically around the bulged disc (Collins, 1949; Vernon-Roberts, 1976). This results in restriction of movement of the spine. In the neck, large osteophytes may cause dysphagia. As the changes are essentially anterior, neurological involvement is extremely rare.

(c) *Neurocentral osteoarthrosis*

In the cervical spine, between the third and seventh vertebrae, there are neurocentral joints which may undergo degenerative disease. This is caused by progressive approximation of the joint surfaces as a result of loss of disc height. Osteophyte formation leads to the radiological appearance of elongation of these joints. The clinical features are related to entrapment of nerve roots and involvement of the vertebral arteries.

(d) *Apophyseal osteoarthrosis*

The vertebral arches are linked by the synovial apophyseal joints (Badgley, 1941). Degenerative disease is invariable after the fifth decade, and stems from stresses associated with trauma or abnormal curvatures. Pain has been attributed to the rich innervation of these joints. Nerve root entrapment and restriction of movement are frequent features of osteoarthrosis of these joints. Other synovial articulations exist in the thoracic spine as costovertebral and costotransverse joints.

(e) *Ligamentous degeneration*

The various spinal ligaments including the anterior longitudinal ligament, posterior longitudinal ligament, ligamenta flava, interspinous ligaments, ligamentum nuchae and iliolumbar ligaments may undergo degenerative change. This may be secondary to changes in the discs, leading to ligamentous laxity and abnormal stresses at the attachments. Pain and tenderness are features as the ligaments are richly supplied with nerves (Wyke, 1976).

13.2.2 Management

(a) *General*

As in peripheral degenerative joint disease, the importance of explanation and reassurance cannot be overemphasized. Radiographs confirm the typical changes of degenerative disease, but also serve to exclude other causes of back pain. In patients with intervertebral disc degeneration and in those with spondylosis, it is better to be pedantic and avoid a reference to *arthritis*, as this has unfortunate connotations.

(b) *Rest*

In most instances of acute back pain, it is wise to rest. Often the pain resolves in a few days. If the pain is severe, the patient should be advised to rest on a firm mattress, with a board underneath, or even on the floor. What most patients regard as rest, is staying off work. Unless the pain is disabling it is difficult to rest completely. Occasionally, it is necessary to admit such patients to hospital. The addition of continuous traction probably confers no extra benefit, apart from enforcing complete rest.

(c) *Drugs*

The principles outlined for osteoarthrosis of peripheral joints apply here. Simple analgesics are useful in most instances where the pain is mild. Narcotic non-addictive drugs are necessary when the pain is more severe. Where the pain is subacute or chronic, NSAIDs taken regularly seem to help. In spinal disease, muscle spasm is a feature and contributes to the pain. Thus, in acute problems with moderate to severe pain, the combination of an analgesic and muscle relaxant has much to offer, even though in general terms polypharmacy is deprecated. This regimen would supplement a programme of strict rest. Patients lying flat on their back may tolerate 20–60 mg diazepam or up to 800 mg chlormezanone per day in divided doses.

In the treatment of long-standing pain in ambulant patients, the combination of an analgesic with meprobamate or chlormezanone is well tolerated. It has been shown to help cervical pain, but in the heterogeneous group of patients in a multicentre study, no benefit was shown for low back pain (Berry *et al.*, 1981).

(d) *Mobilization and manipulation*

These techniques have come under critical scrutiny and had their scientific basis examined (Farfan, 1980) in the past few years. In a large multicentre study (Doran and Newell, 1975), there were four treatment schedules. In the manipulation (rotational) group, a few patients responded well and quickly; patients treated with other forms of physiotherapy responded slowly; those given corsets showed a similar response; patients given analgesics only fared marginally worse. When reviewed after six weeks, there were no differences in the four groups. Two other important clinical trials of rotational manipulation have been published recently, one from an industrial setting (Glover *et al.*, 1974) the other from a hospital setting (Evans *et al.*, 1978). In the report by Glover and colleagues, compared with de-tuned short-wave diathermy, improvement was in favour of the manipulated group but did not achieve statistical significance. However, in the study by Evans *et al.* there was some statistically significant evidence to support the value of manipulation. Studies from a single centre (Sims-Williams *et al.*, 1978, 1979), revealed that in general practice patients, mobilization was superior to placebo physiotherapy at one month, and the difference was less apparent after 3 months; in hospital patients, there were no significant differences in the two groups. It was concluded that the benefits of mobilization and manipulation for low back pain are probably restricted to hastening recovery in patients likely to improve spontaneously. However, diluted in these statistics are the patients who responded very rapidly to manipulative therapy and who were better after one or a few treatments.

(e) Epidural injection

This form of therapy for low back pain and sciatica has been used for over 70 years. Evans (1930) reported the first series of patients with sciatica treated with this method, and Kelman (1944) observed that pain relief outlasted the expected period of activity of the injected local anaesthetic. The method was popularized by Cyriax (1975) who advocated this technique as the treatment of first choice for patients with discogenic pain in whom root symptoms and neurological signs were present. Until recently the only drug was a local anaesthetic, and this was diluted in up to 50 ml of saline. However, the addition of a corticosteroid preparation has now become routine. Many studies have been conducted to establish the value of this treatment and to assess various injected materials. A volume effect is believed to be less important than considered before, and the amounts vary from 20 to 50 ml. In an attempt to derive the longest benefit, the longer-acting drugs are now used widely, 10 or 20 ml of 0.25% plain bupivacaine is diluted in an equal volume of isotonic saline, the injection being carried out using the caudal route, though some favour the lumbar route. Methylprednisolone 80 mg or triamcinolone hexacetonide 60 mg is instilled (Yates, 1978). A testimony to the safety of this procedure is the large number of epidural injections done on out-patients. In addition to being safe the procedure is also very well tolerated (Dilke *et al.*, 1973; Snoek *et al.*, 1977).

(f) Surgery

In a minority of patients, those with intractable nerve root pressure, manifest as persisting severe pain, signs of dural tension and a neurological deficit, surgery brings immediate relief (Harmon, 1963; Freebody *et al.*, 1971). The standard procedure has been a laminectomy, but in recent years a limited operation referred to as fenestration of the disc has been found to be adequate. Most operations involve the L5/S1 or L4/L5 disc. Contrast radiography (radiculography) using water-soluble dye is indicated only as a prelude to surgery, and not for diagnostic reasons only. Occasionally, in the presence of instability, spinal fusion may be necessary; extensive decompression is undertaken to relieve symptoms of spinal stenosis.

(g) *Chemonucleolysis*

Chymopapain is a proteolytic enzyme occurring in papaya latex. It breaks down mucopolysaccharide–protein complexes in the disc. Injection of this substance into a disc shown to be abnormal by discography causes dissolution of part of the disc material, resulting in improvement in the clinical features. Early studies were reported over 15 years ago, but the technique was not taken up widely because of reported side effects such as anaphylaxis, transient rash, delayed urticaria and discitis. The hypersensitivity effects can be overcome with prophylactic measures. There does not seem to be evidence of premature degeneration of the disc from the needling. Several series have been reported and the results are encouraging (Dabezies, 1978). Patients who would otherwise have undergone surgery have been relieved of their symptoms. With proper selection of subjects with the classical features, and little or no psychogenic component, about 70% success rates are reported. Recently, the drug was finally cleared by the American FDA.

In recent years studies of the effect of 'oral chemonucleolytic agents' have been published. In 1971 Gaspardy *et al.* reported their results of chymoral therapy (an oral preparation containing trypsin and chymotrypsin) in 30 patients with lumbar disc prolapse. A systematic benefit was found in favour of the drug compared with placebo, although a much more extensive study by Gibson *et al.* (1975) has failed to support this.

(h) *Physiotherapy*

Mobilization, a technique practised by physiotherapists has been discussed. Other forms of physiotherapy, including ultrasound and short-wave, may give transient relief of pain. Traction, given on an outpatient or inpatient basis, may be helpful when neural symptoms or dural signs are present. However, it is still not clear whether the value of such an approach is derived from the traction forces involved or the simple fact that patients thus harnessed are kept still and at strict rest (Pearce and Moll, 1967; Swezey, 1978). There is some evidence that intermittent traction on an outpatient basis, using heavier loads (50–60 kg) than are conventionally used during continuous inpatient traction, is more effective (Mathews, 1968; Mathews and Hickling, 1975), and epidurographic appearances have been shown to improve after such treatment. Hydrotherapy not only relieves pain in mild acute episodes but is a useful adjunct in recurrent or chronic pain. Back strengthening and abdominal exercises are done routinely.

(i) *Acupuncture*

The principles of this form of treatment have already been discussed. Pain from degenerative spinal disease has been studied in as much as it can be influenced by acupuncture. Pain relief may be instantaneous but transient, with prolonged benefit from each succeeding treatment. MacDonald *et al.* (1983) showed an improvement in pain score and physical signs in a placebo-controlled study of 17 patients with chronic low back pain. In contrast, Mendelson *et al.* (1983) failed to show benefit from acupuncture in a cross-over study of 77 patients. For a review of controlled studies on acupuncture and other heterodox methods, see Liyange (1986).

(j) *Supports*

Spinal supports (collars and corsets) may be invaluable if the sufferer is to remain ambulant. In the case of corsets, it is important that they are fitted properly and are adequately supported front and back (Yates, 1976). Of the many 'instant' corsets available some are useless as they are too shallow and/or too 'floppy'. In general, this is a short-term measure. However, if there are frequent and recurrent episodes of pain, or if the background discomfort is continuous, especially in the elderly, these appliances may be worn over a long period. This may, however, lead to a state of dependence on a corset, and various measures to wean from the corset are doomed to failure, a problem familiar to most clinicians in this field.

A collar may be essential if cervical apophyseal or uncovertebral joint involvement causes vertebro-basilar insufficiency.

(k) *Other measures and factors*

If a lesion can be localized to an apophyseal joint on the basis of clinical or radiographic findings, a direct approach using manipulation or injection of local anaesthetic and corticosteroid may give quick relief.

Psychogenic factors play an important role in many back problems (Grahame, 1977). Clinicians are familiar with surgery/clinic games and may identify these types of patients and a corresponding response in the doctor. A patient who obsessionally conforms, never complaining but never improving, makes the doctor feel more and more inadequate. There may develop a 'battle scenario', the patient scoring points as each remedy fails, causing more and more anger in the doctor. Finally, the attitude of total dependence with an aura of helplessness leading to more and more concern and care.

As Macnab (1977) has pointed out, clouding and confusion of the clinical picture by emotional overtones is more common than a purely psychogenic back pain syndrome. Moreover, clinicians should continually guard against the possibility of organic spinal illness in patients thought to have a purely

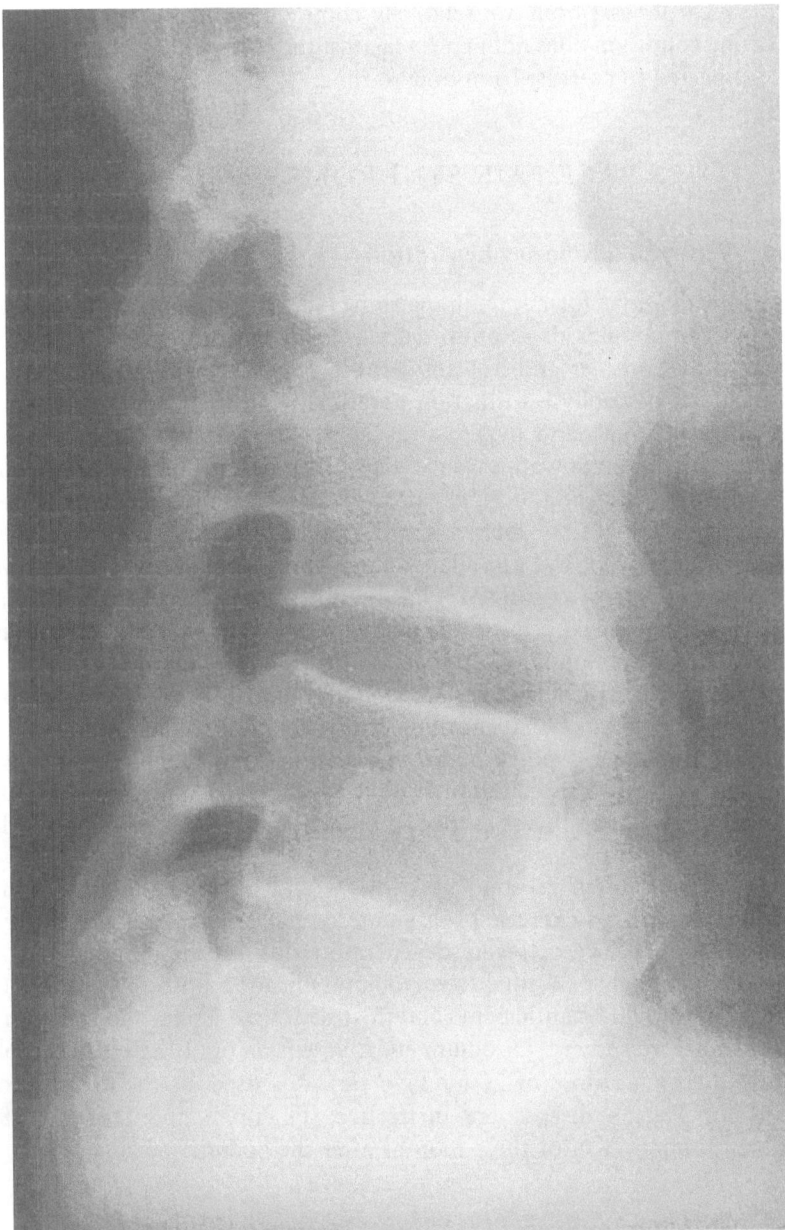

Figure 13.2 Vertebral ankylosing hyperostosis: the large ostophytes give an undulating appearance, and the discs are relatively normal.

psychological illness; both are relatively common in the population at large and, as one condition does not protect against the occurrence of the other, they can be expected to co-exist from time to time.

13.3   OTHER BACK PAIN SYNDROMES

13.3.1   Vertebral ankylosing hyperostosis

Extensive osteophyte formation in the spine has been recognized for nearly 60 years, but the popular description *ankylosing hyperostosis of the spine* was introduced by Forestier and Rotés-Querol in 1950. Typical radiographic features included osteophyte formation anteriorly and on the right side in the lower thoracic spine, and hyperostosis in the cervical and lumbar regions, resulting in an undulating appearance (Fig. 13.2). Diagnostic criteria have now been suggested (Resnick and Niwayama, 1976), stressing the degree of ossification at extra-spinal sites, relative sparing of the discs and apophyseal joints, and lack of erosion of the sacroiliac joints. The alternative title *diffuse idiopathic skeletal hyperostosis* (DISH) has been suggested. The initial pathological changes are in the anterior spinal ligament, and diffuse ossification ensues.

This condition predominates in men, and is usually diagnosed after the age of 65 years, when typical changes are seen after a history which may go back decades. It is interesting that morning stiffness is the commonest symptom. There are conflicting reports of an association with the HLA B27 tissue antigen, but clinically this condition is quite distinct from ankylosing spondylitis. There may be osteophytes at the sacroiliac joints, but bony ankylosis does not occur.

The symptoms often respond to NSAIDs and physical therapy given as hydrotherapy with an exercise programme. If hip arthroplasty is being considered in the presence of severe degenerative disease, these patients should be regarded as 'high risk' for heterotropic ossification post-operatively. This complication should be anticipated and treatment with diphosphonates started one month before surgery. Disodium etidronate is an orally active diphosphonate and the higher dose of 20 mg kg^{-1} day^{-1} is used, as the doses recommended for Paget's disease are ineffective (Finerman and Stover, 1981). Treatment is continued for three months after the operation.

13.3.2   Fibrositis syndrome

This term was originally coined by Gowers (1904), a neurologist, and later taken up by rheumatologists (Stockman, 1920; Copeman, 1943). Fibrositis now refers to conditions with vague musculoskeletal pain usually in the trunk, with no demonstrable clinical or histological abnormality in the spine, peripheral joints or muscles. It became a popular layman's diagnosis when there was no apparent rheumatological disease. However, during the last two decades there has been more interest in this condition. Fourteen easily identifiable sites of exaggerated tenderness have been described (Smythe, 1972), and most of these seem to coincide with distinct acupuncture points, which have been used in the treatment of musculoskeletal disease. Further credence was lent to this syndrome when electroencephalographic abnormalities were described during the phase of stage 4 slow wave (non-REM) sleep, when alpha waves appeared (Moldofsky *et al.*, 1975). In experimental deprivation of slow wave sleep, healthy volunteers developed increase in muscle tenderness. The use of chlorpromazine decreased the subjective pain and dolorimeter scores, and produced increase in slow wave sleep.

Patients may have had symptoms for years, and the severity is variable in that there are painfree days or weeks. Once the diagnosis is established reassurance is essential. The pain-spasm-pain cycle may be broken with NSAID treatment for a few weeks. The propionic acid derivatives appear to be more useful than the other drugs. A convenient dose schedule is naproxen 500 mg twice a day. Occasionally, a tricyclic antidepressant may be necessary. It is not practicable to inject all the tender sites.

13.3.3 Osteoporosis

This is the commonest metabolic bone disease and may lead to vertebral collapse and back pain. About a third of Caucasian women over 65 years are liable to such a fracture in the vertebral body, femoral neck or forearm. There is decreased skeletal mass associated with increased porosity.

All patients with osteoporosis should be provided with supportive measures in addition to drug therapy.

Acute pain from vertebral fracture and associated muscle spasm will require adequate analgesia, bed rest, immobilization and physical treatment such as local deep heat and repeated hot baths. In patients with chronic back pain, posture training, graded spinal extensor muscle exercise carried out in collaboration with the physiotherapist, combined with a back brace are also helpful. The patient should be warned to avoid carrying heavy objects and to avoid sudden or asymmetrical mechanical stress. Care should be exercised when walking in obstructed or poorly lit areas. Care should also be taken to avoid falls and, if necessary, stair rails and a grasp-rail in the bathroom should be provided. Weight reduction, use of a supported mattress and 'gentle' general exercise such as that provided by swimming and walking may also be useful (Seeman and Riggs, 1982). Various drugs have been used in the treatment of osteoporosis and these will now be discussed.

(a) *Oestrogen*

Over the last 40 years studies have firmly supported an important role for oestrogen therapy in postmenopausal osteoporosis. The menopause is associated with a decrease in intestinal calcium absorption and with a more negative calcium balance (Heaney *et al.*, 1978a). Oestrogen deficiency is associated with increased bone resorption measured both by microradiography (Riggs *et al.*, 1969) and by radiocalcium kinetics (Heaney *et al.*, 1978b). Riggs *et al.* (1969) found normalization of bone resorption in 17 patients treated cyclically with conjugated oestrogen (Premarin) 2.5 mg daily. In most patients this occurred within 2–4 months of starting treatment. Similar findings have been reported by Christiansen *et al.* (1980). Oestrogen therapy improves calcium absorption (Gallagher *et al.*, 1979, 1980) and improves calcium balance (Gallagher *et al.*, 1973). Gordon *et al.* (1973) have shown a reduced occurrence of vertebral fracture in patients treated with conjugated oestrogen (Premarin) 1.25–2.5 mg day^{-1} for up to 25 years. Similar findings have been found in terms of reduced loss of height (Wallach and Henneman, 1959) and reduced frequency of Colles' fracture (Burch *et al.*, 1976).

The ideal oestrogen should have the greatest potency regarding decreased bone loss and minimal effect regarding endometrial changes. Gallagher and Nordin (1975) have compared the efficacy of various oestrogen preparations and found that daily administered conjugated oestrogens (Premarin 0.625 mg) and ethinyloestradiol (0.025 mg) were equipotent, and these drugs as well as mestranol (25–50 µg) have been in regular use in clinical practice for some time.

Untoward side effects are as follows: an eightfold increase in the risk of developing endometrial carcinomas (McDonald *et al.*, 1977; Weiss *et al.*, 1979); benign mammary changes, but a suggestion that there may be a protective effect against breast cancer (Wilson, 1962); other complications such as thromboembolism, gallbladder disease, myocardial infarction, hypertension, and clotting factor defects. However, these have been repeated more in the context of contraceptive usage of oestrogens, rather than in their role as therapy for osteoporosis. For minimization of possible endometrial effects oestrogens may be administered at lower doses in conjunction with calcium supplements and given cyclically, with or without a progestational agent in the last 10 days.

(b) *Calcium*

Although no definitive epidemiological evidence is available to show that low dietary calcium intake alone causes osteoporosis, bone mineral content has been found to be lower in those with a more negative calcium balance (Nordin, 1962). Most studies suggest that 0.9–1.5 g day^{-1} of calcium is needed to prevent a negative calcium balance (Hurxthal and Vose, 1969; Heaney *et al.*, 1977; Nordin *et al.*, 1979) and this is more than the 800 mg day^{-1} stipulated as a recommended dietary allowance (National Research Council, Food and Nutrition Board, 1974).

(c) *Vitamin D (1,25(OH)$_2$D$_3$)*

This is currently indicated mainly in the treatment of osteoporosis due to low intestinal calcium absorption. Gallagher *et al.* (1973) have found that the mean dose of vitamin D required to normalize calcium absorption is 20 000 units daily (range 1000–40 000 units daily). Synthetic 1,25(OH)$_2$D$_3$ and 1α-hydroxyvitamin D$_3$ (1α(OH)D$_3$) have both been found to increase intestinal calcium absorption effectively in short-term studies (Davies *et al.*, 1975; Marshall *et al.*, 1977; Sørensen *et al.*, 1977); however the effects are considerably dose-dependent and hypercalcaemia and hypercalciuria often complicate therapy. Vitamin D metabolites, especially in higher doses, have no effect nor detrimental effect on the skeleton.

The use of calcium supplements combined with vitamin D does not appear to enhance the effects of treatment in osteoporosis (Buring *et al.*, 1974; Shapiro *et al.*, 1975).

(d) *Calcitonin*

A definitive role for calcitonin in skeletal remodelling and mineral homeostasis in humans has not yet been confirmed. Raisz *et al.* (1967) showed that calcitonin inhibits bone resorption *in vitro* and the substance has been used to treat osteoporosis with the aim of decreasing bone resorption. However, interpretation of many clinical trials using calcitonin is difficult (short-term analyses, small numbers of patients, lack of controls). Three studies, using total-body neutron activation, have suggested an overall increase in total body calcium after combined treatment with calcium and calcitonin (Cohn *et al.*, 1971; Wallach *et al.*, 1977; Chesnut *et al.*, 1979).

(e) *Microcrystalline hydroxyapatite*

In a study of rheumatoid patients treated with steroids, microcrystalline calcium hydroxyapatite compound had a significant prophylactic effect in preventing the development of osteoporosis (Nilsen *et al.*, 1978).

(f) *Inorganic phosphate*

Limited evidence in humans suggests that phosphate is ineffective in osteoporosis (Hulley *et al.*, 1971; Goldsmith *et al.*, 1976).

(g) *Growth hormone*

The traditional association of osteoporosis with acromegaly has led to study of growth hormone as a possible treatment for osteoporosis. However, results so far are not encouraging (Aloia *et al.*, 1976).

(h) *Other*

Various other therapeutic approaches have been used in osteoporosis, but their usefulness (as with some of the preparations mentioned above) is doubtful or not yet established. Such alternative therapies include: oral sodium fluoride (Jowsey, 1979); anabolic steroids; the newer diphosphonates (Minaire *et al.*, 1980); and various forms of electromagnetic stimulation.

13.3.4 Osteomalacia

Osteomalacia results from decreased mineralization and is associated with the presence of non-mineralized osteoid seams. It results from deficiency of 'vitamin D', which until recently has been regarded as a true vitamin, metabolically stable. It is now known that it is a prohormone (Holick *et al.*, 1977), and hydroxylation at the carbon-25 position occurs primarily in the liver microsomes; 25-hydroxyvitamin D_3 is further hydroxylated at the 1α position exclusively in renal tissue (Haussler and McCain, 1977). The physiologically active metabolite 1,25-dihydroxyvitamin D_3 acts on the intestine to increase the absorption of calcium and phosphorus. It acts on bone in two ways: mobilization of calcium and phosphorus from previously formed bone, and promotion of maturation and mineralization of organic matrix.

The natural source of vitamin D is not dietary, but we depend on the sun's ultraviolet rays to convert a precursor in the skin into the prohormone cholecalciferol. Regardless of the aetiology, the osteomalacic syndromes show abnormalities in mature areas of trabecular and cortical bone. It is characterized by an abnormal increase in the number and width of osteoid seams. Looser's lines or Milkman's pseudofractures seen radiologically are composed of osteoid. The vertebrae show the typical cod fish deformity. Serum alkaline phosphatase is raised and the serum calcium and phosphorus are reduced. Classic dietary vitamin D deficiency is extremely rare in the Western world. However, calcium absorption may be reduced in Asians using chapatti flour. This contains phytate which binds calcium and zinc. Osteomalacia is corrected by exclusion of chapatti flour from the diet or by the addition of vitamin D_2 to the flour. In malabsorption states, vitamin D and probably calcium become deficient from decreased absorption and increased faecal loss. Osteomalacia is not uncommon in the elderly and may coexist with osteoporosis. Prophylaxis and treatment are achieved with the use of calcium and vitamin D tablets (500 units per tablet) or calciferol solution (3000 units per ml).

In severe renal disease, there is inadequate hydroxylation to the active compound. Bone disease may occur. The biochemistry is not classical, as renal failure leads to a rise in serum phosphorus. The low serum calcium may result in secondary hyperparathyroidism and further radiographic appearances typical of this condition. In view of the poor hydroxylation in the kidney, large doses of vitamin D are needed to treat this condition. It is preferable to use the active compound, α-calcidol 0.25–1 µg per day. As hypercalcaemia may ensue, these patients require frequent monitoring of serum calcium levels.

13.3.5 Paget's disease

The aetiology of Paget's disease of bone is uncertain (Singer, 1977). Paget suggested that it was a chronic inflammatory disorder and referred to it as osteitis deformans. Although a few cases have coexisted with hyperparathyroidism, and a subgroup has raised serum parathormone levels, there is no convincing evidence that it is an endocrine disorder. It does not meet the criteria of a neoplasm. There is a distinct family history in some patients, but it is not an inborn error of connective tissue metabolism. In the past few years, interest has focused on a viral aetiology. Electron microscopy has revealed specific inclusions in osteoclasts in tissue from patients with Paget's bone disease. These inclusions present a close morphological analogy with nucleocapsids of paramyxovirus of the measles group. The distribution of the lesions in this disease suggests that skeletal stress may also be an important factor.

The primary abnormality is in the osteoclast. There are increased numbers of osteoclasts which are individually enlarged and contain giant cells. Alterations in osteoclast function are associated with increased rate of bone resorption. This leads to accelerated osteoblastic new bone formation with the production of a mosaic of irregularly formed, incompletely calcified islands of woven bone in place of normal lamellar bone. This eventually leads to structurally weak and deformed bone with a tendency to fracture, and pain ensues. Radiologically, there is disruption of the normal trabecular pattern and bone expansion. Figure 13.3 shows typical spinal changes. The serum alkaline phosphatase is invariably raised, as is the urinary excretion of hydroxyproline.

Simple analgesics and NSAIDs often relieve pain. Specific therapy is indicated only in a small group of patients with Paget's disease, who experience more severe bone pain or have involvement in sites where the likelihood of future disability exists. Calcitonin is a polypeptide which decreases bone resorption by acting at specific receptors in osteoclasts, leading to an alteration of cell function through cyclic AMP-mediated systems. Salmon calcitonin is the usual preparation employed as it causes much less resistance than porcine calcitonin, and it is more potent than human calcitonin. Calcitonin 100 units by subcutaneous or intramuscular injection daily, or at least three times a week, leads to a fall in the excretion of hydroxyproline. Within a month, the serum alkaline phosphatase also declines.

Bone pain may be relieved for years with calcitonin treatment, and the benefit may be maintained for a year longer without therapy. Histologically, there is a reversal towards normal bone architecture; spontaneous fractures heal satisfactorily; and there may be radiological improvements as well.

Diphosphonates are analogues of pyrophosphate and inhibit the growth and dissolution of hydroxyapatite crystals, and directly impair osteoclast function (Russell and Fleisch, 1975). Disodium etidronate is an oral diphosphonate and used at a dose of $5 \text{ mg kg}^{-1} \text{ day}^{-1}$. Lowering of serum alkaline phosphatase is

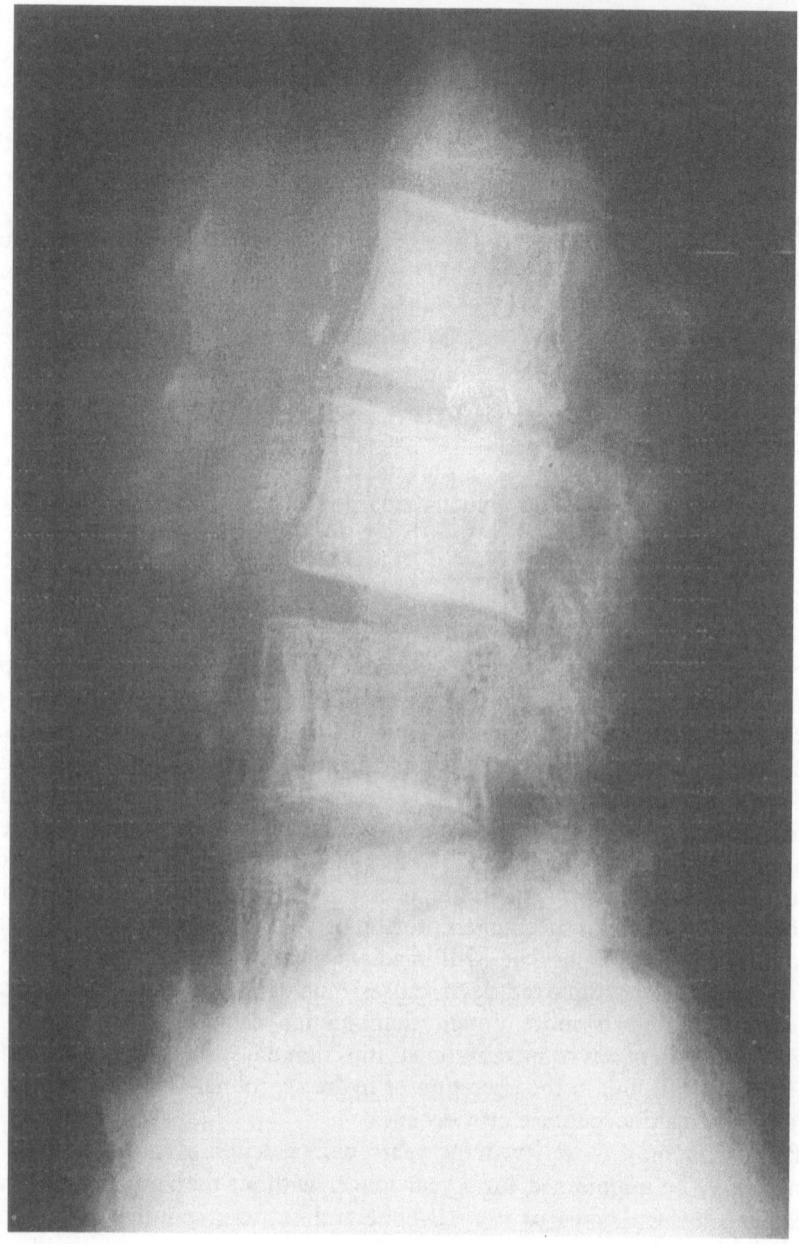

Figure 13.3 Paget's disease showing expansion of bone and increased trabecular pattern.

noted in the first month, and it continues to fall to about half the pretreatment value by six months. It is recommended that a course of treatment be for six months only. Continued use may lead to excessive suppression of bone re-modelling causing more bone pain and possibly a higher risk of fracture. Some patients experience a sustained response after a single six-month course of therapy. Most will continue to have alkaline phosphatase levels above the normal range, and they require further six-month courses after an interval of 3–6 months. If a pathological fracture is present, it is best to delay the use of diphosphonates until healing has occurred, possibly with the use of calcitonin. Where the response to the standard dose of etidronate is poor, 10 mg kg^{-1} day^{-1} may be tried for three months. Side effects such as nausea and diarrhoea may occur but are uncommon.

Mithramycin is a cytotoxic antibiotic, observed to lower serum calcium probably through an action on osteoclasts (Ryan *et al.*, 1970). It is adminis-tered as an intravenous infusion over 4–6 hours. The higher doses used in earlier studies were associated with nausea and gross elevation of serum aspartate transaminase, which were rarely encountered when a dose of 10 µg kg^{-1} day^{-1} was used during the 10-day course. Pain relief is noted by the third to fifth day. Thus, this form of treatment is indicated for severe incapacitating bone pain or impending neurological damage. Long-term treatment with calcitonin or etidronate must follow the course of mithramycin. This treatment may also help in differentiating the cause of pain when Paget's disease coexists near a joint affected by osteoarthrosis.

13.3.6 Infections

Pritchard (1975) has recently reviewed granulomatous infections of bones and joints and the reader is referred to this source for details. The distribution of bone and joint infection is influenced by the causative organism and the age of the patient. Thus, involvement of the spine is commoner in adults than in infants and children; tuberculous bone disease affects the spine more than the long bones; in brucellosis of the spine, sacroiliac involvement is common.

Haematogenous spread of organisms to the vertebral body is facilitated by a rich arterial network, and in about half the patients a remote septic focus such as in the pharynx or a toe can be identified. Spread from pelvic infection probably occurs through a valveless venous plexus (Batson's vertebral venous plexus) linked to the spinal and paraspinal tissues. Initial involvement of a disc is rare except in children whose discs are vascularized. Direct infection may result from local procedures like needling a disc, surgery, or rarely from an adjacent suppurative focus.

In the early stages when the infection is in the subchondral regions of the vertebral body, the radiographs may be normal. Indeed, the X-rays lag about 3–4 weeks behind clinical signs, and may remain normal during this time. When the disc becomes involved, X-rays show reduction of disc height and loss of normal definition of the bone plate. After 2 months there may be reactive changes.

Pain is the most consistent feature; it becomes continuous and especially troublesome at night. Muscle spasm is marked and often there is a list to one side. The rigidity of the spine differentiates infective spondylitis from mechanical spinal derangements. The white cell count may be normal or raised, but the ESR is invariably raised.

In infective disease of the bones and joints, as for meningitis, attempts should be made to identify the causative organism before starting antibiotic therapy. Blood culture is positive in some. If not, needle aspiration or even open biopsy may be necessary. When antibiotic therapy is begun, it is customary, though not for validated reasons, to start treatment intravenously.

Oral therapy may be just as effective and is certainly the route for continuation of treatment. The choice of antibiotic is of course dependent on the organism identified. Streptococcal and pneumococcal infections are unusual and best treated with benzylpenicillin. Staphylococcal infections may need flucloxacillin and fusidic acid; clindamycin, too, is effective against this organism as well as against many anaerobes, but its use is limited by serious side effects such as pseudomembranous colitis. Ampicillin and amoxycillin are broad-spectrum penicillins effective against some Gram-positive and Gram-negative organisms. As almost all staphylococci, one-third of *E. coli*, and one-tenth of *H. influenzae* are resistant, these broad spectrum drugs should not be used blindly. Augmentin consists of amoxycillin with the beta-lactamase inhibitor clarulanic acid which inactivates penicillinases, making the product active against penicillinase-producing bacteria that are resistant to amoxycillin. The cephalosporins are broad spectrum drugs, and the many preparations available have a similar antibacterial spectrum; some are administered by injection, but a few are orally active. Pseudomonas infections respond to the penicillin drugs – carbenicillin, ticarcillin and azlocillin, and to the amnioglycoside drugs – gentamicin and tobramycin. When an infection is treated 'blindly', the combination of gentamicin with a penicillin or metronidazole is recommended.

Gentamicin is widely used for the treatment of serious infections. It has a broad spectrum but is inactive against anaerobes. Blood levels ought to be estimated just before and 1 hour after an injection to ensure that these are under 2 μg ml^{-1} and 10 μg ml^{-1} respectively. It is ototoxic and nephrotoxic. Small doses are sufficient in renal disease.

Estimates vary regarding the optimal duration of antibiotic treatment, but it should be continued for some weeks after clinical evidence of eradication of infection and the return of the ESR to normal. The patient should be immobilized in bed when the infection is still active. During early mobilization, a spinal support is recommended. Repeat X-ray examination reveals healing with sclerosis; there may be a kyphosis; ankylosis occurs in about half the patients at one year.

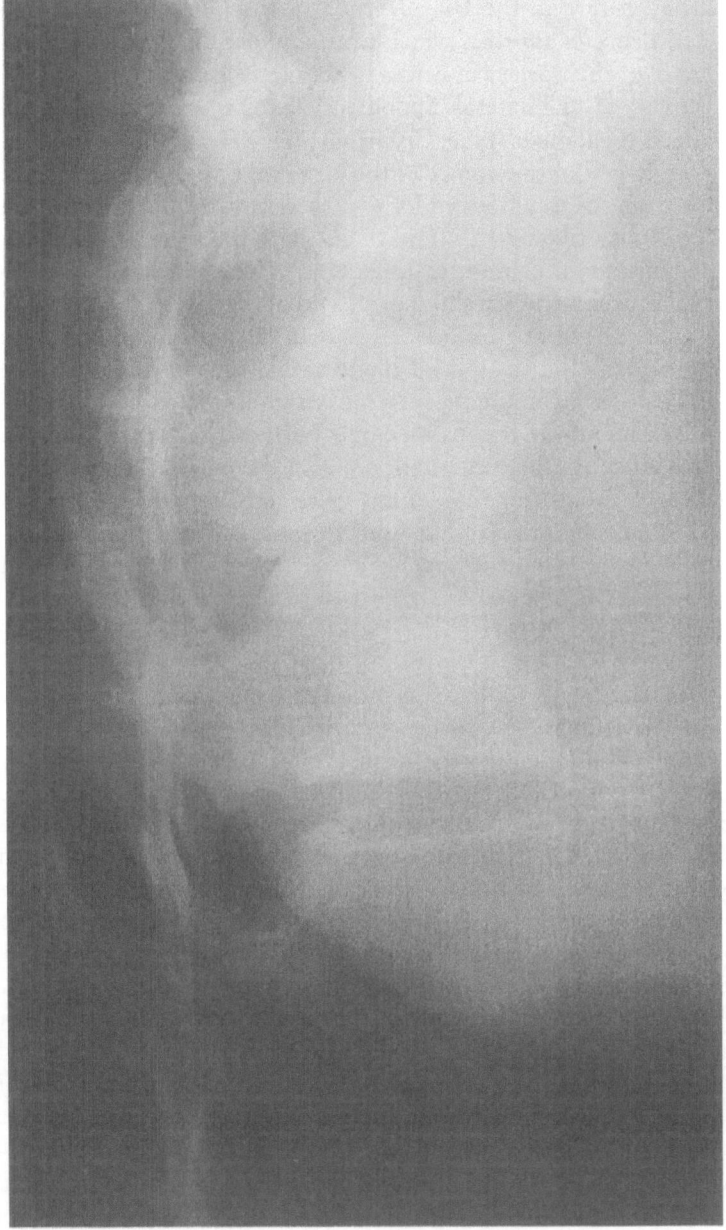

Figure 13.4 Tuberculosis of T11 and L1 with destructive changes in contiguous vertebral surfaces and the adjacent disc.

Brucellosis is rare in the UK. *Brucella suis* is likely to cause suppurative lesions, but *Brucella abortus*, which causes milder disease, is the only significant member of this species in Britain. Sacroiliitis is seen in about a third, and may be unilateral or bilateral. Spondylitis tends to occur in older men, and mainly affects the lumbar spine. Classically, there is marginal erosive change at the upper or lower anterior angle of the vertebral body, with disc involvement. Tetracycline 2 g per day is given for 6–10 weeks to eradicate the infection.

In tuberculous osteomyelitis (Hodgson, 1975) the lower thoracic and upper lumbar regions are often affected (Fig. 13.4). There is debate on the choice of antimicrobial drugs and on the role of early surgery. In the initial phase of treatment, it is best to use three drugs, so that the population of viable bacteria is reduced rapidly and the risk of ineffective treatment minimized. Isoniazid and rifampicin as a combination tablet is supplemented by ethambutol and given for 2–3 months. Pyrazinamide may be added to give the most intensive bactericidal effect. In the continuation phase, the first two drugs may be used for a total of 9 months or three drugs given for 6 months. Anterior debridement and immediate grafting has been suggested as the treatment of choice, but controlled studies indicate that chemotherapy alone may be more effective.

13.3.7 Tumours

Primary benign tumours of the spine include plasmacytoma (Fig. 13.5), haemangioma (McAllister, 1975), osteoid osteoma (Maclellan and Wilson, 1967), osteoblastoma – including benign forms (Immemkamp, 1971; Gelberman and Olson, 1974), eosinophilic granuloma (Baraffaldi *et al.*, 1972), aneurysmal bone cyst (Slowicj *et al.*, 1968), and giant cell tumour (Fors and Stenkvist, 1966). Most of these present with back pain, and clues to diagnosis come from a history of persistent pain, the age of the patient, and radiographic appearances. One of the characteristic features of an osteoid osteoma is the response of the pain to aspirin. In general, if the pain is severe, surgery may be indicated.

Myelomatosis is a malignant tumour of plasma cell origin. The ESR is very high, there is an excess of globulin in the blood, with a monoclonal immunoglobulin, and there may be Bence Jones protein in the urine. A localized lesion responds to radiotherapy. Generalized disease is treated with combination chemotherapy. The alkylating agent cyclophosphamide, or melphalan, is employed in pulse therapy. Melphalan 10–15 mg and prednisolone 30–40 mg per day for 3 days is a popular regimen, and the courses are repeated every 4–6 weeks. The maximal effect on the blood forming cells occurs after about 14 days when the white cell and platelet counts may be low. Hyperuricaemia is common. If the level is well above normal, or if there is clinical evidence of gout, it would be wise to lower the uric acid level using allopurinol. The usual dose is 300 mg as a single tablet daily, and treatment is 'covered' for some weeks with a NSAID, to avoid precipitating an attack of gout.

Metastatic disease of the spine is an important problem in the differential

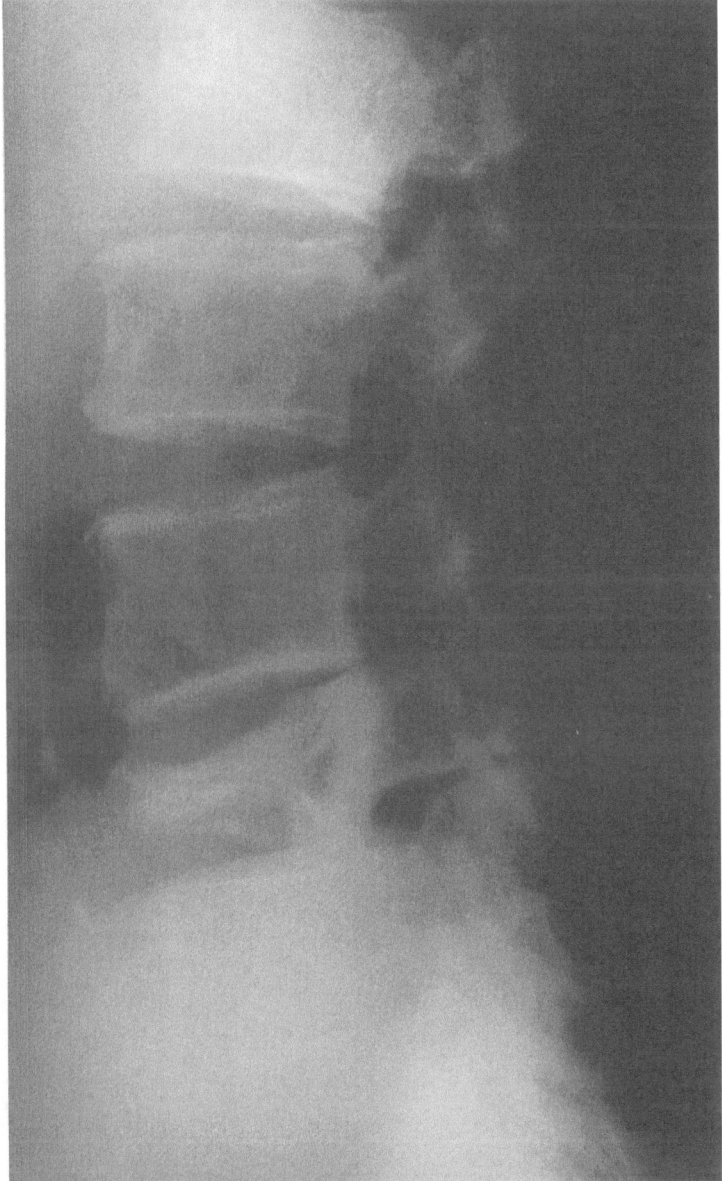

Figure 13.5 Vertebral collapse from a plasmacytoma; note the normal disc spaces.

diagnosis of back pain, a subject reviewed by Young and Funk (1953) and Bhalla (1970). The spine is the commonest site of metastatic spread in the skeleton, and the lumbar vertebrae are the most frequently involved. The early

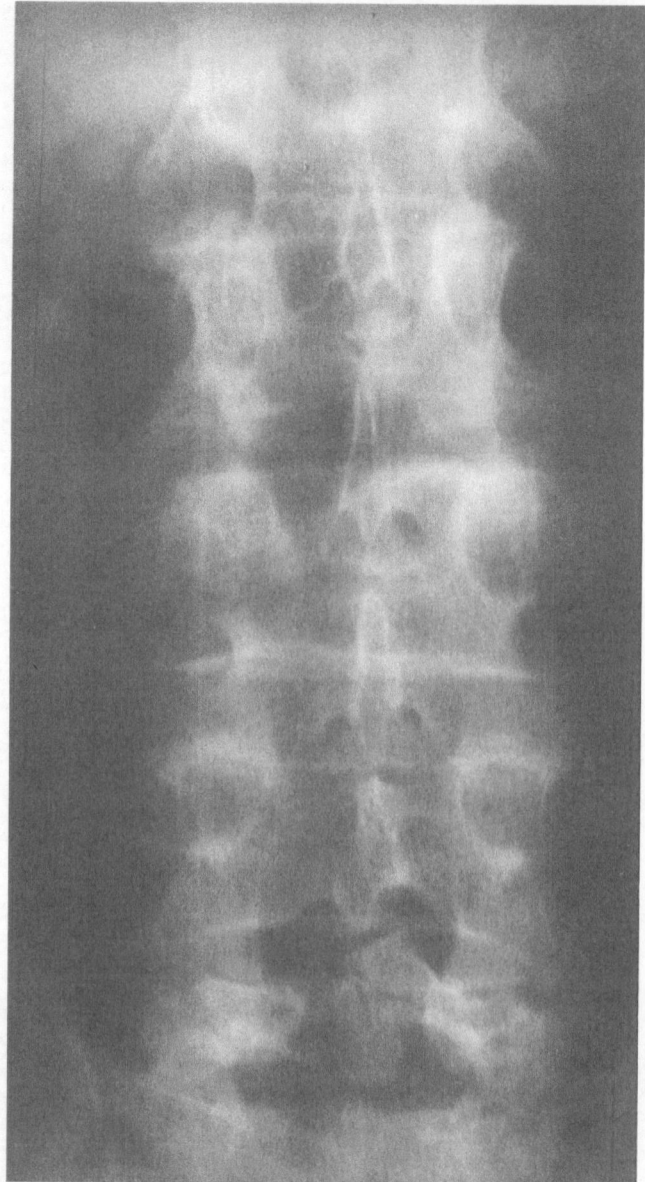

Figure 13.6 Early metastatic spread of carcinoma, with poor definition of the right pedicle of the third lumbar vertebra. The lateral view was normal at this stage.

lesion is in the pedicle (Fig. 13.6). The primary tumour is usually in the breast, bronchus, thyroid, kidney or prostate, or rarely in the colon. The secondary deposit appears radiographically as an osteolytic lesion and may cause vertebral collapse. About 30% of the osseous mass of a bone must be destroyed before a lesion is radiologically apparent. Thus, a radioisotope scan is much more sensitive in assessing the presence and extent of bony metastases. Secondary deposits from carcinoma of the prostate appear sclerotic, sometimes giving rise to difficulty in differentiation from Paget's disease, but there is no expansion of the bone.

For pain relief paracetamol is not adequate, and the narcotic, non-addictive drugs are often necessary. They are used as in peripheral degenerative joint disease. Codeine, dihydrocodeine, meptazinol or nefopam are often prescribed. Drugs that may cause tolerance and dependence must be reserved for patients with more advanced disease, and the usual practice is to adjust the dose and frequency to give satisfactory and continued pain relief. Morphine, diamorphine and pethidine are available as tablets for regular use. Morphine sulphate (MST Continus) 10 or 30 mg tablet given twice a day is a satisfactory regimen. Where the pain is more severe, an injection of one of these agents or nalbuphine 10 mg may be offered; alternatively dextromoramide 5–20 mg by mouth may give short-lived pain relief. Also available are elixirs containing morphine or diamorphine.

In malignant bone pain, calcitonin 200 IU by intramuscular injection, 6 hourly for 48 hours may give relief of pain for a week or more. The course of treatment may be repeated. Serum calcium levels may fall. Where hypercalcaemia is a problem, the patient should be adequately rehydrated by intravenous infusion. Steroids may be given in moderate doses for a short time.

In secondary bone disease from carcinoma of the prostate, hormonal therapy is of value. Stilboestrol is the most widely used oestrogen and gives good control in up to 80% of patients. Cyproterone is a progestogen and anti-androgen. It is effective at a dose up to 300 mg per day in divided doses. In the palliative treatment of breast cancer, the anti-oestrogen drug tamoxifen is often used, the initial dose being 20–40 mg a day. It probably acts by blocking receptor sites in target organs.

13.4 REFERENCES

Adams, P. and Muir, H. (1976) Qualitative changes with age of proteoglycans of human lumbar disks. *Ann. Rheum. Dis.*, 35, 289–96.

Aloia, J. F., Zanzi, I., Ellis, K., Jousey, J., Roginsky, M., Wallach, S. and Cohn, S. H. (1976) Effects of growth hormone in osteoporosis. *J. Clin. Endocrinol. Metabolism*, 43, 992–9.

Apley, A. G., Millner, W. F. and Porter, D. S. (1969) A follow-up study of Moore's arthroplasty in the treatment of osteoarthrosis of the hip. *J. Bone Jt Surg.*, 51B, 638–47.

Badgley, C. E. (1941) The articular facets in relation to low back pain and sciatic radiation. *J. Bone Jt Surg.*, 23, 481–96.

Balch, H. W., Gibson, J., El-Ghobarey, A. F., Bain, L. S. and Lynch, M. P. (1977) Repeated corticosteroid injections into knee joints. *Rheumatol. Rehabil.*, 16, 137–40.

Baraffaldi, O., Oero, G. and Serra, E. (1972) Two cases of eosinophilic granuloma. *Minerva Ortopedica*, 23, 446–53.

Bentley, G. and Goodfellow. J. W. (1969) Disorganisation of the knee following intra-articular hydrocortisone injections. *J. Bone Jt Surg.*, 51B, 498–502.

Berry, H., Liyanage, S. P., Durance, R. A., Goode, J. D. and Swannell, A. J. (1981) A double blind study of benorylate and chlormezanone in musculoskeletal disease. *Rheumatol. Rehabil.*, 20, 46–9.

Bhalla, S. K. (1970) Metastatic disease of the spine. *Clin. Orthopaed.*, 73, 52–60.

Bollet, A. J. (1969) An essay on the biology of osteoarthritis. *Arthr. Rheum.*, 12, 156–63.

Bonica, J. J. (1953) *The Management of Pain*, Lea and Febiger, Philadelphia.

Burch, J. C., Byrd, B. F. and Vaughn, W. K. (1976) Results of oestrogen treatment in one thousand hysterectomized women for 14318 years, in *Consensus on Menopause Research: A Summary of International Opinion* (eds P. A. Van Keep, R. B. Greenblatt and M. Albeaux-Fernet), University Park Press, Baltimore, pp. 164–9.

Buring, K., Julth, A. G., Nilsson, B. E., Westlin, N. E. and Wiklund, P. E. (1974) Treatment of osteoporosis with vitamin D. *Acta Med. Scand.*, 195, 471–2.

Carson, D. J. L. and Carson, E. D. (1977) Fatal dextropropoxyphene poisoning in Northern Ireland. Review of 30 cases. *Lancet*, i, 894–7.

Chang, Hsiang-tung (1978) Neurophysiological basis of acupuncture analgesia. *Scientia Simica*, 21, 829–46.

Chesnut, C. H., Baylink, D. J. and Nelp, W. B. (1979) Bone mass change with calcitonin therapy in osteoporosis as assessed by total body activation analysis (abstract). *J. Nucl. Med.*, 20, 677.

Chrisman, O. D., Fessel, J. M. and Southwick, W. O. (1965) Experimental production of synovitis and marginal articular exostoses in the knee joints of dogs. *Yale J. Biol. Med.*, 37, 409–12.

Christiansen, C., Christiansen, M. S., McNair, P., Hagen, C., Stockland, E. and Transbol, I. (1980) Prevention of early postmenopausal bone loss, controlled 2 year study in 315 normal females. *Eur. J. Clin. Invest.*, 10, 237–9.

Clark, R., Thompson, R. P. H., Borirakchanyavat, V., Widdop, B., Davidson, A. R., Goulding, R. and Williams, R. (1973) Hepatic damage and death from overdose of paracetamol. *Lancet*, i, 66–9.

Cohn, S. H., Dombrowski, C. S., Hanser, W., Klopper, J. and Atkins, H. L. (1971) Effects of porcine calcitonin on calcium metabolism in osteoporosis. *J. Clin. Endocrinol. Metab.*, 33, 719–28.

Collins, D. H. (1949) *The Pathology of Articular and Spinal Diseases*. Edward Arnold, London.

Copeman, W. S. C. (1943) Arthology of the fibrositic nodule: a clinical contribution. *Br. Med. J.*, 2, 263.

Crain, D. C. (1961) Interphalangeal osteoarthritis. *J. Am. Med. Assoc.*, 175, 1049–53.

Cyriax, J. (1975) Diagnosis of soft tissue lesions in *Textbook of Orthopaedic Medicine*, 6th edn, Ballière Tindall, London, pp. 469–86.

Davies, M., Mawer, E. B. and Adams, P. H. (1975) Vitamin D metabolism and the response to 1,25-dihydroxycholecalciferol in osteoporosis. *J. Clin. Endocrinol. Metab.*, 45, 199–208.

Dabazies, E. J. (1978) Chemonucleolysis vs Laminectomy. *Orthopaedics*, 1, 26–9.

Dieppe, P. and Calvert, P. (1983) *Crystals and Joint Disease*, Chapman and Hall, London, pp. 207–8.

Dilke, T. F. W., Burry, H. C. and Grahame, R. (1973) Extradural corticosteroid injection in the management of lumbar nerve root compression. *Br. Med. J.*, 2, 635–7.

Doran, D. M. L. and Newell, D. J. (1975) Manipulation in treatment of low back pain: a multicentre study. *Br. Med. J.*, 2, 161–4.

Evans, W. (1930) Intrasacral epidural injections in the treatment of sciatica. *Lancet*, ii, 1225–9.

Evans, D. P., Birk, M. S., Lloyd, K. M., Roberts, E. E. and Roberts, G. N. (1978) Lumbar spinal manipulation on trial. Part I – Clinical assessment. *Rheumatol. Rehabil.*, 17, 46–53.

Farfan, H. F. (1980) The scientific basis of manipulative procedures, in *Low Back Pain, Clinics in Rheumatic Diseases*, Vol. 6, No 1 (ed. R. Grahame), Saunders, London, pp. 159–77.

Finerman, G. A. M. and Stover, S. L. (1981) Heterotopic ossification following hip replacement or spinal cord injury. Two clinical studies with EHDP. *Metab. Bone Dis. Related Res.*, 4 & 5, 337–42.

Forestier, J. and Rotes-Querol, J. (1950) Senile ankylosing hyperostosis of the spine. *Ann. Rheum. Dis.*, 9, 321–30.

Fors, B. and Stenkvist, B. (1966) Giant-cell tumour of thoracic vertebra. *Acta Orthopaed. Scand.*, 37, 191–6.

Freebody, D., Bendall, R. and Taylor, R. D. (1971) Anterior transperitoneal lumbar fusion. *J. Bone Jt Surg.*, 53B, 617–27.

Gallagher, J. C., Aaron, J., Horsman, A., Marshall, D. H., Wilkinson, R. and Nordin, B. E. C. (1973) The crush fracture syndrome in postmenopausal women. *Clinics Endocrinol. Metab.*, 2, 293–315.

Gallagher, J. C. and Nordin, B. E. C. (1975) Effects of oestrogen and progestogen therapy on calcium metabolism in postmenopausal women. *Frontiers Hormone Res.*, 3, 150–76.

Gallagher, J. C., Riggs, B. L. and DeLuca, H. G. (1980) Effect of oestrogen on calcium absorption and serum vitamin D metabolites in postmenopausal osteoporosis. *J. Clin. Endocrinol. Metab.*, 51, 1359–64.

Gallagher, J. C., Riggs, B. L., Elsman, J., Hamstra, A., Arnand, S. B. and DeLuca, H. F. (1979) Intestinal calcium absorption and serum vitamin D metabolites in normal subjects and osteoporotic patients: effects of age and dietary calcium. *J. Clin. Invest.*, 64, 729–36.

Gaspardy, G., Balint, G., Mitusova, M. and Lorincz, G. (1971) Treatment of sciatica due to intervertebral disc herniation with chymoral tablets. *Rheumatol. Phys. Med.*, 11, 14–19.

Gelberman, R. H. and Olson, C. O. (1974) Benign osteoblastoma of the atlas: a case report. *J. Bone Jt Surg.*, 56A, 808–10.

Gibson, T., Dilke, T. F. W. and Grahame, R. (1975) Chymoral in the treatment of lumbar disc prolapse. *Rheumatol. Rehabil.*, 14, 186–90.

Glover, J. R., Morris, J. G. and Khosla, T. (1974) Back pain: a randomised clinical trial of rotational manipulation of the trunk. *Br. J. Ind. Med.*, 31, 59–64.

Godfrey, C. M. and Morgan, P. (1978) A controlled trial of the theory of acupuncture in musculo-skeletal pain. *J. Rheumatol.*, 5, 121–4.

Goldsmith, R. S., Jowsey, J., Dubé, W. J., Riggs, B. L., Arnaud, C. D. and Kelly, P. J. (1976) Effects of phosphorus supplementation on serum parathyroid hormone and bone morphology in osteoporosis. *J. Clin. Endocrinol. Metab.*, 43, 523–32.

Gordon, G. S., Picchi, J. and Roof, B. S. (1973) Antifracture efficacy of long-term estrogens for osteoporosis. *Trans. Assoc. Am. Phys.*, 86, 326–31.

Gower, W. E. and Pedrini, V. (1969) Age related variations in protein-polysaccharides from human nucleus pulposus, annulus fibrosus, and costal cartilage. *J. Bone Jt Surg.*, 51A, 1154–62.

Gowers, W. R. (1904) Lumbago: its lessons and analogues. *Br. Med. J.*, 1, 117.

Grahame, R. (1977) Cruralgie d'origine discale: aspects cliniques, thérapeutiques et progurstique. Actualites en rééducation fonctionelles et réadaptation. 2 eme series pp. 91–95 Plasson, Paris.

Harmon, P. H. (1963) Anterior excision and vertebral body fusion operation for intervertebral disk syndromes of the lower lumbar spine. *Clin. Orthopaed.* 26, 107–27.

Hart, F. D. (1978) *Drug Treatment of the Rheumatic Diseases,*. ADIS Press, Sydney.

Hart, F. D. (1980) Rheumatic disorders. in *Drug Treatment: Principles and Practice of Clinical Pharmacology and Therapeutics* (ed. G. S. Avery), 2nd edn, ADIS Press, Sydney, pp. 846–88.

Haussler, M. R. and McCain, T. A. (1977) Basic and clinical concepts related to vitamin D metabolism and action. *N. Engl. J. Med.*, 297, 974–83.

Heaney, R. P., Recker, R. R. and Saville, P. D. (1977) Calcium balance and calcium requirement in middle-aged women. *Am. J. Clin. Nutr.*, 30, 1603–11.

Heaney, R. P., Recker, R. R. and Saville, P. D. (1978a) Menopausal changes in calcium balance performance. *J. Lab. Clin. Med.*, 92, 953–63.

Heaney, R. P., Recker, R. R. and Saville, P. D. (1978b) Menopausal changes in bone remodelling. *J. Lab. Clin. Med.*, 92, 964–70.

Hodgson, A. R. (1975) Infectious disease of the spine in *The Spine* (eds R. H. Rothman and F. A. Simeone), Saunders, Philadelphia.

Holick, M. F., Frommer, J. E., McNeill, S. C., Richtand, N. M., Henley, J. W. and Potts, J. T. (1977) Photometabolism of 7-dehydrocholesterol to previtamin D_3 in skin. *Biochem. Biophys. Res. Commun.*, 76, 107–14.

Hulley, S. B., Vogel, J. M., Donaldson, C. L., Bayers, J. H., Friedman, R. J. and Rosen, S. N. (1971) The effect of supplemental oral phosphate on the bone mineral changes during prolonged bed rest. *J. Clin. Invest.*, 50, 2506–18.

Hurxthal, L. M. and Vose, G. P. (1969) The relationship of dietary calcium intake to radiographic bone density in normal and osteoporotic persons. *Calcified Tiss. Res.*, 4, 245–56.

Huskisson, E. C. (1978) Non-steroidal anti-inflammatory analgesics: basic clinical pharmacology and therapeutic use. *Drugs*, 15, 387–92.

Immemkamp, M. (1971) Benign osteoblastoma of the fourth lumbar vertebra with lumbosacral stiffness. *Z. Orthopaed.*, 109, 616–25.

Jowsey, J. (1979) The long-term treatment of osteoporosis with fluoride, calcium and vitamin D, in *Osteoporosis II.* (ed. U. S. Barzel), Grune and Stratton, New York, p. 123.

Kellgren, J. G. (1961) Osteoarthrosis in patients and populations. *Br. Med. J.*, 2, 1–6.

Kelman, H. (1944) Epidural injection therapy for sciatic pain. *Am. J. Surg.*, 64, 183–90.

Lee, P., Rooney, P. J., Sturrock, R. D., Kennedy, A. C. and Dick, W. C. (1974) The aetiology and pathogenesis of osteoarthrosis, a review. *Seminars Arthr. Rheum.*, 3, 189–218.

Lindsay, R., Hart, D. M., Purdie, D., Ferguson, M. M., Clark, A. S. and Kraszewski, A. (1978).

Livingstone, W. K. (1943) *Pain Mechanisms*. Macmillan, New York.

Liyanage, S. P. (1986) The orthodox/heterodox fringe in rheumatological management in *Recent Advances in Rheumatology*, 4 (ed. J. M. H. Moll and R. D. Sturrock), Churchill Livingstone, Edinburgh, London, Melbourne, New York, pp. 235–48.

Macdonald, A. J. R., Macrae, K. D., Master, B. R. and Rubin, A. P. (1983) Superficial acupuncture in the relief of chronic low back pain. *Ann. R. Coll. Surg of Eng.*, 65, 44–6.

MacLellan, D. I. and Wilson, F. C. (1967) Osteoid osteoma of the spine. *J. Bone Jt Surg.*, **49A**, 111–21.

Macnab, I. (1977) *Backache*, Williams & Wilkins, Baltimore, p. 18.

Man, S. C. and Baragar, F. D. (1974) Preliminary clinical study of acupuncture in rheumatoid arthritis. *J. Rheumatol.*, 1, 126–9.

Marshall, D. M., Gallagher, J. C., Guha, P., Hanes, F., Oldfield, W. and Nordin, B. E. C. (1977) The effect of 1α-hydroxycholecalciferol and hormone therapy on the calcium balance of post-menopausal osteoporosis. *Calcified Tiss. Res.*, **22**, 78–84.

Mathews, J. A. (1968) Dynamic discography: a study of lumbar traction. *Ann. Phys. Med.*, 9, 275–9.

Mathews, J. A. and Hickling, J. (1975) Lumbar traction: a double-blind controlled study for sciatica. *Rheumatol. Rehabil.*, **14**, 222.

McAllister, V. L. (1975) Symptomatic vertebral haemangiomas. *Brain*, **98**, 71–80.

McDonald, T. W., Annegers, J. F., O'Fallon, W. M. *et al.* (1977) Exogenous estrogen and endometrial carcinoma: case-control and incidence study. *Am. J. Obs. Gynacol.*, **127**, 572–80.

McKee, G. K. (1971) McKee–Farrar total prosthetic replacement of the hip. in *Total Hip Replacement* (ed M. Jayson), Sector, London, pp. 47–67.

Melzack, R. (1978) *The Puzzle of Pain*. Basic Books, New York.

Melzack, R. and Wall, P. D. (1965) Pain mechanisms: a new theory. *Science*, **150**, 971–9.

Mendelson, G., Selwood, T. S., Kranz, H., Loh, T. S., Kidson, M. A. and Scott, D. S. (1983) Acupuncture treatment of chronic back pain. *Amer. J. Med.*, **74**, 49–55.

Minaire, P., Meunier, P. J., Berard, E., Edouard, C., Goedert, G. and Pilonchery, G. (1980) Effects du dichloromethylene diphosphonate sur la perte osseuse précoce du paraplégique. *Ann. Méd. Phys.*, **23**, 37–43.

Mitchell, J. R., Jollow, D. J., Potter, W. Z., Davies, D. C., Gillette, J. R. and Brodie, B. B. (1973) Acetaminophen-induced hepatic necrosis – I. Role of drug metabolism. *J. Pharmacol. Exp. Ther.*, **187**, 185–94.

Moldofsky, H., Scarisbrick, P. and England, R. (1975) Musculoskeletal symptoms and non-REM sleep disturbance in patients with 'fibrositis syndrome' and health subjects. *Psychosomat. Med.*, **37**, 341–51.

Moll, J. M. H. (1976) Investigation of osteoarthrosis in *Osteoarthrosis. Clinics in Rheumatic Diseases*, Vol. 2, No 3 (ed V. Wright), Saunders, London, pp. 587–613.

Moll, J. M. H. (1983) *Management of Rheumatic Disorders*, Chapman and Hall, London.

National Research Council, Food and Nutrition Board (1974) *Recommended Dietary Allowances*, 8th revised edn, National Academy of Sciences, Washington DC.

Nesterov, A. L. (1964) The clinical course of Kashin–Beck disease. *Arthr. Rheum.*, 7, 29–40.

Nilsen, K. H., Jayson, M. I. V. and Dixon, A. St. J. (1978) Microcrystalline calcium hydroxyapatite compound in corticosteroid-treated rheumatoid patients: a controlled study. *Br. Med. J.*, 2, 1124.

Nogen, A. G. and Bremner, J. E. (1978) Fatal acetaminophen overdosage in a young child. *J. Paediatr.*, **92**, 832–3.

Nordin, B. E. C. (1962) Calcium balance and calcium requirement in spinal osteoporosis. *Am. J. Clin. Nutr.*, **10**, 384–90.

Nordin, B. E. C., Horsman, A., Marshall, D. H., Simpson, M. and Waterhouse, G. M. (1979) Calcium requirement and calcium therapy. *Clin. Orthopaed. Relat. Res.*, **140**, 216–39.

Owens, R. (1971) The Charnley arthroplasty, in *Total Hip Replacement* (ed. M. Jayson), Sector, London, pp. 68–85.

Pearce, J. M. S. and Moll, J. M. H. (1967) Conservative treatment and natural history of acute lumbar disc lesions. *J. Neurol. Neurosurg. Psychiat.*, 30, 13–17.

Pritchard, D. J. (1975) Granulomatous infections of bones and joints. *Orthopaed. Clinics N. Am.*, 6, 1029–47.

Raisz, L. G., Au, W. Y. W., Friedman, J. and Niemaun, I. (1967) Thyrocalcitonin and bone resorption: studies employing a tissue culture bioassay. *Am. J. Med.*, 43, 684–690.

Reeve, J., Meunier, P. J., Parsons, J. A., Bernat, M., Bijvoet, O. L. M., Courpron, P. *et al.* (1980) Anabolic effect of human parathyroid hormone fragment on trabecular bone in involutional osteoporosis: a multicentre trial. *Br. Med. J.*, 280, 1340–4.

Resnick, D. and Niwayama, G. (1976) Radiographic and pathologic features of spinal involvement in diffuse ideopathic skeletal hyperostosis (DISH). *Radiology*, 119, 559–68.

Riggs, B. L., Jawsey, J., Kelly, P. J., Jones, J. D. and Mahen, F. T. (1969) Effect of sex hormones on bone in primary osteoporosis. *J. Clin. Invest.*, 48, 1065–72.

Robinson, W. D. (1981) Management of degenerative joint disease, in *Textbook of Rheumatology*, Vol. II (eds W. N. Kelley, E. D. Harris, S. Ruddy and C. B. Sledge), Saunders, Philadelphia, pp. 1491–9.

Russell, R. G. G. and Fleisch, H. (1975) Pyrophosphate and diphosphonates in skeletal metabolism. Physiological, clinical and therapeutic aspects. *Clin. Orthopaed. Relat. Res.*, 108, 241–63.

Ryan, W. G., Schwartz, T. B. and Northrop, G. (1970) Experiences in the treatment of Paget's disease of bone with mithramycin. *J. Am. Med. Assoc.*, 213, 1153–7.

Saville, P. D. and Heaney, R. (1972) Treatment of osteoporosis and diphosphonates. *Seminars Drug Treat.*, 2, 47–50.

Schmorl, G. and Junghanns, J. (1971) *The Human Spine in Health and Disease*, 2nd American edn, Grune and Stratton, New York.

Seeman, E. and Riggs, B. L. (1982) The treatment of postmenopausal and senile osteoporosis, in *Calcium Disorders* (eds D. Heath and S. J. Marx), Butterworth, London, pp. 69–91.

Shah, K. D. and Wright, V. (1967) Intra-articular hydrocortisone in osteoarthrosis. *Ann. Rheum. Dis.*, 26, 316–18.

Shapiro, J. R., Moore, W. T., Jorgensen, H., Reid, J., Epps, C. H. and Whedon, D. (1975) Osteoporosis: evaluation of diagnosis and therapy. *Arch. Intern. Med.*, 135, 563–67.

Simmons, D. P. and Chrisman, O. D. (1965) Salicylate inhibition of cartilage degeneration. *Arthr. Rheumatol.*, 8, 960–9.

Sims-Williams, H., Jayson, M. I. V., Young, S. M. S., Baddeley, H. and Collins, E. (1978) Controlled trial of mobilization and manipulation for patients with low back pain in general practice. *Br. Med. J.*, 2, 1338–40.

Sims-Williams, H., Jayson, M. I. V., Young, S. M. S., Baddeley, H. and Collins, E. (1979) Controlled trial of mobilization and manipulation for low back pain in hospital patients. *Br. Med. J.*, 2, 1318–20.

Singer, F. R. (1977) *Paget's Disease of Bone*, Plenum, New York.

Slowicj, F. A., Campbell, C. J. and Kettelkamp, D. B. (1968) Aneurysmal bone cyst: an analysis of 13 cases. *J. Bone Jt Surg.*, 50A, 1142–51.

Smythe, H. A. (1972) Non-articular rheumatism and the fibrositis syndrome. *Arthritis and Allied Conditions*. 8th edn (eds J. L. Hollander and D. J. McCarty), Lee and Febiger, Philadelphia, pp. 874–84.

Snoek, W., Webber, H. and Jorgensen, B. (1977) Double-blind evaluation of extradural corticosteroid methylprednisolone for herniated lumbar discs. *Acta Orthopaed. Scand.*, 48, 635–41.

Sola, A. E. and Williams, R. L. (1956) Myofascial pain syndromes. *Neurology*, 6, 91–5.

Sørensen, O. H., Andersen, R. B., Christensen, M. S., Friis, T., Hjorth, L., Jorgensen, F. S., Lund, B., Melsen, F. and Mosekilde, L. (1977) Treatment of senile osteoporosis with 1 α-hydroxyvitamin D$_3$. *Clin. Endocrinol. (Oxford)*, 7, 1695–775.

Stecher, R. M. (1955) Heberden's nodes: a clinical description of osteoarthritis of the finger joints *Ann. Rheum. Dis.*, 14, 1–10.

Stockman, R. (1920) *Rheumatism and Arthritis*, Green, Edinburgh.

Swezey, R. L. (1978) *Arthritis: National Therapy in Rehabilitation*, Philadelphia, Saunders, p. 140.

Travell, J. and Rinzler, S. H. (1952) The myofascial genesis of pain. *Postgrad. Med.*, 11, 425–34.

Turban, E. and Urlich, S. (1978) The evaluation of therapeutic acupuncture. *Social Sci. Med.*, 12, 39.

Urban, J. P. G. and Maroudas, A. (1979) Measurement of fixed charge density in the intervertebral disc. *Biochim. Biophys. Acta*, 586, 166–78.

Vernon-Roberts, B. (1976) Pathology of degenerative spondylosis, in *The Lumbar Spine and Back Pain* (ed M. Jayson), Sector, London, pp. 55–75.

Vismans, F. I. F. E. and Bijvoet, O. L. M. (1985) Biphosphonates – do they have a role in osteoporosis? *Bone*, 2, 2–3.

Wallach, S., Cohn, S. H., Atkins, H. L., Ellis, K. J., Kohberger, R., Aloia, J. F. and Zanzi, I. (1977) Effect of salmon calcitonin on skeletal mass in osteoporosis. *Curr. Ther. Res.*, 22, 556–72.

Wallach, S. and Henneman, P. H. (1959) Prolonged estrogen therapy in postmenopausal women. *J. Am. Med. Assoc.*, 171, 1637–42.

Weiss, N. S., Szekely, D. R., English, D. R. and Schweid, A. I. (1979) Endometrial cancer in relation to patterns of menopausal estrogen use. *J. Am. Med. Assoc.*, 242, 261–4.

Wilson, R. A. (1962) The roles of estrogen and progesterone in breast and genital cancer. *J. Am. Med. Assoc.*, 182, 327–31.

Wood, P. H. N. (1976) Osteoarthrosis in the community, in *Osteoarthrosis Clinics in Rheumatic Diseases* Vol. 2, No 3 (ed V. Wright), Saunders, London, pp. 495–507.

Wyke, B. (1976) Neurological aspects of low back pain, in *The Lumbar Spine and Back Pain* (ed M. Jayson), Sector, London, pp. 189–256.

Yates, A. (1976) Treatment of back pain, in *The Lumbar Spine and Back Pain* (ed M. Jayson), Sector, London, pp. 341–53.

Yates, D. W. (1978) A comparison of the types of epidural injection commonly used in the treatment of low back pain and sciatica. *Rheumatol. Rehabil.*, 17, 181–6.

Young, J. M. and Funk, F. J. (1953) Incidence of tumor metastasis to the lumbar spine. *J. Bone Jt Surg.*, 35A, 55–64.

CHAPTER 14

Gout and other

crystal-deposition disorders

J. M. H. Moll

14.1 INTRODUCTION

The three main crystal-deposition disorders encountered in clinical practice are those associated with urate, pyrophosphate, and hydroxyapatite. The three types of crystal deposited in relation to tissues of the locomotor system are characterized by somewhat different clinical presentations and therapeutic needs. Although this chapter will be largely devoted to the 'classical' crystal deposition disease, urate gout, brief comments will also be made on the management of other crystal-deposition states the rheumatologist is likely to encounter in clinical practice.

14.2 GOUT

Gout has featured prominently in medical and social circles for over 2000 years and has been variously termed 'The King of Diseases' and the 'Disease of Kings', the former reflecting its dramatic clinical expressions, the latter its tendency to affect personages rather than persons.

There are three main points of therapeutic relevance in the context of hyperuricaemic individuals. The first is the treatment of acute attacks of gout (if present) – generally agreed by patients and doctors to be one of the most painful experiences known to man. The second is the long-term management of gouty patients, and the decision regarding the institution of hypouricaemic therapy. The third, over which there is not total agreement, is what to do when asymptomatic hyperuricaemia is detected.

This section will endeavour to deal with the points individually, although in practice overlap may exist between these issues.

14.2.1   Acute gout

The acute episode of gout should be regarded as a rheumatological emergency, demanding immediate treatment. The degree of the patient's discomfort is such that therapy cannot be left to the next day.

The management of the acute attack is along the following lines:

1. Advise the patient to rest in bed or in a chair with the limb protected and raised. (The patient may intuitively have adopted this position in view of the need to avoid physical contact with the affected part.)
2. Cold compresses may provide some relief while drug therapy is taking effect.
3. *Avoid using hypouricaemic drugs in the acute episode.* This is a common error and may well prolong the attack.

TABLE 14.1
NSAIDs found to be useful in acute gout

NSAID	*References*
Phenylbutazone (now withdrawn for use in gout in UK)	Wallace (1972) Kuzell *et al.* (1952) Kidd *et al.* (1953) Johnson *et al.* (1954)
Indomethacin	Smyth *et al.* (1963) Hart and Boardman (1963) Norcross (1963)
Naproxen	Cuq (1973) Willkens and Case (1973) Sturge *et al.* (1977)
Fenoprofen	Wallace (1975) Wanasukapunt *et al.* (1976)
Ibuprofen	Schweitz *et al.* (1978)
Indoprofen	Caruso *et al.* (1977)

4. Analgesic/anti-inflammatory drugs (Table 14.1). *Colchicine* is the classical remedy, although more modern drugs are equally effective. *Phenylbutazone* enjoyed a vogue for many years, but a recent recommendation by the CSM stipulates that in view of dangerous toxic effects the drug should be reserved for ankylosing spondylitis. *Indomethacin* has for many years been considered a reasonable substitute for phenylbutazone in acute gout. More recently marketed NSAIDs such as naproxen have also been shown to be beneficial. These drugs and their handling will now be discussed in further detail.

(a) Colchicine

The drug can be given orally or intravenously. The most common route of administration is by mouth in repeated small doses in order to minimize gastrointestinal side effects. Patients vary as to their reaction to the drug, and it is important that when taken for the first time, the dose at which side effects appear is recorded, as this dose will lead to the same toxic effects next time the drug is taken. If titrated in this way, it may be possible to achieve a therapeutic effect with a smaller dose that is non-toxic.

The usual dose is 0.5 mg (one tablet) every hour or 1 mg every 2 hours, with a dose of 1 mg given at the start of the attack. This regime is continued until either (1) the attack subsides or (2) gastrointestinal side effects call for the drug to be stopped.

If there is a delay or seeming non-response to treatment, it is wise to bear in mind the maximum recommended dose. This depends on body weight, and the range for colchicine given orally is 8–16 mg.

About 75% of unselected patients with acute gout respond briskly to colchicine (Wallace *et al.*, 1967), non-response being attributable in some patients to delay in initiating therapy.

In view of the high frequency of gastrointestinal side effects with oral colchicine (80% in those receiving full therapeutic doses), the intravenous route is a useful alternative means of administration. It is preferable (and as effective) in patients known to react adversely to the oral preparation, or for those in whom it is not desirable to run the risk of gastrointestinal side effects.

A single dose of 3 mg intravenously is as effective as full amounts of oral colchicine, and this dose is usually sufficient to halt the attack within 6–24 hours. This raises the other benefit of intravenous administration, its rapidity of response which is substantially greater than treatment via the oral route (in which response takes 12–48 hours). However, intravenous colchicine administration is not without problems, the main one being extravenous infiltration due to inaccurate venepuncture. Local tissue necrosis ensues as the colchicine solution is a powerful irritant. This toxic effect may also manifest as phlebitis after intravenous injection.

The gastrointestinal effects of colchicine may display biochemical as well as clinical features, and the site of action of the drug is largely at jejunal and ileal levels (Webb *et al.*, 1968; Race *et al.*, 1970; Rubulis *et al.*, 1970), with consistent increases in faecal fat, nitrogen, sodium and potassium, and decreases in D-xylose and vitamin B_{12} absorption. Such malabsorption effects are only observed with oral colchicine.

Other toxic effects are unusual with colchicine. One man has been reported to have developed azoospermia while taking 0.6 mg twice daily as prophylaxis (Merlin, 1972), although other evidence is against significant effects of long-term colchicine on sperm counts, testosterone, LH or FSH levels (Brenner and Paulsen, 1976), or on fertility (Yü and Gutman, 1961).

In addition to its therapeutic effect, colchicine has a useful diagnostic value in that acute gout is the only disorder in which a dramatic, objective response to the drug occurs consistently (Wallace *et al.*, 1967). However, although characteristic, this effect is not pathognomic as the response has been reported in sarcoid arthritis (Kaplan, 1960), hydroxyapatite deposition disease (Thompson *et al.*, 1968), and in pyrophosphate arthropathy (McCarty, 1976).

(b) *Phenylbutazone*

Phenylbutazone (its equally effective analogue, oxyphenbutazone, has recently been withdrawn in the UK) is a highly effective drug in the treatment of acute gout, some would say even more effective than colchicine.

The drug used to be the drug of first choice in treating acute gout in suitable patients but recent CSM recommendations have placed its further use in this disorder *sub judice*, and at present it is advised that phenylbutazone be restricted to ankylosing spondylitis.

However, whether or not phenylbutazone survives current restrictions it is of historic and therapeutic interest to consider its anti-gout effects in some further detail.

The optimal dose of the drug in the treatment of acute gout was about 600 mg day^{-1}. Higher doses gave no additional advantage. The drug was usually administered orally 200 mg three times daily, and 3–5 days of treatment was usually sufficient to halt an acute attack of gout. Although too high for long-term management of other disorders such as rheumatoid arthritis, these short courses were relatively safe providing the drug was not given for more than a few days (Scott, 1978). However, even in the short term, serious toxic effects could occur, the most likely being aggravation of an already existing peptic ulcer. For this reason gastric or duodenal ulceration contraindicated phenylbutazone therapy. Fluid retention was another side effect that could occur in the short term, and the drug was withheld in those with congestive heart failure.

Marrow depression (the main source of current opposition to continuing phenylbutazone in disorders other than ankylosing spondylitis), hepatocellular damage, and rashes are very rare during brief therapy (Wallace, 1977).

The question of interaction between phenylbutazone and other drugs has been considered elsewhere in this book.

(c) *Indomethacin*

Indomethacin in substantial dosage is acknowledged as an effective treatment for acute gout. A usual dosage is 50 mg four times daily. Its efficacy in this disorder is comparable to that of phenylbutazone (Smyth, 1970). The main drawback to large-dose indomethacin therapy is the frequency of side effects, particularly CNS and gastrointestinal effects. Boardman and Hart (1967), for example, found that 60% of patients on relatively high doses of indomethacin developed side effects, usually within 48 hours of starting treatment. A particularly unpleasant side effect is headache, which can be so severe as to incapacitate the patient for 2–3 days.

(d) Other drugs

Naproxen has been shown to be a useful NSAID in acute gout (Cuq, 1973; Willkens and Case, 1973; Willkens et al., 1976). Dosages of up to 1.5 g in the first 24 hours, with lesser dosages for 3–4 days have provided satisfactory relief in about 75% of patients.

Fenoprofen has also been shown to be effective in acute gout, 14 of 19 patients in one study exhibiting an 'excellent' or 'good' response (Wallace, 1975). Doses averaged 3200 g per day for 3–8 days.

Salicylates are less effective than the drugs already mentioned. Like phenylbutazone, salicylate (in large dosage) is uricosuric. In low dosage, however, it causes urate retention.

Systemic corticosteroids or corticotrophins are effective in the treatment of acute gout but are rarely indicated. They are, however, useful in the occasional patient who remains refractory to non-steroidal drugs.

Acute gout is sometimes associated with a large joint effusion. This is particularly so when the knee is affected and immediate relief can be obtained by fluid drainage and injection of a corticosteroid preparation.

14.2.2 Long-term management

(a) Indications

Although swift control of the acute attack of gout is important, a more compelling issue is long-term control of the gouty diathesis with hypouricaemic drugs. It is this long-term control of hyperuricaemia that eventually controls the manifestations of this biochemical disorder, although in view of its genetic provenance a 'cure' cannot be achieved.

In general, if long-term management is thought indicated the aim is to reduce the serum uric acid to below 6.0 mg %, which is below the 6.4 mg % concentration level at which uric acid saturates the extracellular fluid.

The question of long-term management can be divided into two issues. First, whether hypouricaemic treatment should be given at all? Second, if indicated, which type of drug should be used – uricosuric or xanthine oxidase inhibitor?

Indications for lowering the serum urate are not absolute, but a reasonable practical guide is as follows:

1. Gout with chronic joint manifestations.
2. The presence of tophi.

3. Evidence of renal damage.
4. Joint manifestations associated with a much raised serum urate level – 8.0 mg % or over.

In the treatment of uncomplicated gout, usually the form in which the condition presents at the initial diagnosis, the choice between uricosuric therapy and allopurinol depends largely on personal preference. Both drugs are effective in lowering the serum uric acid, although allopurinol is rather more potent. However, uricosurics have been in clinical use for longer than allopurinol and have been shown to be relatively free from harmful effects. Some clinicians therefore continue to use uricosuric therapy as a first choice, although the current swing is slightly in favour of allopurinol.

However, there are some special indications for using allopurinol, and not one of the uricosurics. These are as follows (Scott, 1978):

1. Extensive tophaceous gout.
2. Gout associated with massive over production of urate, with high renal excretion of this substance.
3. Failed uricosuric therapy. (However, before pronouncing therapeutic failure ensure that this is not due to lack of compliance.)
4. Intolerance or hypersensitivity to uricosuric drugs.
5. Gout attended by severe renal failure. (Uricosurics depend on the kidney for their action, and cannot therefore operate when significant renal disease is present.)
6. Uric acid stone formation.
7. Acute uric acid nephropathy. (This occurs during treatment of leukaemia or reticuloses with cytotoxic agents, when massive amounts of uric acid are produced from nucleoprotein breakdown.)
8. Hypoxanthine–guanine phosphoribosyltransferase (HGPRT) deficiency.

The most widely used uricosuric agents are probenecid and sulphinpyrazone. Benzbromarone, benziodarone, and zoxazolamine have also been used in Europe. Attention has been drawn recently to some combined-action drugs, such as halofenate (uricosuric + hypolipidaemic) (Hutchison and Wilkinson, 1973), and ticrynafen (uricosuric + diuretic) (Jain *et al.*, 1976). However, these novel drugs have somewhat limited clinical indications in routine gout therapy and have been received with reserved acceptance. Ticrynafen (Tienilic acid) has (unfortunately) been withdrawn in the UK and USA because of severe liver damage associated with a number of deaths.

The alternative to uricosuric therapy is to achieve hypouricaemia by decreasing urate synthesis, as opposed to increasing its excretion (Kelley and Wyngaarden, 1971; Wyngaarden and Kelley, 1972; Yü, 1974; Kelley, 1975a, b). Allopurinol was the first drug introduced into clinical practice as a uric acid lowering agent, and achieves this by inhibiting xanthine oxidase (Elion *et al.*, 1966). Thiopurinol also inhibits uric acid synthesis (this is achieved by a different mechanism), but the drug has only enjoyed limited clinical usage (Delbarre *et al.*, 1968; Carter and Hamet, 1973).

The hypouricaemic drugs will now be considered in some further detail.

(b) *Uricosuric agents* (Table 14.2)

In the UK the two uricosuric drugs in current usage are probenecid (the related compound ethebenecid was withdrawn some years ago) and sulphinpyrazone.

The dose of probenecid is 0.5–1.0 g twice daily, and that of sulphinpyrazone 100 g three times daily. Minor dose adjustments may be necessary in order to maintain the plasma uric acid within normal levels.

TABLE 14.2
Uricosurics

Preparations available in UK	Tablets	Relative cost (BNF price bands)
Probenecid (Benemid, MSD)	500 mg	C
Sulphinpyrazone (Anturan, Geigy)	100 mg	C
	200 mg	D

The benzofuran compounds, benzbromarone and benziodarone are more powerful uricosurics and appear to possess in addition a uricostatic effect (Begemann and Neu, 1975). As stated previously these compounds are not in use in the UK but are popular on the Continent.

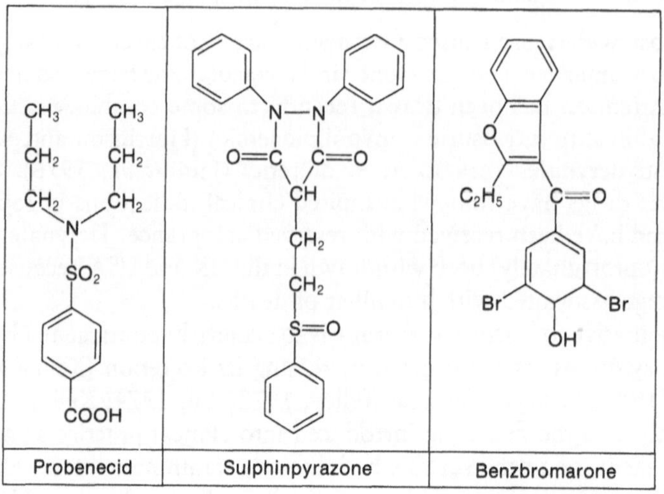

Figure 14.1 Comparison of structural formulae of uricosuric agents (after Fox, 1977).

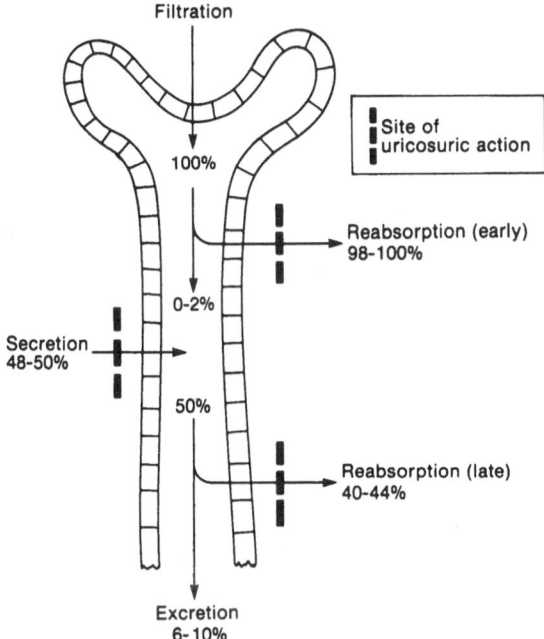

Filtration

100%

Site of
uricosuric action

Reabsorption (early)
98-100%

0-2%

Secretion
48-50%

50%

Reabsorption (late)
40-44%

Excretion
6-10%

Figure 14.2 Hypothetical mode of action of uricosuric agents – inhibition of initial absorption and secretion, and probably an important inhibiting effect at a distal reabsorptive site (after Rieselbach and Steele, 1974; Fox, 1977).

The structures of the different uricosurics is shown in Fig. 14.1. As can be seen there are considerable variations in their chemical constitution. The drugs act by inhibiting the renal tubular reabsorption of uric acid. This probably takes place at two sites (Fig. 14.2) although the precise mechanism of reabsorption blockade is not yet clear (Rieselbach and Steele, 1974). The increased urinary output of urate, if sustained, is accompanied by a decrease in the frequency of gouty attacks (not a sudden cessation of attacks) and eventually complete freedom from further attacks. Tophi became smaller and may disappear.

It is important to cover the first few months of interval treatment with a NSAID. Colchicine remains popular for this purpose at a relatively low dose of 0.5 mg three times daily. The duration of NSAID cover varies between clinicians, but most would continue NSAID therapy for 6 months and some for as long as a year.

Uricosurics are well tolerated although dyspepsia and rashes are seen occasionally. The nephrotic syndrome has been reported as a rare complication with probenecid (Ferris *et al.*, 1961; Sokol *et al.*, 1967; Scott and O'Brien, 1968).

TABLE 14.3
Metabolic effects of allopurinol (after Kelley, 1975)

Clinical effect	Mechanism	Effector
Hypouricaemia	Xanthine oxidase inhibition	Allopurinol Oxipurinol
Decreased total purine production	Inhibition of PP-ribose-P amidotransferase PP-ribose-P depletion	Allopurinol-1-*N*-ribosylphosphate IMP Allopurinol
Orotidinuria	Inhibition of orotidine 5'-phosphate decarboxylase	Oxipurinol-7-*N*-ribosylphosphate Oxipurinol-1-*N*-ribosylphosphate Allopurinol-1-*N*-ribosylphosphate
Orotic aciduria	Inhibition of orotate-phosphoribosyl transferase PP-ribose-P depletion	OMP Allopurinol
Apparent increased activity of orotate phosphoribosyl transferase and orotidine 5'-phosphate decarboxylase	Stabilization of enzymes by shift to higher molecular weight	Allopurinol-1-*N*-ribosylphosphate Oxipurinol-7-*N*-ribosylphosphate

(c) *Allopurinol*

Allopurinol is the most commonly used hypouricaemic agent in the UK (Table 14.3). The drug competitively inhibits xanthine oxidase, and also suppresses overall purine biosynthesis (Fig. 14.3). The net effect is a reduction of the serum and urine uric acid, and an accumulation of urine hypoxanthine and xanthine. (The formation of xanthine stones, a complication expected on theoretical grounds, is in fact very rare.)

The maintenance dose of allopurinol is usually between 300 and 400 mg/ day, although for patients who do not respond to this dosage up to 1000 mg/ day have been used. When there is renal impairment, smaller dosages may be indicated.

The fall in serum uric acid is very rapid with allopurinol therapy, and, as mentioned for uricosuric therapy, it is essential to employ concurrent anti-inflammatory therapy for several months to avoid precipitating fresh attacks of acute gout. Some clinicians reduce this risk by starting with a smaller daily dose of 100 mg and increasing this gradually. There is evidence that single daily dose administration is effective in producing a sustained fall in serum urate (Brewis *et al.*, 1975).

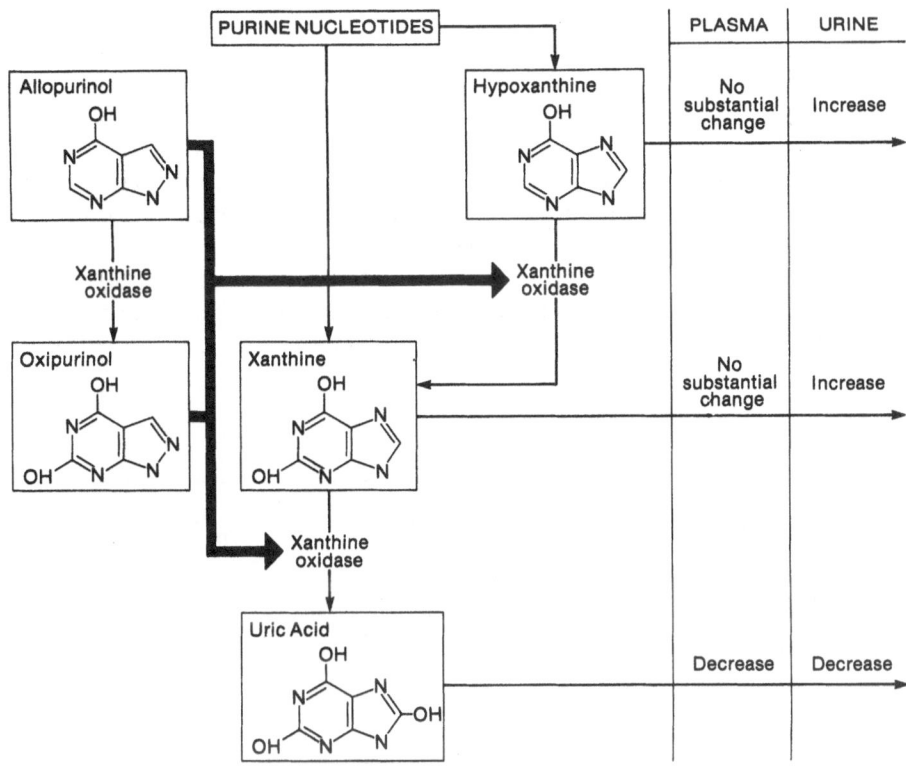

Figure 14.3 Effect of allopurinol on uric acid formation in man. The final steps of nucleotide degradation are catalysed by xanthine oxidase. Allopurinol is converted into oxipurinol by this enzyme, and both of these compounds inhibit xanthine oxidase. The effect on plasma and urine concentrations are included (after Fox, 1977).

TABLE 14.4
Allopurinol toxicity

Toxic effect	Reference
*Rash	Straitigos *et al.* (1972)
Gastrointestinal intolerance	Kantor (1970)
Alopecia	Auerbach and Orentrich (1968)
Bone marrow suppression with leukopenia and thrombocytopenia	Irby *et al.* (1966)
Agranulocytosis	Greenberg and Zambarano (1972)
Hepatitis	Lidsky and Sharp (1967)
	Simmons *et al.* (1972)
Vasculitis	Jarzobski *et al.* (1970)
Fatality	Mills (1971)
	Kantor (1970)
Total 20%	Tjandramaga *et al.* (1972)

*Most common side effect

The pattern of improvement with allopurinol is similar to that observed with uricosurics; the gouty attacks gradually became less frequent and ultimately stop altogether. In parallel with this, tophi diminish in size and eventually disappear.

If allopurinol is stopped, uric acid levels return to pretreatment levels (Loebl and Scott, 1974). However, acute gouty attacks may not return. Despite this, the usual policy is to continue urate-lowering drugs – whether uricosuric or xanthine oxidase inhibitor – indefinitely.

Allopurinol, like the uricosurics, is relatively free from side effects (see Table 14.4). Rashes are seen occasionally, and these are more common in patients with renal failure. Very rarely an acute hypersensitivity reaction occurs (Scott, 1980).

TABLE 14.5
Allopurinol

Preparations available in UK	Tablets	Relative cost (BNF price bands)
Allopurinol tablets (BP)	100 mg	D
(BNF)	300 mg	G
Aluline (Steinhard)	100 mg	E
	300 mg	H
Caplenal (Berk)	100 mg	E
	300 mg	H
Cosuric (DDSA)	100 mg	E
	300 mg	G
Zyloric (Calmic)	100 mg	F
	300 mg	I

(d) *Combination therapy*

Allopurinol and a uricosuric drug may be used in combination (Kelley and Wyngaarden, 1971; Wyngaarden and Kelley, 1972; Yü, 1974; Kelley, 1975a, b), and such an approach is sometimes tried in patients in whom either drug used singly is without effect. This combined therapy usually results in a further increase of urine uric acid excretion and a further diminution in the serum urate level.

(e) *Other measures*

(i) Diet

Severe dietary restriction by limiting purine intake is no longer regarded necessary since the advent of effective hypouricaemic agents. However, it is still worth advising the average gouty patient to avoid excessive purine intake. Although some clinicians doubt the effectiveness of purine restriction, there is evidence to show that, properly adhered to, a diet limited in purine content will reduce the urinary excretion of uric acid by 200–400 mg per day, with a lowering of mean serum urate level by 1 mg % (Gutman and Yü, 1952) or even more (Rieselbach *et al.*, 1970).

Severe dietary restriction of purine, although not generally necessary, may be useful in: (1) patients in whom renal function is very limited and the control of hyperuricaemia with drugs ineffective; (2) patients who are averse to taking drugs of any kind.

Foodstuffs can be divided into three main categories according to their purine content (Smyth, 1972):

1. High (150–1000 mg purine/100 g food) (e.g. sweetbreads, anchovies, sardines, liver, kidney, meat extracts).
2. Medium (50–150 mg/100 g) (e.g. meats, fish, seafood, beans, peas, lentils, spinach).
3. Low (0–15 mg/100 g) (e.g. vegetables, fruits, milk, cheese, eggs, cereal).

Other dietary considerations are as follows:

1. *Calorie restriction.* Many gouty patients are overweight and should attempt to restore this to ideal weight, although severe restriction as part of 'crash' dieting should be avoided as acute gout may be precipitated.
2. *Alcohol restriction.* Alcohol over indulgence is relatively common among gouty patients. Chronic overconsumption may increase purine production (MacLachlan and Rodnan, 1967) and patients should be advised about this. Particular alcoholic beverages appear to carry a greater gout-triggering effect, notably beers, heavy wines, and champagnes. Spirits, perhaps surprisingly, seem to be less provocative.
3. *Avoiding 'idiosyncratic' items.* The differential effect of alcohol drinks could be included here. Some foods appear to trigger acute gout in some individuals by an idiosyncratic effect. Asparagus is one example, and several of the author's patients have commented on the seeming effect of strawberries in this respect.
4. *Caution at times of dietary indiscretion.* Whether or not this advice will be heeded is another matter, but gouty patients should be warned that the 'binge eating' during 'high days and holidays' and on other feasting occasions can be against their interests, if they haven't previously experienced this!

(ii) Uricase

Increased destruction of uric acid by the use of uricase (an enzyme that degrades uric acid to allantoin and carbon dioxide) remains experimental, but may eventually find a place in controlling hyperuricaemia in patients with renal failure caused by acute uric acid nephropathy (Brogard et al., 1973; Kissel et al., 1975).

14.2.3   Asymptomatic hyperuricaemia

It is important not to confuse hyperuricaemia per se with gout – the latter being defined as 'a clinical disease manifest by acute inflammatory arthritis and induced by the deposition of urate crystals' according to Seegmiller and Howell (1962). There are many causes for hyperuricaemia (a biochemical abnormality defined solely by the serum urate concentration), and primary gout is only one of these conditions. The management of asymptomatic hyperuricaemia therefore requires special considerations.

In order to clarify the therapeutic approach to a patient with asymptomatic hyperuricaemia it is perhaps helpful to divide hyperuricaemia as follows:

1. Hyperuricaemia associated with clinical gout;
2. Hyperuricaemia associated with some other disease (e.g. psoriasis) or physiological state (e.g. starvation) – secondary hyperuricaemia; and
3. Hyperuricaemia of unknown aetiology (asymptomatic hyperuricaemia) – a finding usually discovered by chance.

It is with the last category that this section is concerned. The first consideration embraces the risks of developing gout in hyperuricaemic individuals. The Framingham study (Hall et al., 1967) found that 90% of individuals with a serum uric acid over 540 μmol 1^{-1} (9.0 mg %) developed gout. However, only smaller numbers with this level of hyperuricaemia were observed and other work has not supported risks of this level. For instance, Fessel's study (Fessel, 1972) reported only 3 of 66 men with subsequent gout in the face of such high levels of hyperuricaemia.

A second consideration is the risk of renal disease in hyperuricaemic individuals. Here again the risks have probably been exaggerated. For example, Fessel (1979) found that azotaemia due to hyperuricaemia is usually mild and occurs no more often than azotaemia in people with a normal uric acid. It was also felt that the risk of urolithiasis was also small. It is likely therefore that unless serum concentrations of uric acid are very high the risks of renal disease are more theoretical than practical.

A further concern about asymptomatic hyperuricaemia is the suggested association with atheroma (Dreyfuss, 1960; Eidlitz, 1961; Hansen, 1966). Here again, however, current experience fails to support such a link, whether judged by clinical studies (Graham and Scott, 1970) or by epidemiological surveys (Hall, 1965; Myers et al., 1968). Looking at this more recent evidence, it does not appear that hyperuricaemia carries a special risk in respect of coronary disease, and there are no grounds for believing that hypouricaemic therapy will reduce the risk of cardiovascular disease (Scott, 1980).

What then should be done when the clinician is faced by an incidental finding of hyperuricaemia? There is imperfect concurrence as to the policy to adopt, but there is some agreement about the following:

1. If a detailed assessment should reveal concomitant disease, such as hypertension, obesity, excessive alcohol consumption, appropriate measures should be taken to treat and advise the patient as in the normouricaemic individual. Hypouricaemic therapy is not necessarily indicated in these patients unless the level of serum urate is very high (see 3 below).
2. If there is clear evidence of recurrent uric acid calculi, hypouricaemic therapy with allopurinol is called for, regardless of the level of hyperuricaemia. However, previously static calculi may become dislodged and lead to ureteric impaction.
3. If serum concentrations of uric acid are high, say 540 µmol 1^{-1} (9.0 mg/ 100 ml) or more, these patients should probably be treated with allopurinol, even if no concomitant disease is present. Despite the lack of unequivocal evidence to support this line of management, it is offered in a spirit of giving patients the benefit of the doubt.
4. Mild degrees of hyperuricaemia, on the other hand, may be left untreated, although such patients should be kept under observation.

For further details the reader is referred to the excellent reviews by Klinenberg (1977), Scott (1980) and Bayliss *et al.* (1984).

14.2.4   Diuretic-induced hyperuricaemia

The arrival of the benzothiadiazines and related orally effective diuretics rapidly led to the discovery that hyperuricaemia, and in some cases clinical gout, could arise as side effects in patients on long-term therapy with these agents (De Martini, 1965). Soon after, similar complications were reported with the chronic administration of the newer 'loop-active' diuretics – ethacrynic acid (Cannon *et al.*, 1965) and furosemide (Stason *et al.*, 1966). These complications of diuretic therapy occasionally call for the advice of a rheumatologist on a general medical ward, and this cause of hyperuricaemia is an important though neglected area of management.

Criteria for treating diuretic-induced hyperuricaemia, though not entirely agreed, are according to the lines suggested for managing asymptomatic hyperuricaemia.

The *degree* of hyperuricaemia, as well as its *duration* may be important in deciding which patients to treat (Steele, 1977). However, high levels of serum urate are rarely reached with diuretics, unless the patient is additionally predisposed to this biochemical abnormality. A history of articular gout is a sufficient reason for treating hyperuricaemia in these patients.

The therapy of diuretic-induced hyperuricaemia is rationally achieved with uricosuric drugs since the pathogenesis of the raised serum urate level is related to sluggish renal urate clearance. Currently available diuretics known to cause hyperuricaemia do not appear significantly to interfere with the uricosuric efficacy of probenecid or sulphinpyrazone (Steele, 1977).

The criteria for using allopurinol in these patients have been discussed by Kelley (1975). One indication is when the rate of urinary urate output exceeds 1000 mg/24 hours. However, these levels would be exceptional in 'uncomplicated' diuretic-induced hyperuricaemia, and would be more likely in patients with malignancies undergoing treatment with cytotoxic agents. A more common indication for using allopurinol rather than uricosurics in diuretic-induced hyperuricaemia is failure to tolerate or failure to respond to uricosurics. Allopurinol would also be the preferred hypouricosuric agent if renal insufficiency were present in moderate or severe degree.

A comment has already been included about a novel approach to prevent diuretic-induced hyperuricaemia by means of drugs combining anti-hypertensive/diuretic function with uricosuric activity.

14.2.5   Other hyperuricaemic states

There are many causes of hyperuricaemia other than primary gout (Table 14.6). In general these disorders or physiological conditions (secondary hyper-

TABLE 14.6
Conditions associated with hyperuricaemia (after Klinenberg, 1977)

Primary gout
Myeloproliferative disorders
Lymphoproliferative disorders
Chronic haemolytic anaemia
Pernicious anaemia
Psoriasis
Sarcoidosis
Renal dysfunction
Drugs (low-dose salicylates, diuretics, pyrazinamide)
Lead toxicity
Acute alcoholism
Diabetic ketoacidosis
Lactic acidosis
Starvation
Toxaemia of pregnancy
Glycogen storage disease – Type 1
Obesity
Congestive heart failure
Down's syndrome
Hyperparathyroidism
Hypoparathyroidism
Hypothyroidism
Acromegaly

uricaemic states) are not associated with clinical gout, and there is rarely an indication to treat them. Notable examples of secondary hyperuricaemia requiring treatment are those associated with malignant disorders under treatment with cytotoxic agents and patients with renal insufficiency.

When a patient has *stable* renal function with decreased creatinine clearance and a persistently raised but stable serum urate, no treatment for the hyperuricaemia is necessary. However, if renal function is deteriorating, the subsequent further increase in serum urate may give rise to a superimposed gouty nephropathy. In these circumstances the hyperuricaemia should be treated with allopurinol. However, it is interesting that patients with chronic azotaemia tend not to have acute gouty attacks, and it has been suggested that this is related to the reduced inflammatory response occurring in uraemia (Buchanan *et al.*, 1965).

14.2.6 Hypouricaemic applications in children

(a) *The Lesch–Nyhan syndrome*

In 1964 Lesch and Nyhan described a childhood disorder characterized by choreoathetosis, striking growth and mental retardation, spasticity, self-mutilation, and marked hyperuricaemia, with excessive urate production and uric acid crystals in the urine. Three years later Seegmiller *et al.* (1967) reported an enzyme deficiency in erythrocyte lysates and fibroblasts of children with this syndrome, the lacking enzyme being hypoxanthine-guanine phosphoribosyltransferase (HGPRT). Since then adolescent and adult patients with partial rather than complete forms of the syndrome have been reported (Kelley *et al.*, 1967, 1969). These patients present with uric acid calculi or gouty arthritis and fail to show the advanced neurological and behavioural features of children with the complete enzyme defect.

Allopurinol is useful to treat these patients, benefiting the arthritis, tophi and renal calculi, and normalizing the urate levels. However, it does not appear to benefit the neurological manifestations (Wyngaarden and Kelley, 1976). Uricosuric drug therapy should probably not be used in these patients, unless allopurinol is also given, because of the very heavy load of uric acid already confronting the kidneys.

Allopurinol may also be useful to treat the hyperuricaemia of patients with glycogen storage disease (glucose 6-phosphatase deficiency). Uricosurics, on the other hand, appear to be less beneficial in this condition, perhaps because substances such as lactic acid interfere with the pharmacological effects of protein acids in a way similar to that of salicylates (Jakovcic and Sorensen, 1967).

The dose of allopurinol in children is 10–20 mg/kg body weight per day.

(b) *In the management of malignant disorders*

Excess urate may be found in association with neoplastic diseases and during their treatment. In children, leukaemia is the malignancy most often requiring treatment, and allopurinol may be used in the dosage shown above to prevent gouty episodes resulting from the massively increased purine metabolism that occurs in these patients from breakdown of nucleic acids.

In addition, cytoproliferative and lymphoproliferative disorders and some carcinomas, multiple myeloma, secondary polycythaemia, pernicious anaemia, haemoglobinopathies (including thalassaemias), other haemolytic anaemias, and infectious mononucleosis may be associated with increased turnover of nucleic acids sufficient to cause hyperuricaemia and hyperuricaciduria.

14.2.7   Concomitant drug therapy

(a) *Other uricosuric drugs*

Several drugs possess uricosuric activity. Most of these are not used primarily for this effect, but at least for theoretical considerations it is valuable to know which drugs have this property, as concomitant therapy with 'primary' uricosuric agents might lead to potentiation of hypouricaemia. Some of the substances with uricosuric properties are shown in Table 14.7.

TABLE 14.7
Drugs with uricosuric effects (after Kelley, 1979)

Drugs with uricosuric effects	References
Acetohexamide	Yü *et al.* (1968)
ACTH	Friedman and Byers (1950)
Cinchophen	Nicolaier and Dohrn (1980)
Dicoumarol	Hansen and Hotten (1958)
Ethyl biscoumacetate	Sougin-Mibashan and Horwitz (1973)
Oestrogens	Nicholls *et al.* (1973)
Mersalyl	Combs *et al.* (1940)
Phenolsulfonphthalein	Talbott (1943)
Salicylates	Dixon (1963)
Zoxazolamine	Burns *et al.* (1958)

(b) *Other drug–drug effects*

It is beyond the scope of this chapter to discuss interactions between NSAIDs and other drugs, as this subject has been covered in detail elsewhere (Chapter 3).

However, among drugs with hypouricaemic properties, several potential interactions should be considered in the long-term management of gouty patients, often in an age range when drug co-administration can be expected to be more frequent.

(i) Probenecid (Table 14.8)

This influences the renal excretion, volume of distribution, and hepatic uptake of several drugs. Caution should therefore be exercised when combining certain drugs with probenecid. For example, dapsone and indomethacin should be given in lower dosage with this drug. Acetylsalicylate blocks the uricosuric effect of probenecid and most other uricosurics. The anticoagulant effect of heparin is considerably enhanced by probenecid. Probenecid may prolong or enhance the action of oral sulphonylureas and thereby increase the risk of hypoglycaemia. If the drug is given with methotrexate, the dosage of the latter should be reduced. Enhancement of blood levels of ampicillin, penicillin and other antibiotics can be therapeutically beneficial. However, certain antibacterial agents are unaffected by this effect, e.g. gentamicin, sulphonamides, streptomycin, chloramphenicol, tetracycline.

TABLE 14.8
Probenecid toxicity

Toxic effects	Reference
* Gastrointestinal intolerance	Boger and Strickland (1955)
	Gutman and Yü (1951)
	De Seze *et al.* (1963)
	Reynolds *et al.* (1957)
Hypersensitivity	Boger and Strickland (1955)
	Gutman and Yü (1951)
	Boger and Strickland (1955)
Fever	Boger and Strickland (1955)
Rash	Boger and Strickland (1955)
	Boger and Strickland (1955)
Hepatic necrosis	Ferris *et al.* (1961)
Nephrotic syndrome	Hertz *et al.* (1972)
Overall withdrawals 2%	Talboth (1964)
12%	Gutman and Yü (1955)
30%	De Seze *et al.* (1964)
	Kuzell *et al.* (1964)

* Most common side effect

(ii) Sulphinpyrazone (Table 14.9)

Though likely, it is not known precisely whether this drug shares all the drug–drug effects of probenecid. However, from the practical standpoint potentia-

TABLE 14.9
Sulphinpyrazone toxicity

Toxic effects	Reference
* Gastrointestinal intolerance	De Seze *et al.* (1964)
	Emmerson (1963)
	Kaegi *et al.* (1974)
	Kuzell *et al.* (1964)
Hypersensitivity	Glick (1961)
Bone marrow suppression	Kaegi *et al.* (1974)
	Perd *et al.* (1969)

* Most common side effect

tion of oral coumarin-type anticoagulants (e.g. warfarin) may occur and frequent estimation of prothrombin time should be undertaken when these drugs are given concurrently. Sulphinpyrazone may also potentiate the action of plasma protein-binding drugs such as oral hypoglycaemic agents, and this may require modification of dosage of the latter.

(iii) Allopurinol

Several potentially important drug interactions involve allopurinol. These include potentiation of cytotoxic agents (e.g. 6-mercaptopurine, azathioprine, which are both inactivated by xanthine oxidase, and cyclophosphamide by a mechanism that is still unresolved). The effect of probenecid is prolonged by 50% and is thought to be due to inhibition of the microsomal drug oxidizing system. For further details of these drug–drug effects, and of those affecting the previously mentioned hypouricaemic agents, see Kelley (1979).

14.3 PSEUDOGOUT

Pseudogout (or calcium pyrophosphate dihydrate crystal deposition disease) poses different therapeutic problems compared with its more biochemically studied sister, true gout. Treatment of pseudogout is entirely empirical, as there is yet no therapy available to halt or reverse the progressive deposition of pyrophosphate crystals in cartilage.

In general, therapy of pseudogout may be divided into:

1. Treatment of chronically symptomatic osteoarthrotic joints associated with pyrophosphate deposition. This is identical to that of uncomplicated osteoarthrosis (see Chapter 13).

2. Treatment of acute attacks. As the knee joint is commonly affected and the acute episode attended by synovial effusion, aspiration of crystal-laden fluid often provides much relief (McCarty *et al.*, 1962; Skinner and Cohen, 1969). If symptoms persist after 24 hours, repeated arthrocentesis, combined with injection of an intra-articular corticosteroid preparation, will usually halt the inflammatory episode rapidly. However, if weight-bearing joints are unstable, or are the site of advanced degenerative disease, steroid injection should be withheld.

The response of pseudogout to colchicine is less predictable than that of gout, but occasionally the response in pseudogout can be dramatic. More usually, one of the NSAIDs is used to control the acute attack. Indomethacin is effective, as are the newer non-steroidal agents. These are given in large dosage initially, being reduced gradually as the attack settles. It is worth bearing in mind that the attack may take weeks rather than days to subside, although the degree of pain and inflammation is often less than in gout. It is rarely necessary to employ systemic corticosteroids or corticotrophins in this condition.

As with any weight-bearing joint affected by acute arthritis, the general principles of rest and gentle passive exercises apply, together with the administration of physical agents (e.g. cold compresses).

14.4 OTHER CRYSTAL-DEPOSITION DISORDERS

14.4.1 Calcium apatite deposition in soft tissues

Soft tissue hydroxyapatite deposition occurs in a wide spectrum of rheumatic disorders and disorders usually covered by other specialties. For example, it occurs in association with connective tissue diseases (e.g. scleroderma, dermatomyositis), in generalized soft tissue calcification (e.g. tumoral calcinosis, myositis ossificans progressiva), and in localized soft tissue calcification (e.g. diffuse idiopathic skeletal hyperostosis, acute calcific periarthritis).

No specific therapy is available and treatment is along the general lines appropriate for the disease in which apatite deposition has occurred (see relevant sections in other chapters).

14.4.2 Corticosteroid synovitis

Most long-acting steroid preparations used for intra-articular therapy are crystalline and are visible under polarized light microscopy. They may cause confusion with other crystals and may also be responsible for a transient synovitis after intra-articular injection. The frequency of post-injection synovitis is variable. It probably depends on the batch characteristics of the preparation, which probably vary in the size and nature of the crystals in suspension. It is impossible to anticipate post-injection synovitis and all that can be done is to warn patients of the possibility of such a reaction after an injection. When such flares are reported, reassurance is all that is necessary; but if the episode seems unduly prolonged the question of post-injection infection should be raised.

14.5   DIAGNOSTIC PROBLEMS AND PITFALLS

The management of any rheumatic disorder includes (and indeed demands) accurate diagnosis, as well as therapy. In the crystal-deposition disorders, and particularly in urate gout, diagnosis can be hampered by several mimicking disorders and states.

Diagnostic difficulty can face the clinicians in the following ways:

1. Disorders which, because of acute 'gouty' modes of presentation and a tendency to be associated with raised serum urate levels, are diagnosed as 'gout'. Notable in this group is psoriatic arthritis in which the rash or nail involvement is overlooked, minimal, or non-existent (psoriatic arthritis *sine* psoriasis). However, although hyperuricaemia of slight or moderate degree may be present, urate crystals are not found in joint aspirates. The referring clinician may offer a tentative diagnosis of 'gout' in young females in whom the first manifestation of psoriatic arthritis is in the big toe. However, the Hippocratic maxim that true gout usually appears after the menopause should draw attention to the true diagnosis.

2. Acute painful non-gouty events occurring in patients with established gout. In these patients, acute episodes resulting from fortuitously associated *infection, trauma* (particularly fracture), or *haemarthrosis* may be ascribed to gout because of the history of previous acute episodes due to the gouty diathesis itself. However, the patients will often realize the difference between their true gouty attack and any circumstantial episodes, and failure to respond to treatment for acute gout should add to the diagnostic suspicion.

3. 'The borderline serum urate'. In patients with painful episodes in the big toe, such as those that occur in hallux valgus associated with trauma (e.g. osteophyte fracture), confusion can arise if the serum urate approaches the upper limit of normal. Serum urate estimations may throw further light on whether to regard the urate level as normal.

4. Mixed arthritis. Occasionally true gout is associated with nodular rheumatoid arthritis. Only biopsy will reveal whether or not the nodules are tophaceous. The author has seen two patients in whom both tophi and rheumatoid nodules coexisted.

5. Patients previously under the care of another clinician in whom seemingly borderline clinical and biochemical features led to hypouricaemic treat-

ment. The decision will have to be made whether or not to withdraw the long-term agent in order to examine the effect of this on the serum uric acid, and thereby enable a re-evaluation of the diagnosis.

6. Pseudogout and other crystal arthropathies (e.g. corticosteroid synovitis) may generate diagnostic difficulty (hence the name of the former) but the attendant features/circumstances of their presentation will usually lead to their correct diagnosis.

14.6 SUMMARY AND CONCLUSIONS

Most of this chapter has been concerned with the main crystal-deposition disorder encountered in rheumatological practice – urate gout. The importance of this disease lies not only in the devastatingly painful nature of its acute attacks, but, even more important, its potential for causing systemic disease, notably renal effects.

The following comments summarize the main features of gout therapy:

1. The acute attack is readily amenable to control with high-dosage NSAIDs. The classical therapy with colchicine has now become largely superseded by less toxic anti-inflammatory agents such as indomethacin and certain propionic acid derivatives such as naproxen and fenoprofen. (Phenylbutazone is now restricted to the treatment of ankylosing spondylitis. However, its effectiveness in halting the acute episode of gout remains undoubted.)

2. Long-term therapy with hypouricosurics is an effective method to prevent further attacks. Lowering of serum urate levels is also accompanied by a decrease in the size of tophi and eventually in their disappearance. The choice between uricosurics and xanthine oxidase inhibitors is governed by firm criteria and these have been discussed.

3. The special cases posed by asymptomatic hyperuricaemia, diuretic-induced hyperuricaemia, and the control of hyperuricaemia in children have received separate consideration.

4. The chapter is concluded by considering some pitfalls and problems in diagnosis. Particular challenges are presented by infection, trauma, and haemorrhage. These can closely mimic acute gouty episodes, particularly if they occur in patients with established gout.

14.7 REFERENCES

Auerbach, R. and Orentrich, N. (1968) Alopecia and ichthyosis secondary to allopurinol. *Arch. Dermatol.*, **98**, 104.

Bayliss, R., Clarke, C., Whitehead, T. P. and Whitfield, A. G. W. (1984) The management of hyperuricaemia. *J. R. Coll. Phys. Lond.*, **18**, 144–6.

Begemann, H. and Neu, I. (1975) Die behandlung der urikopathie mit benz bromaronum unter besonderer berucksichtigune der neireninsuffizienz. *Therapie*, 25, 2184–94.

Boardman, P. L. and Hart, F. D. (1967) Side effects of indomethacin. *Ann. Rheum. Dis.*, 26, 127–32.

Boger, W. P. and Strickland, S. C. (1955) Probenecid (Benemid). *Arch. Intern. Med.*, 95, 83–92.

Brenner, W. J. and Paulsen, C. A. (1976) Colchicine and testicular function in man. *N. Engl. J. Med.*, 294, 1384–5.

Brewis, I., Ellis, R. M. and Scott, J. T. (1975) Single daily dose of allopurinol. *Ann. Rheum. Dis.*, 34, 256–9.

Brogard, J. M., Frankhauser, J. and Stahl, A. (1973) Application de l'uricolyse enzymatique au traitement des hyperuricemies d'origine renal. *Schweizer. Med. Wochens.*, 103, 404–10.

Buchanan, W. W., Klinenberg, J. R. and Seegmiller, J. E. (1965) The inflammatory response to injected microcrystalline monosodium urate in normal, hyperuricaemic, gouty and uremic subjects. *Arth. Rheum.*, 8, 361.

Burns, J. J., Yü, T-F. and Berger, L. (1958) Zoxazolamine: physiological disposition, uricosuric properties. *Am. J. Med.*, 25, 401–8.

Cannon, P. J., Heinemann, H. O., Stason, W. B. and Laragh, J. H. (1965) Ethacrynic acid. Effectiveness and mode of diuretic action in man. *Circulation*, 31, 5–18.

Cartier, P. H. and Hamet, M. (1973) Mechanism of antiuric action of 4-oxy and 4-thiopyrazolopyrimidines. *Biochem. Pharmacol.*, 22, 3061–75.

Caruso, I., Fumagalli, M., Marcolongo, R. and Sacchetti, G. (1977) Indoprofen for acute gouty arthritis (letter). *Arthr. Rheum.*, 20, 1438–9.

Coombs, F. S., Pecora, L. J., Thorogood, E. *et al.* (1940) Renal function in patients with gout. *J. Clin. Invest.*, 19, 525–35.

Cuq, P. (1973) Experience française du traitement de la crise de goutte aigue par le naproxen-C1674. *Scand. J. Rheumatol.*, (Suppl.) 2, 64–8.

Delbarre, F., Auscher, C., Gery, A., Brouilheb, H. and Olivier, J. L. (1968) Le traitement de la dyspurinie goutteuse par la mercaptopyrazolopyrimidine (MPP: thiopurinol). *Presse Med.*, 76, 2329–32.

Demartini, F. E. (1965) Hyperuricaemia induced by drugs. *Arthr. Rheum.*, 8, 823–9.

De Seze, S., Ryckewaert, A., Caroit, M. *et al.* (1964) Congres International de la Goutte et de la Lithiase Urique. Sept. 4, Evian, p. 297.

Dixon, A. St. J. (1963) Salicylates and uric acid excretion, in *Salicylates. An International Symposium* (eds A. St. J. Dixon, B. K. Martin, M. J. H. Smith and P. H. N. Ward), Churchill Livingstone, London, p. 38.

Dreyfuss, F. (1960) The role of hyperuricaemia in coronary heart disease. *Dis. Chest*, 38, 332–4.

Eidlitz, M. (1961) Uric acid and arteriosclerosis. *Lancet*, ii, 1046–7.

Elion, G. B., Kovensky, A. and Hitchings, G. H. *et al.* (1966) Metabolic studies of allopurinol, an inhibitor of xanthine oxidase. *Biochem. Pharmacol.*, 15, 863–80.

Emmerson, B. T. (1963) A comparison of uricosuric agents in gout, with special reference to sulphinpyrazone. *Med. J. Austr.*, 50, 839–44.

Ferris, T. F., Morgan, W. S. and Levitin, H. (1961) Nephrotic syndrome caused by probenecid. *N. Engl. J. Med.*, 265, 381–3.

Fessel, W. J. (1972) Hyperuricaemia in health and disease. *Seminars Arthr. Rheum.*, 1, 275.

Fessel, W. J. (1979) Renal outcomes of gout and hyperuricaemia. *Am. J. Med.*, 67, 74–82.

Fox, I. H. (1977) Hypouricaemic agents in the treatment of gout, in *Clinics in Rheumatic Diseases*, Vol. 3, No. 1. *Crystal Induced Arthropathies* (ed W. N. Kelley), Saunders, London, p. 148.

Glick, E. N. (1961) Sulphinpyrazone in the treatment of arthritis associated with hyperuricaemia. *Proc. R. Soc. Med.*, 54, 423–6.

Graham, R. and Scott, J. T. (1970) Clinical survey of 354 patients with gout. *Ann. Rheum. Dis.*, 29, 461–8.

Greenberg, M. S. and Zambarano, S. S. (1972) Aplastic agranulocytosis after allopurinol therapy. *Arthr. Rheum.*, 15, 413–6.

Gutman, A. B. and Yü, T-F. (1951) Benemid (*p*-(di-*n*-propylsulfamyl)-benzoid acid) as uricosuric agent in chronic gouty arthritis. *Trans. Assoc. Am. Phys.*, 64, 279–88.

Gutman, A. B. and Yü, T-F. (1952) Gout, a derangement of purine metabolism. *Adv. Inter. Med.*, 5, 227.

Gutman, A. B. and Yü, T-F. (1955) Prevention and treatment of chronic gout. *J. Am. Med. Assoc.*, 157, 1096–102.

Hall, A. P. (1965) Correlations among hyperuricaemia, hypercholesterolism, coronary disease and hypertension. *Arthr. Rheum.*, 8, 846–52.

Hall, A. P., Barry, P. E., Dawber, T. R. and McNamara, P. M. (1967) Epidemiology of gout and hyperuricaemia. A long-term population study. *Am. J. Med.*, 42, 27–37.

Hansen, O. E. (1966) Hyperuricaemia, gout and atherosclerosis. *Am. Heart J.*, 72, 570–3.

Hensen, O. E. and Holten, C. (1958) Uricosuric effect of dicoumarol. *Lancet*, i, 1047–8.

Hart, F. D. and Boardman, P. L. (1963) Indomethacin: a new non-steroid anti-inflammatory agent. *Br. Med. J.*, 2, 965–70.

Hertz, P., Yager, H. and Richardson, J. A. (1972) Probenecid-induced nephrotic syndrome. *Arch. Pathol.*, 94, 241.

Holmes, E. W. (1977) Pathogenesis of hyperuricaemia in primary gout, in *Clinics in Rheumatic Diseases*, Vol. 3, No. 1. *Crystal-Induced Arthropathies* (ed. W. N. Kelley), Saunders, London, p. 15.

Hutchinson, J. C. and Wilkinson, W. H. (1973) The uricosuric action of halofenate (MK-185) in patients with hyperuricaemia or uncomplicated primary gout and hyperlipidemia. *Atherosclerosis*, 18, 353–62.

Irby, R., Toone, E. and Owen, D. (1966) Bone marrow depression associated with allopurinol therapy. *Arthr. Rheum.*, 9, 860.

Jain, A. K., Ryan, J. R. and McMahon, F. G. (1976) Comparison of ticrynafen and probenecid in treatment of hyperuricemia. *Clin. Res.*, 24, 43A.

Jakovcic, S. and Sorensen, C. B. (1967) Studies of uric acid metabolism in glycogen storage disease associated with gouty arthritis. *Arthr. Rheum.*, 10, 129–34.

Jarzobski, J., Ferry, J., Wombolt, D., Fitch, D. M. and Egan, J. D. (1970) Vasculitis with allopurinol therapy. *Am. Heart J.*, 79, 116–21.

Johnson, H. P., Engleman, E. P., Forsham, P. H. *et al.* (1954) Effects of phenylbutazone in gout. *N. Engl. J. Med.*, 250, 665.

Kaegi, A., Pineo, G. F., Shimizu, A., Trivedi, H., Hirsh, J. and Gent, M. (1974) Arteriovenous-shunt thrombosis: prevention by sulfinpyrazone. *N. Engl. J. Med.*, 290, 304–6.

Kantor, G. L. (1970) Toxic epidermal necrolysis, azotemia, and death after allopurinol therapy. *J. Am. Med. Assoc.*, 212, 478–9.

Kaplan, H. (1960) Sarcoid arthritis with a response to colchicine. *N. Engl. J. Med.*, 263, 778–81.

Kelley, W. N. (1975a) Effects of drugs on uric acid in man. *Ann. Rev. Pharmacol.*, 15, 327–50.

Kelley, W. N. (1975b) Pharmacologic approach to the maintenance of urate homeostasis. *Nephron*, **14**, 99–115.

Kelley, W. N. (1979) Treatment of hyperuricemia, in *Arthritis and Allied Conditions. A Textbook of Rheumatology* (ed D. J. McCarty), 9th edn, Lea and Febiger, Philadelphia, p. 1231.

Kelley, W. N., Greene, M. L., Rosenbloom, F. M., Henderson, J. F. and Seegmiller, J. E. (1969) Hypoxanthine-gnomic phosphoribosyltransferase deficiency in gout. *Ann. Intern. Med.*, **70**, 155–206.

Kelley, W. N., Rosenbloom, E. M., Henderson, J. F. *et al.* (1967) A specific enzyme defect in gout associated with overproduction of uric acid. *Proc. Nat. Acad. Sci. USA*, **57**, 1735.

Kelley, W. N. and Wyngaarden, J. B. (1971) Drug treatment of gout. *Seminars Drug Treat.*, **1**, 119–47.

Kidd, E. G., Boyce, K. C. and Freyberg, R. H. (1953) Clinical studies of phenylbutazone (Butazolidin) and butapyrine (Irgapyrine) in rheumatoid arthritis, rheumatoid spondylitis and gout. *Ann. Rheum. Dis.*, **12**, 20–4.

Kissel, P., Mauuary, G., Royer, R. and Toussain, P. (1975) Treatment of malignant haemopathies and urate oxidase. *Lancet*, **1**, 229.

Klinenberg, J. R. (1977) The management of asymptomatic hyperuricaemia, in *Clinics in Rheumatic Diseases*, Vol. 3, No. 1. *Crystal-Induced Arthropathies* (ed W. N. Kelley), Saunders, London, p. 159.

Kuzell, W. C., Glover, R. P., Gibbs, J. O. *et al.* (1964) Effect of sulfinpyrazone on serum uric acid in gout. A long-term study. *Genetics*, **19**, 894–909.

Kuzell, W. C., Schaffarzick, R. W., Brown, B. and Mankle, E. A. (1952) Phenylbutazone (Butazolidin) in rheumatoid arthritis and gout. *J. Am. Med. Assoc.*, **149**, 729–34.

Lesch, M. and Nyhan, W. L. (1964) A familial disorder of uric acid metabolism and central nervous system function. *Am. J. Med.*, **36**, 561–70.

Lidsky, M. D. and Sharp, J. T. (1967) Jaundice with the use of 4-hydroxypyrazolo (3, 4-D) pyrimidine (4-HPP) (Abstract). *Arthr. Rheum.*, **10**, 294.

Loebl, W. Y. and Scott, J. T. (1974) Withdrawal of allopurinol in patients with gout. *Ann. Rheum. Dis.*, **33**, 304–7.

MacLachlan, M. J. and Rodnan, G. P. (1967) Effects of food and alcohol in serum uric acid and acute attacks of gout. *Am. J. Med.*, **42**, 38–57.

McCarty, D. J. (1976) Calcium pyrophosphate dihydrate crystal deposition disease – 1975. *Arthr. Rheum.*, **19**, 275–85.

McCarty, D. J., Kohn, N. N. and Faires, J. S. (1962) The significance of calcium phosphate crystals in the synovial fluid of arthritis patients: the 'pseudogout syndrome'. 1. Clinical aspects. *Ann. Intern. Med.*, **56**, 711–37.

Merlin, H. E. (1972) Azoospermia caused by colchicine. *Fertil. Steril.*, **23**, 180–1.

Mills, R. M. (1971) Severe hypersensitivity reactions associated with allopurinol. *J. Am. Med. Assoc.*, **216**, 799–802.

Myers, A. R., Epstein, F. H., Dodge, H. J. and Mikkelsen, W. M. (1968) The relationship of serum uric acid to risk factors in coronary heart disease. *Am. J. Med.*, **45**, 520–8.

Nicholls, A., Snaith, M. L. and Scott, J. T. (1973) Effect of oestrogen therapy on plasma and urinary levels of uric acid. *Br. Med. J.*, **1**, 449–51.

Nicolaier, A. and Dohrn, M. (1908) Ueber die Wirkung von Chinolincarbonsäure und ihrer Derivate auf die Ausscheidung der Harnsaüre. *Deutsch Arc. Klin. Med.*, **xciii**, 331–5.

Norcross, B. M. (1963) Treatment of connective tissue diseases with a new non-steroid compound (indomethacin) (Abstract). *Arthr. Rheum.*, **6**, 290.

Perd, J. M., Dayton, P. G., Snell, M. M., Yü, T-F. and Gutman, A. B. (1969) Studies of interactions among drugs in man at the renal level: probenecid and sulfinpyrazone. *Clin. Pharmacol. Ther.*, 10, 834–40.

Race, T. F., Paes, I. C. and Falcon, W. W. (1970) Intestinal malabsorption induced by oral colchicine. *Am. J. Med. Sci.*, 259, 32–41.

Reynolds, E. S., Schlant, R. C., Gonick, H. and Dammin, H. C. (1957) Fatal massive necrosis of the liver as a manifestation of hypersensitivity to probenecid. *N. Engl. J. Med.*, 256, 592–6.

Rieselbach, R. E. and Steel, T. H. (1974) Influence of the kidney upon urate haemostasis in health and disease. *Am. J. Med.*, 56, 665–75.

Rieselbach, R. E., Sorensen, L. B., Shelp, W. D. and Steele, T. H. (1970) Diminished renal urate secretion per nephron as a basis for primary gout. *Ann. Intern. Med.*, 73, 359–66.

Rubulis, A., Rubert, M. and Faloon, W. W. (1970) Cholesterol lowering, fecal bile and sterol changes during neomycin and colchicine. *J. Clin. Nutr.*, 23, 1251–9.

Schweitz, M. C., Nashel, D. J. and Alepa, F. P. (1978) Ibuprofen in the treatment of acute gouty arthritis. *J. Am. Med. Assoc.*, 239, 34–5.

Scott, J. T. (1978) Gout, in *Copeman's Textbook of the Rheumatic Diseases* (ed J. T. Scott), 5th edn, Churchill Livingstone, Edinburgh, pp. 647–91.

Scott, J. T. (1980) Long-term management of gout and hyperuricaemia. *Br. Med. J.*, 281, 1164–6.

Scott, J. T. and O'Brien, P. K. (1968) Probenecid, nephrotic syndrome and renal failure. *Ann. Rheum. Dis.*, 27, 249–52.

Seegmiller, J. E. and Howell, R. R. (1962) The old and new concepts of acute gouty arthritis. *Arthr. Rheum.*, 5, 616–23.

Seegmiller, J. E., Rosenbloom, R. M. and Kelley, W. N. (1967) An enzyme defect associated with a sex-linked human neurological disorder and excessive purine synthesis. *Science*, 155, 1682.

Simmons, F., Feldman, B. and Gerety, D. (1972) Granulomatous hepatitis in a patient receiving allopurinol. *Gastroenterology*, 62, 101–4.

Skinner, M. and Cohen, A. S. (1969) Calcium pyrophosphate dihydrate crystal deposition disease. *Arch. Intern. Med.*, 123, 636–64.

Sokol, A., Bashner, M. H. and Okun, R. (1967) Nephrotic syndrome caused by probenecid. *J. Am. Med. Assoc.*, 199, 43.

Smyth, C. J. (1970) Indomethacin – its rightful place in treatment. *Ann. Intern. Med.*, 72, 430–2.

Smyth, C. J. (1972) Diagnosis and treatment of gout, in *Arthritis and Allied Conditions* (eds J. L. Hollander and D. J. McCarty), 8th edn, Lea and Febiger, Philadelphia, pp. 1112–39.

Smyth, C. J., Velayos, E. E. and Amorosa, C. (1963) A method for measuring swelling of hands and feet. II. Influence of new anti-inflammatory drug, indomethacin in acute gout. *Acta Rheumatol. Scand.*, 9, 306.

Sougin-Mibashan, R. and Horwitz, M. (1955) The uricosuric action of ethyl biscoumacetate. *Lancet*, i, 1191–7.

Stason, W. B., Cannon, P. J., Heinemann, H. O. and Laragh, J. H. (1966) Furosemide. A clinical evaluation of its diuretic action. *Circulation*, 34, 910–20.

Steele, T. H. (1977) Diuretic-induced hyperuricaemia, in *Clinics in Rheumatic Diseases*, Vol. 3, No. 1. *Crystal-Induced Arthropathies* (ed W. N. Kelley), Saunders, London, p. 44.

Straitigos, J. D., Bartosokas, S. K. and Capetanakis, J. (1972) Further experiences of toxic epidermal necrolysis incriminating allopurinol, pyrazolone and derivatives. *Br. J. Dermatol.*, 86, 564–7.

Sturge, R. A., Scott, J. T., Hamilton, E. B. D., Liyanage, S. P., Dixon, A. St. J., Davies, J. and Engler, C. (1977) Multicentre trial of naproxen and phenylbutazone in acute gout. *Ann. Rheum. Dis.*, **36**, 80–2.

Talbott, J. H. (1943) *Gout*, Oxford University Press, London.

Talbott, J. H. (1964) *Gout*, 2nd edn, Grune and Stratton, New York, p. 206.

Thompson, G. R., Ting, Y. M., Riggs, G. A., Fenn, M. E. and Denning, R. M. (1968) Calcific tendinitis and soft tissue calcification resembling gout. *J. Am. Med. Assoc.*, **203**, 464–72.

Tjandramaga, T. B., Cucinell, S. A., Israile, Z. H. *et al.* (1972) Observations on the disposition of probenecid in patients receiving allopurinol. *Pharmacology*, **8**, 259–72.

Wallace, S. L. (1972) The treatment of gout. *Arthr. Rheum.*, **15**, 317–23.

Wallace, S. L. (1975) Colchicine and new antiinflammatory drugs for the treatment of acute gout. *Arthr. Rheum.*, **18**, 847–51.

Wallace, S. L. (1977) The treatment of the acute attack of gout, in *Clinics in Rheumatic Diseases*, Vol. 3, No. 1. *Crystal-Induced Arthropathies* (ed W. N. Kelley), Saunders, London, p. 138.

Wallace, S. L., Bernstein, D. and Diamond, H. (1967) Diagnostic value of the colchicine therapeutic trial. *J. Am. Med. Assoc.*, **199**, 525–8.

Wanasukapunt, S., Lertratanakul, Y. and Rubinstein, H. M. (1976) Effect of fenoprofen calcium on acute gouty arthritis. *Arthr. Rheum.*, **19**, 933–8.

Webb, D. I., Chodos, R. B., Mahar, C. Q. and Faloon, W. W. (1968) Mechanism of vitamin B_{12} malabsorption in patients receiving colchicine. *N. Engl. J. Med.*, **279**, 845–50.

Willkens, R. F. and Case, J. B. (1973) Treatment of acute gout with naproxen. *Scand. J. Rheumatol.* (Suppl.) **2**, 69–72.

Willkens, R. F., Case, J. B. and Huix, F. J. (1976) Treatment of acute gout with naproxen. *J. Clin. Pharmacol.*, **16**, 363–7.

Wyngaarden, J. B. and Kelley, W. N. (1972) Gout, in *The Metabolic Basis of Inherited Disease*, 3rd edn (eds J. B. Stanbury, J. B. Wyngaarden and D. S. Fredrickson), McGraw Hill, New York, p. 889.

Wyngaarden, J. B. and Kelley, W. N. (1976) Clinical syndromes associated with hypoxanthine-guanine phosphoribosyltransferase deficiency, in *Gout and Hyperuricemia*, Grune and Stratton, New York, pp. 309–44.

Yü, T. (1974) Milestones in the treatment of gout. *Am. J. Med.*, **56**, 676–85.

Yü, T-F. and Gutman, A. B. (1961) Efficacy of colchicine prophylaxis in gout. *Ann. Intern. Med.*, **55**, 179–92.

Yü, T-F., Berger, L. and Gutman, A. B. (1968) Hypoglycemia and uricosuric properties of acetohexamide and hydroxyhexamide. *Metabolism*, **17**, 309–16.

CHAPTER 15

Miscellanea and rarities

F. Dudley Hart

15.1 GENERAL COMMENT

The central place of rheumatology within general (internal) medicine is reflected by the wide spectrum of rheumatic conditions arising as 'co-diseases' or 'complications' of essentially non-rheumatic disorders, e.g. malignant, haematological, and endocrine diseases.

Although not commonly encountered by the rheumatologist, these rheumatoses, loosely referred to here as 'Miscellanea and rarities', are seen often enough to warrant special consideration of their various treatments.

15.2 CONNECTIVE TISSUE DISORDERS (COLLAGEN DISORDERS)

15.2.1 Systemic lupus erythematosus (SLE)

Systemic lupus erythematosus is a systemic disorder of connective tissue that has become more widely recognized in recent years. It is characterized by general organ involvement, and a rich variety of clinical manifestations which, because of their wide spectrum, often cause diagnostic difficulty. The disease typically displays exacerbations and remissions. A large proportion of patients (about 95%) manifest musculo-articular features. Other common manifestations are: cutaneous (81%), fever (77%), neuropsychiatric (59%), renal (53%), pulmonary (48%), and cardiac (38%).

There are well-developed immunological features, evidenced by the presence in the serum of various antinuclear antibodies. Those directed against DNA are the most constant, and are thus used as the diagnostic hallmark of the disease.

(a) Therapy

There is no evidence that treatment of patients in remission improves the long-term prognosis. These patients therefore probably require no treatment. A conservative approach should probably also be applied to patients in whom raised titres of anti-DNA antibodies are found despite clinical absence of disease activity. However, it should be borne in mind that abnormal DNA-binding values generally precede disease flares (Lightfoot and Hughes, 1976). On the other hand, the finding of a lowered serum complement implies renal involvement, and this serological feature should demand corticosteroid therapy.

(b) General measures

Patients with Raynaud's phenomenon should avoid exposure to cold, and wear gloves in cold weather. If these patients are smokers they should be encouraged to stop. Patients should be advised to avoid excess sunlight (sun barrier creams may be useful), and certain chemicals or drugs should be avoided. Agents that may potentiate the disease include oral contraceptives, penicillin, and sulphonamides. Drug-induced lupus is a separate matter, and drugs known to be associated with this syndrome (e.g. hydralazine and isoniazid) are not necessarily contraindicated in SLE.

(c) Drugs

(i) Salicylates

Although of help in patients with predominant joint involvement, as are other NSAIDs such as indomethacin, these drugs are usually relegated to second or third choice. It is worth remembering, too, that prolonged high-dose salicylates may be hepatotoxic (Rich and Johnson, 1973), particularly in children.

(ii) Chloroquine

This drug binds to DNA, although its precise action in SLE is not known. In patients with predominant skin or joint disease, chloroquine salts are still in vogue, and are particularly indicated in discoid LE (Winkelmann et al., 1961). The effect of antimalarials tends to be symptomatic rather than remission-inducing.

(iii) Corticosteroids

These drugs continue to be the bedrock of management. Patients with severe disease are usually given 40–80 mg prednisolone daily. Even higher starting doses (>200 mg) may be necessary, particularly in patients with CNS complications (Dubois, 1974). Corticosteroids are always indicated in those with haemolytic anaemia and in active renal disease. Aseptic necrosis of the hip is a troublesome complication in these patients on long-term steroid therapy, and other complications of steroid treatment are those also described under the management of rheumatoid arthritis. Recently there has been a trend towards combining steroid therapy with an immunosuppressive drug.

(iv) Immunosuppressives

No clear differentiation emerges from this group of drugs as to which is most effective. The most tried in SLE are azathioprine, cyclophosphamide, and chlorambucil, and their application has been predominantly in patients with renal lupus. A combination of azathioprine or cyclophosphamide with prednisolone appears to be better than either drug alone, as mentioned above. Cade *et al.* (1973) showed a significant reduction in death rate, and improvement in renal function tests, complement levels, and side effects. However, other work has suggested that after three-year follow up there were no clear differences between prednisolone used alone or in combination with azathioprine (Donadio *et al.*, 1974).

(v) Other therapies

These include thoracic duct cannulation, plasmapheresis, DNAase treatment of serum, and the avoidance of antigenic challenge using special diets. None of these treatments can be deemed specific, and the evidence for each of them remains equivocal.

More recently danacrine, a novel androgen, has been evaluated in SLE, and in mild disease appears to have an ameliorating effect. It is also potent in reversing thrombocytopenia.

Nifedipine (a potent calcium antagonist and peripheral vasodilator, usually used for the treatment and prophylaxis of angina pectoris and for the treatment of hypertension) has recently been used to treat Raynaud's phenomenon and peripheral ischaemic disease (Douglas Smith and McKendry, 1982; Rodeheffer *et al.*, 1983; Rustin *et al.*, 1983), and pulmonary hypertension (Camerini *et al.*, 1980; Ocken *et al.*, 1983), some of these patients having concomitant systemic sclerosis. The encouraging results with this agent contrast with the disappointing effects of other vasodilators in this disease.

Another novel vasodilator approach that exhibits some potential in patients in whom Raynaud's phenomenon is prominent is prostaglandin (PG) infusion

(Dowd *et al.*, 1982; Belch *et al.*, 1983; Kahan *et al.*, 1983; Kennerly, 1983). Prostacyclin has been the agent used in these studies. It is a highly potent vasodilator, inhibitor of platelet aggregation and of thromboxane and serotonin release, and it increases red cell deformability. Dowd *et al.* (1982) reported an 80–88% benefit in symptoms in 25 patients with severe Raynaud's phenomenon and systemic sclerosis. These workers used a 72-hour intravenous infusion of prostacyclin 10 ng kg^{-1} min^{-1}. The marked side effects can be minimized according to Belch *et al.* (1983) by giving 5-hour infusions intermittently and slowly building up the dose to 7.5 ng kg^{-1} min^{-1}.

Doubtless, further therapies will emerge in the next few years, but this field is likely to be more active in the USA where the disease appears to be more common and less benign than the SLE encountered in the UK.

15.2.2 Progressive systemic sclerosis (PSS) (scleroderma)

This generalized disorder of unknown aetiology involves not only skin and subcutaneous structures but also kidneys, lungs, gastrointestinal tract, and other organs. Joints are affected only secondarily, though in the early stages of the disease there may be articular features that may lead to the misdiagnosis of rheumatoid arthritis. As the aetiology is unknown, therapy is empirical and symptomatic, and not curative. Drug therapy is perhaps less important than physical measures such as avoidance of extremes of heat and cold, avoidance of injury, and suitable inunctions with gentle massage and appropriate physiotherapy.

(a) *Therapy*

(i) Drugs acting on blood vessels

Reserpine 0.25–1 mg by mouth four times daily has been used in an attempt to produce a better circulation to the tissues, but without demonstrably dramatic effect. A dose of 0.5–1 mg has been used intra-arterially when severe digital ulceration is threatening, but effects are variable and usually transient, and the same was true of surgical sympathectomy in the past. Methyldopa 500–2000 mg by mouth four times daily and guanethidine 10–50 mg by mouth four times daily have also been used but without impressive effect on the disease in the hands and feet. Two percent glyceryl trinitrate ointment applied to the fingers 3 times daily has been shown to be of benefit. These agents may assist in preventing tissue necrosis from Raynaud's phenomenon in certain circumstances at certain times, but do not appear to have a long-term beneficial effect. See also under (v) p. 443.

(ii) Antihypertensive drugs

Hypertension is usually due either to generalized arterial changes (atherosclerosis) or to intimal hyperplasia, which is characteristic of this disease. Antihypertensive drugs that inhibit renin release have therefore a reasonable rationale. Propranolol, methyldopa, reserpine, clonidine, hydralazine, and a number of other antihypertensive agents have been used, more in the hope of helping the renal rather than the peripheral circulation, but sometimes with beneficial effects on both. Diuretics that increase plasma renin levels may in theory (and sometimes in practice) aggravate renal disease. If malignant hypertension sets in, rapid deterioration of the clinical condition with renal failure may call for intensive antihypertensive therapy, such as intravenous sodium nitroprusside, diazoxide or even dialysis. In special circumstances renal transplantation may be indicated.

(iii) Anti-inflammatory drugs

Anti-inflammatory drugs do not have a profound effect, but do ease pain and reduce early inflammatory changes. Corticosteroids, corticotrophin or tetracosactrin produce short-term benefit and symptomatic ease, but do not appear to affect the long-term course of the disease in the peripheries or in the viscera. They may also aggravate hypertension and increase the risk of side effects such as cross-infection. A dose of 40–60 mg of prednisolone by mouth initially, gradually reducing over several weeks or months, may be used for symptomatic control in the early stages, or smaller doses, such as 5 mg prednisolone daily, for its 'tonic' effect in increasing appetite and well-being and decreasing fatigue. As with corticosteroid therapy in any chronic condition, the clinical benefits wear off and undesired effects tend in time to wear on. It is therefore perhaps wiser in general to avoid corticosteroid therapy, though it helps early acute myositis and other inflammatory features, and increases the sense of well being more dramatically than the NSAIDs in the early stages of the disorder. In the later stages, corticosteroids are of little help and may only produce unwanted side effects.

(iv) Other agents

Many agents have been used experimentally in the hope of improving or delaying progress in PSS, but none has been proved to be efficient. These agents include: penicillamine, colchicine, *para*-aminobenzoic acid (POTABA), azathioprine, tocophenols, relaxin, and several other substances. Dimethylsulphoxide (DMSO), when applied locally, may lead to softening and healing of digital ulcers. In general, systemic drug therapy plays only a small part in this unpleasant chronic disease, though local applications may help temporarily and general physical supportive commonsense measures, such as warm double (inner and outer) gloves, warm footwear, etc. Drugs to avoid are vasconstrictors such as amphetamines, nicotine, ergotamine, coffee, tea, and tobacco.

15.2.3   Polyarteritis nodosa

This is a relatively rare and serious disorder. The concept of polyarteritis has broadened over the last decade and many rheumatologists now regard the condition as one of a group including Wegener's granulomatosis, Takayasu's arteritis, and allergic and cutaneous vasculitis. Some even include polymyalgia and giant cell arteritis in this category.

The disease is characterized by widespread focal panarteritis, with fibrinoid necrosis of the vessel wall. This produces clinical manifestations in many systems, and particularly causes renal disease, heart failure, and peripheral neuropathy. The association of arthritis and involvement of other systems usually suggests the diagnosis, and this can be confirmed by biopsy. 'Overlap' with the vasculitis of rheumatoid disease is a relatively common feature.

(a) *Therapy*

(i) Corticosteroids

These drugs remain the standard therapy in polyarteritis (Johnsson and Leon-hardt, 1957; Shick, 1958). Doses of more than 80 mg/day may be necessary in severe forms of the disease. The main factor in governing the prognosis is the presence of renal disease and hypertension. There is some evidence that steroids have a beneficial effect in these patients (Moskowitz *et al.*, 1963; Barzel, 1963), although renal failure and hypertension are often irreversible. The neuropathy is particularly resistant to steroid therapy, as is the closely related condition Wegener's granulomatosis. However, the latter can now be controlled with immunoactive drugs, particularly cyclophosphamide (Wolff *et al.*, 1974).

(ii) Other drugs

The rarity of this condition has limited trials and experience with immunosup-pressives, compared with our knowledge of these drugs in SLE. Penicillamine and gold are particularly ineffective in polyarteritis nodosa.

15.2.4   Dermatomyositis and polymyositis

These are chronic non-suppurative inflammatory conditions of muscle with (dermatomyositis) or without (polymyositis) skin involvement. The aetiology is obscure: underlying several cases of dermatomyositis is a malignant condi-tion of which the dermatomyositis may be the presenting sign. Treatment lies in control of the condition rather than cure, the aims being to maintain or improve function and to improve or normalize laboratory tests and improve the clinical state. Physical measures such as graded rest, exercise and exercises, and physiotherapy and occupational therapy are important in preventing contractures and improving function and morale. Laboratory guides are measurement of serum enzyme activity, creatinine kinase, glutamic oxalacetic transaminase and lactic dehydrogenase, and sedimentation rate estimations. However these are affected by muscle trauma, exertion and injections as well as by disease activity. Electromyograph studies and muscle biopsies are initial diagnostic measures rather than indicators of the progress of the disease.

(a) *Corticosteroid therapy*

Corticosteroids are used in most patients, for though they do not cure or alter basically the long-term results of the disease, they improve the clinical condition in most individuals. If there is no improvement, or even a worsening, on corticosteroid therapy in an adult of middle age or beyond, an underlying malignant process is likely. However, as any of the side effects of corticosteroid therapy may occur, the possibility of steroid myopathy should be borne in mind in such patients. Because of reports of dexamethasone and triamcinolone causing muscle weakness these substances are usually not used. According to Pearson (1979), response to corticosteroids may be:

1. Satisfactory with clinical improvement and a decline in serum enzyme levels. This is most often seen in patients where such treatment has been started within 2 months of onset;
2. A slower and less dramatic improvement in clinical and laboratory indices in patients with more chronic, long-standing disease. Such improvement may not be apparent for several weeks or months;
3. A worsening after initial improvement in patients with malignancy or Sjøgren's syndrome.

Dosage of corticosteroids

Usually prednisolone or prednisone is started 40–50 mg daily in divided dosage until a remission is effected or maximal improvement occurs, when the dose is very gradually lowered. The initial high dosage period is usually 4–6 weeks, reductions being 5 or 2.5 mg daily every 1–2 weeks. These reductions are monitored clinically and by enzyme estimations, reductions being halted or slowed if relapse occurs. The aim is to reach a dosage below 20 mg daily which keeps clinical and enzymatic control, preferably 5–15 mg daily. For children the initial dose range is from 1 to 2 mg/kg body weight/day given in divided dosage with the same programme of gradual slow reduction where possible. The same total dosage as alternate-day therapy may be used to reduce adrenocortical hypophyseal suppression in adults and children, i.e. 2 days' dosage given on alternate days. In adults, supplements of calcium (500 mg daily) and vitamin D (50000 U once or twice weekly) may delay or possibly lessen corticosteroid-induced osteoporosis. While corticosteroid therapy does not appear to prolong or shorten survival times in most patients it does produce worthwhile symptomatic improvement.

(b) *Immunoregulatory ('immunosuppressive') agents*

Where life-threatening disease has not responded to full dosage corticosteroids, or side effects are becoming intolerable, one of the so called immunoregulatory agents may be employed, though how, or even if, they affect the disease process is debatable. The choice lies between the following.

(i) Methotrexate

10–15 mg i.v. weekly, with a gradual increase to 30–50 mg, the frequency of administration being reduced to 2, 3 or 4 weekly later, when improvement occurs. Toxic reactions are pneumonitis, stomatitis, hepatotoxicity, pruritus, rashes, bone marrow suppression, lowered resistance to infection, nephropathy and gastrointestinal haemorrhage. Under its cover, steroid therapy may be reduced to better tolerated levels. In children, methotrexate has been given 2–3 mg kg body weight fortnightly in conjunction with steroid therapy.

(ii) Azathioprine

This is given at 100–500 mg day^{-1} by mouth, reducing to 50–75 mg day^{-1} when definite improvement occurs. Toxic reactions are bone marrow suppression, infections such as herpes zoster, pneumonia, fungal infections, gastrointestinal intolerance (nausea, vomiting and diarrhoea occur in about 15% of patients), rash, alopecia, hypersensitivity reactions, which include muscle weakness and tenderness which may be thought to be due to the disease, and fever. Children have been given 50–125 mg daily. In a recent study (Bunch *et al.*, 1980) azathioprine did not appear to add any therapeutic advantage when used with prednisone in the initial treatment of polymyositis, but a later follow up (Bunch, 1981) found the group given prednisone and azathioprine did better than the groups with prednisone and control over a longer period of time than the initial 3 months, and the patients required less prednisone for symptomatic control.

(iii) Cyclophosphamide

Dosage of 100–200 mg/day/month has been used, but results are awaited. Toxic effects are bone marrow depression, infections, alopecia and haemorrhage from the urinary bladder.

Overall, steroid-sparing substantial effects have been found in 42–50% of patients treated with immunoregulatory agents, but against this have to be put the side effects, sometimes serious and occasionally fatal, that may arise. Prolonged high dosage of corticosteroids is in itself, however, dangerous therapy, but we need to know far more of the late effects of immunoregulatory agents and their clinical worth in these disorders.

(c) *Other drug treatment*

Analgesics and NSAIDs have only a modest pain-relieving role in these disorders, and calcinosis has so far proved resistant to various forms of therapy.

15.2.5 Polymyalgia rheumatica and giant cell arteritis

Polymyalgia rheumatica (Barber, 1957) is now the accepted name for this disorder, previously known as senile rheumatic gout, anarthritic rheumatoid syndrome, and polymyalgia arteritica. The condition is identical with the prodromal phase of giant cell arteritis (temporal arteritis, cranial arteritis, senile arteritis) and may be defined as a protracted general illness of the elderly with central pain on movement, marked limb stiffness, muscle tenderness and a raised (often markedly so) ESR or raised plasma viscosity.

About one-third of patients with polymyalgia rheumatica develop at some time symptoms and signs of giant cell arteritis. Conversely, about half the patients with temporal arteritis can remember a polymyalgic prodromal phase. For this reason the conditions, if indeed they are separate, are considered together.

Therapy

(i) Corticosteroids

The crucial element in management is adequate corticosteroid therapy. As observed by Gordon (1960) this has a dramatic effect on polymyalgic symptoms within 1–3 days. For polymyalgia rheumatica a usual starting dose is 10 mg daily (5 mg b.d.). In patients with giant cell arteritis twice this dose is given. However, no hard and fast rules can be given and the dose should be titrated to both the clinical manifestations of the disease and the ESR. The minimal dose will therefore be the lowest dose that will both relieve stiffness and keep the ESR below 20–30 mm h^{-1}. Caution should be exercised in this disease (compared with, say, rheumatoid arthritis) to take particular note of the ESR, as patients with good clinical control but with a raised ESR are still liable to develop serious complications (Kogstad, 1965).

In order to avoid the tragedy of avoidable blindness, it is a wise precaution to give a corticosteroid first, *then* arrange for temporal artery biopsy if giant cell arteritis is suspected.

(ii) Other drugs

NSAIDs such as phenylbutazone have been reported to relieve pain but do not prevent serious complications (Wadman and Werner, 1967). Salicylates and paracetamol are ineffective. Corticotrophin, although as effective as corticosteroids are best avoided in these elderly patients because of the risk of fluid retention and heart failure.

15.2.6 Sjögren's syndrome

This syndrome is the triad of keratoconjunctivitis sicca, xerostomia, and a connective tissue disorder. The combination of dry eyes and dry mouth constitutes the sicca syndrome. Often rheumatoid arthritis is the connective tissue disorder, but any of the 'collagenoses' may be a part of this complex. Sjögren's syndrome probably represents an overlap with rheumatoid arthritis (in which about 30% have the syndrome), SLE, dermatomyositis, scleroderma, and fibrosing alveolitis.

(a) *Therapy*

Treatment is symptomatic.

(i) Eyes

Methylcellulose (0.5 or 1%) eye drops 4–5 times daily and treatment of bacterial superinfection of the conjunctiva. Rarely electrocoagulation of the lower lacrimal punctum may prevent the escape of the remaining tears. Glasses fitted with side shields may be useful in windy weather.

(ii) Mouth

The dry mouth is more difficult to manage. However, regular small drinks, chewing gum, or sucking acid drop sweets, together with meticulous attention to dental care are of some help. Methylcellulose is of no value in the treatment of xerostomia. Salivix lozenges, a new saliva-promoting preparation, may be beneficial.

(iii) Vaginal or vulva dryness

This may require topical preparations to alleviate dyspareunia.

(iv) Corticosteroids

Topical steroids may help the conjunctivitis, but long-term usage should be avoided in view of the dangers of superadded bacterial or fungal infection, or glaucoma. Systemic steroids in small doses are used by some clinicians. However, more potent drugs such as cytotoxic agents, rightly or not, are not usually considered justifiable in this condition.

(v) Drugs should be given cautiously to Sjögren's patients as undue hypersensitivity occurs, particularly to penicillin and other antibiotics (Henderson, 1950; Bloch *et al.*, 1965; Talal, 1966).

15.3 INFECTIVE ARTHRITIDES

15.3.1 General

In the infective arthropathies one or sometimes more than one infective agent reaches the joint from the blood stream, from adjacent tissues, or from foreign bodies introduced from outside, such as plant thorns or needles. Joints affected by inflammatory arthropathies, such as rheumatoid arthritis, are more liable to become infected than normal joints, and surgical joint prostheses may become infected at the time of operation or later from the blood stream. It would seem logical, therefore, in such patients to give appropriate antibiotics in the face of systemic infections to protect the joints at risk. Since the first report by Kellgren and his colleagues in Manchester in 1958 there have been over 100 case reports in the English literature of septic arthritis complicating rheumatoid disease, and about a third of these patients have died. As Sturrock *et al.* noted in Glasgow in 1975, the prognosis seems largely dictated by the speed of initiating antibiotic therapy; the longer the delay, the worse the prognosis. As these cases are often missed in the early stages, the answer to the problem is, 'when in doubt, aspirate'.

15.3.2 Septic arthritis

When diagnostic aspiration of the affected joint is done, it is wise to set up blood cultures at the same time as joint cultures, particularly if there are features suggesting systemic disease, such as high fever and rigors. Therapy should be started with the antibiotic most likely to be appropriate as soon as cultures have been set up; this can be changed if necessary when the results of cultures and drug sensitivities are available. The most common invaders are *Staphylococcus aureus*, *Streptococcus pyogenes* or *Strep. faecalis*, occasionally *Strep. viridans*, *Gonococcus* (see p. 455), *Pneumococcus*, *Meningococcus*, more rarely *H. influenzae*, *E. coli*, and several other organisms. The smear from the joint fluid may show the infecting organism.

(a) *Therapy*

The patient should be on bed rest, the joint immobilized, sometimes with pillows or sandbags, sometimes in plaster casts. Traction may be necessary. If no organism is seen on smears from the joint of an adult patient, and there is no lead as to the likely infecting agent, or if a Gram negative coccus is seen, benzylpenicillin (penicillin G) 50 000 to 75 000 units per kg may be given by continuous or 6 hourly i.v. administration; this drug penetrates the joint rapidly. Alternatively, ampicillin 50 mg kg^{-1} i.v. or 6-hourly i.m. Infections due to sensitive staphylococci, pneumococci or gonococci will usually respond satisfactorily but many strains of the commonest cause, *Staph. aureus*, are insensitive to these agents, so other agents have to be tried. These include flucloxacillin 250 mg 6 hourly i.m. with or without ampicillin, 250 mg ampicillin 6 hourly i.m., or ampicillin + cloxacillin 250–500 mg of each by injection 4–6 hourly i.m. or i.v., diethanolamine fusidate by i.v. infusion, or sodium fusidate 500 mg orally with meals 8 hourly. Intravenous or intramuscular administration is preferred initially and, since these agents reach the joint effectively in most cases, intra-articular injections are usually unnecessary; they may also cause synovial irritation if injected into the joint space. Most orthopaedic surgeons favour surgical drainage, but some prefer needle aspiration repeated as required. In the most common staphylococcal septic arthritis some surgeons prefer arthrotomy with drainage and thorough perfusion with fluid containing the appropriate antibiotic. Gentamicin is effective but tends to cause ototoxicity; it may be given as a loading dose of 5 mg kg^{-1} i.v. over 10 minutes or by i.m. injection in divided doses 8 hourly. If renal function is normal and there is no ototoxicity or drug sensitivity, gentamicin may be continued, monitoring blood levels to keep peak levels about 8 µg ml^{-1}, but checking urine for protein casts and serum creatinine levels. Peak concentrations greater than 10 µg ml^{-1} and minimal pre-dose levels over 2 µg ml^{-1} for 10 days or more may prove nephrotoxic. Carbenicillin may be effective in some infections, for instance those caused by pseudomonas resistant to other antibiotics. Intensive antibiotic therapy is maintained for 10–14 days then continued orally for a further 6–12 weeks. In infections with penicillin-resistant staphylococci, penicillinase-resistant penicillin (nafcillin or methicillin) may be necessary. The latter is more painful than other preparations when given by i.m. injection. Patients with diabetes mellitus, severe nodular seropositive rheumatoid arthritis, sufferers from Felty's syndrome, alcoholics, and narcotic 'main-liners' are at particular risk, as are patients on high doses of corticosteroids or immunosuppressive agents.

Ball (1982), in a recent review, states that 75% or more of bone and joint infections are caused by *Staph. aureus* and half the remainder by *Strep. pyogenes*. He recommends clindamycin, a combination of erythromycin and fusidic acid, cloxacillin, or flucloxacillin, and points out that 90% of *Staph. aureus* strains in Great Britain to-day are pencillin resistant. He advises that acute infections of bone and joint be treated for at least 6 weeks, chronic infections for 3–6 months.

Currently available oral and parenteral antibiotics, and antibiotic mixtures are listed in Tables 15.1, 15.2 and 15.3 respectively. (Kellgren *et al.*, 1958; Sturrock *et al.*, 1975; Ball, 1982.)

TABLE 15.1
Oral antibiotics currently available in Great Britain

Antibiotic	Usual maintenance daily dosage
Amoxycillin + clavulanic acid	250–500mg t.d.s.
Ampicillin	250–1000mg q.i.d.
Amoxycillin trihydrate	250–500mg t.d.s.
Bacampicillin	400–800mg b.d. or t.d.s.
Benzathine penicillin G	458mg 6–8 hourly
Cefaclor	750–2000mg daily
Cefadroxil	500–1000mg b.d.
Cephalexin	250–500mg q.i.d.
Cephradine	1–2g daily in 2 or 4 divided doses
Chlortetracycline hydrochloride	250–500mg q.i.d.
Clindamycin	150–450mg q.i.d.
Clomocycline	170–340mg t.d.s. or q.i.d.
Cloxacillin	500mg q.i.d.
Demeclocycline hydrochloride	150mg q.i.d. or 300mg b.d.
Doxycycline hydrochloride	200mg day 1 then 100mg daily
Erythromycin	250mg 4–6 hourly
Flucloxacillin sodium	250mg q.i.d.
Lincomycin hydrochloride	500mg t.d.s. or q.i.d.
Lymecycline	408mg b.d.
Neomycin sulphate	15mg-kg^{-1} daily in 4 divided doses
Oxytetracycline dihydrate	250–500mg q.i.d.
Penicillin G	250–500mg q.i.d.
Penicillin V Potassium	250–500mg 4 hourly
Phenethicillin potassium	250mg q.i.d.
Pivampicillin	500mg b.d.
Pivmecillinam	1.2–2.4 g daily
Sodium fusidate	500mg t.d.s.
Talampicillin hydrochloride	250mg t.d.s.
Tetracycline hydrochloride	250–500mg q.i.d.
Vancomycin	500mg q.i.d.

The above doses, taken from the current Monthly Index of Medical Specialities (MIMS) are for adults only and should be checked before use. For children's doses MIMS should be consulted.

TABLE 15.2
Parenteral antibiotics available in Great Britain, 1986

Antibiotic	Usual maintenance daily dosage
Amikacin	15mg kg^{-1} i.m. or i.v. in 2 divided doses
Amoxycillin sodium + clavulanic acid	1.2g i.v. 6–8 hourly
Amoxycillin	500mg i.m. 5 hourly or 1g i.v. 6 hourly
Ampicillin sodium	500mg 4–6 daily i.m. or i.v.
Azlocillin	2–5g 8 hourly i.v. or i.v. infusion
Carbenicillin sodium	up to 30g i.v. or 8g i.m. in divided doses
cefamandole	500mg–2g i.m. or i.v. 4–8 hourly divided doses
Cefotaxime	1g i.v. or i.m. every 12 hours up to daily 12g in 3 or 4 hourly divided doses in severe cases
Cefoxitin	1–2g 8 hourly i.m. or i.v.
Cefsulodin	1–4g i.m. or i.v. in divided dosage
Cefuroxime sodium	750mg t.d.s. i.m. or i.v., max. 6g daily
Cephalothin sodium	6–12g i.v. in divided doses
Cephazolin sodium	500mg–1g i.m. or i.v. in 3 or 4 divided doses
Cephradine	2–4g i.m., i.v. or i.v. infusion
Chloramphenicol	1g i.v. 6–8 hourly
Clindamycin phosphate	600mg–2.7g i.m. or i.v. inf. in divided dosage
Cloxacillin	250mg i.m. 4–6 hourly
Diethanolamine fusidate	580mg i.v. t.d.s.
Erythromycin	100mg i.m. 4–8 hourly
Erythromycin lactobionate	i.v. 300mg 6 hourly or 600mg 8 hourly
Flucloxacillin	250mg i.m or i.v. q.i.d.
Gentamicin	up to 5mg kg^{-1} i.m. or i.v. daily in 3 divided doses
Lincomycin	600mg i.m. 12–24 hourly or i.v. inf. 8–12 hourly
Mecillinam	15mg kg 6 hourly i.m. or i.v.
Methicillin sodium	1g i.m. or i.v. 4–6 hourly
Mezlocillin	2–5g i.v. 6–8 hourly or i.v. inf., 1–2g deep in 6–8 hourly
Netilmicin	150mg b.d. i.m. or i.v. inf. 4–6mg kg^{-1} 3–4 times daily
Oxytetracycline	200–500mg i.m.
Piperacillin sodium	100–300mg kg^{-1} i.v. inf. or i.m. or i.v. in divided dosage
Procaine penicillin G	300mg i.m. 1–2 daily
Soluble penicillin G sodium	1–2 mega units i.m. or i.v. in 2 or 4 divided doses
Tetracycline	200–500mg i.m.
Ticarcillin	15–20g i.v. or i.v. infusion
Tobramycin	3–5mg kg^{-1} in divided dosage i.m. or i.v. or i.v. infusion
Vancomycin	2g i.v. in divided dosage

The above doses, taken from the current Monthly Index of Medical Specialities (MIMS) are for adults only and should be checked before use. For children's doses MIMS should be consulted.

TABLE 15.3
Antibiotic mixtures

Mixture	Contents	Dosage
Ampiclox (Beecham)	Ampicillin 250mg Cloxacillin 250mg	1–2 vials i.m. or i.v. 4–6 hourly
Magnapen (Beecham)	Ampicillin 250mg Flucloxacillin 250mg	1 capsule by mouth q.i.d.
Triplopen (Glaxo)	Benethanine penicillin G 475mg Procaine penicillin 250mg Penicillin G sodium 300mg	1 dose by deep i.m. injection every 2–3 days
Augmentin (Beecham)	Clavulanic acid 125mg Amoxycillin 250mg	1–3 tablet t.d.s. by mouth
Deteclo (Lederle)	Chlortetracycline hydrochloride 115.4mg Tetracycline hydrochloride 115.4mg Demeclocycline hydrochloride 69.2mg	1 tablet b.d. by mouth
Bicillin (Brocades)	Procaine penicillin G 300mg Penicillin G sodium 60mg	1 ml i.m. 1–2 daily

The above doses, taken from the current Monthly Index of Medical Specialities (MIMS) are for adults only and should be checked before use. For children's doses MIMS should be consulted.

15.3.3 Gonococcal arthritis

Once a common disorder, the advent of sulphonamides and penicillin made gonococcal arthritis a rarity, but now it is seen rather more often. It is a pyarthrosis which occurs more commonly in females than males, usually aged 15–40, starting about 10–14 days after infection. There may be associated vesicopustular skin lesions from which the gonococcus may be isolated. It may also be isolated from the joint fluid, blood, genital tract, pharynx or rectum. The gonococcal complement test is unreliable and of no real diagnostic value. In women, the source of the infection may easily be missed as genital manifestations may be minimal or absent; arthritis in them often appears during menstruation or pregnancy, though the reason is not known. The modern concept of disseminated gonorrhoea is that there are two stages – (1) the initial bacteriaemic stage and (2) a subsequent septic joint stage (the first stage, the 'new' gonococcal dermatitis and the second, the 'old' gonococcal arthritis). Fortunately, the bacteria responsible for these infections are nearly always very penicillin-sensitive strains, and the initial stage of bacteriaemia, which may settle down without the joints ever being involved, responds very well to the usual dosages of penicillin.

(a) *Therapy*

Therapy (summarized in Table 15.4) is to eradicate the infection as soon as possible, as delay leads to destructive changes in the joint. Procaine penicillin G 1.2 mega units + benzylpenicillin G 1 mega unit daily for 5 days may be given but, if the gonococcus is resistant, tetracycline 500 mg q.d.s. should be given for a week to 10 days. For disseminated gonococcal infection some clinicians recommend 10 mega units of penicillin G i.v. daily at first until acute symptoms subside, followed by oral ampicillin 2 g daily in divided dosage for up to 10 days. However, other workers recommend oral ampicillin alone. Penicillin G 60 000u i.m. twice daily for 10 days appears as satisfactory as higher dosage in most instances. If endocarditis or meningitis is present more prolonged intravenous penicillin G 10–20 mega units i.v. is usually necessary until all symptoms subside. The joint is aspirated for diagnostic purposes and may be injected with penicillin, but intra-articular injections are usually not necessary and may cause a synovial reaction. It is advisable to aspirate repeatedly rather than drain surgically if fluid collects. Analgesics and NSAIDs may be used as required, and all potentially infected cases, particularly genital, should be carefully checked before a cure is assumed. The affected joint or joints should be rested and immobilized in the acute stages. As bacterial endocarditis can result from gonococcal infection, blood cultures should be done if fever, rigors, systemic upset or other evidence of septicaemic infection is present. Surgical drainage is rarely necessary. Probenecid 1 g may be given by mouth daily, 0.5–1 hour before injections, or in conjunction with penicillin taken by mouth to

TABLE 15.4
Treatment of gonococcal arthritis or periarthritis

INITIALLY
    Procaine penicillin 1.2 mega units + benzyl penicillin (penicillin G) 1 mega unit daily for 5 days, both intramuscularly
    OR
    Benzyl penicillin G 1 mega unit i.m. 6–12 hourly for 5–7 days + probenecid 500mg by mouth 6 hourly in both cases

FOR PENICILLIN-RESISTANT ORGANISMS
    Co-trimoxazole 2g 12 hourly by mouth for 5–7 days
    OR
    Tetracycline 250mg 6 hourly by mouth for 7 days
    OR
    Spectinomycin 2g daily i.m. for men for 3 days or
    Spectinomycin 4g daily i.m. for women for 3 days.
    For severely ill patients 10–20 mega units penicillin G i.v. daily until acute symptoms subside, then ampicillin 500mg + probenecid 0.5g 6 hourly for 10 days.

raise blood penicillin levels. The therapeutic response to antibiotic therapy in gonococcal arthritis is brisk and usually occurs within 48 hours. Skin infection with gonococci often responds to 250 mg ampicillin q.i.d. but procaine penicillin + benzyl penicillin i.m. as outlined above, given over a period of 5 days, is probably more reliable. Such skin infections are often para-articular rather than intra-articular.

Many gonococcal infections, particularly if acquired in Africa or the Far East, are penicillinase producers, i.e. are penicillin resistant. In such patients co-trimoxazole 2 g 12 hourly by mouth for 5–7 days or spectinomycin 2 g daily i.m. for 3 days for men, or twice this dose for women for 3 days, is advocated by Dr J. K. Oates of Westminster Hospital, to whom I am grateful for much of the information in this section. Infections from the Far East and Africa that are penicillinase producers are rare causes of septicaemic gonorrhoea. The treatment for those is either co-trimoxazole or spectinomycin, the dosage usually given being 2g i.m., and twice the dose for women, for 3 days. For severe gonococcal pyarthrosis treatment could be continued for a week, but spectinomycin 4 g a day for a week is extremely painful. An alternative for penicillinase-producing organisms is cefuroxime 1.5 g 8 hourly for 3–4 days.

15.3.4 Tuberculous arthritis

Tuberculous infection of joint or spine should be suspected in any low-grade inflammatory condition which is not apparently due to the usual infective agents. Histological appearances on joint biopsy may resemble those of rheumatoid arthritis: bacteriological confirmation is required, if necessary by culture. The main hazard in treatment is the emergence of resistant strains of tubercle bacilli. For this reason drugs are given in combination, the most effective initial combinations being:

1. ethambutol   + isoniazid   + rifampicin
   15 mg kg^{-1} daily   3–5 mg kg^{-1} 600 mg daily
   by mouth   by mouth   by mouth

or

2. streptomycin   + isoniazid   + rimfampicin
   0.5–1 g daily   as above

   by i.m. injection

If drug sensitivities are not known it is wiser to start with the second combination of drugs.

Treatment should be continued for 12 months. In severe disseminated disease, it is wise to use streptomycin in full doses daily initially, after 2–3 months reducing to twice a week for a further 2–4 months. Surgical measures, debridement or fusion, should be deferred until the infection is controlled, which usually takes 3–4 weeks. If the spine is affected, it is initially immobilized by a plaster bed for a month or more.

A few practical points might be made regarding the drugs used in the treatment of tuberculous disease of bone and joint.

Isoniazid (isonicotinylhydrazide) is both tuberculostatic and tuberculocidal *in vitro*, the last action is exerted only against actively growing tubercle bacilli. Over 75% of a dose is excreted in the urine in 24 hours, entirely as metabolites of the drug. It is usually given as one oral dose, maximum 300 mg daily; after 1–4 months of daily dosage isoniazid may be given twice weekly 15 mg kg^{-1}. Pyridoxine 10 mg daily may be given to diminish side effects, especially in malnourished patients and in diabetics and alcoholics, i.e. those predisposed to neuropathy. Dosage is usually 3 mg kg^{-1} day^{-1}, an average of 200 mg daily, and may be increased in certain cases to 5 mg kg^{-1} day^{-1}. Patients may be fast or slow acetylators; this is an inborn and racial characteristic and is unaffected by age or sex. Those who metabolize the drug rapidly (fast acetylators) may need slightly larger doses of the drug, particularly if therapy is given once or twice a week. For those receiving the drug daily, therapeutic efficacy and side effects appear much the same in both fast and slow acetylators.

Side effects: rash and fever (1–2%); jaundice and peripheral neuritis are rare (under 1%), but at high dosage, over 300 mg daily, peripheral neuritis is more common unless pyridoxine is given concurrently. Agranulocytosis is rare, as are a number of other side effects, such as psychoses and convulsions.

Rifampicin is rapidly absorbed from the gastrointestinal tract and is rapidly eliminated in the bile, giving an enterohepatic circulation. It is distributed widely throughout the body and may give an orange–red colour to sweat, urine, faeces, saliva, sputum and tears. About 600 mg (10 mg kg^{-1} day^{-1}) is given once daily by mouth 1 hour before or 2 hours after a meal. Side effects are uncommon, occurring in less than 4% of patients. These include rash, fever, nausea and vomiting. At higher dosage a pyrexial illness and thrombocytopenia have been reported. Hepatitis and jaundice rarely occur in patients with normal hepatic function, but are a risk in alcoholics, the elderly, or those with pre-existent chronic liver disease.

Ethambutol. About 80% of an oral dose of ethambutol is absorbed from the gastrointestinal tract, plasma concentrations being maximal in 2–4 hours; 50% is excreted unchanged in the urine within 24 hours. 15 mg kg^{-1} is taken once a day, though some physicians prefer a higher daily dose of 25 mg kg^{-1} initially for several weeks. If renal function is impaired dosage should be reduced. Toxic effects are few, diminished visual acuity, rash or drug fever occurring in under 1% of patients. Pruritus, joint pains and gastrointestinal upsets are rare. The loss of visual acuity is due to optic neuritis; loss of ability to perceive green colours is common. The frequency of this side effect parallels dosage, 15% in patients on 50 mg kg^{-1} day^{-1}, 5% on 25 mg kg^{-1} day^{-1}, but only about 0.8% on 15 mg kg^{-1} day^{-1}. Recovery usually follows on stopping the drug. It is wise to perform ophthalmic examination before, and periodically during, therapy. Uric acid levels rise in 50% of patients due to diminished renal excretion of urate. Because of its lower frequency of toxic reactions, ethambutol has largely replaced aminosalicylic acid.

The above three agents are best given together to avoid the emergence of drug resistance, but in many cases the first two (isoniazid and rifampicin) suffice in combination. Even so, drug resistance may still occur in some cases.

Streptomycin. The action of streptomycin *in vivo* is essentially suppressive, i.e. bacteriostatic. It is used in the more severe cases of disseminated disease or meningitis, together with other agents. It is largely excreted in the urine. It is given by deep i.m. injection. Side effects include rashes, fever, blood dyscrasias, stomatitis, and anaphylactic shock. Local reactions may occur at the sites of injection. Nearly 75% of patients receiving 2 g daily of streptomycin for 2–4 months have detectable vestibular disturbances; reducing the dose to 1 g daily lowers the frequency to around 25%. Intense headaches may precede the labyrinthine disturbances which are manifested by nausea and vomiting, dizziness and vertigo. This acute labyrinthitis is followed by chronic ataxia and, less commonly, defects in hearing. Though the vestibular toxic effects are more common than the acoustic, 4–15% of patients receiving the drug for more than a week have a measurable decrease in hearing, particularly with high tones. A high-pitched tinnitus is often the first sign of trouble and streptomycin therapy should then be stopped immediately. Optic neuritis with enlargement of the blind spot, peripheral neuritis, and renal toxicity may occur but are less common. Dosage is 0.5–1 g daily, depending on age and weight, and the drug is given by deep i.m. injection, reducing to twice weekly after 2 months. If the patient is over 40 years of age, or there is evidence of renal insufficiency, streptomycin should be given on alternate days and the dosage monitored by serum streptomycin levels (Hart, 1982).

15.4 MALIGNANT DISEASE AND ARTHRITIS

Malignant disease may arise primarily in joint tissues, as with osteogenic sarcoma, chondrosarcoma, primary lymphoma of bone, lymphoma, leukaemia, primary synovioma, or as metastatic involvement from a tumour elsewhere in the body. In all these cases the disease is usually localized to the joint in question. It is as well to note however, that the association may be indirect and less obvious, as in Table 15.5. The underlying malignant process, if carcinomatous, resides most commonly in bronchus, breast or prostate. In such cases a polyarthritis is the rule. Certain indirect associations between musculoskeletal syndromes and malignancy are summarized in Table 15.5.

TABLE 15.5
Indirect associations between musculoskeletal syndromes and malignancy

1. Pseudohypertrophic osteoarthropathy
2. Dermatomyositis; less commonly polymyositis and scleroderma
3. Secondary gout and pyrophosphate arthropathy
4. Carcinoma polyarthritis
5. Amyloidosis
6. Haemorrhagic manifestations (as in acute leukaemia)
7. Carcinoid syndrome
8. Systemic lupus syndrome
9. Cryoglobulinaemia
10. Erythema nodosum and arthritis
11. Necrotizing vasculitis and polyarteritis
12. Pseudo-polymyalgia rheumatica
13. Immune complex disease
14. Steinbrocker syndrome (reflex sympathetic dystrophy)
15. Panniculitis
16. Relapsing polychondritis
17. Pancreatic carcinoma syndrome

15.4.1 Therapy

In both groups, primary or secondary (indirect) involvement of joints, the basic treatment is of the primary malignant condition. When this can be removed the secondary arthropathy often rapidly settles. This is often seen quite dramatically in pseudo-hypertrophic pulmonary osteoarthropathy, carcinoma polyarthritis, and the pancreatic carcinoma syndrome, and sometimes with some of the other malignant arthropathic syndromes. The treatment is otherwise symptomatic and palliative with analgesics and NSAIDs, rest, and, in some cases, splintage, and occasionally corticosteroids, corticotrophin or tetracosactrin. Many of these syndromes are associated with a bronchial carcinoma. Even if this cannot be removed, ligation of the major artery or vagotomy may improve symptoms; this has been seen particularly in pseudo-hypertrophic pulmonary osteoarthropathy. In some patients, as is usual in the pancreatic carcinoma syndrome, arthritic symptoms may spontaneously subside with little or no therapy.

15.5   HAEMATOLOGICAL CAUSES OF JOINT DISEASE

15.5.1 Arthropathies secondary to haemorrhage

Haemorrhage may occur into a joint as a result of trauma, disease, or therapy, or due to combinations of these three. The treatment of *misuse of anticoagulants*, sometimes due to using excessive dosage, sometimes to using drugs that potentiate the action of the anticoagulant, an example being warfarin and phenylbutazone, is essentially: (1) to discontinue the offending drug or drugs, and later to modify the dosage of anticoagulant; (2) to aspirate the haemarthrosis and rest the affected joint, usually a knee; and (3) if necessary, to give blood transfusions and possibly an antidote such as an intravenous very slow injection of protamine sulphate in heparin overdosage and 20–40 mg of oral or 50 mg or more of intravenous vitamin K_1 (phytonadione). In the case of oral anticoagulants such as warfarin or dicoumarol, the intravenous route is used for serious bleeding in the CNS or pericardium.

In *haemophilia* blood clotting is defective by reason of 'deficiency' of factor VIII (haemophilia A), inherited as an X-linked recessive character or in Christmas disease factor IX (haemophilia B). Deficiency in these factors leads to coagulation defects and haemorrhage. Haemophilia A and B occur almost always in males. In Von Willebrand's disease or pseudohaemophilia there is a mild to moderate deficiency of factor VIII, plus an abnormality of platelet adhesiveness, leading to a prolonged bleeding time. The disease is inherited as an autosomal dominant trait.

Therapy

(a) *The acute bleed in haemophilia*

As soon as possible after the first symptoms of haemarthrosis the patient should receive an infusion of factor VIII or factor IX as appropriate. A dose of 5–15 u kg^{-1} factor VIII will lead to control of the bleeding within 6 hours, but if severe pain continues a repeat dose may be necessary. A large percentage of young haemophiliacs with severe (<1% normal factor VIII level) or moderately severe (1–5% normal level) with frequent spontaneous bleeds have now been started on home therapy. The patient or his parent will then give the treatment at the earliest possible stage. If home treatment is not possible the patient should attend a designated haemophilia centre where treatment can be given quickly on an outpatient basis without the need to pass through accident and emergency departments, and other sites of delay. In addition, a proportion of children and young adults receive factor VIII of IX on a prophylactic basis – factor VIII two or three times per week and factor IX once or twice, with additional doses as required. This method has greatly reduced the number of spontaneous bleeds in patients, increased their independence, and only slightly increased the total usage of factor. While there are encouraging preliminary reports, it has not yet been proven that this method of treatment prevents the establishment of chronic arthritis, which was previously expected in most adults with severe haemophilia.

In the acute bleed the joint should be put in a position of minimal discomfort and, in the case of severe bleeds, splinted or bandaged. Analgesics up to narcotic strength may be required for pain control, but administration of the factor itself is the most beneficial form of achieving analgesia. When pain becomes less, passive physiotherapy should be started, and thereafter active physiotherapy to regain full range of movement in the joint and to repair muscle bulk. In severe bleeds some workers recommend a short course of oral steroids to reduce the synovial inflammation that results from the bleed and so regain full mobility earlier, but this is not usual or universal practice. Aspiration of the joint, which was often done in the past, has been almost completely superseded by factor replacement.

(b) *Subacute arthritis in haemophilia*

After one or more bleeds into the same joint, a self-perpetuating inflammatory synovial reaction may set in, pathologically not unlike rheumatoid arthritis. This may be accompanied by a marked effusion and a boggy synovium. This state predisposes to further bleeds and may of itself be chronically painful, but in some patients is painless. Untreated, this phase progresses to cartilage and bone destruction, with clinical and radiological features similar to severe osteoarthrosis. If painful, NSAIDs are used by most clinics. Although theoretically contraindicated, as they may compromise platelet aggregation, in practice this does not seem to be a problem. All clinics (and textbooks) advise against aspirin, but most NSAIDs are used and ibuprofen seems most widely so, perhaps because it is a relatively weak inhibitor of prostaglandin synthetase and is said to be less of a gastric irritant. If the subacute arthritis does not settle, a period of regular prophylactic factor replacement and rest of the limb will lead to settling of the synovitis in most patients. In some centres, steroids are used for this problem. If this programme fails, progressive joint damage is likely and a direct attack on the synovium is recommended in most centres. Radioactive gold has been injected locally, mostly in Scandinavia, with much benefit. Recurrence may occur after 2–3 years, and the procedure is not recommended in children because of potential oncogenesis. This technique has not gained widespread acceptance outside Scandinavia. Intra-articular osmic acid has also been used with little benefit, and intra-articular steroids have been disappointing. All these procedures are naturally carried out under cover of factor replacement. Regular physiotherapy is also recommended, especially for knee disease, as weakened quadriceps and ligaments cause an unstable joint which is more likely to be traumatized and bleed. A number of centres have now reported on the use of surgical synovectomy in subacute arthritis. Performed under factor cover, this will reduce the frequency of bleeding dramatically for two or more years. Loss of range of movement and post-operative mobilization may be a problem, and the operation should probably not be done in children.

(c) *Chronic arthritis in haemophilia*

Many adults with severe haemophilia have chronically painful and deformed joints. Bleeding may be less at this stage of the illness. Muscle bleeds leading to contractures may further compromise joints and also put additional strain on adjacent joints, leading to increased bleeding in them. NSAIDs and analgesics are used but the results are unimpressive. Orthopaedic appliances and serial splinting can correct contractures and improve function. In the chronically painful joint, surgery may be undertaken. Osteotomy and arthrodesis are favoured by conservative orthopaedic surgeons, but a number of successful total joint replacements have been carried out on the hip and about 40 total knee replacements reported from America; several knee replacements performed in Glasgow are currently under review.

(d) *Complications of therapy in haemophilia*

Antibodies or inhibitors to factor VIII develop in up to 10% of patients. Allergic reactions, urticaria, pruritus and fever may occur, and rarely bronchospasm and severe anaphylactic reactions. Hepatitis either A, B or non-A, non-B types occur rarely. Venous thrombosis may occur with factor IX infusions, particularly with large infusions.

In *Von Willebrand's disease* the defect is less well worked out, but, in spite of combined platelet and haemostatic defects and deficiency of factor VIII, spontaneous bleeds are rare and arthritis unusual though haemorrhages may follow injuries or surgical procedures. The treatment is with infusions of factor VIII to raise the haemostatic levels. Alternatively, the administration of fresh plasma or suitable cryoprecipitates of plasma can be given if available. Transfusion of normal plasma has a more prolonged effect on factor VIII levels in Von Willebrand's disease than it has in haemophilia (Kisker and Burke, 1970; Duthie *et al.*, 1972; Biggs, 1976).*

15.5.2 Haemoglobinopathies

Patients with sickle cell disease, a condition in which haemoglobin A is replaced most often by haemoglobin S as an inherited autosomal intermediate characteristic, have thrombotic crises which cause local bone infarcts leading to arthritis. Similar episodes occur in thalassaemia. Avascular necrosis occurs in about 10%, most commonly in the head of femur, rarely knee, shoulder or vertebrae. Negroes are most commonly affected wherever they are in the world, but most often in Africa. Analgesics are needed during crises, and i.v. fluids such as bicarbonate infusions may help, as may oxygen when oxygen tension is lowered. However, blood transfusions, iron preparations, tourniquets, and periods of anoxia and hypotension should be avoided if possible. Folic acid 1 mg daily is given for the anaemia. These patients are very susceptible to infection, and osteomyelitis is caused by various organisms, more often

* My thanks are due to Dr Malcolm Steven of the Glasgow Centre for Rheumatic Diseases for the above practical first-hand account of the treatment of this group of disorders.

Salmonella than staphylococci. Treatment includes splinting of involved bones to prevent fracture, appropriate antibiotics (e.g. chloramphenicol for infections due to *Salmonella*). Corticosteroids have been claimed to modify the disorder (Thomas *et al.*, 1982) by inhibiting sickling and by marrow stimulation (De Ceular *et al.*, 1982). Surgical drainage can usually, but not always, be avoided. In beta thalassaemia aseptic necrosis and infection is much less likely. There is thinning of bone and microfractures occur in the legs and feet. Such patients have often received multiple transfusions. No therapy except rest has proved effective. Recently, successful marrow transplantation has been reported in thalassaemia major (Isaacs and Hayhoe, 1967; Alexanian and Nadell, 1975; De Ceular *et al.*, 1982; Thomas *et al.*, 1982).

15.5.3   Drug-induced blood dyscrasias

In any anaemia or blood dyscrasia in an arthritic subject it is as well to consider whether any previously given drug therapy has been a contributory factor.

15.5.4   Leukaemic arthropathy

(a) *Acute leukaemia*

In *acute leukaemia* of any type, arthritis is due to haemorrhage in or around the joint or to leukaemic infiltration of bone or soft tissue. Septic arthritis may be associated. Arthritis occurs more often in children than in adults, most commonly in the lymphoblastic type, and is often misdiagnosed as Still's disease.

Therapy

Treatment is of the leukaemia with corticosteroids and cytotoxic drugs, with analgesics and anti-inflammatory agents as required.

(b) *Chronic leukaemia*

In *chronic leukaemia* large numbers of lymphocytes or myelocytes infiltrate the synovium and haemorrhagic and/or thrombotic changes may complicate the clinical picture. Knees are the commonest joints to be affected. Hyperuricaemia and acute gout may occur, particularly during antileukaemic treatment.

Therapy

Treatment is of the leukaemia with cytotoxic drugs and possibly radiotherapy. Blood transfusions may be necessary, as may allopurinol to prevent a rise in serum uric acid levels and precipitation of renal damage or future episodes of acute gout. The treatment otherwise is palliative with analgesics, NSAIDs and supportive physical measures, graded rest and exercises.

15.6   ENDOCRINE ARTHROPATHIES

Arthropathies may be associated with acromegaly, hypothyroidism, hyperparathyroidism and hypoparathyroidism, and several articular clinical features may be associated with diabetes mellitus and hyperthyroidism. In the first two conditions, carpal tunnel median nerve compression may be seen.

Therapy

(a) *Acromegaly*

The basic treatment of the pituitary condition, whether by hypophysectomy, irradiation or bromocriptine, has little or no effect on the arthropathy, which affects spine, girdle, peripheral and intermediate joints. However, bromocriptine, which suppresses secretion of growth hormone in the pituitary, may improve some soft tissue changes. Once acromegalic arthropathy has developed, it is irreversible, though carpal tunnel compression is often relieved immediately by successful surgery on the pituitary. The treatment is therefore of osteoarthrosis of spine and other joints by the usual medical and surgical measures, surgical total hip and knee replacements usually giving entirely satisfactory results. Deposition of calcium pyrophosphate may cause pseudogout, which may be treated in the usual ways with NSAIDs and possibly intra-articular corticosteroids.

(b) *Hypothyroidism*

One of the most pleasant therapeutic results in medicine is to see the features of myxoedema resolve, the original person gradually re-emerging from the myxoedematous state. Thyroxine therapy should be gradual and the patient and his tissues should be normalized gradually over a month or more. Sodium-l thyroxine 0.05 mg daily is very gradually increased by 0.05 mg every 10–20 days to the usual adult maintenance dose of 2–3 mg daily. More rapid increase in dosage may precipitate angina or heart failure. A further problem may arise from falls and injuries due to the cerebrally awakened patient attempting more activities more rapidly than his joints can perform. Phenylbutazone, which can exert an antithyroid and water loading effect, should be avoided. Carpal tunnel compression will probably respond to this therapy. Analgesics and NSAIDs may be used for osteoarthrotic features and for secondary gout, though this is not common, the true frequency of hyperuricaemia and gout in hypothyroidism being uncertain. Chondrocalcinosis is often apparent in X-rays, but pseudogout is uncommon though treated in the usual way. A residual thickening and tenderness of the flexor tendon sheaths in hands and wrists may persist in some patients after a euthyroid state is achieved; for these, local injections of corticosteroids may be given. Apart from permanent osteoarthrotic changes, and the unexplained destructive changes in the tibial plateaux seen in this disease, response to thyroid therapy should be complete, though it is necessary to maintain such therapy for life.

(c) Hyperparathyroidism

Excessive production of parathyroid hormone, usually from a parathyroid adenoma, more rarely from hyperplasia or a carcinoma, may result in: (1) osteogenic synovitis from softening and collapse of subchondral bone; (2) pyrophosphate arthropathy, with attacks of pseudogout, due to hypercalcaemia; (3) true gout. Treatment is to remove the parathyroid tumour (10% are multiple). Successful removal of the tumour may have no effect on chondrocalcinosis, and may therefore not entirely prevent future attacks of pseudogout. Hyperparathyroidism secondary to renal disease (renal osteodystrophy) may lead to similar changes and to ectopic calcification, including calcium hydroxyapatite deposits in and around tendon sheaths, sometimes with considerable disruption or even complete avulsion. Therapy here is symptomatic and palliative. Long-term haemodialysis therapy is comparatively ineffective in reversing either calcium malabsorption or the associated skeletal lesions.

(d) Hypoparathyroidism

This leads to various osseous changes and to ectopic soft-tissue calcification and new bone formation, the clinical picture resembling ankylosing spondylitis or hyperostotic spondylosis (Forestier's disease). Treatment is palliative and symptomatic.

(e) Pancreas

Pancreatic *exocrine* failure may result in steatorrhoea, malabsorption, and metabolic bone disease. With modern therapy children with chronic cystic fibrosis are now sometimes able to survive to adult life. It there have been recurrent bronchopulmonary infections these patients may develop pseudohypertrophic pulmonary osteoarthropathy. Therapy of this is symptomatic.

(f) Endocrine haemochromatosis (bronzed diabetes)

This may manifest in joints as a chronic arthropathy, mostly affecting the hands, or as a pyrophosphate arthropathy. Treatment is by analgesics or NSAIDs, by aspiration and injection of affected joints as required, and by rest. Insulin to control the diabetes and repeated venesections for the haemochromatosis have, however, no direct effect on the arthropathy. Treatment for the chronic changes is as for osteoarthrosis, medical and possibly surgical.

(g) *Diabetes mellitus*

A very common disorder, it is said to occur more often in patients with true and pseudogout, bursitis and periarthritis of the shoulders, the stiff hand (pseudoscleroderma) syndrome, Dupuytren's contracture, hypertrophic ankylosing hyperostosis (Forestier's syndrome), neuropathic (Charcot) foot, and resorptive arthropathy (diabetic osteopathy) of the forefoot. The treatment in general lies in diabetic and dietetic control, in great care of the feet, and in general health measures with avoidance of smoking and alcohol. There is no specific treatment of these various locomotor diseases, but a disciplined control of all health measures is essential in these patients whose resistance to infection is diminished and whose tendency to arteriosclerotic changes renders their feet highly vulnerable to ischaemic and infective complications. Good chiropodic care is essential in such patients.

15.7 MISCELLANEOUS ARTHROPATHIES

15.7.1 Rheumatic fever

Rheumatic fever used to be very common in this country and every paediatric ward contained a child with rheumatic carditis before 1939. The incidence had been falling for some years, and it is probable that the advent of the sulpha drugs and penicillin and the fall in haemolytic streptococcal infections in the community hastened its almost complete disappearance. But, though this is true of Europe and the USA, it is not true of other parts of the world, and rheumatic fever, rheumatic chorea and rheumatic carditis are still present in most communities elsewhere.

(a) *Therapy*

The flitting polyarthritis, so typical of the condition, is often absent or modified, and the child may present to his doctor for the first time with acute carditis. Clinically, rheumatic fever develops 10–18 days after a sore throat due to a group A haemolytic streptococcus. The drug of choice to eliminate this infection is benzylpenicillin (penicillin G) 1 mega unit daily for 10 days or more, and if the child is allergic to penicillin, erythromycin 250 mg q.i.d. for 10 days. For fever and joint symptoms aspirin 100 mg kg^{-1} day^{-1} is the drug of choice, but if there is already a carditis this high dosage of salicylate may cause cardiac embarrassment, particularly if mitral valvular disease is already present with left ventricular enlargement. In these patients, prednisolone

TABLE 15.6
Treatment of rheumatic fever

ACUTE ATTACK

Benzylpenicillin (penicillin G) 1 mega daily for 10–15 days
OR
Erythromycin 250×4 daily by mouth for 10 days
+
Aspirin 100mg kg^{-1} day^{-1} by mouth
OR
Prednisolone 2mg kg^{-1} day^{-1} by mouth

FOLLOWED BY

Oral penicillin 250mg b.d.
OR
Benzathine penicillin i.m. 1.2 mega i.m. monthly
OR
Oral erythromycin 125mg b.d.
OR
Sulphadiazine 0.5–1g daily by mouth
For several years.

2 mg kg^{-1} day^{-1} is to be preferred, with diuretics and possibly digitalis when the acute inflammation is controlled by the prednisolone. Full dosage treatment with either salicylate or prednisolone is continued for 4–6 weeks, then gradually reduced and discontinued. There is no evidence that either drug prevents or modifies cardiac damage. The therapeutic regime for rheumatic fever is summarized in Table 15.6.

(b) *Prophylaxis*

To prevent streptococcal infection sulphonamides, i.e. sulphadiazine 0.5–1 g daily depending on whether the child's weight is under or over 27 kg (60 lbs) may be given, or oral penicillin 250 mg b.d. or benzathine penicillin i.m. 1.2 mega units monthly. If there is penicillin allergy, erythromycin 125 mg b.d. may be substituted. This prophylaxis should be continued for several years, but opinions vary as to how many. The greatest risk of recurrence after re-infection is within a year of the initial attack, and as the risk appears to diminish after the age of 20 it is wise to continue prophylactic therapy until then, if not longer. Should streptococcal infection break through this prophylactic therapy, full treatment as for a fresh acute attack should be given. When there is a likelihood of penicillin-resistant streptococcal infection occurring in a child with valvular changes, sulphadiazine is to be preferred in long-term prophylactic therapy. There is a risk of children with damaged valves developing bacterial endocarditis, and any operations on teeth or mouth, dental extractions or tonsillectomy, or instrumentation of the genito-urinary tract should be covered by penicillin prophylaxis, penicillin i.m. being given 1–2 hours before the procedure and continued in full dosage for 2–5 days subsequently. Erythromycin can be substituted for penicillin if patients are penicillin sensitive. Before instrumentation of the genito-urinary tract streptomycin 50 mg kg^{-1} (dosage not to exceed 1 g daily) may be added; this is started 1–2 hours previously and continued for 2 days.

15.7.2 Sarcoidosis

Two types of arthritis occur in sarcoidosis: (1) early acute transient type; (2) chronic persistent variety.

(a) *Early acute transient variety*

This is usually associated with erythema nodosum. The arthritis is usually symmetrical, affecting knees and ankles most often. The hands, wrists, elbows and shoulders are affected less often. The arthritis usually starts in one joint and spreads to involve several joints within a few days. The joint symptoms and signs usually subside completely within 3–6 months without any residual disability. X-rays of the chest usually show typical bilateral hilar lymph node enlargement. Tuberculin tests tend to be negative. Kveim tests are positive.

Therapy

Treatment is essentially symptomatic and palliative, with rest, aspirin or some other NSAID being all that is required – time being the essential component for natural healing.

(b) *Chronic persistent type*

This affects about 10% of patients with sarcoidosis. The joints affected are the knees and ankles most commonly; elbows, wrists, hands and shoulders less commonly; feet, hands and spine more rarely. It is usually polyarticular and usually symmetrical, lasts for years with relapses and remissions, but usually subsides completely with minimal or no deformity. The tuberculin test is usually negative; the Kveim test is positive in 70% of patients. X-rays of chest usually show enlarged hilar glands. Iritis occurs in about 30% of patients, cutaneous sarcoid in 50%, a peripheral lymphadenopathy in the majority. Carpal tunnel compression and tenosynovitis may be present. A biopsy of joint or lymph node, skin or liver shows granulomata and inflammatory changes, synovial effusions (if present) showing an inflammatory polymorphonuclear leucocytosis.

Therapy

Therapy is symptomatic with analgesics and NSAIDs, graded rest and local therapy. In patients with hypercalcaemia (about 10%) or with severe iritis corticosteroids may be needed. Prednisolone 40–60 mg daily initially is given in severe cases where a rapid effect is required. However, 15–20 mg daily is given for maintenance therapy or 30 mg on alternate days, the dosage being reduced to 5–10 mg daily or 10–20 mg alternate days for long-term therapy (which may have to last for weeks, months and sometimes years). When severe skin lesions are present, hydroxychloroquine 400–800 mg by mouth daily may be useful initially, dosage being reduced to 200–400 mg daily, and if possible discontinued after 6 months or given as alternate-day or intermittent therapy.

15.7.3 Palindromic rheumatism

In 1944 Hench and Rosenberg described a relapsing remitting type of arthritis characterized by multiple afebrile attacks of arthritis, periarthritis, and sometimes para-arthritis. Thirty four cases had been studied in the Mayo Clinic since 1928. Ages ranged from 21 to 73 and age at onset varied from 13 to 68 years. Originally suspecting an allergic background, the authors came to no firm conclusion about aetiology. A follow up of 27 patients reviewed 'not a single one' to be crippled permanently, but only 15% had recovered completely. One patient had died of unrelated causes, the rest continued with their symptoms. Mattingley studied 20 such patients over a 10 year period, 1955–65, in London (Mattingley, 1966); over half the patients developed signs and symptoms of a low grade polyarthritis, and in a later study of 35 patients 19 developed a low grade rheumatoid arthritis, but 16 had no residual arthropathy. The latex test usually became weakly positive. In 1981, in his last follow up of 63 patients observed for over 10 years, 21 were in remission, 51 appeared to be in remission due to drugs and 18 still had episodic arthritis; 41 of the 45 seropositive patients had developed rheumatoid arthritis (Mattingley *et al.*, 1981).

Today the syndrome would appear in most instances in Great Britain to be a variant of rheumatoid arthritis. Many cases subside spontaneously, often after many years; others become established rheumatoid arthritis, and a few develop into systemic lupus erythematosus. Attacks occur at irregular intervals, averaging 20 a year. Such attacks last a few hours or days, seldom more than a week, and may cease completely for many months. The patient is normal between attacks. The joints most commonly affected are hands, wrists, knees and feet; the shoulders, elbows and ankles are affected less commonly, and the hips and jaws occasionally. The joints are tender, painful and swollen. The sedimentation rate may be raised during an attack; the rheumatoid factor may or may not be present in the serum.

Therapy

Mattingley *et al.* believe that weekly intramuscular injections of as little as 5–10 mg of sodium aurothiomalate (Myocrisin) weekly by i.m. injections may be enough to suppress or modify the acute attacks, though they used doses varying from 5 to 50 mg 1–4 weekly. They concluded that relapses occurred more often if intervals between injections exceeded 2 weeks. Chrysotherapy appeared to suppress or modify acute attacks in 53 of 62 patients.

Huskisson (1976) found that in 5 patients D-penicillamine 250 mg daily appeared to prevent attacks if taken regularly as prophylaxis; I personally have not found indomethacin or phenylbutazone effective as prophylactic agents. Based on experience with colchicine in the prevention of gout and familial Mediterranean fever this might be worthy of more extensive trials in the future. However, so far only gold salts and penicillamine have any claim to be accepted as possibly effective prophylactic agents. The treatment of the acute episode is symptomatic with analgesics and NSAIDs in full doses and possibly intraarticular injections of corticosteroid. If, as seems likely, most of these patients have mild rheumatoid arthritis which 'switch off' repeatedly, they would seem to be good material for clinical trials of prophylactic and thera-peutic agents in the future (Hench and Rosenberg, 1944; Mattingley, 1966; William *et al.*, 1971; Huskisson, 1976; Mattingley *et al.*, 1981).

15.7.4 Familial Mediterranean fever

Familial Mediterranean Fever (FMF, recurrent polyserositis) is an odd disorder of uncertain origin in which recurrent bouts of abdominal pain and fever occur. Seventy percent have joint pain at some time, and pleurisy affects more than half the patients. The disorder is familial, transmitted by a recessive autosomal gene, most of the reported patients being Sephardic Jews, Arme-nians or Levantine Arabs. The disease occurs also in these and other groups of patients in Greece, the USA, France, Russia, Israel, the Lebanon, and else-where. The joint involvement is usually monarticular, the knee being the most commonly involved by arthralgia or arthritis, but the ankle, hip, shoulder and elbow may also be affected. The hands and feet are seldom affected. The onset is usually but not invariably in childhood. Pains may be severe or moderate, come on acutely with tenderness and muscle spasm and may be precipitated by trauma or exertion. Erysipeloid rashes may occur, as may small effusions in the joints. Males are affected more often than females in a 3:2 ratio. Attacks occur at irregular intervals, days, months or years apart, lasting up to a week. Sacroiliac involvement may occur, and occasionally the clinical picture of ankylosing spondylitis is seen. Amyloidosis occurs in about a quarter of patients leading to renal failure in 5–10 years; this complication is said to be more common in Sephardic Jews. Frequent attacks may lead to physical crippling and mental disturbances.

The cause is obscure, the underlying pathological lesion being hyperaemia and a non-bacterial inflammation.

Therapy

A large variety of drugs were tried with no great results until Goldfinger in 1972 reported that small doses of colchicine prevented attacks in five patients. Soon afterwards Eliakim and Licht (1973) published similar results in 10 patients observed for up to 12 months. Since then, double-blind trials have shown that colchicine in a prophylactic regular daily dose of 1–1.5 mg will prevent attacks in most patients. It is of interest that this same drug, colchicine, is now largely used in gout to prevent rather than to treat attacks. The correct use of colchicine in FMF is therefore prophylactic to prevent attacks but not to treat them. In FMF, as in gout, it has been used as a diagnostic aid, but this is somewhat unreliable in both disorders. How it works in either disorder is still not known, though theories abound. It appears to inhibit the migration of polymorphonuclear leucocytes into the inflamed areas, reducing the release of lactic acid and pro-inflammatory enzymes, so breaking the cycle that leads to the inflammatory response. However, the basis of its prophylactic action in FMF is obscure. Stopping therapy is usually followed by a return of attacks. Long-term prophylactic dosage of 1–2 mg daily in gout and FMF has not to date been shown to have adverse effects on chromosomes or spermatogenesis, though it would seem to be wise to discontinue therapy at the start of pregnancy. Bremner and Paulsen (1976) found no apparent toxic effect on testicular function in normal adults aged 20 to 25 who had taken colchicine for 3–6 months, but this does not necessarily apply to younger patients with FMF. It would seem on present evidence that if started early it may prevent the onset of amyloidosis. Treatment of the acute attack is otherwise symptomatic and relatively unsatisfactory. Steroids have not proved effective (Goldfinger, 1972; Eliakim and Licht, 1973; Leading Article, 1975; Bremner and Paulsen, 1976; Huskisson and Hart, 1978).

15.7.5   Paget's disease of bone (osteitis deformans)

In most patients this disorder of unknown aetiology is symptomless and the result of a chance radiological discovery. However, in some patients pains arise from bone, from secondary osteoarthrosis and occasionally from malignant (sarcomatous) change. The disorder has two basic phases: (1) an initial phase of osteolysis and bone resorption; (2) an osteoblastic phase with new bone formation. Both activities run parallel in time in adjacent sections of bone. In the first phase X-rays show characteristic expanding V-shaped osteolytic lesions. Later new bone formation leads to an irregular pattern of increased and decreased bone density. Pains may appear and, weeks or months later, disappear. Bone deformity occurs, particularly in the skull, tibiae and spine, and pseudofractures are observed in the femora and tibiae. There is increased vascularity of the areas, sometimes resulting in diversion of circulation from non-affected areas. These and minor traumata and periosteal changes may contribute to the painful phase.

Therapy

(i) Etidronate

No treatment is indicated in mild asymptomatic cases, which form the large majority. Analgesics and NSAIDs may be used as required. In the past, oestrogens, androgens, fluoride and deep X-ray therapy have been used to relieve painful symptoms, but these are now outdated. Etidronate (disodium ethane-l-hydroxydiphosphonate (EHDP) inhibits bone resorption *in vivo* and stabilizes hydroxyapatite crystals *in vitro*. Given by mouth in doses usually 2.5–10 mg kg^{-1} daily but if necessary up to 20 mg kg^{-1} daily, it accumulates in bone and is only slowly removed. Absorption is poor and it should be taken before meals as its absorption is decreased by food and by antacids. Under treatment, bone turnover decreases, serum alkaline phosphatase levels fall, as does urinary total hydroxyproline excretion.

Vitamin D intake in the diet should be adequate. Six months of continuous daily treatment results in remission lasting up to 2 years, when second courses can be given; but in some patients symptoms are only relieved for a few months. About 80% of patients with Paget's disease improve biochemically, but only about 50% improve clinically to a satisfactory degree. Peripheral nerve entrapment, secondary osteoarthrosis, and hearing loss are not affected. Prolonged treatment beyond six months does not generally improve the biochemical indices to any greater extent than shorter courses of therapy, although isotope (radionuclide) bone scans may show improvement. On dosages above 10 mg kg^{-1} day^{-1} bone pains may occur, as may spontaneous fractures. The latter are probably related to defective mineralization and are rarely seen with the lower dose of 5 mg kg^{-1} day^{-1}. Etidronate therapy is effective, easier to administer and cheaper than calcitonin, and it is not antigenic. It may be effective when calcitonin has proved unhelpful and *vice versa*; to avoid demineralization, low dosage of etidronate may be combined with calcitonin in selected cases.

Side effects. Nausea, diarrhoea and/or hyperphosphataemia may occur at doses over 10 mg daily. Etidronate is excreted without metabolic change in the urine and dosage should therefore be reduced when there is impaired renal function. Hyperphosphataemia does not appear to be harmful.

Preparations. Etidronate disodium (disodium etidronate) (Didronel, Brocades) is put up in 200 mg tablets. Therapy is usually started at 5 mg kg^{-1} d^{-1} given as a single dose 2 hours before food for periods not longer than 6 months at a time. However, courses may be repeated if symptomatic relapse occurs. Adequate calcium and vitamin D intake should be maintained. If diarrhoea occurs at higher doses, the daily dosage may be divided. High dosage over 10 mg daily should not be used unless lower dosage is ineffective and should not be continued for more than 3 months.

(ii) Calcitonin

Calcitonin inhibits osteoclastic activity in bone and reduces bone turnover. It is a hypocalcaemic hormone with effects in general the opposite of parathyroid hormone. It is produced by the parafollicular 'C' cells of the thyroid, which in man are probably also present in thymus and parathyroid glands. Human secretion is regulated by the levels of calcium in the plasma, rising when plasma levels rise and *vice versa*. The hypocalcaemic and hypophosphataemic effects of calcitonin are due to direct inhibition of bone resorption.

Three preparations are available, synthetic salmon calcitonin, given in doses of 100 units daily by intramuscular or subcutaneous injection for 3 to 6 months, then at a maintenance dose of 50 units thrice weekly. Extracted porcine calcitonin is given in a dose of 160 units daily for 3–6 months, then 80 units thrice weekly. Some patients develop high antibody titres to these preparations (though synthetic salmon calcitonin is less immunogenic than porcine calcitonin) and for such resistant patients human calcitonin, which is non-immunogenic, may be helpful. Biochemical improvement with all three preparations is usual, but pain relief only occurs in about a third of patients within 2–6 weeks: if no response occurs in 6 weeks it may be discontinued as no response is likely to occur later. However, if helpful, treatment should be continued for a year then stopped; a further course being given if there is a response. Side effects are nausea, anorexia, and allergic reactions. An initial test dose of calcitonin can be given intradermally.

Side effects. Side effects occur in about a third of patients on calcitonin. These include nausea, vomiting, shivering, flushing, anorexia, urticarial skin reactions, metallic tastes, swelling and tenderness of the hands. Because of the resemblance to the effect of 5-hydroxytryptamine (serotonin), Crisp (1981) gave the serotonin antagonist, pizotifen, in a dose of 0.5 mg by mouth thrice daily with benefit in 3 patients.

Available preparations of calcitonin. Porcine calcitonin (Calcitare) (Armour) 160 units per vial: synthetic salmon calcitonin, salcatonin (Calsynar) (Armour) 100 units per ml. The latter is most used.

(iii) Mithramycin

Mithramycin is a cytotoxic antibiotic which, though highly toxic, appears to have a relatively specific effect on osteoclasts. In Paget's disease striking reduction in plasma alkaline phosphatase levels with relief in bone pain have been reported. It may inhibit osteoblast activity and thereby new bone formation. Serum calcium and liver function tests should be monitored daily. Nausea, thrombocytopenia, bone-marrow, nephro- and hepatotoxic reactions may occur, as may hypocalcaemia. It may produce a severe haemorrhagic diathesis apparently independent of its thrombocytopenic effect, and this may prove fatal. Adverse gastrointestinal, neurological and cutaneous reactions often occur. The raised alkaline phosphatase and increased hydroxyproline excretion improves slowly, but pain is often relieved within a few days of initiating treatment. Recurrence of pain is unusual within 5 years.

Administration. Dosage is 15 µg kg^{-1} daily once or twice a week by i.v. infusion in 5% dextrose over a 6-hour period. Because of its toxicity its use is confined only to patients with intolerable pain not controlled by other measures.

As stated above, only a small minority – probably less than 5% of patients with Paget's disease of bone – need any therapy, and then mostly only analgesics. It is my experience that quite severe pain may arise spontaneously in a few weeks rather reminiscent of crush fractures in osteoporotic vertebral bodies, so simple analgesics or NSAIDs suffice in most cases. Mithramycin is highly toxic, and calcitonin expensive and unpleasant. If more than symptomatic control is needed, as in patients with increasing pain not responding to NSAIDs and analgesics, patients with deformity, or those with complications such as fracture, early signs of nerve compression, or high output failure, the easiest to administer and the least toxic is disodium etidronate. Other indications are: osteolytic lesions, particularly of long bones; immobilization hypercalcaemia, preparation for orthopaedic surgery, and prevention of disease spread in young persons in whom progression of the disease is the rule rather than the exception. It may be very difficult to separate bone pains from Paget's disease from those of osteoarthrosis arising in nearby joints. Healing of fractures in bones affected by Paget's disease may be normal or delayed and may in theory be delayed further by calcitonin or etidronate therapy. However, both drugs effectively reduce cardiac output when this is increased, and calcitonin encourages sodium loss. Therefore, both agents should improve heart failure due to Paget's disease. Progress in the disease is judged by (a) symptoms, (b) X-ray changes, (c) measurement of urinary hydroxyproline, and, (d) reduction in plasma alkaline phosphatase levels. If long-term therapy is needed with other than symptomatic agents, it would seem best to refer to a special centre (Crisp, 1981; Huskisson, 1982; Smith, 1982).

15.8 SUMMARY AND CONCLUSIONS

This chapter has considered rheumatoses loosely labelled 'Miscellanea and rarities'. It has included discussions concerning the treatment and management of a diverse spectrum of disorders that may be regarded as much within the province of general (internal) medicine as within rheumatology. After the 'collagenoses', the various infective arthritides have been described (septic (pyogenic), gonococcal, and tuberculous); this section has been followed by comments on the therapy of rheumatic conditions associated with malignancy, blood disorders, and endocrine conditions. The chapter finishes with a consideration of a miscellaneous collection of rheumatic and related diseases – rheumatic fever, sarcoidosis, palindromic rheumatism, familial Mediterranean fever, and Paget's disease of bone.

The importance of this rather heterogeneous collection of rheumatic conditions, in addition to highlighting the strong links between rheumatology and general medicine, is as follows:

1. Treatment of the primary disease will often lead to control of the rheumatic condition (e.g. endocrine arthropathies), and thus obviate the need of long-term and potentially toxic antirheumatic drug therapy.
2. Awareness that rheumatological repercussions arise 'secondarily' in certain diseases may lead to the diagnosis of the primary disorder (e.g. malignancy).
3. Regarding one of the most commonly encountered arthropathies discussed here – septic arthritis – *immediate* diagnosis is mandatory as severe joint damage occurs rapidly without antibiotic treatment.

15.9 REFERENCES

Alexanian, R. and Nadell, J. (1975) Oxymetholone treatment for sickle cell anaemia. *Blood*, 45, 769–77.

Ball, A. P. (1982) Clinical use of penicillins. *Lancet*, ii, 197.

Barber, H. S. (1957) Myalgic syndrome with constitutional effects. *Ann. Rheum. Dis.*, 16, 230.

Barzel, U. S. (1973) Polyarteritis nodosa and hypertension: treatment with corticoids with complete remission. *N. Y. State J. Med.*, 63, 2263.

Belch, J. J. F., Newman, P., Drury, J. K., McKenzie, F., Capell, H., Lieberman, P., Forber, C. D. and Prentice, C. R. N. (1983) Intermittent epoprostenol (prostacyclin) infusion in patients with Raynaud's syndrome. *Lancet*, i, 313–15.

Biggs, R. (ed.) (1976) *The Treatment of Haemophilia A and B and Von Willebrand's Disease*, 2nd edn, Blackwell, Oxford.

Bloch, K. J., Buchanan, W. W., Wohl, M. T. and Bunim, J. J. (1965) Sjøgren's syndrome. A clinical, pathological and serological study of sixty-two cases. *Medicine (Baltimore)*, 44, 187.

Bremner, W. J. and Paulsen, C. A. (1976) Colchicine and testicular function in man. *N. Engl. J. Med.*, 294, 1384–5.

Bunch, T. W. (1981) Prednisone and azathioprine for polymyositis. *Arthr. Rheum.*, 24, 45.

Bunch, T. W., Worthington, J. W., Commbs, J. J., Duane, M., Ilstrup, M. and Engel, A. G. (1980) Azathioprine with prednisone for polymyositis. *Ann. Intern. Med.*, 92, 365.

Cade, R., Spooner, G., Schlein, E., Pickering, M. *et al.* (1973) Comparison of azathioprine, prednisone and heparin alone or combined in treating lupus nephritis. *Nephron*, 10, 37.

Camerini, F., Alberti, E., Klugmann, S. and Salvi, A. (1980) Primary pulmonary hypertension: effects of nifedipine. *Br. Heart J.*, 44, 352–6.

Crisp, A. J. (1981) Pizotifen to prevent side effects of calcitonin. *Lancet*, i, 775.

De Ceular, K., Gruber, C., Hayes, R. and Sarjeant, G. R. (1982) Medroxyprogesterone acetate and homozygous sickle-cell disease. *Lancet*, ii, 229–31.

Donadio, J. V., Holley, K. E., Wagener, R. D., Ferguson, R. H. and McDuffie, F. C. (1974) Further observations on the treatment of lupus nephritis with prednisone and combined prednisone and azathioprine. *Arthr. Rheum.*, 17, 573.

Douglas Smith, C. and McKendry, R. J. R. (1982) Controlled trial of nifedipine in the treatment of Raynaud's phenomenon. *Lancet*, ii, 1299–301.

Dowd, P. M., Martin, M. F. R. and Cooke, E. D. (1982) Treatment of Raynaud's phenomenon by intravenous infusion of prostacyclin (PGI_2). *Br. J. Dermatol.*, 106, 81–9.

Dubois, E. L. (1974) *Lupus Erythematosus*. University of Southern California Press, Los Angeles.

Duthie, R. B., Matthews, J. M., Rizza, C. H. and Steel, W. M. (1972) *The Management of Musculo-skeletal Problems in the Haemophilias*, Blackwell, Oxford.

Eliakim, M. and Licht, A. (1973) Colchicine–aspirin for recurrent polyserositis (F.M.F.). *Lancet*, ii, 1333.

Franks, A. G. (1982) Topical glyceryl trinitrate as adjunctive therapy in Raynaud's disease. *Lancet*, i, 76.

Goldfinger, S. E. (1972) Colchicine for F.M.F. *N. Engl. J. Med.*, 287, 1302.

Gordon, I. (1960) Polymyalgia rheumatica. *Q. J. Med.*, 29, 473.

Gratwick, G. (1982) Progressive systemic sclerosis in *Drug Treatment of the Rheumatic Diseases* (ed. F. D. Hart), 2nd edn, Adis Press, Australasia, p. 172.

Hart, F. D. (1982) *Drug Treatment of the Rheumatic Diseases*, 2nd edn, Adis Press, Australasia.

Hench, P. S. and Rosenberg, E. F. (1944) Palindromic rheumatism. *Arch. Intern. Med.*, 73, 293–321.

Henderson, J. W. (1950) Keratoconjunctivitis sicca – a review with a survey of 121 additional cases. *Am. J. Ophthalmol.*, 33, 197.

Huskisson, E. C. (1976) Treatment of palindromic rheumatism with d-penicillamine. *Br. Med. J.*, 2, 979.

Huskisson, E. C. (1982) Less common arthropathies in *Drug Treatment of the Rheumatic Diseases* (ed F. D. Hart), 2nd edn, Adis Press, Australasia.

Huskisson, E. C. and Hart, F. D. (1978) *Joint Disease*, 3rd edn, Wright, Bristol, p. 32.

Isaacs, W. A. and Hayhoe, F. G. J. (1967) Steroid hormones in sickle-cell disease. *Nature*, 215, 1139–42.

Johnsson, S. and Leonhardt, T. (1957) Polyarteritis nodosa and its treatment with ACTH or cortisone. *Acta Med. Scand.*, 157, 479.

Kagen, L. (1982) Dermatomyositis and Polymyositis in *Drug Treatment of the Rheumatic Diseases* (ed F. D. Hart), 2nd edn, Adis Press, Australasia, pp. 166–71.

Kahan, A., Weber, S., Amor, B. and Menkes, C. J. (1983) Epoprostenol (prostacycline) infusion in patients with Raynaud's syndrome (Letter). *Lancet*, i, 538.

Kellgren, J. H., Ball, J., Fairbrother, R. W. and Barnes, K. L. (1958) Suppurative arthritis complicating rheumatoid arthritis. *Br. Med. J.*, 1, 1193–200.

Kennerly, D. (1983) Raynaud's disease and prostacycline (Letter). *Ann. Intern. Med.*, 98, 258.

Kisker, C. T. and Burke, C. (1970) Double blind studies in the use of steroids in the treatment of acute haemarthrosis in patients with haemophilia. *N. Engl. J. Med.*, 282, 639–42.

Kogstad, O. A. (1965) Polymyalgia rheumatica and its relation to arteritis temporalis. *Acta Med. Scand.*, 178, 591.

Leading Article (1975) *Br. Med. J.*, 3, 60.

LeRoy, E. C. (1981) Scleroderma (systemic sclerosis), in *Textbook of Rheumatology* (eds W. N. Kelley, E. D. Harris, S. Ruddy and C. B. Sledge), Saunders, Philadelphia, London, Toronto, p. 1211.

Lightfoot, R. W. and Hughes, G. R. V. (1976) Significance of persisting serologic abnormalities in SLE. *Arthr. Rheum.*, 19, 837.

Mattingley, S. (1966) Palindromic rheumatism. *Ann. Rheum. Dis.*, 25, 307–17.

Mattingley, S., Jones, D. W., Robinson, W. M., Williams, R. A. and Dunn, E. C. (1981) Palindromic rheumatism. *J. R. Coll. Phys.*, 15, 119.

Moskowitz, R. W., Baggenstoss, A. H. and Slocumb, C. H. (1963) Histopathologic classification of periarteritis nodosa: a study of 56 cases confirmed at necroscopy. *Proc. Mayo Clinic*, 38, 345.

Ocken, S., Reinitz, E. and Strom, J. (1983) Nifedipine treatment for pulmonary hypertension in a patient with systemic sclerosis. *Arthr. Rheum.*, 26, 794–6.

Pearson, C. M. (1979) Polymyositis and dermatomyositis in *Arthritis and Allied Conditions* (ed. D. J. McCarty), 9th edn, Lea and Febiger, Philadelphia, pp. 742–61.

Rich, R. R. and Johnson, J. S. (1973) Salicylate hepatotoxicity in patients with juvenile rheumatoid arthritis. *Arthr. Rheum.*, 16, 1–9.

Rodeheffer, R. J., Rommer, J. A., Wigley, F. and Smith, C. R. (1983) Controlled double-blind trial of nifedipine in the treatment of Raynaud's phenomenon. *N. Engl. J. Med.*, 308, 880–3.

Rodnan, G. P. (1979) Progressive systemic sclerosis (scleroderma) in *Arthritis and Allied Conditions* (ed D. J. McCarty), 9th edn, Lea and Febiger, Philadelphia, p. 762.

Rustin, M. H. A., Cooke, E. D., Bowcock, S. A. and Kirby, J. D. T. (1983) Nifedipine for Raynaud's phenomenon (Letter). *Lancet*, i, 130.

Shick, R. M. (1958) Periarteritis nodosa and temporal arteritis: treatment with adrenal corticosteroids. *Med. Clinics N. Am.*, 42, 959.

Smith, R. (1982) Modern treatment of Paget's disease of bone. *Prescribers' J.*, 22, 25–31.

Sturrock, R. D., Cowden, E. A., Howie, E., Grennan, D. M. and Buchanan, W. W. (1975) The forgotten nodule: complications of sacral nodules in rheumatoid arthritis. *Br. Med. J.*, 4, 92–3.

Talal, N. (1966) Sjøgren's syndrome. *Bull. Rheum. Dis.*, 16, 404.

Thomas, E. D., Buckner, C. D., Sanders, J. E., Papayannopoulou, T., Borgna-Pignatti, C., De Stefano, P., Sullivan, K. M., Clift, R. A. and Storb, R. (1982) Marrow transplantation for thalassaemia. *Lancet*, ii, 227–9.

Wadman, B. and Werner, I. (1967) Therapeutic hazards of phenylbutazone and oxyphenbutazone in polymyalgia rheumatica. *Lancet*, i, 597.

William, M. H., Sheldon, P. J. H. S., Torrigiani, G., Eisen, V. and Mattingley, S. (1971) Palindromic rheumatism. *Ann. Rheum. Dis.*, 30, 375–80.

Winkelmann, R. K., Merwin, C. F. and Brunsting, L. A. (1961) Antimalarial therapy of lupus erythematosus. *Ann. Intern. Med.*, 55, 772.

Wolff, S. M., Fauci, A. S., Horn, R. G. *et al.* (1974) Wegener's granulomatosis. *Ann. Intern. Med.*, 81, 513.

CHAPTER 16

Drug-induced syndromes and drug toxicity

B. L. Hazleman

16.1 INTRODUCTION

Aches and pains in joints and muscles may be caused or precipitated by drugs, and the management of some of the more severe conditions will be discussed in this chapter together with a discussion of their pathogenesis. The emphasis will be on conditions such as systemic lupus erythematosus which may be exacerbated or precipitated by a large number of drugs, and the management of this will be discussed in detail. Ill-defined conditions such as the arthralgia caused by barbiturates will be discussed in less detail as the management usually consists of withdrawing the drug. Indeed, in any patient with an unexplained arthralgia or arthritis it is worth stopping any non-steroidal drug the patient is taking.

The management of the side effects arising from the drugs used in the management of rheumatic disease will of course be considered in detail. Crush fractures in osteoporotic vertebrae arising from the use of corticosteroids are difficult to treat, whereas the management of analgesic nephropathy is more successful, since cessation of analgesic 'abuse' often leads to stabilization or improvement in renal function. It should be remembered that symptoms and signs involving bones, joints, tendons and subcutaneous tissues may be the earliest indication of an adverse drug reaction.

16.2 RHEUMATIC DRUGS CAUSING DISEASE

16.2.1 Analgesic nephropathy

(a) *Definition*

In 1953 Spühler and Zollinger recognized that many patients with the combination of chronic interstitial nephritis and papillary necrosis had taken large quantities of analgesic drugs, and they suggested that phenacetin might be nephrotoxic. Analgesic nephropathy is now considered to be a major cause of chronic renal failure, but there is considerable geographical variation in reported cases. In Australia (Ferguson, 1974) it accounts for up to a third of cases referred for dialysis and transplantation. In the USA and Britain the frequency is lower and accounts for 7–13% of patients with chronic renal failure (Murray and Goldberg, 1975; Cove-Smith and Knapp, 1978). There are several reasons for this difference; analgesic consumption is the most important. Other factors that may affect the incidence include climate, genetic susceptibility, and the form in which the analgesics are taken: powders may cause more renal damage than tablets, whereas mixtures of analgesics are more nephrotoxic than single preparations (Prescott, 1976).

The total quantity consumed is thought to be of importance in determining the degree of renal damage, and most patients have consumed 1–2 kg of analgesics, equivalent to six tablets daily for 3–5 years, by the time the diagnosis is made. Most series have included patients with arthritis (Burry *et al.*, 1974; Cove-Smith and Knapp, 1978), and recent studies suggest that severe renal damage only develops in those who have taken analgesic mixtures containing aspirin, phenacetin and caffeine, or aspirin, phenacetin and codeine (APC).

(b) *Pathogenesis*

Analgesic drugs cause renal damage by leading first to papillary necrosis, and cortical changes occur as a secondary event (Burry, 1965). It is thought that the kidney is vulnerable to the toxic effects of drugs because of its large blood flow and the hypertonicity of the renal medulla, where many drugs and their metabolites are concentrated. Our knowledge of the pathogenesis of the renal lesion comes largely from studies in rats and from clinical studies in man. However, the rat has only a single renal papilla, and there are structural differences that affect the handling of drugs and susceptibility to damage (Shelley, 1978). Burry considers that the renal changes follow from a direct toxic effect on the tubules, but Nanra *et al.* (1973) feel that interference with the papillary blood supply is the primary event. The exact cause of analgesic nephropathy remains unknown, largely because the agent or agents responsible for the damage have not been identified.

There is little evidence that paracetamol taken alone is nephrotoxic in man, and chronic ingestion appears to have few effects on the kidney (Edwards *et al.*, 1971). Phenacetin may also not be nephrotoxic, and most attempts to produce papillary necrosis in animals have been unsuccessful, and the lesion differs from that seen in man. However, it was the common constituent of many widely used analgesic mixtures, and there is now substantial evidence in both animals and man that mixtures containing aspirin and phenacetin result in a higher frequency of renal damage than when each drug is given individually. If rats are given a dose equivalent to that given to patients with analgesic nephropathy, papillary necrosis is seen in 55% (Saker and Kincaid-Smith, 1969). Dehydration increased the frequency of medullary and cortical lesions, which were identical to those seen in man.

Despite the large amounts of aspirin taken by patients with rheumatoid arthritis, few cases of analgesic nephropathy have been attributed to aspirin alone. The New Zealand Rheumatism Association reported that of 763 patients with rheumatoid arthritis only five had renal papillary necrosis, and all had taken mixtures of analgesics (New Zealand Rheumatism Association study 1974).

It is currently thought that the papillary lesion is caused by phenacetin and/ or its metabolites producing direct oxidative damage to the renal papillary cells. Salicylates potentiate this damage by inhibiting the synthesis of renal prostaglandins, and by reducing medullary blood flow. They also inhibit glucose-6 phosphate dehydrogenase, an enzyme which aids the defence of tissues against oxidative damage. The high concentrations of both drugs in the renal papilla makes this site prone to necrotic damage. There is no evidence that the replacement of phenacetin by paracetamol in analgesic mixtures reduces the frequency of analgesic nephropathy (Nanra *et al.*, 1978). However, when phenacetin and paracetamol-containing preparations have been withdrawn from wide consumption the frequency of analgesic nephropathy appears to decline (Nordenfelt, 1972).

There is little evidence that other NSAIDs are a major cause of analgesic nephropathy, although minor degrees of interstitial damage may be seen on renal biopsy, and they can cause fluid retention and a rise in plasma creatinine. There is no way of predicting which patients are susceptible to papillary necrosis, and all patients receiving drug treatment for rheumatoid arthritis should probably have their renal function intermittently examined. There have been extensive studies, but we still cannot explain the geographical variation of analgesic nephropathy, nor why some patients are more susceptible to analgesic damage. We also do not know why combinations of analgesics are more nephrotoxic than single preparations.

(c) *Management of analgesic nephropathy*

It is important to make the diagnosis, as analgesic nephropathy is one of the few preventable causes of chronic renal failure. Furthermore, cessation of the analgesic often leads to stabilization or improvement in renal function. Diagnosis depends on a high index of suspicion and a careful drug history. Apart from the history of analgesic abuse, there may be little to distinguish the clinical picture from other forms of renal disease, and renal papillary necrosis is seen radiologically in only 20–30% of patients. In the early stages, intravenous urography may be normal, but later the changes can be distinguished from the changes of chronic pyelonephritis which they resemble (Hare and Poynter,

1973). However, it is important to emphasize the need of an accurate analgesic intake history.

The main principles of management are, in addition to total exclusion of analgesics, the careful long-term supervision of hypertension, treatment of urinary tract infection, and salt and water imbalance. Moreover, it is necessary to detect complications such as urinary tract obstruction and transitional cell carcinoma.

The avoidance of analgesics is essential if renal function is to be preserved. Many analgesic abusers may still take tablets and deny that they are continuing to consume them. It therefore may be necessary to test urine for analgesic metabolites. Serum creatinine provides an accurate guide to glomerular filtration rate and should be estimated regularly. The maintenance of hydration and the use of salt supplements may be necessary to improve renal function. Sodium requirements may change with time, but there is a tendency to sodium depletion, which may cause pre-renal uraemia and even further papillary necrosis. Care is necessary to minimize haemorrhage and to avoid hypotension and saline depletion during and after surgery, for this may cause acute deterioration in renal function. Surgery may be necessary to relieve obstruction from an impacted renal stone or papilla, or from peri-ureteric fibrosis. Nephro-ureterectomy may be needed for complicating carcinoma.

In rheumatoid arthritis patients, analgesic therapy should be kept to a minimum and analgesic mixtures forbidden. A small dose of corticosteroids may be preferable to continued treatment with NSAIDs; there is no evidence as to which of these drugs is least nephrotoxic. If analgesia is essential, codeine or an acetate derivative, e.g. pentazocine, may be used, and paracetamol may also be safe if prescribed in small amounts and without the addition of a prosta-glandin synthetase inhibitor.

16.2.2 Gold and D-penicillamine renal disease

Gold and D-penicillamine treatment often lead to side effects, amongst which renal damage, presenting as proteinuria, is common.

(a) Gold

Proteinuria develops in less than 10% of patients, and nephrotic syndrome occurs less often. The nephropathy is unrelated to other side effects of gold, may present at any time and at any dose, and cannot be predicted from serum or urine gold concentrations.

A clear association has now been described between the presence of the B cell autoantigens HLA DR3 and/or HLA B8 and the development of proteinuria during gold or penicillamine treatment (Wooley et al., 1980). An association has also been described between the presence of the DR3 antigen and idiopathic membranous glomerulonephritis (Klouda et al., 1979).

(b) *Penicillamine*

Proteinuria develops in up to 20% of patients. It occurs most often in the first year of treatment, but it can occur at any time and at any dose, and even after 5 years of otherwise uncomplicated treatment (Bacon *et al.*, 1976). There is some evidence that there is a lower frequency of proteinuria in patients treated with less than 500 mg daily.

(c) *Pathology*

Renal biopsy shows a membranous glomerulonephritis, and electron and immunofluorescence microscopy of the glomeruli show subepithelial electron-dense deposits and granular deposition of immunoglobulins and complement. In comparison with idiopathic membranous glomerulonephritis, the changes are often segmental and mild under light microscopy. Follow-up renal biopsies after discontinuing therapy have shown decreasing amounts or complete absence of IgG and C3 on immunofluorescence.

(d) *Prognosis*

Proteinuria may persist or increase initially after stopping therapy. It then decreases gradually and resolves completely in more than 80% of patients within two years. In those with persistent proteinuria, moderate impairment of renal function may occur, and there is evidence that a small number of patients may develop a persistent membranous glomerulonephritis. This has not yet been shown to progress to chronic renal failure (Huskisson, 1979).

(e) *Management*

Renal function should be assessed before gold or penicillamine treatment is started. Proteinuria present before treatment is begun requires full investigation, and is a contraindication to treatment as it makes the detection of gold- or penicillamine-induced renal damage difficult.

During therapy, at least monthly urine samples should be tested for protein. If the urine contains 30 mg % (0.3 g l) or more of protein, a 24-hour urine sample should be collected to quantitate the proteinuria, together with a midstream specimen for microscopy to exclude urinary infection. Some clinicians would consider a renal biopsy if there were significant proteinuria. This is done partly to substantiate the diagnosis, as renal amyloid or coincidental glomerulonephritis could be present, and also to avoid depriving the patient unnecessarily of the benefits of treatment, especially if there has been a good clinical response.

Gold should be stopped if there is significant proteinuria. Although the proteinuria may resolve if gold is continued (Skrifvars *et al.*, 1977), it is much more usual for it to increase and reach nephrotic levels, and death can occur (Silverberg *et al.*, 1970). Renal vein thrombosis can be the cause of death (Nelson *et al.*, 1979).

Penicillamine need not be discontinued if proteinuria develops, and it seems that as long as the proteinuria and creatinine clearance are monitored at monthly intervals, and as long as the creatinine clearance does not deteriorate, penicillamine may be continued with a proteinuria of up to 2 g day. The decision to stop treatment must be made on an individual basis, balancing the benefits against the risks of continuing treatment. Thus, for the patient with aggressive disease who has responded to treatment, treatment may continue in the presence of the nephrotic syndrome, provided that the creatinine clearance does not deteriorate. However, the dose of penicillamine should not be increased. If response to therapy has been poor, most clinicians would stop penicillamine even in the presence of mild proteinuria.

In the presence of marked proteinuria, conservative management is the treatment of choice, since in nearly all cases proteinuria decreases to low levels when treatment with gold or penicillamine is stopped. A high protein, high calorie, and low salt diet should be given, and diuretics should be given if oedema develops.

D-penicillamine has been used in the treatment of gold-induced proteinuria on the grounds that it chelates gold, and may mobilize tissue deposits. However, there is no evidence that it helps, and it can produce a membranous glomerulonephritis, similar to that of gold. Penicillamine is therefore contraindicated for gold-induced proteinuria.

There are no controlled studies of the use of prednisolone alone, or in combination with immunosuppressive drugs, in the treatment of proteinuria, but there have been several reports of the use of steroids in the treatment of gold-induced proteinuria. It would seem that dosages of 40–60 mg daily do help in reducing proteinuria in severe cases of nephrotic syndrome (Silverberg *et al.*, 1970; Skrifvars *et al.*, 1977); whereas prednisone in doses of 10–30 mg daily over periods of 1–6 months was not effective in abolishing proteinuria. Dosages higher than 60 mg of prednisone, or the combination of prednisone with immunosuppressive therapy, do not seem to offer advantages over the dose of 40–60 mg of prednisone. However, the author has used bolus intravenous injections of methylprednisolone (500–1000 mg) in the presence of massive proteinuria and hypovolaemia that has not responded to other therapy, and this was associated with improvement.

16.2.3 Drug-induced bladder damage

Haemorrhagic cystitis is a major complication of cyclophosphamide therapy, and may occur within several hours of a large intravenous dose. This acute cystitis usually abates with drug cessation, but prolonged cyclophosphamide administration can lead to hyperplastic changes affecting both the epithelial and muscular layers of the bladder, and may occur in the absence of an episode of acute cystitis.

Carcinoma of the bladder has been reported as a late complication of treatment (Plotz *et al.*, 1979). These tumours may be difficult to diagnose when bladder tissue is already oedematous from chronic cyclophosphamide therapy. Prophylactic mesnum (sodium-2-mercapto-ethane sulphonate) may reduce the severity of haemorrhagic cystitis (Scheef *et al.*, 1979). Maintenance of adequate hydration and urine flow may help to prevent episodes of acute cystitis.

16.2.4　Drug-induced pulmonary disease

(a) *Asthma*

Although aspirin-induced asthma has long been recognized, its mechanism remains uncertain. Most patients who are sensitive to aspirin react also to other NSAIDs. Although a reaction may be produced by a very small dose (30 mg aspirin), individual patients vary and an immunological basis seems unlikely. All the agents are inhibitors of prostaglandin synthetase, and the present explanation is based on this action (Szczeklik and Czerniawska-Mysik, 1976). However, since both prostaglandin $F_2\alpha$, which is a broncho-constrictor, and prostaglandin E_2, which is a bronchodilator, are found in the lungs, selective inhibition of the latter would be required to provoke an asthma attack. However, this explanation is probably not correct as sodium cromoglycate has been shown to have a protective effect in aspirin-induced asthma, and it is known to have no effect in preventing bronchoconstriction due to prostaglandin $F_2\alpha$. In addition, whereas all asthmatics are unduly sensitive to inhaled prostaglandin $F_2\alpha$, aspirin-sensitive subjects are less affected than many non-sensitive atopic asthmatics. It is possible that the histamine may be released from mast cells due to a reduction in prostaglandin levels which lower cyclic AMP. Aspirin-sensitive individuals may be abnormally dependent on the prostaglandin regulatory mechanism and less influenced by sympathetic regulation.

About 2% of asthmatics appear to be intolerant of aspirin. Females predominate in a ratio of 3:2, and the symptoms usually begin at 30–40 years of age. Intermittent watery nasal discharge is subsequently associated with the development of nasal polyps and chronic nasal blockage. Avoidance of anti-inflammatory drugs is the mainstay of treatment, but of course this is often difficult and treatment of the asthma may be necessary, although deaths have been reported and exacerbations of asthma can persist for up to three weeks. Paracetamol seems least likely to produce asthma, although occasional reports are well documented.

Many patients with analgesic-induced asthma are sensitive to benzoic acid and to the azo dye, tartrazine, a commonly used colouring agent in drugs (especially those coloured yellow, orange or red) and also in food, e.g. orange juice or custard. Usually reactions to tartrazine are not as severe as with aspirin.

(b) *Alveolar reactions*

Cytotoxic and immunosuppressive drugs, particularly bulsulphan, bleomycin and methotrexate, have increasingly been associated with pulmonary complications. Histologically most of the drugs produce diffuse alveolar damage, with destruction of lining cells, formation of hyaline membranes, a variable inflammatory infiltrate, and fibrosis. Azathioprine has been associated with the development of a restrictive defect, impaired gas transfer, and radiological signs of basal atelectasis or infiltration, all of which disappear after withdrawal (Rubin *et al.*, 1972). Diffuse alveolitis may be caused by penicillamine (Eastmond, 1976), and Goodpasture's syndrome has complicated penicillamine therapy. Phenylbutazone has also been implicated in diffuse pulmonary reactions in isolated instances.

Eosinophilic reactions in the lung occur with aspirin and gold. The pulmonary eosinophilia seen with aspirin appears to be separate from aspirin-induced asthma. Gold can produce a number of pulmonary reactions (Gould *et al.*, 1977). Symptoms develop 5–16 weeks after the start of treatment, with development of cough, dyspnoea and sometimes pleurisy. Diffuse reticulonodular shadowing occurs on X-ray. The pulmonary reaction improves on cessation of gold therapy and with corticosteroid therapy, but there may be permanent impairment of pulmonary function. There is a prompt relapse on re-exposure to gold injections.

Analgesics given during labour have been implicated in the development of pulmonary hypertension in the newborn: drugs such as aspirin, indomethacin, and naproxen delay premature labour but may also, by their inhibitory effects on prostaglandin synthesis, cause constriction of the ductus arteriosus *in utero* leading to postnatal pulmonary hypertension and respiratory distress.

16.2.5 Drug eruptions of the skin

(a) *Clinical features*

The 1975 Boston Collaborative Program of Drug Surveillance found that 3% of hospital admissions, 14% of medical resources and 30% of hospital patients developed adverse reactions. It is wise to assume that any drug can cause any rash, but the diagnosis depends on clinical judgement as there are no *in vitro* tests that are reliable and specific. Drug rashes often have a symmetrical urticarial, erythematous, or purpuric and ischaemic pattern determined by vascular anatomy.

Scaling or the vesiculation of eczema is less likely to be seen as the first manifestation of a drug rash. If a rash looks like eczema it is probably not caused by a drug. If it is erythematous and urticarial it may well be. Later stages of a rash are often complicated by a secondary epidermal reaction so diagnosis should be made on the initial manifestation. One exception to this of course is the intra-epidermal immunologically induced 'pemphigus' rash of penicillamine. Paracetamol and steroids seldom cause drug rashes. In general, drug rashes do not persist after withdrawal of the drug – exceptions include pemphigus from penicillamine.

When examining a list of drugs taken by a patient, drugs added within the previous month are the most likely cause of the rash. In the absence of a previous reaction to drugs, and especially if a drug is new to the patient, it is unlikely to cause a rash within the first few days of administration.

An urticarial rash may be triggered by prostaglandin synthetase inhibitors such as aspirin. A toxic urticated erythema develops as a red indurated papular eruption which later involves the epidermis and produces scales. This type of rash is usually not seen for 8–10 days after the ingestion of a drug. Fever and arthropathy may be associated. Exfoliative dermatitis is the end result and is seen with gold, phenylbutazone and indomethacin.

The antimalarials lead to pigmentary changes in the skin which slowly resolves when the drug is discontinued. Mepacrine produces a lemon-yellow

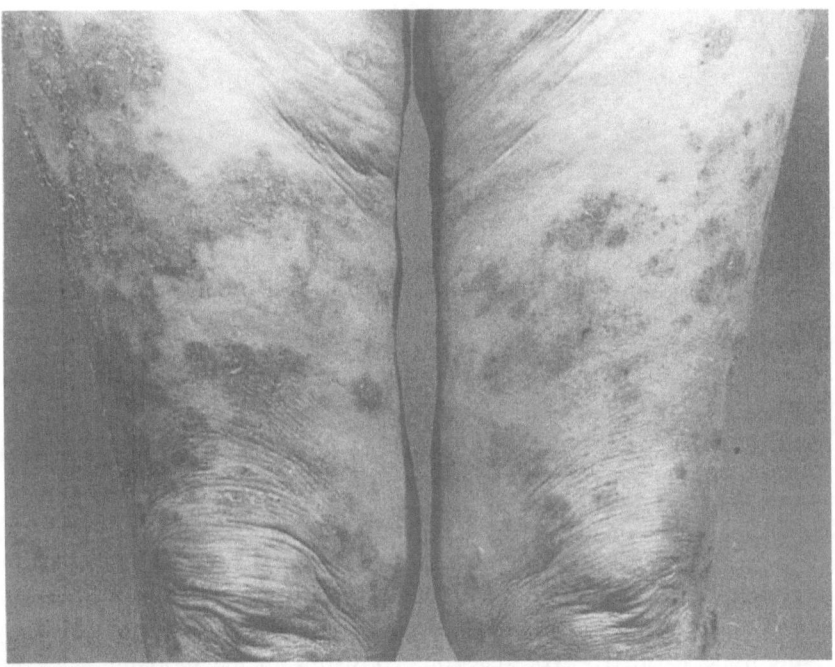

Figure 16.1 Erythema and purpura and superficial scaling with erythematous features as seen in gold sensitivity.

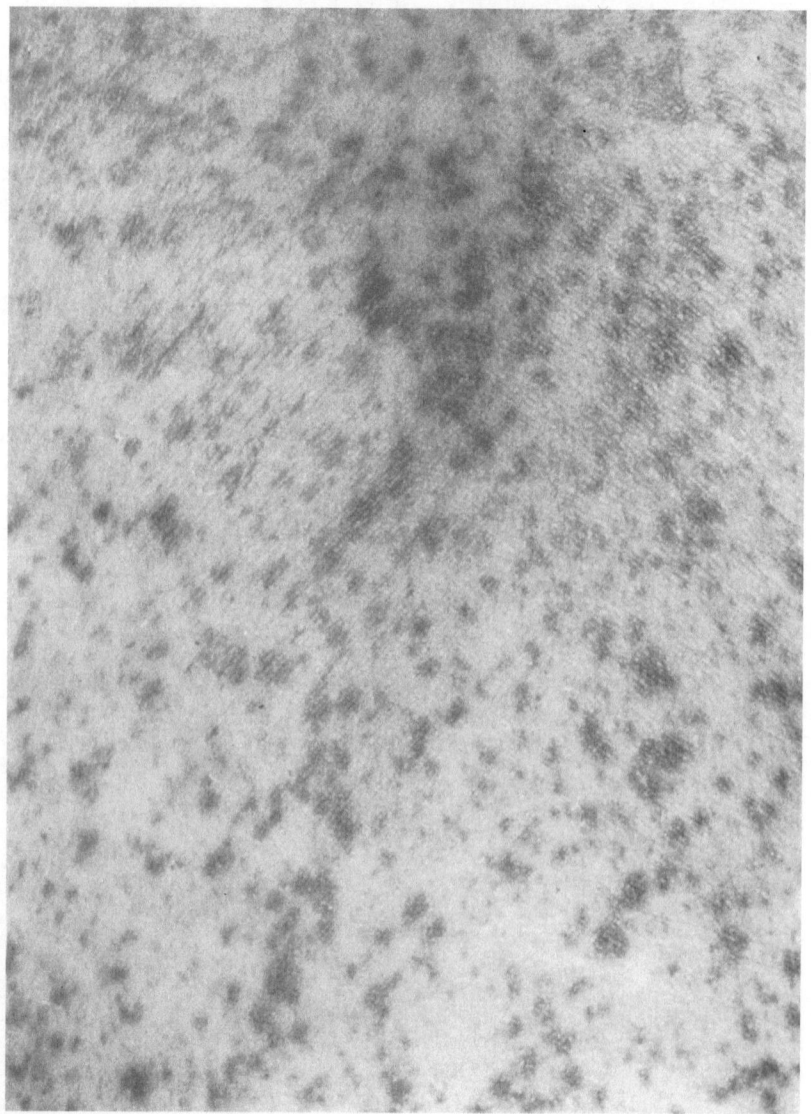

Figure 16.2 Purpura due to gold toxicity.

discoloration. They may also produce a similar picture to lichen planus. Exacerbations of psoriasis have been reported with the antimalarials and, although usually not severe, an exfoliative dermatitis can occur.

Acute hypersensitivity-type reactions consisting of maculopapular lesions, urticaria and pruritus occur in the first month of treatment with penicillamine. Less common, but of more significance, is the association of penicillamine with pemphigus. Lichen planus may occur, and there have been reports of elastosis perforans serpiginosa-like lesions.

The most common cutaneous reaction with gold is a non-specific erythematous maculopapular eruption. Therapy must be discontinued or a much more severe generalized exfoliative dermatitis may ensue. A rash identical to pityria-

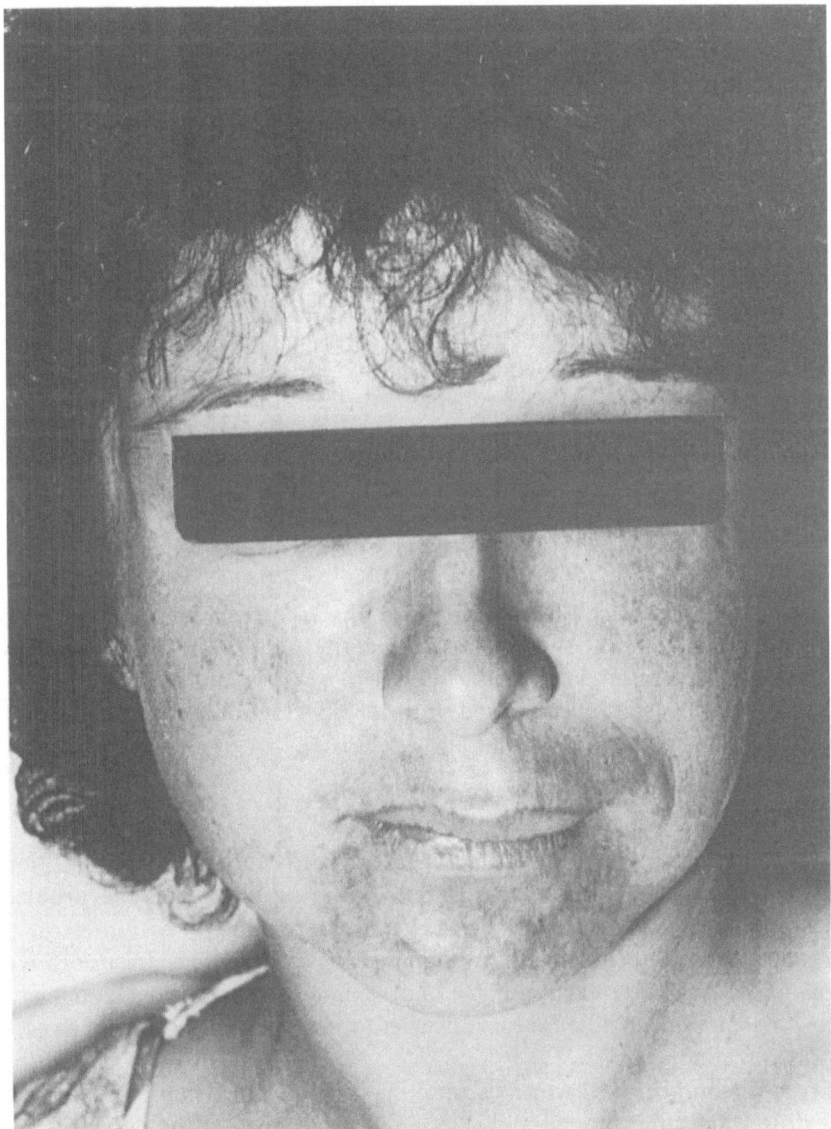

Figure 16.3 Assymetry of the face with wealing of the chin and swelling of the left upper lip due to NSAID therapy.

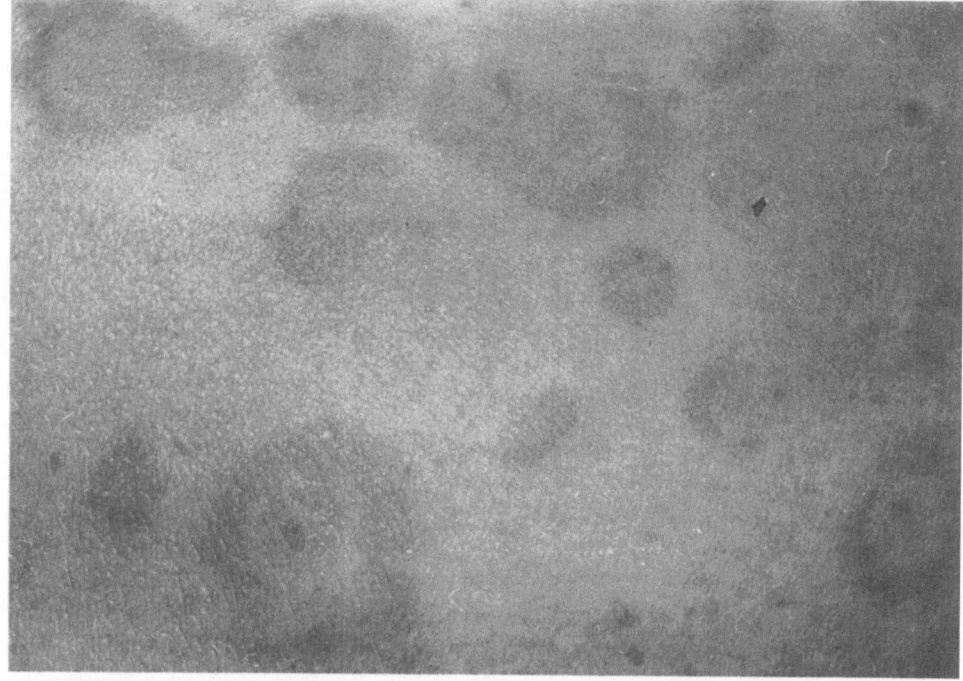

Figure 16.4 Erythema with a target lesion in the lower field as seen in drug eruption.

sis rosea may also occur. Most gold eruptions are self-limited and regress on discontinuation of gold therapy. Gold therapy may be re-instated in most patients after the rash has cleared.

Some typical rashes encountered with NSAIDs and long-term therapy for rheumatoid arthritis are shown in Figs 16.1–16.4.

(b) Management

The best way is to stop the use of all drugs likely to cause the eruptions. Blood tests are of no help in trying to find which drug is causing the problem. Eosinophilia may suggest that an eruption is due to a drug.

Skin tests are not helpful, as a risk of dangerous anaphylaxis, false negatives, and lack of knowledge of the antigen make skin testing useless. Re-administration of the drug is possible for most drug eruptions, but it is usually at a risk of considerable morbidity.

Erythema multiforme can result from the treatment of rheumatoid arthritis. The drug should be stopped and systemic steroids given if the patient is very uncomfortable and toxic.

Pemphigus vulgaris, a blistering condition affecting the mucosa as well as the skin can be caused by penicillamine therapy. Corticosteroids are life saving; prednisolone 120 mg daily is a common starting dose and failure to control the eruptions within a week merits doubling this very high dose. As soon as there are no new blisters the steroids are reduced quickly to 30 mg daily and then with slower reduction. An immunosuppressive drug is usually added as a steroid-sparing agent.

16.2.6 Anti-inflammatory drugs and the gastrointestinal tract

(a) *Pathogenesis*

Gastrointestinal ulceration and haemorrhage often occur from the ingestion of aspirin and other NSAIDs. The development of gastric mucosal damage by these drugs has a multi-factorial basis resulting from their various biological effects. The impairment of prostaglandin production could be one important factor in affecting the vascular and/or secretory functions in the gastric mucosa. This leads to mucosal ischaemia, stimulation of acid and pepsin production, mast cell degranulation, and increased membrane permeability. Rainsford and Willis (1982) showed that whereas ulcerogenic drugs reduce the mucosal and plasma prostaglandin levels in parallel with their ulcerogenicity, this relationship does not always hold for drugs with low ulcerogenic activity. Gastric mucosal damage may result from the direct effect of an acidic drug on membrane permeability (which in turn is influenced by the rate of absorption of the drug).

(b) *Management of upper gastrointestinal haemorrhage*

Any patient with melaena or haematemesis within the preceding 48 hours should be admitted to hospital because of the risk of further haemorrhage. There are three phases in the management of a patient with an acute gastrointestinal haemorrhage: resuscitation, diagnosis, and treatment.

(c) *Resuscitation*

A rapid clinical assessment must be made before resuscitation is begun. Pulse, respiratory rate, blood pressure, and the state of the peripheral circulation must be noted and recorded. Blood should be taken for cross-matching and for determination of haemoglobin, haematocrit, platelet count, and prothrombin time. Assessment must be made by the physician and surgeon together so that joint decisions on management can be made.

An intravenous line is set up immediately. Patients who are shocked or who are elderly should have central lines so that central venous pressure can be monitored during subsequent transfusion. A patient should be transfused for shock or anaemia. Before blood is available, plasma or a colloid volume expander may be necessary. It is usual to treat anaemia by transfusion until the patient's haemoglobin is at least 10 g dl^{-1}. It is important to remember that the haemoglobin may initially be normal after a bleed, before there is haemodilution of a depleted red cell mass.

The use of a nasogastric tube is controversial, but it adds to the discomfort of the patient and may cause fresh bleeding.

(d) Diagnosis

Either endoscopy or a barium meal can be used 12–24 hours after hospital admission. Prospective studies have shown that emergency endoscopy does not influence the clinical outcome. Endoscopy has two main advantages: first, it provides the highest rate of correct diagnosis and, secondly, it can detect continuing haemorrhage or predict the likelihood of a rebleed.

(e) Treatment

About 10% of patients die, but this is partly explained by the increasing age of patients. Emergency surgery is considered if there is continuing severe haemorrhage or if there is a combination of factors that make major re-haemorrhage likely. Elderly patients, those with gastric ulceration, and those who have suffered a major initial bleed, are all more liable to recurrent haemorrhage. There are no medical treatments that decrease the frequency or severity of rebleeding. H_2 receptor antagonists do not help.

Little has been published on treatment with cimetidine during anti-inflammatory treatment. Mitchell and Sturrock (1982) found that dyspeptic symptoms were relieved rapidly with cimetidine, but the ulcers did not heal, and continued use resulted in perforation.

16.2.7 Drugs and liver damage

The liver is a major site of drug metabolism and many drugs or their metabolites are excreted in the bile. In addition, many drugs affect the liver cell's metabolism, which can lead to irreversible cell damage or the changes may revert on stopping the drug.

Paracetamol is a cause of hepatic necrosis. Phenylbutazone and allopurinol can cause granulomatous hepatitis. The detection of liver damage is important as the changes may become chronic and irreversible if the drug is continued. If a drug is not suspected as a cause of liver damage, and if a laparotomy is carried out, this can precipitate liver failure in patients with pronounced cholestasis. Re-exposure to a toxic drug may produce a more serious or fatal illness when initial exposure may have produced only a brief, trivial illness.

Paracetamol produces hepatic necrosis only in high doses when toxic metabolites are formed. The severity of liver damage can be reduced by infusions of cysteamine acetylcysteine or methiamine. These substances alter the relative amounts of the drug metabolized by different routes and thus reduce the amount of toxic metabolites produced.

Hepatotoxicity from paracetamol almost always accompanies the ingestion of 15 g or more, and some indication of the likely outcome can be obtained from single estimates of plasma paracetamol concentrations at a known time after overdose. Recently, reports have been published of six patients showing a relationship between ingestion of lower doses of paracetamol and liver damage. Barker *et al.* (1977) described a toxic hepatitis after 5.2–7.5 g per day for 7 days to 3 weeks. In some of the patients there was pre-existing liver damage.

Hepatocellular necrosis or cholestatic hepatitis can occur with NSAIDs. Elevations in serum transaminases have been reported in 20–66% of patients receiving high doses of aspirin. Histology shows hepatocellular damage, with focal necrosis and portal tract infiltration. Recovery is prompt if the drug is stopped. Salicylate hepatotoxicity is dose-related and is not seen unless more than 2 g per day are taken. Abnormalities in liver function tests correlate generally with plasma concentrations of the drug. Current evidence suggests that salicylates are mildly hepatotoxic and that this hepatotoxicity is increased especially in systemic lupus erythematosus and juvenile rheumatoid arthritis. The mechanism for this hepatocellular damage is unknown.

16.2.8   Corticosteroids

(a) *Side effects and complications*

Side effects and complications of treatment with corticosteroids or ACTH can be divided into two main categories – those that arise from continued use of large doses and those that, on stopping treatment, occur as a result of a suppressed hypothalamo-pituitary-adrenal axis.

The frequency, severity, and importance of side effects depend mainly on the duration of treatment and the size of the dosage used, as well as on the patient's response. Side effects on the musculoskeletal system include: osteoporosis with crush fracture of vertebrae, aseptic necrosis of the femoral head, myopathy with wasting and weakness, and retardation of growth in children.

A more detailed list of steroid-induced effects, including both musculoskeletal changes and changes in other systems, can be summarized thus (Hart, 1978):

1. Endocrine: Adrenal suppression; hypotension; lack of
                      energy; hyperglycaemia and glycosuria ('steroid
                      diabetes mellitus'); hirsutism; amenorrhoea;
                      growth retardation in children.

2. Electrolyte   Hypokalaemia; sodium and fluid retention;
   disturbances: hypertension.
3. Muscles: Myopathy.
4. Bones and joints: Infection; aseptic necrosis; osteoporosis.
5. C.N.S.:   Headaches; mental and mood changes;
                           intracranial hypertension.
6. Eye: Posterior subcapsular cataract; glaucoma;
                           papilloedema.
7. Gastrointestinal: Gastroduodenal upsets; peptic ulcer exacerbation
                           and perforation; intussusception; perforated
                           diverticula.
8. Skin and subcutaneous   Atrophy; 'steroid purpura'; moon face; acne;
   tissues: redistribution of body fat; 'buffalo hump';
                           increased tendency to infection.

(See also Chapter 8 for further details.)

(b) *Corticosteroid-induced osteoporosis*

The relation between corticosteroid therapy and osteoporosis is complex, and is governed by the dose and duration of treatment, and by the underlying state of bone turnover and balance (which may vary with age and may be modified by disease). It seems that osteoporosis seldom develops in patients receiving up to 10–15 mg of prednisone or its equivalent each day. Children and postmenopausal women appear to be most likely to develop osteoporosis, and the most severely affected bones are the ribs and vertebral bodies. In both groups, more trabecular bone is lost than compact bone. Fractures of the ribs seem to occur more commonly in corticosteroid osteoporosis than in osteoporosis from other causes. It is of interest that patients with bronchial asthma lose little or no bone, compared with rheumatoid patients, despite receiving similar amounts of corticosteroid (Mueller *et al.*, 1973).

Corticosteroids affect bone and mineral metabolism in several ways, and their combined effect leads to a negative calcium balance and accelerated bone loss. Bone biopsy shows reduced bone formation and increased bone resorption (Riggs *et al.*, 1966). Reduced formation is thought to be a direct inhibitory effect of corticosteroids on the functional activity of osteoblasts. Increased resorption is regarded as a secondary phenomenon mediated by parathyroid hormone, and Jee *et al.* (1970) have suggested that this can be prevented by parathyroidectomy. In man, the administration of corticosteroids is followed by a brisk but transient increase in the serum parathyroid hormone circulation (Fucik *et al.*, 1975), and this may be sustained with long-term therapy. This apparent secondary hyperparathyroidism is thought to arise from a tendency to hypocalcaemia caused by a reduction of intestinal absorption, which is unexplained. There is also an increased urinary excretion of calcium (which may be associated with renal stone formation) reflecting in part the net increase in bone resorption. There is no firm evidence of an abnormality of vitamin D metabolism.

The treatment of corticosteroid-induced osteoporosis is unsatisfactory. Relief of Cushing's syndrome does not restore bone mass (Riggs *et al.*, 1966). The same is likely to be true for corticosteroid-induced osteoporosis, and attempts have been made to improve calcium balance by increasing intestinal absorption of calcium with vitamin D. Gallagher *et al.* (1973) found that the extra calcium gained by this route was excreted promptly in the urine. Hahn *et al.* (1979) gave 25-(OH)D$_3$ and observed similar responses; modest gains in bone mass occurred during the first year of treatment, but there was little change afterwards. There is no evidence that vitamin D or 25-hydroxy-vitamin D reduces the risk of fracture, and both forms of treatment carry the risk of vitamin D intoxication.

Nilsen *et al.* (1978) claimed that microcrystalline hydroxyapatite protects patients with rheumatoid arthritis from the usual accelerated loss of bone produced by corticosteroid therapy. Compared with controls, the patients treated with microcrystalline hydroxyapatite had a small but significant reduction in loss of radial bone density when calculated as bone mineral content/bone width, but not when calculated as percentage of initial density. Since there was no difference in loss of ulnar bone density between treated patients and controls, it is very difficult to draw any meaningful conclusions.

Sheagren *et al.* (1977), in an attempt to prevent osteoporosis, found that alternate-day therapy causes less bone loss than the same dose of corticosteroid given on a daily basis.

(c) *Muscle weakness*

This is a feature of an excess of corticosteroids. The muscles of the pelvic girdle are primarily affected. Tolerance to corticosteroids is variable and not related to age, nor does it appear to be related to the size of the dose or the duration of treatment. 9α-fluorinated steroids, such as dexamethasone and triamcinolone, appear to be particularly harmful to muscle. Usually the myopathy is insidious, and muscle enzyme activity is usually normal. Creatine excretion in the urine is increased, its extent correlating well with the extent of muscle weakness. Electromyography reveals no specific features. Histochemistry shows atrophy of type 2b fibres and an increase in the numbers of lipid droplets without cellular infiltration.

When myopathy occurs, corticosteroids should be stopped or the dose reduced, and, if it is essential to continue treatment, alternate-day administration may be preferable. The muscle atrophy induced by fludrocorticoids in rats may be partially prevented by endurance training (Hickson and Davis, 1981), which suggests that patients at risk of developing steroid myopathy should be encouraged to take exercise.

(d) *Retardation of growth*

Children treated for long periods with corticosteroids show retarded linear growth due to inhibition of the skeletal effect of growth hormone. This leads to depression of epiphyseal cartilage cell proliferation. Harvard (1965) has suggested that one can predict the critical daily dose of steroid above which suppression of growth may be expected. This is 5.1 mg of prednisone or 45 mg of cortisone per square metre of body surface. Oliver (1970) feels that rigid guidelines cannot be given.

Substitution of a single dose early in the morning at 48 hour intervals, reduction of the daily dosage, or withdrawal of therapy is followed by normal or accelerated growth rate, provided that fusion of the epiphyses has not occurred.

(e) *Suppression of the hypothalamo-pituitary-adrenal axis (HPA)*

By increasing the plasma steroid level, systemic corticosteroids suppress the secretion of corticotrophin releasing factor (CRF) from the hypothalamus and the output of ACTH from the anterior pituitary. The degree of this suppression depends on the dosage and duration of corticosteroid administration, and the time of day when the steroid is given; physiological dosages of corticosteroids completely suppress ACTH release if given at midnight. The decreased secretion of ACTH causes physiological and eventually anatomical atrophy of the adrenal cortex.

ACTH and its analogues increase cortisol secretion from the cortex of the adrenal gland. This and ACTH suppress the release of CRF from the hypothalamus and of corticotrophin from the pituitary. Therefore, the corticosteroid-treated patient may fail to respond to stress because of adrenocortical atrophy, and the ACTH-treated patient may also fail to respond because of hypothalamo-pituitary suppression.

Although suppression cannot be avoided when prolonged treatment in high dosage is given, side effects can largely be avoided by withdrawing treatment gradually, particularly when treatment has been prolonged. A reduction in steps of 5.0 mg prednisone every 2–4 days is recommended until the total daily dose is 5.0 mg. Then the dosage can be reduced at the rate of 1.0 mg every 2–4 weeks. The earliest one may expect some biochemical changes in HPA function would be one week after beginning therapy with 20 mg or more of prednisone, but the time is variable and cannot be easily pinpointed. A precise correlation between the clinical and biochemical status of the HPA system does not exist. The most sensitive indices of steroid-induced HPA axis suppression are the insulin-induced hypoglycaemia and metyrapone tests. On present evidence there is a relatively slight adrenal-suppressive effect with alternate-day treatment if less than 40 mg of prednisone are given. This compares well with similar effects achieved by ACTH.

Suppression of the HPA axis leads to hypotension and collapse when patients are subjected to stress (infective, traumatic, or occasionally psychological). About 10% of deaths in patients receiving corticosteroids are due to this cause, and this emphasizes the importance of giving additional corticosteroids to patients under stress and to the slow withdrawal of steroids to allow recovery of the HPA axis.

There may be a delay of several months after stopping corticosteroid or corticotrophin treatment before the atrophic adrenal glands respond normally to stress. Both the dose and duration of therapy modulate the process. The recovery takes the following course:

1. The suppressed plasma level of ACTH returns to normal.
2. The circadian variation in ACTH level is resumed, with higher levels in the early morning and lower levels at midnight.
3. The plasma cortisol concentrations return to normal and show a circadian rhythm.
4. The HPA system then responds normally to a neurogenic stimulus, such as insulin-induced hypoglycaemia.

(f) *Prevention of adrenocortical insufficiency*

Patients on steroids will require an increased dose to cover stress or a surgical operation. Minor procedures can be covered by doubling the daily dose, but larger doses will be required for major surgery. Patients who have been off treatment for 12 months usually respond normally to stress. When possible, an insulin tolerance test should be carried out to assess the responsiveness of the HPA axis.

Patients who have been off steroids for over a year should be watched during the operative and postoperative period, and, if hypotension develops, should receive 200 mg hydrocortisone sodium succinate intravenously, followed by intramuscular and then oral hydrocortisone, beginning with 100–150 mg daily. Those patients requiring cover for surgery should receive 100–200 mg hydrocortisone sodium succinate by intramuscular injection with the premedication and then 50–100 mg six hourly until the patient is able to take prednisone orally. A major operation normally stimulates the adrenal cortex to secrete 200–400 mg cortisol, and it is safer to give too much cover than too little.

(g) *Replacement steroid therapy*

Patients should carry a steroid card and should double their dose if there should be fever over 38 °C, intermittent infection or an accident. In the event of vomiting they should receive their cortisol parenterally.

If these precautions are not taken the patient may require treatment for acute adrenal insufficiency. The shocked patient requires circulatory support, and normal saline should be given initially at a rate of 1 litre for the first hour and then according to the patient's condition. Blood should be taken for glucose infusion. Cortisol hemisuccinate should be given intravenously. After an initial 100 mg, 200 mg of cortisol should be given over 24 hours. Cortisol, 100 mg, should then be given in divided doses orally or intramuscularly over the next two days.

There should be obvious improvement, especially in the blood pressure, within 4–6 h if the correct diagnosis has been made. The underlying cause, such as septicaemia, must of course be treated.

16.2.9   Thyroid disease

Drugs used in the treatment of rheumatic diseases may alter thyroid function tests e.g. fenclofenac, leading to a mistaken impression of thyroid dysfunction. Salicylates, for example, decrease the binding capacity of thyroid binding globulin. Steroids reduce the level of thyroid-binding globulin and also affect reverse T_3 levels.

Conversely, drugs used in treatment of thyroid disease have been reported to cause rheumatological conditions. Amrhein *et al.* (1970) studied 38 patients aged between 2 and 18 years under treatment with propylthiouracil for hyperthyroidism. One boy developed an SLE-like syndrome with positive antinuclear factor, which responded to treatment with steroids. Other similar cases with propylthiouracil have been reported, and thionamides have led to symptoms suggesting both rheumatoid arthritis and SLE (Librik *et al.*, 1970).

16.2.10   Antirheumatic drugs and pregnancy

There are divergent views concerning the mortality and teratogenicity risk to the fetus from corticosteroid therapy taken during pregnancy. Hart (1978) has reviewed this subject and his general policy is echoed by the one supported here – continue corticosteroids in pregnancy in patients who need it – ensuring, as in general with this drug, that the minimal effective dose is given. Prednisolone is excreted in very small amounts in breast milk, and appears to be of no consequence to the nursing infant. The natural amelioration of rheumatic symptoms during pregnancy may enable some reduction in steroid dosage, but clinicians should be alert to the symptomatic 'rebound' in the puerperium when the steroid dose may have to be increased to or slightly above the usual maintenance level.

16.2.11   Iatrogenic eye disease

A number of drugs used for the treatment of the rheumatic diseases can themselves cause eye lesions. Drugs shown to cause ocular damage include mepacrine (Dame, 1946), allopurinol (Pinnas, 1968; Laval, 1968), indometha-cin (Burns, 1968) and ibuprofen (Collum and Bowen, 1971). These complications may be insidious and the consequences far reaching.

(a) Corticosteroids

(i) Infection

Local steroids may suppress the reaction of the eye to infection, and they should never be given until an accurate diagnosis has been made. In particular, patients with dry eyes are prone to infection of the conjunctiva and cornea because of the destruction of the normal lysosome content of the tears in Sjøgren's syndrome. Infections in these patients must always be taken very seriously, and no intra-ocular surgery undertaken without antibiotic cover. Single-dose containers or often replaced dropper bottles must be used by these patients because dirty drops can be a source of infection.

(ii) Cataract

Cataracts complicate corticosteroid therapy and are more likely to occur if high doses over prolonged periods have been given. Steroid cataract is most commonly produced by local therapy because of the high concentration given locally to the eye. If the steroid is given systemically, cataract is unlikely with doses of less than 10 mg prednisone daily; however, 5% of patients developed steroid cataracts when treated with 10–15 mg prednisolone for 2–8 years, and 20% suffered this complication when treated with more than 15 mg for the same period (Williamson et al., 1969). Children are particularly susceptible to this complication.

Steroid-induced cataract is almost always bilateral and occupies the polar region of the posterior cortex. It has sharply defined edges and, because of its position near the nodal points of the eye, causes early visual impairment. It can be differentiated from senile cataracts, which start peripherally, have diffuse edges, and do not cause early interference with vision. Regular slitlamp examination should be undertaken in all patients on long-term high steroid doses, especially children. A typical steroid cataract is shown in Fig. 16.5.

The opacities may be graded according to their severity from I to IV (Crews, 1963). However, visual symptoms are minimal up to Grade III. Cessation of therapy, except in grade IV, results in clear lens fibres being laid down around the opacities (Williamson et al., 1969), but the opacities will continue to increase if steroid therapy is continued. Cataract extraction is no more hazardous than usual.

Exudative macular lesions have been described after corticotrophin therapy, and a non-specific conjunctivitis has been observed after sudden withdrawal of steroids.

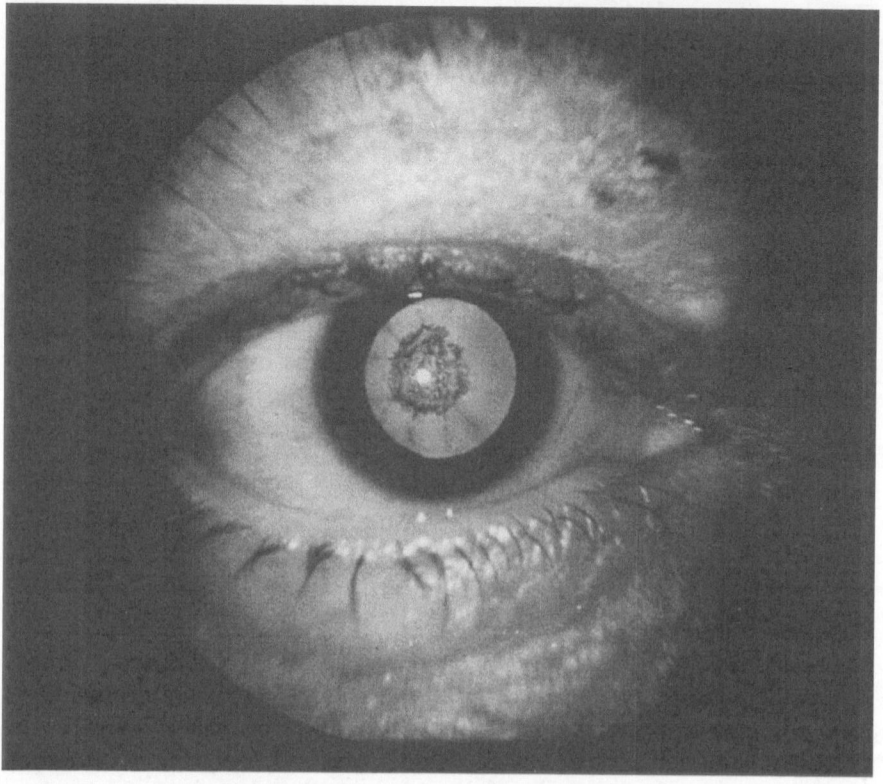

Figure 16.5 Cataract from steroid therapy.

(iii) Glaucoma

Glaucoma may develop with local or systemic steroid therapy. If drops are used, 30% of patients show a rise in intra-ocular pressure after a few weeks. It occurs less commonly with systemic therapy and takes months to develop. Patients are usually receiving very large doses, in the range of 40 mg of pred-nisolone a day (Williamson *et al.*, 1969). It is thought that the rate of aqueous humour formation is increased, and drainage is impaired as a result of alter-ation in the collagen fibres of the trabecular meshwork. It is probably also commoner in people with an hereditary tendency to primary open-angle glau-coma and in myopes (Armally, 1966). Although it may resemble acute angle-closure glaucoma, with pain, red eye and blurring of vision from corneal oedema, the acute onset is uncommon and pain is not usually a feature, nor is the eye red. The raised intra-ocular pressure results in cupping of the optic disc and insidious loss of visual field, which contracts slowly until only a tubular visual field is left. A further feature of steroid-induced glaucoma is that it is unusually resistant to conventional glaucoma treatment. Most intra-ocular pressures return to baseline levels within 10 days after cessation of therapy, although some patients may have persistent glaucoma.

All patients given corticosteroid therapy should have their intra-ocular pressures checked periodically.

(b) *Chloroquine and hydroxychloroquine*

About 4% of patients treated with these drugs develop disturbance of vision. In one series 16% had retinopathy, although the frequency of severely affected vision is less (Nylander, 1967). Although reversible in its early asymptomatic phase, it becomes irreversible once it is severe enough to cause symptoms. Once established, the retinopathy often progresses, even if medication is discontinued, and may progress to blindness (Okum *et al.*, 1963).

The earliest detectable sign is a pigmentary mottling of the macular (Henkind and Rothfield, 1963), which is not easy to detect and regresses if therapy ceases. If the drug is continued it concentrates in the pigment epithelium of the retina, which degenerates particularly around the fovea. The fovea loses its reflex, the area around this becomes depigmented and this is surrounded

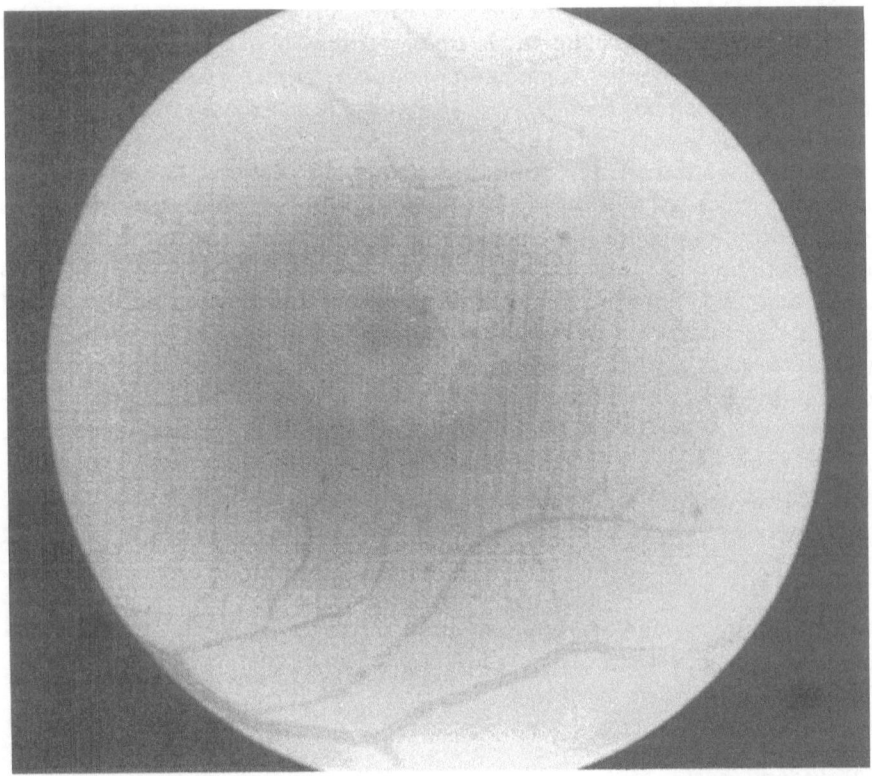

Figure 16.6 Bull's-eye macula due to chloroquine therapy.

peripherally by a hyperpigmented region, the classical 'bull's-eye' macula (Fig. 16.6). This change is highly characteristic, if not pathognomic, of over-dosage of chloroquine, and is not reversible.

The earliest detectable changes are in the electroretinogram in which the 'A' wave is enlarged and the 'B' wave reduced. At one time extra-oculography (EOG) was thought to be a reliable method for the early detection of chloroquine retinopathy (Copeman *et al.*, 1964). However, retinopathy may co-exist with apparently normal EOGs in some patients (Henkind *et al.*, 1964), and marked variations in EOG readings can occur in normal subjects (Kelsey, 1967).

A battery of tests is now employed, but no single screening test for retinal toxicity is adequate. Examination of the paracentral visual fields using low intensity red targets shows reduced sensitivity in the 'bull's-eye' type of retinopathy (Percival and Berkman, 1969) and peripheral constriction in the generalized retinal pigmentary disturbance. Later, the central visual acuity begins to fail. Sometimes blurring of vision or haloes around lights may be seen very shortly after the start of treatment because of deposition of chloroquine in the cornea. These symptoms disappear if the drug is withdrawn. Other complications include bleaching of the eyelashes, decreased corneal sensitivity, increased sensitivity to light, and extra-ocular muscle palsies.

While there are reports of patients developing significant chloroquine retinopathy after taking less than 100 g (Bernstein, 1976), most affected individuals have received a total dose of 400 g or more. Although most reports on retinopathy concern chloroquine phosphate, this may be due to the high dosage at which it has been used. Mepacrine is probably not retinotoxic. Rynes *et al.* (1979) have studied the ocular safety of hydroxychloroquine in a daily dose of 400 mg in 79 patients who had taken a medium dose of 365 g – no significant loss of vision was recorded. Marks and Power (1979) reached similar conclusions about the safety of chloroquine phosphate but felt that toxicity was dose-related, particularly in the older patient. It follows that if a critical threshold daily dose could be established, below which retinal accumulation of the drug did not occur, then the necessity for screening would cease. Alternatively, if toxicity is determined by total dose, then screening should be directed towards those individuals who had consumed the highest total dose.

(c) *Aspirin*

Ocular complications are unusual. Rare instances of allergic keratitis and conjunctivitis may occur and overdose may cause temporary blindness (Grant, 1962).

(d) *Indomethacin*

There are several recorded complications – corneal deposits, blurred vision, constricted visual fields, night blindness, and pigment changes in the fundus. Most disappeared on withdrawal of the drug (Burns, 1968; Henkes *et al.*, 1972).

(e) *Phenylbutazone*

Phenylbutazone occasionally causes blurred vision (Woodbury, 1965), retinal haemorrhages, and peripheral stromal corneal vascularization (Walsh and Hoyt, 1969).

(f) *Ibuprofen*

Centrocaecal field defects have been reported in 3 of 38 patients receiving this drug in all of whom vision improved after withdrawal (Collum and Bowen, 1971).

(g) *Gold*

A generalized gold reaction may include blepharitis and conjunctivitis, and rarely keratitis, corneal ulcers and iritis (Goldstein, 1971). These settle gradually after stopping therapy. If more than 2 g of gold salts are given, chrysiasis (corneal deposition of gold) may occur.

It is important to be aware of the ocular complications of rheumatoid arthritis because many are potentially blinding, particularly in children with juvenile chronic polyarthritis, who can lose their vision from virtually asymptomatic, progressive anterior uveitis.

16.3 DRUGS CAUSING RHEUMATIC DISEASES

16.3.1 Myalgia and cramps

Severe and widespread myalgia and joint pains may occur on steroid withdrawal in patients who have been taking daily doses of corticosteroids equivalent to at least 10 mg of prednisone for at least 30 days. Kriegel and Muller (1972) described patients with features that resembled systemic lupus erythematosus, and it is possible that the disease became unmasked when steroid therapy was withdrawn. However, a more benign condition is common on steroid withdrawal and is best managed by re-introducing steroids and withdrawing them by small amounts (1 mg) over several days or weeks, depending on the severity of symptoms. Rest and analgesia may be required as well. Conversely, arthralgia and arthritis can be a rare adverse side effect of steroid therapy (Bennet and Strong, 1975).

Severe muscle pain often follows the use of the muscle-relaxant suxamethonium. It is commoner in adults and in women, and less common in pregnant women. Various suggestions for these differences include better muscular fitness in men, the time between surgery and resumption of activity, position during surgery, and the increased concentration of progesterone in the tissue during pregnancy (Leatherdale *et al.*, 1959). Less severe myalgia, sometimes accompanied by muscle cramps, has occurred with a number of other drugs including clofibrate and penicillamine, and, in addition, muscle twitching has been reported with the β_2 adrenoceptor stimulant, terbutaline. Some hypotensive drugs, particularly guanethidine, can cause unpleasant aching in the legs, and severe discomfort in the back, buttocks and calves can occur as a rare adverse reaction to digitalis glycosides.

In drug-induced deficiency of sodium, magnesium and potassium, muscle pains and cramps may be early symptoms. Slight muscle aching in women on the contraceptive pill may be due to fluid retention, and several other drugs can cause myalgia in this way. The contraceptive pill can also cause myalgia, arthralgia and swelling affecting only the hands (Spiera and Plotz, 1969), and, less commonly, aching of the calves whilst walking may occur.

Myalgia and muscle cramps may be an early symptom of drug-induced polyneuropathy, myopathy, or disorders of the extrapyramidal system, but it is usually overshadowed by other features of these conditions. The same is true of the aching in the legs produced by retroperitoneal fibrosis occurring as a complication of methysergide therapy.

Drug-induced weakness of the proximal limb muscles is well described by Lane and Mastalgia (1978), and the symptoms are usually of gradual onset. Corticosteroids produce myopathy by an unknown mechanism. Electromyography shows a myopathic pattern, and discontinuation of the steroid results in clinical improvement.

Chloroquine causes a neuromyopathy affecting the lower limbs more severely, and usually in patients taking 500 mg or more daily. Improvement is slow after withdrawal of the drug (Whisnant *et al.*, 1963). Penicillamine may cause myasthenia which requires the appropriate treatment. Penicillamine should be discontinued, but the syndrome does not invariably resolve when the drug is withdrawn. There is a significant increase in the titre of circulating antibodies to acetylcholine receptor.

16.3.2 Drug-induced arthralgia and arthritis

Mild arthralgia and arthritis may accompany almost any type of generalized drug-induced skin eruption. More severe joint pain and swelling occurs in 'serum sickness' induced by drugs. Drug-induced systemic lupus is discussed separately.

Acute vasculitis, predominantly affecting small vessels, may be caused by drugs, particularly penicillamine, sulphonamides and thiouracils. Histological changes vary from mild cellular infiltration to acute necrosis. Prolonged administration of these drugs and others may produce chronic vasculitis. Rose and Spencer (1957) doubted the aetiological relationship of drugs to polyarteritis nodosa. It is also unlikely that a short period of drug administration produces a vasculitis that continues months after the drug has been withdrawn. However, it is possible that acute vasculitis may become a chronic condition due to a self-perpetuating mechanism.

The treatment of anaemia in rheumatoid arthritis with iron–dextran (Imferon) as a total dose infusion may cause an acute exacerbation of the disease and an arthralgia in patients without arthritis.

Levamisole has produced an acute synovitis when used in the treatment of Crohn's disease and Behçet's syndrome.

16.3.3 Shoulder–hand syndrome

This was first described as a complication of treatment with phenobarbitone (Maillard and Renard, 1925). It is not clear how phenobarbitone produces these changes. The drug had been given in daily doses between 100 and 300 mg for a few weeks to up to 20 years. In most patients the condition was bilateral, and there were acute symptoms of burning pain, oedematous swelling, and decreased sweating, followed after 3–9 months by dystrophic changes in the hand and contractures of the fingers (Van der Korst *et al.*, 1960).

Kriegel and Müller (1972) describe the shoulder–hand syndrome as a side effect of antituberculous therapy, isoniazid seeming to be the main drug responsible. Ethionamide has been suspected as a cause or a contributory factor, but the available evidence does not allow any firm conclusion.

The mechanism by which isoniazid produces symptoms is unclear. It has been suggested that as isoniazid interferes with serotinin metabolism an excess of this substance may induce fibrosis. The symptoms suddenly develop and consist of pain, tenderness, and stiffness in the finger joints and shoulder, together with widespread myalgia and arthralgia. The symptoms are commonest in men between 40 and 50 years of age. When the pain subsides it leaves restricted movement of the shoulder, flexion deformity of the elbow, and tendon contractures of the hand. The lower limb may also be involved.

The frequency of the syndrome falls when the daily dosage is reduced from 600 mg to 300 mg. Affected patients should therefore be treated by reducing the daily dose to this level. The cause of this condition has not been clearly determined and its treatment remains empirical. Intensive physical therapy, sympathetic blockade, or systemic corticosteroids have been recommended as therapy but the assessment of the results is difficult since partial or complete remission of the condition may occur spontaneously.

16.3.4   Aseptic (avascular, ischaemic) necrosis

Aseptic necrosis is associated with corticosteroid therapy, with trauma, or very rarely after arteriography or radiotherapy. It occurs particularly in rheumatoid arthritis and systemic lupus erythematosus. Of 95 patients with corticosteroid-induced aseptic necrosis of bone, 91 had involvement of the femoral head, 16 of the humeral head, 18 of the distal femur or proximal tibia, 6 of the talus, and 3 of the capitulum. In this series the risk of developing bone involvement correlated with the total steroid dosage (Cruess, 1977). The pain may be intermittent at onset, but it later becomes constant and may markedly limit the patient's activities.

The most characteristic features are seen on radiography. The initial finding is an apparent increase in the density of the affected area; this presumably arises because of hyperaemia of bone next to the lesion (Bohr and Heerfordt, 1977). Subsequently, there is a subchondral fracture with a radiolucent line. At the time of the first symptoms, radiographic features may be absent, and a bone scan may reveal changes at an early stage. There is initially decreased uptake of the radionuclide in the area of the joint, followed by increased uptake by the bone surrounding the necrosis.

The pathogenesis of aseptic necrosis is unclear; it has been suggested that steroids induce a vasculitis of the small vessels affecting that area of bone, or that steroids lead to a fat embolus. Large variations in steroid dosage and the use of large doses for long periods may be factors; but once evidence of aseptic necrosis appears, the ultimate outlook does not vary with steroid dosage.

The management of aseptic necrosis is far from satisfactory. During the early stages, a reduction of weight bearing and analgesia may help symptoms. However, as the disease progresses, surgery may be necessary. Recently it has been suggested that pulsed electromagnetic field therapy may be of value.

16.3.5   Fibrous tissue and drugs

Migrainous patients receiving vasoconstrictor drugs, particularly methysergide, have developed proliferation of fibrous tissue. This mainly affects retroperitoneal fibrous tissue, but fibrotic changes have also developed in mediastinum, pleura, lungs and pericardium, and myalgia can occur.

Retroperitoneal fibrosis tends to regress when methysergide should be used at the lowest effective dose, and treatment should not exceed 6 months and then should be withheld for at least 1 month. A scleroderma-like syndrome has been described in association with ethosuximide, the changes regressing after withdrawing the drug and returning after re-introducing therapy (Teoh and Can, 1975).

A clinical syndrome comprising Raynaud's phenomenon and dermal thickening occurs in men exposed to monomeric vinyl chloride during the manufacture of polyvinyl chloride. Further features such as acro-osteolysis, thrombocytopenia and liver and pulmonary abnormalities have been described. Recent studies have shown that the syndrome is a multi-system disorder, and immunological abnormalities have been revealed in some cases paralleling the clinical severity (Ward *et al.*, 1976).

16.3.6 Drug-induced lupus

This is rare, possibly ten times less common than systemic lupus erythematosus. Many drugs can produce the condition. Some require prolonged ingestion before SLE develops, whereas others may trigger the disease after a brief period.

(a) *Drugs implicated in drug-induced LE*

> *Frequent*
> Hydralazine
> Procainamide
> Isoniazid
> Chlorpromazine
> Anticonvulsants (phenytoin, hydantoins, primidone)
> Oral contraceptives (may exacerbate pre-existing SLE)
> *Less frequent*
> D-Penicillamine
> L-Dopa
> Methyldopa
> Aminosalycilic acid
> Methylthiouracil
> Quinidine
> Reserpine
> Penicillin and sulphonamides

The disease appears to be dose related to the drugs that often cause lupus and may be the result of an allergic mechanism in the second group. The frequency of a positive antinuclear antibody (ANA) is higher with the first group, being several times greater than the frequency of clinical lupus.

The clinical features resemble those of SLE, but important differences exist between the two forms of SLE, including differences in age, race, sex, organ involvement, and antibody specificity.

The main features are:

1. Resolves on withdrawing drugs.
2. Renal and central nervous system involvement rare; rash uncommon.
3. Polyarthritis, polyserositis, pulmonary infiltrates, rash, lymphadenopathy.
4. Hypergammaglobulinaemia, leucopenia, positive ANA but DNA antibodies negative, complement normal.

While blacks account for 30% of the cases of idiopathic SLE, few blacks develop drug-induced lupus. Idiopathic SLE is a disease of the young, with a mean age of onset of 29 years. Drug-induced lupus occurs in an older age group, 50–60 years.

DNA antibodies are usually absent, or present in low titre, and the ANA does not appear to be complement fixing, which may explain the low frequency of renal involvement. It is thought that drugs act as haptens, leading to the disease in genetically predisposed individuals. Slow acetylators of a particular drug are more likely to develop the syndrome. The disease usually improves on discontinuing the drug, but may persist for years, or become irreversible in a few patients. In these patients the drug may merely unveil latent disease.

Hughes *et al* (1981) reported hydralazine-induced lupus in about 5–10% of patients on mean daily doses of less than 150 mg. The frequency of the lupus syndrome is greater in women, in slow acetylators, and in people of the HLA type DR4. Positive antinuclear antibody tests far outnumber clinical side effects. A rising antinuclear antibody titre provides an 'early warning', but is not necessarily a reason for withdrawing the drug in the absence of symptoms.

A positive antinuclear antibody develops in about 25% of patients treated with isoniazid. Unlike that of procainamide and hydralazine, the acetylation of isoniazid appears to play no role in the development of antinuclear antibodies.

The molecular structure of certain drugs is sufficiently similar to that of purine bases to suggest a possible role of cross-reactivity in the induction of antibodies to DNA. Several drugs also have the capacity to interact with nuclear antigens, and several lupus-inducing drugs may impair immune function by interacting with lymphocytes or by eliciting antilymphocyte antibodies, or both.

Hydralazine, procainamide, isoniazid, and anticonvulsants should be used with great caution in patients with SLE. Although these drugs are to be avoided if possible, patients have been treated with these agents without undergoing clinical exacerbation of the disease (Reza *et al.*, 1975).

(b) *Management*

In all patients with manifestations of SLE, it is wise to discontinue any drugs that the patient was taking at the time of onset of the first symptoms of the disease. Once the drug has been withdrawn the patient should be followed carefully. If clinical symptoms do not improve or are severe, corticosteroids should be given. In general, the decision to treat or to await spontaneous resolution of the symptoms depends on the severity of the illness and whether the patient is at home or in hospital. The continued presence of antinuclear antibodies in the serum after the clinical manifestations have disappeared should be expected, and treatment should not be given for presence or persistence of antinuclear antibodies in the absence of clinical disease.

16.3.7   Contraceptive pill

A syndrome of persistent arthralgias, myalgias, and morning stiffness, with occasional development of polyarticular synovitis, has been described in women in the third decade of life taking oral contraceptives (Bole *et al.*, 1969). Positive tests for antinuclear antibodies are common, and several patients have circulating rheumatoid factor. Symptoms resolve after the medication is discontinued. The contraceptive pill can also cause myalgia, arthralgia, and swelling of the hands (Spiera and Plotz, 1969), and discomfort of the calves has been described. These earlier reports have largely been discounted, and some work implies that oral contraceptives are beneficial. It has also been suggested that oral contraceptives were protective against the development of rheumatoid arthritis (Wingrave and Kay, 1978).

16.4   REFERENCES

Amrhein, J. A., Kenny, F. M. and Ross, D. (1970) Granulocytopenia, lupus-like syndrome and other complications of propylthiouracil therapy. *J. Paediatr.*, 76, 54–63.

Armally, M. F. (1966) Heritable nature of dexamethasone-induced ocular hypotension. *Arch. Ophthalmol.*, 75, 32–5.

Bacon, P. A., Tribe, C. R., Mackenzie, J. C., Verrier-Jones, J., Cumming, R. H. and Amer, B. (1976) Penicillamine nephropathy in rheumatoid arthritis. *Q. J. Med.*, 45, 661–84.

Barker, J. D., De Carle, D. J. and Anuras, S. (1977) Chronic excessive acetaminophen use and liver damage. *Ann. Intern. Med.*, 87, 299.

Batchelor, J. R., Welsh, K. I., Tinoco, R. M., Dollery, C. T., Hughes, G. R. V., Bernstein, R., Ryan, P., Naish, P. F., Ager, G. M., Burry, R. F. and Russell, G. I. (1980) Hydralazine-induced systemic lupus erythematosus: influence of HLA-DR and sex in susceptibility. *Lancet*, i, 1107–9.

Bennet, W. M. and Strong, D. (1975) Arthralgia after high-dose steroids. *Lancet*, i, 1332.

Bernstein, M. (1976) Chloroquine ocular toxicity. *Surv. Ophthalmol.*, 12, 415–18.

Bohr, H. and Heerfordt, J. (1977) Autoradiography and histology in a case of idiopathic femoral head necrosis. *Clin. Orthopaed. Rel. Res.*, 129, 209–12.

Bole, G. G., Friedlaender, M. H. and Smith, C. K. (1969) Rheumatic symptoms and serological abnormalities induced by oral contraceptives. *Lancet*, i, 323.

Burns, C. A. (1968) Indomethacin, reduced retinal sensitivity and corneal deposits. *Am. J. Ophthalmol.*, 66, 825–35.

Burry, A. F. (1965) The evolution of analgesic nephropathy. *Nephron*, 5, 185–201.

Burry, A. F., Axelsen, R. A. and Trolove, P. (1974) Analgesic nephropathy: its present contribution to the renal mortality and morbidity profile. *Med. J. Aust.*, 1, 31–6.

Burry, H. C., Dieppe, P. A., Bresnihan, F. B. and Brown, C. B. (1976) Salicylates and renal function in rheumatoid arthritis. *Br. Med. J.*, 1, 613–15.

Collum, L. M. T. and Bowen, D. I. (1971) Ocular side-effects of ibuprofen. *Br. J. Ophthalmol.*, 55, 472.

Copeman, P. W., Cowell, T. K. and Dallas, N. L. (1964) Screening test for chloroquine retinopathy. *Lancet*, i, 1369.

Cove-Smith, J. R. and Knapp, M. S. (1978) Analgesic nephropathy: an important cause of chronic renal failure. *Q. J. Med.*, **47**, 49–69.

Crews, S. J. (1963) Posterior subscapular lens opacities in patients on long-term corticosteroid therapy. *Br. Med. J.*, **1**, 1644.

Cruess, R. L. (1977) Cortisone-induced avascular necrosis of the femoral head. *J. Bone Jt Surg.*, **59B**, 308.

Dame, L. R. (1946) The effects of atebrine on the human visual system. *Am. J. Ophthalmol.*, **29**, 1432.

Eastmond, C. J. (1976) Diffuse alveolitis as a complication of penicillamine treatment for rheumatoid arthritis. *Br. Med. J.*, **1**, 1506.

Edwards, O. M., Edwards, P., Huskisson, E. C. and Taylor, R. T. (1971) Paracetamol and renal damage. *Br. Med. J.*, **2**, 87–9.

Ferguson, I. (1974) How safe are analgesics? The Queensland experience. *Aust. N. Z. J. Med.*, **4**, 603.

Fucik, R. F., Kukreya, S. C., Hargis, G. K., Bowsher, E. N., Henderson, W. J. and Williams, G. A. (1975) Effect of glucocorticoids on function of the parathyroid glands in man. *J. Clin. Endocrinol. Metab.*, **40**, 152–5.

Gallagher, J. C., Aaron, J., Horsman, A., Wilkinson, R. and Nordin, B. E. C. (1973) Corticosteroid osteoporosis. *Clinics Endocrinol. Metab.*, **2**, 355–68.

Goldstein, J. H. (1971) Effects of drugs on cornea, conjunctiva and lids. *Int. Ophthalmol. Clinics*, **11**, 13.

Gould, P. W., McCormack, P. L. and Palmer, D. G. (1977) Pulmonary damage associated with sodium aurothiomalate therapy. *J. Rheumatol.*, **4**, 252.

Grant, W. M. (1962) *Toxicology of the Eye*. Thomas, Springfield.

Hahn, T. J., Halstead, L. R., Teitelbaum, S. L. and Hahn, B. H. (1979) Altered mineral metabolism in glucocorticoid-induced osteopenia. *J. Clin. Invest.*, **64**, 655–65.

Hare, W. S. C. and Poynter, J. D. (1973) The radiology of renal papillary necrosis as seen in analgesic nephropathy. *Clin. Radiol.*, **25**, 423–43.

Hart, F. D. (ed) (1978) *Drug Treatment of the Rheumatic Diseases*, MTP Press, Lancaster.

Harvard, C. W. H. (1965) Corticosteroid therapy, in *Fundamentals of Current Medical Treatment* (ed C. W. H. Harvard), Staples Press, London.

Henkes, H. E., Van Lith, G. H. M. and Canta, L. R. (1972) Indomethacin retinopathy. *Am. J. Ophthalmol.*, **73**, 846.

Henkind, P., Carr, R. and Siegel, I. E. (1964) Early chloroquine retinopathy (American Medical Association). *Arch. Ophthalmol.*, **71**, 157–65.

Henkind, P. and Rothfield, N. F. (1963) Ocular abnormalities in patients treated with synthetic anti-malarial drugs. *N. Engl. J. Med.*, **269**, 433.

Hickson, R. C. and Davis, J. R. (1981) Partial prevention of glucocorticoid-induced muscle atrophy by endurance training. *Am. J. Physiol.*, **241E**, 226–32.

Hughes, G. R. V., Rynes, R. I., Gharain, A., Ryan, P. F. J., Sewell, J. and Mansilla, R. (1981) The heterogeneity of serological findings and predisposing factors in drug-induced lupus erythematosus. *Arthr. Rheum.*, **24**, 1071–3.

Huskisson, E. C. (1979) Renal diseases and penicillamine. *Eur. J. Rheumatol. Inflamm.*, **3**, 156–9.

Jee, W. S. S., Park, H. Z., Roberts, W. E. and Kenmer, G. H. (1970) Corticosteroid and bone. *Am. J. Anat.*, **129**, 477–9.

Kelsey, J. H. (1967) Variations in the normal electro-oculogram. *Br. J. Ophthalmol.*, **51**, 44–9.

Klouda, P. T., Manos, J., Acheson, E. J., Dyer, P. A., Golby, F. S., Harris, R., Lawler, W., Mallick, N. P. and Williams, G. (1979) Strong association between idiopathic membranous nephropathy and HLA–DRW8. *Lancet*, **ii**, 770–1.

Kreigel, W. and Müller, W. (1972) Drug-induced diseases of the bones, joints and connective tissue, in *Drug-induced Diseases*, Vol. 4 (eds L. Meyler and H. M. Peck) Associated Scientific Publishers, Amsterdam.

Lane, R. J. M. and Mastalgia, F. L. (1978) Drug-induced myopathies in man. *Lancet*, ii, 562.

Laval, J. (1968) Allopurinol and macular lesions. *Arch. Ophthalmol.*, 80, 415.

Leatherdale, R. A. L., Mayhew, R. A. J. and Hayton-Williams, D. S. (1959) Incidence of 'muscle pain' after short-acting relaxants; a comparison between suxamethonium chloride and suxamethonium bromide. *Br. Med. J.*, 1, 904.

Librik, L., Sussman, L., Bejar, R. and Clayton, G. W. (1970) Thyrotoxicosis and collagen-like disease in three sisters of American Indian extraction. *J. Paediatr.*, 76, 64–8.

Maillard, G. and Renard, G. (1925) Un nouveau traitment de l'epilepsie la phenolyl-methyl-malonyluree (Rutonal). *Press. Med.*, 33, 315.

Marks, J. S. and Power, B. J. (1979) Is chloroquine obsolete in treatment of rheumatic disease. *Lancet*, i, 371–3.

Mitchell, W. S. and Sturrock, R. D. (1982) Ulcers and anti-inflammatory agents. *Br. Med. J.*, 284, 731.

Mueller, M. W., Mazess, R. B. and Cameron, J. R. (1973) Corticosteroid therapy accelerated osteoporosis in rheumatoid arthritis, in *Int. Conf. Bone Mineral Measurement* (ed R. B. Mazess), US Department of Health, Education and Welfare No. 75, 685.

Murray, T. G. and Goldberg, M. (1975) Chronic interstitial nephritis: etiologic factors. *Ann. Intern. Med.*, 82, 453–9.

Nanra, R. S., Chirawong, P. and Kincaid-Smith, P. (1973) Medullary ischaemia in experimental analgesic nephropathy: the pathogenesis of renal papillary necrosis. *Aust. N. Z. Med. J.*, 3, 580–6.

Nanra, R. S., Stuart-Taylor, J., de Leon, A. H. and White, V. H. (1978) Analgesic nephropathy: etiology, clinical syndrome and clinico-pathological correlations in Australia. *Kidney Int.*, 13, 79–92.

Nelson, D. C., Birchmore, D. A. and Birchmore, D. A. (1979) Renal vein thrombosis associated with nephrotic syndrome and gold therapy in rheumatoid arthritis. *South. Med. J.*, 72, 1616–18.

New Zealand Rheumatism Study (1974) Aspirin and the kidney. *Br. Med. J.*, 1, 593–6.

Nilsen, K. H., Jayson, M. V. and Dixon, A. St. J. (1978) Microcrystalline calcium hydroxyapatite compound in corticosteroid-treated rheumatoid patients: a controlled study. *Br. Med. J.*, 12, 1124.

Nordenfelt, O. (1972) Deaths from renal failure in abusers of phenacetin-containing drugs. *Acta Med. Scand.*, 191, 11–16.

Nylander, V. (1967) Ocular damage in chloroquine therapy. *Acta Ophthalmol.*, 45 (Suppl. 92), 1.

Okum, E., Gouvas, P., Bernstein, H. and Von Sallman, L. (1963) Chloroquine retinopathy (American Medical Association). *Arch. Ophthalmol.*, 69, 59–71.

Oliver, W. J. (1970) Recent advances in paediatrics, in *The International Handbook of Medical Progress*, 2nd edn (ed R. H. Mose), Thomas, Springfield.

Percival, S. P. B. and Berkman, J. (1969) Ophthalmological safety of chloroquine. *Br. J. Ophthalmol.*, 53, 101–9.

Pinnas, G. (1968) Possible association between macular lesions and allopurinol. *Arch. Ophthalmol.*, 79, 786.

Plotz, P. H., Klippel, J. H. and Decker, J. L. (1979) Bladder complications in patients receiving cyclophosphamide for systemic lupus erythematosus or rheumatoid arthritis. *Ann. Intern. Med.*, 91, 221–3.

Prescott, L. F. (1976) Analgesic nephropathy – the international experience. *Aust. N. Z. J. Med.*, (Suppl. 1), 6, 44–8.

Rainsford, K. D. and Willis, C. (1982) Relationship of gastric mucosal damage induced in pigs by anti-inflammatory drugs to their effects on prostaglandin production. *Digest. Dis. Sci.*, 27, 624–35.

Reza, M. J., Dornfeld, L. and Goldberg, L. S. (1975) Hydralazine therapy in hypertensive patients with idiopathic systemic lupus erythematosus. *Arthr. Rheum.*, 18, 335–8.

Riggs, B. L., Jowsey, J. and Kelly, P. J. (1966) Quantitative microradiographic study of bone remodelling in Cushing's syndrome. *Metabolism*, 15, 773–80.

Rose, G. A. and Spencer, H. (1957) Polyarteritis nodosa. *Q. J. Med.*, 24, 43.

Rubin, G., Baume, P. and Vanderberg, R. (1972) Azathioprine and acute restrictive lung disease. *Aust. N. Z. J. Med.*, 2, 272.

Rynes, R. J., Krohel, G., Falbo, A., Reinecke, R. D., Wolfe, B. and Bartholomew, L. E. (1979) Ophthalmological safety of long-term hydroxychloroquine treatment. *Arthr. Rheum.*, 22, 32–6.

Saker, B. M. and Kincaid-Smith, P. (1969) Papillary necrosis in experimental analgesic nephropathy. *Br. Med. J.*, 1, 161–662.

Scheef, W., Klein, H. O. and Brock, N. (1979) Controlled clinical studies with an antidose against urotoxicity of oxazophosphamides: preliminary results. *Cancer Treat. Rep.*, 63, 501–5.

Sheagren, J. N., Jowsey, J., Bird, D. C., Gurton, M. E. and Jacobs, J. B. (1977) Effect on bone growth of daily versus alternate-day corticosteroid administration: an experimental study. *J. Lab. Clin. Med.*, 89, 120–30.

Shelley, J. H. (1978) Pharmacological mechanisms of analgesic nephropathy. *Kidney Int.*, 13, 15–26.

Silverberg, D. S., Kidd, E. G., Shnitka, T. H. and Vlan, R. A. (1970) Gold nephropathy: a clinical and pathological study. *Arthr. Rheum.*, 13, 812, 825.

Skrifvars, B. V., Tornroth, T. S. and Tallquist, G. N. (1977) Gold-induced immune complex nephritis in sero-negative rheumatoid arthritis. *Ann. Rheum. Dis.*, 36, 549–56.

Spiera, H. and Plotz, C. M. (1969) Rheumatic symptoms and oral contraceptives. *Lancet*, i, 571.

Spuhler, O. and Zollinger, H. V. (1953) Die Chronisch-interstitielle nephritis. *Z. Klin. Med.*, 151, 1–50.

Szczeklik, A. and Czerniawska-Mysik, G. (1976) Prostaglandins and aspirin-induced asthma. *Lancet*, i, 488.

Teoh, D. C. and Can, H. L. (1975) Lupus scleroderma syndrome induced by ethosuximide. *Arch. Dis. Child.*, 50, 658–61.

Van Der Korst, J. K., Colenbrauer, H. and Cats, A. (1960) Phenobarbitol and the shoulder–hand syndrome. *Ann. Rheum. Dis.*, 25, 553.

Walsh, F. B. and Hoyt, W. F. (1969) *Clinical Neuro-ophthalmology*, Williams and Wilkins, Baltimore.

Ward, A. M., Udnoon, S. and Watkins, J. (1976) Immunological mechanisms in the pathogenesis of vinyl chloride disease. *Br. Med. J.*, 1, 936–8.

Williamson, J., Paterson, R. W., McGavin, D. D., Jasani, K. K., Boyle, J. A. and Doig, W. M. (1969) Posterior subscapular cataracts and glaucoma associated with long-term corticosteroid therapy. *Br. J. Ophthalmol.*, 53, 361–72.

Wingrave, S. J. and Kay, C. R. (1978) Reduction in incidence of rheumatoid arthritis associated with oral contraceptives. *Lancet*, i, 569–71.

Whisnant, J. P., Espinosa, R. E., Kierland, R. R. and Lambert, E. H. (1963) Chloroquine neuromyopathy. *Proc. Staff Meetings Mayo Clinic*, 38, 501.

Woodbury, D. M. (1965) in *The Pharmacological Basis of Therapeutics* (eds L. S. Goodman and A. Gilman), 3rd edn, MacMillan, New York, pp. 336–9.

Wooley, P. A., Griffen, J., Panayi, G. S., Batchelor, J. R., Welsh, K. I. and Gibson, T. J. (1980) HLA-DR antigens and toxic reactions to sodium aurothiomalate and D-penicillamine in patients with rheumatoid arthritis. *N. Engl. J. Med.*, 303, 300–2.

International glossary of proprietary antirheumatic drugs*

Compiled by J. M. H. Moll

SIMPLE ANALGESIC DRUGS

(excluding powerful narcotic analgesics used for severe pain)

Paracetamol (including compound preparations)

United Kingdom

Cafadol	Paracodol
Calpol	Parahypon
Cosalgesic	Parake
Delimon	Paralgin
Distalgesic	Paramax
Femerital	Paramol
Fortagesic	Pardale
Lobak	Pharmidone
Medised	Pholcolix
Medocodene	Propain
Midrid	Rinurel
Migraleve	Safapryn
Myolgin	Safapryn-Co
Neurodyne	Salzone
Norgesic	Solpadeine
Paedo-sed	Sudafed-Co
Paldesic	Syndol
Panadeine	Triogesic
Panadol	Unigesic
Panasorb	

*Drugs selected primarily by their availability in the United Kingdom. Data largely based on Martindale: *The Extra Pharmacopoiea*, 28th edn (ed. J. E. F. Reynolds), (The Pharmaceutic Press, London, 1982) with supplementary information from BNF (*British National Formulary*, British Medical Association and The Pharmaceutical Society of Great Britain, London, 1985); *MIMS* (*Monthly Index of Medical Specialities*, Medical Publications, London, 1985–6 issues): and *ABPI Data Sheet Compendium 1985–6* (Datapharm Publications, London, 1984).

Eire

Cetamol
Ticelgesic
Tinol

Sweden

Alvedon
Panodil
Termidor

United States of America

Anuphen
Apamide
Capital
Can-Apap
Dolanex
Febrigesic
Febrogesic
Korum
Liquiprin
Lyteca

Nebs
Neopap
Phendex
Proval
SK-Apap
Tapar
Temlo
Tempra
Tylenol
Valadol

Canada

Atasol
Campain
Chemcetaphen
Pediaphen
Rounox
Tempra
Tylenol

Germany

Ben-u-ron

Australia

Ceetamol
Dolamin
Dymadon
Nevrol
Paracet

Parasin
Parmol
Placemol
Tempra

France

Doliprane

South Africa

Napamol   Tempra
Panado   Valadol
Restin Elixir

New Zealand

Pacemol

Codeine phosphate

Most proprietary preparations of codeine phosphate are in the form of compound preparations – usually with paracetamol and aspirin or other substances (antidiarrhoeals and cough mixtures excluded).

United Kingdom

Antoin (with aspirin and caffeine)
Codis (with aspirin)
Hypon (with aspirin and caffeine)
Medocodene (with paracetamol)
Myolgin (with paracetamol, aspirin and caffeine)
Neurodyne (with paracetamol)
Panadeine Co (with paracetamol)
Paracodol (with paracetamol)
Parahypon (with paracetamol and caffeine)
Parake (with paracetamol)
Paralgin (with paracetamol)
Pardale (with paracetamol and caffeine hydrate)
Pharmidone (with diphenhydramine hydrochloride, paracetamol and caffeine)
Propain (with diphenhydramine hydrochloride, paracetamol and caffeine)
Safapryn-Co (with paracetamol and aspirin)
Solpadeine (with paracetamol and caffeine)
Syndol (with paracetamol doxylamine succinate and caffeine)

Spain

Codeinfos
Codeisan
Solcodein

Australia

   Codlin

Canada

   Paveral

Germany

   Tricodein

Dextropropoxyphene (including compound preparations)

United Kingdom

   Cosalgesic (hydrochloride)
   Distalgesic (hydrochloride)
   Dolasan (napsylate)
   Doloxene (napsylate)
   Doloxene Compound (napsylate)
   Napsalgesic (napsylate)

Australia

   Algaphan

France

   Antalvic

United States of America

   Darvon
   Dolene
   Dolocap
   Mardon
   Propoxychel
   Proxagesic
   Darvon-N (napsylate)

Sweden

   Dolotard (hydrochloride)

Canada

Pro-65 (hydrochloride)
Darvon-N (napsylate)
Progesic (hydrochloride)

Ethoheptazine citrate

United Kingdom

Equagesic (with mebrobamate and aspirin)
Zactirin (with aspirin and calcium carbonate)

Italy

Panalgin

Several Countries

Ecuagesica
Zactane
Zactrin

Pentazocine

Fortagesic (with paracetamol) Fortral }	United Kingdom
Fortral {	Australia, Austria, Belgium, Denmark, France, Germany, Iceland, Netherlands
Algopent	Italy
Fortalgesic	Sweden, Switzerland
Fortralin	Finland, Norway
Fortwin	India
Leticon Pentafen Pentalgina }	Italy
Sosegon	Argentina, South Africa, Spain
Talwin	Canada, Italy, USA

Nefopam hydrochloride

Acupan {	United Kingdom, Argentina, Belgium, Switzerland
Ajan	Germany
Sinalgio	Argentina

Dihydrocodeine

DF118
Paramol (with paracetamol)   } United Kingdom

Bicodein
Paracodina   } Spain

Paracodin   { Australia, Germany, South Africa,
                Switzerland

Remedacen   Germany

Rikodeine
Tuscodin   } Australia
Fortuss

ANALGESIC/ANTI-INFLAMMATORY DRUGS

Aspirin (including its salts and complexes)

Antoin
Aspav
Aspellin
Breoprin
Caprin
Claradin
Codis
Dolasan
Doloxene Compound
Equagesic
Hypon
Laboprin
Levius   } United Kingdom
Migravess
Myolgin
Napsalgesic
Nu-Seals aspirin
Paynocil
Robaxisal forte
Safapryn
Safapryn-Co
Solprin
Trancoprin
Zactirin

Other proprietary names of aspirin, its salts and its complexes

AAS
Adiro
Aspirinetas
Bayaspirina   } Argentina
Enteretas
Rhonal

Bi-prin
Codral Junior
Ecotrin
Elsprin
Novosprin
Prodol
Provoprin   } Australia
Rhusal
Sedalgin
Solusal
SRA
Winsprin

Acenterine
Adiro
Aspegic (lysine acetylsalicylate)
Dispril
Dolean pH 8
Enterosarin   } Belgium
Primaspan
Rhodine
Rhonal
Soparine

Acetophen
Asadrine C-200
Astrin
Coryphen
Ecotrin
Entrophen
Neopirine-25
Nova-Phase   } Canada
Novasen
Rhonal
Sal-Adult
Sal-Infant
Supasa
Triaphen-10

Acetard
Albyl
Albyl-Selters
Globentyl
Idotyl　　　　　　　　} Denmark
Kalcatyl
Magnyl
Reumyl
Aspegic (lysine acetylsalicylate)
Aspirisucre
Aspisol (lysine acetylsalicylate)
Catalgine
Claragine　　　　　　} France
Ivepirine
Juvepirine
Rhonal
Acetylin
Colfarit
Contrheuma retard
Delgesic (lysine acetylsalicylate)
Godamed
Halgon　　　　　　　} Germany
Monobeltin (with aluminium
　　salicylate)
Pyracyl (magnesium
　　acetylsalicylate)
Trineral 600
Istopirine　　　　　　　Hungary
Asatard
Aspegic (lysine acetylsalicylate)
Cemirit
Dolean pH 8
Domupirina　　　　　} Italy
Endydol
Flectadol (lysine acetylsalicylate)
Kilios
Longasa
Rectosalyl
Rhonal　　　　　　　} Japan
Salitison

Acenterine ⎫
Acetyl   ⎪
Adiro   ⎪
Aspegic (lysine acetylsalicylate) ⎬ Netherlands
Chefarine-N ⎪
Enterosarine ⎪
Rhonal   ⎭

Albyl   ⎫
Dispril   ⎪
Globentyl ⎬ Norway
Licyl   ⎪
Magnyl   ⎪
Novid   ⎭

Aquaprin ⎫
Aspasol   ⎬ South Africa
Aspegic (lysine acetylsalicylate) ⎭

AAS   ⎫
Adiro   ⎪
Calmo Yer Analgesico   ⎪
Casprium Retard   ⎪
Codalgina Retard   ⎪
Dolmega (lysine acetylsalicylate) ⎬ Spain
Lafena   ⎪
Mejoral Infantil   ⎪
Rhonal   ⎪
Riane (arginine acetylsalicylate) ⎪
Salicilina   ⎪
Solusprin (lysine acetylsalicylate) ⎭

Acetard   ⎫
Albyl   ⎪
Albyl-Selters ⎪
Apernyl   ⎪
Bamyl S   ⎬ Sweden
Dispril   ⎪
Magnecyl   ⎪
Premaspin   ⎪
Reumyl   ⎭

Acenterine	Switzerland
Acetylo	Switzerland
Aspegic (lysine acetylsalicylate)	Switzerland
Asrivo	Switzerland
Bebesan	Switzerland
Dispril	Switzerland
Dolean pH 8	Switzerland
Enterosarine	Switzerland
Rhonal	Switzerland
Aluprin	USA
Ecotrin	USA
Empirin	USA

Newer salicylate preparations

Benorlylate

Benoral	United Kingdom
Benoral	Australia
Benortan	Belgium, Denmark, Finland, France, Germany, Iceland, Netherlands, Switzerland
Benotamol	Argentina
Salipran	France
Winolate	South Africa

Salsalate

Disalcid	United Kingdom
Disalcid	USA
Arcylate	USA
Nobegl	Denmark

Choline magnesium trisalicylate

Trilisate	United Kingdom
Trilisate	USA

Diflunisal

Dolobid	United Kingdom
Dolobid	Australia, Italy
Dolisal	Peru
Donobid	Costa Rica, Denmark, Finland
Dopanone	Greece
Dorbid	Brazil
Unisal	Switzerland

Sulindac

Clinoril	United Kingdom, Argentina, Australia, Belgium, Canada, Denmark, Italy, Netherlands, South Africa, Switzerland, USA
Arthrocine	France
Artribid	Portugal
Citireuma	Italy
Imbaral	Germany

Indomethacin

Artracin	
Imbrilon	
Indocid	
Indocid R	
Indoflex	United Kingdom
Indolar	
Indomod	
Mobilan	
Indocid	Argentina, Australia, Belgium, Canada, Denmark, France, Italy, Netherlands, Norway, South Africa, Switzerland, USA
Agilex	Argentina
IM-75	
Rheumacin	Australia
Infrocin	Colombia
Indren	Czechoslovakia
Confortid	Denmark
Amuno	Germany
Algometacin	
Artrobase	
Artrocid	
Boutycin	
Cidalgon	
Imet	
Indium	Italy
Liometacen (meglumine salt)	
Metacen	
Metartril	
Peralgon	
Sadoreum	

Indacia	Japan
Confortid	Norway
Arthrexin	South Africa
Artrinovo	
Artrivia	Spain
Inacid	
Confortid	
Indomee	Sweden
Confortid	Switzerland

Etodolac

Lodine	United Kingdom

Tolmetin sodium

Tolectin	United Kingdom
Tolectin	Belgium, Canada, Denmark, Germany, USA, Italy, Netherlands, South Africa, Switzerland
Tolmex	Italy

Diclofenac sodium

Voltarol	United Kingdom
Aflamin	Italy
Blesin	
Dichronic	
Neriodin	
Prophenatin	Japan
Seecoren	
Sofarin	
Tsudohmin	
Voltaren	Argentina, Belgium, Denmark, Germany, Italy, Japan, Netherlands, Spain, Switzerland
Voltarene	France

Ibuprofen

Apsifen	
Brufen	
Ebufac	
Fenbid Spansule	United Kingdom
Ibumetin	
Motrin	
Paxofen	

Emodin	Argentina
Inflam	Australia
Amersol	} Canada
Motrin	
Algofen	
Focus	} Italy
Rebugen	
Andran	
Anflagen	
Bluton	
Brufanic	
Donjust B	
Epobron	
IB-100	
Ibuprocin	
Lamidon	} Japan
Liptan	
Mynosedin	
Nagifen-D	
Napacetin	
Nobfelon	
Nobgen	
Pantrop	
Roidenin	
Inza	South Africa
Motrin	USA

Naproxen

Naprosyn	} United Kingdom
Synflex	
Naprosyn	{ Argentina, Australia, Canada, Denmark, Germany, Italy, Norway, South Africa, Spain, Sweden, Switzerland, USA
Anaprox	USA
Flanax	Brazil, Mexico
Floginax	
Gibixen	
Laser	} Italy
Leniartril	
Naixan	Japan
Naproxyne	Belgium, France, Netherlands
Proxen	Germany, Switzerland
Proxine	} Italy
Xenar	

Tiaprofenic acid

Surgam   United Kingdom, France

Fenoprofen

Fenopron   ⎫
Progesic   ⎬   United Kingdom
Fepron   Belgium, Italy, Netherlands
Feprona   Germany
Nalfon   Denmark, Spain, Switzerland, USA
Nalgesic   France

Ketoprofen

Alrheumat   ⎫
Orudis   ⎬   United Kingdom
Oruvail   ⎭
Profenid   France
Alreumun   ⎫
Anaus   ⎪
Kevadon   ⎬   Argentina
Lertus   ⎪
Profenid   ⎭
Alrhumat   ⎫
Rofenid   ⎬   Belgium
Alreumat   Denmark
Artosilene (asylsinate)
Alrheumun
                        Germany

Fastum   ⎫
Flexen   ⎪
Iso-K   ⎪
Kefenid   ⎪
Ketalgin   ⎬   Italy
Keto   ⎪
Salient   ⎪
Sinketol   ⎭
Capisten   Japan
Remauric   Spain
Alrhumat   ⎫
Profenid   ⎬   Switzerland

Flurbiprofen

Froben	United Kingdom
Froben	South Africa, Switzerland
Cebutid	France

Fenbufen

Lederfen	United Kingdom
Bufemid	Brazil
Cinopal	Italy, South Africa, Switzerland

Suprofen

Suprol	United Kingdom
Surfrex	Belgium

Flufenamic acid

Meralen	United Kingdom (recently withdrawn)
Alfenamin Parlef	} Argentina
Ansatin	Japan
Arlef	{ Australia, Belgium, France, Germany, Italy, South Africa, Switzerland
Sastridex Surika	} Germany

Mefenamic acid

Ponstan	} United Kingdom, Australia, Belgium, Canada, South Africa, Switzerland
Bafameritin-M Bonabol Pontal	} Japan
Coslan	Spain
Lysalgo Mefedolo Parke-Med	} Italy
Parkemed	Germany
Ponstil	Argentina
Ponstyl	France
Ponstel	USA

Phenylbutazone

Butazolidin Butacote	United Kingdom (restricted to hospital use for ankylosing spondylitis)
Tibutazone	Eire
Butazolidina	Argentina
Butacal Butalan Butarex Butoroid Butoz Buzon	Australia
Butazolidine Glycyl	Belgium
Algoverine Butagesic Intrabutazone Malgesic Nadozone Neo-Zoline Phenbutazone	Canada
Artrizin	Denmark
Butazolidine	France
Praecirheumin Rheumaphen Spondyril	Germany
Artropan Butartril Butazina Butazolidina Diossidone Fenilbutina (diethylaminoethyl derivative) Kadol Reumilene (aminopropyl derivative) Ticinil	Italy
Artricin	Norway
Butapirazol	Poland
Butrex Panazone	South Africa

Butadiona
Butalgina
Butazolidina
Butial (benzidamine enolate
   derivative)
Fenibutasan ⎫ Spain
Pirarreumol-P
Sintobutina (aminopropyl
   derivative)
Todalgil

Butadion
Butaphen
Dibuzon
Elmedal ⎬ Switzerland
Mepha-Butazon
Ticinil Calcio (calcium derivative)

Azolid   USA

Azapropazone

Rheumox	United Kingdom
Cinnamin	Japan
Pentosol	Spain
Prolix	South Africa
Prolixan	Belgium, Denmark, France, Germany, Hungary, Italy, Netherlands, Switzerland
Prolixana	Sweden

Feprazone

Methrazone	United Kingdom (recently withdrawn)
Zepelin	Switzerland, Italy
Analud	Argentina

Brotazona
Danfenona
Grisona
Naloven
Nilatin ⎬ Spain
Prenazon
Rangozona
Represil
Tabrien

Piroxicam

Feldene   United Kingdom

PURE ANTI-INFLAMMATORY DRUGS

Prednisolone

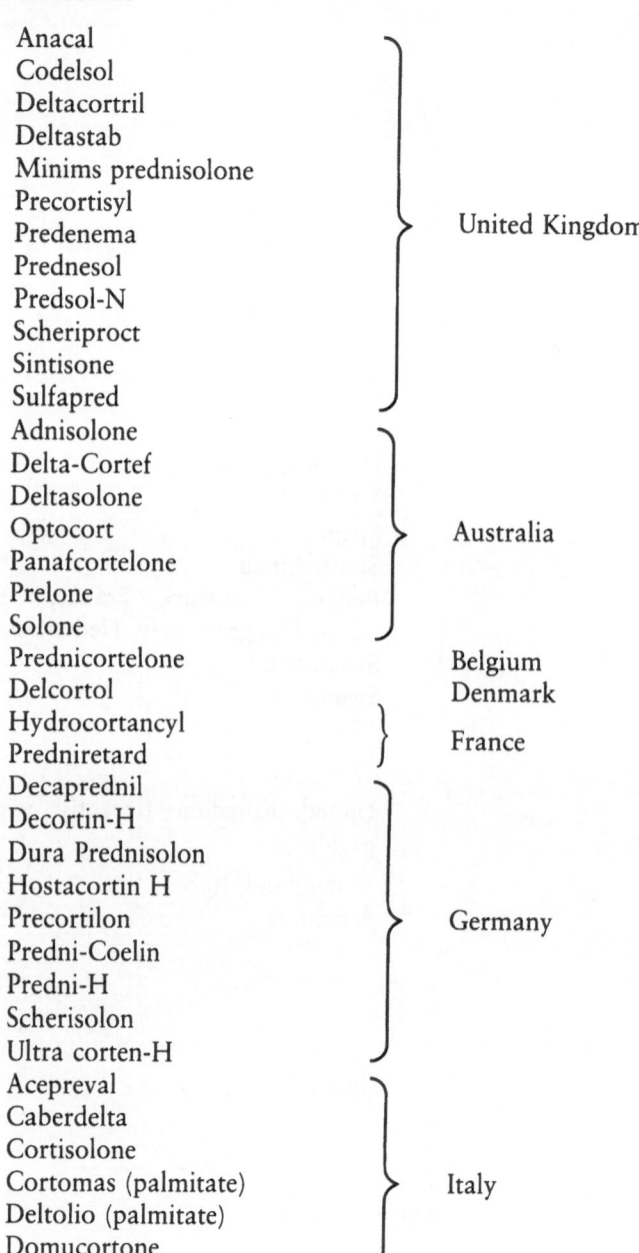

Anacal
Codelsol
Deltacortril
Deltastab
Minims prednisolone
Precortisyl
Predenema   United Kingdom
Prednesol
Predsol-N
Scheriproct
Sintisone
Sulfapred

Adnisolone
Delta-Cortef
Deltasolone
Optocort   Australia
Panafcortelone
Prelone
Solone

Prednicortelone   Belgium
Delcortol   Denmark
Hydrocortancyl
Predniretard   France

Decaprednil
Decortin-H
Dura Prednisolon
Hostacortin H
Precortilon   Germany
Predni-Coelin
Predni-H
Scherisolon
Ultra corten-H

Acepreval
Caberdelta
Cortisolone
Cortomas (palmitate)   Italy
Deltolio (palmitate)
Domucortone
Predartrina

Derpo PD	
Donisolone	} Japan
Prednine	
Encortolone	Poland
Lenisolone	
Meticortelone	
Predeltilone	} South Africa
Normonsona	
Scherisolona	
Dacortin	
Meprisolon	} Switzerland
Predni-Helvacort	
Delta-Cortef	
Meti-Derm	
Prednis	
Ropredlone	} USA
Sterane	
Ulacort	

Corticotrophin

Long-acting

Acthar Gel	United Kingdom
Acthar Gel	{ Australia, Canada, Italy, South Africa, USA
Acthelea	
Actonar	} Argentina
Cortrophin ZN	Australia
Durackin	Canada
Acortan Prolongatum	
Depot-Acethropan	} Germany
Acton prolongatum	Sweden
Reacthin	
Cortrophine-2	} Switzerland
Cortigel	USA

Tetracosactrin

Synacthen	
Synacthen Depot	} United Kingdom
Synacthen and/or	{ Argentina, Australia, Belgium,
Synacthen Depot	Canada, Denmark, Germany, Italy,
	Netherlands, Norway, South Africa,
	Sweden, Switzerland

Cortrosinta Depot	Spain
Cotrosyn	Belgium, Canada, Italy, Netherlands
Cotrosyn Depot	Australia, Belgium, Italy, Netherlands, Norway, South Africa, Sweden, Switzerland
Nuvacthen	Spain
Nuvacthen Depot	
Synacthene	France

LONG-TERM RHEUMATOID SUPPRESSANTS

Gold salts

Sodium aurothiomalate

Myocrisin	United Kingdom
Myochrysine	Canada, USA
Tauredon	Germany, Switzerland

Sodium aurothiosulphate

Sanocrysin	Denmark

Antimalarials

Chloroquine phosphate

Avloclor	United Kingdom
Niraquine	
Aralen	Australia, Canada, USA
Chlorochin	Switzerland
Chlorquin	Australia
Dichinalex	Italy
Resochin	Australia, Denmark, Netherlands, Norway, Spain, Switzerland
Resochine	Belgium

Hydroxychloroquine sulphate

Plaquenil	United Kingdom
Ercoquin	Denmark, Norway, Sweden
Quensyl	Germany

D-Penicillamine

Distamine Pendramine	} United Kingdom
D-Penamine	Australia
Kelatin	Belgium
Dimetylcystein	Denmark
Trolovol	France
Metalcaptase Trolovol	} Germany
Premine	Italy
Metalcaptase	Japan
Kelatin	Netherlands
Cuprenil	Poland
Metalcaptase	South Africa
Cupripen Sufortanon	} Spain
Artamin Mercaptyl	} Switzerland
Depen	USA

Azathioprine

Imuran	United Kingdom
Imuran (injectable)	{ Argentina, Australia, Belgium, Canada, Italy, Netherlands, South Africa, USA
Azanin	Japan
Imurek	Australia, Germany, Switzerland
Imurel	{ Denmark, France, Norway, Spain, Sweden

Cyclophosphamide

Endoxana	United Kingdom
Cytoxan	USA, Canada
Endoxan	{ Belgium, Denmark, Germany, Netherlands, South Africa
Endoxan-Asta	{ Argentina, Australia, France, Italy, Switzerland
Enduxon	Brazil
Genoxal	Spain
Procytox	Canada
Sendoxan	Norway, Sweden

Chlorambucil

Leukeran	United Kingdom
Chloraminophene	France

Methotrexate

Emtexate	United Kingdom
Emthexate	Netherlands
Ledertrexate	Belgium, France, Netherlands
Methotrexat	Germany
Metotrexato	Argentina
Mexate	USA

ANTI-GOUT DRUGS

Colchicine

Colcin Colgout Coluric	} Australia
Colchineos	France, South Africa
Colchicum-Dispert (colchicum corn) Colchysat Burger (flower juice)	} Germany

Probenezid

Benemid	United Kingdom
Benemid	{ Australia, Belgium, Canada, Germany, Italy, Netherlands, South Africa, Switzerland, USA
Procid	Australia
Probenid	Belgium
Benuryl	Canada
Benemide	France
Panuric Proben	} South Africa
Probemid	Spain
Probecid	Sweden

Sulphinpyrazone

Anturan	United Kingdom
Anturan	Argentina, Australia, Belgium, Canada, Denmark, South Africa, Spain, Switzerland
Anturane	USA
Anturano	Germany
Enturen	Italy, Netherlands
Zynol	Canada

Benzbromarone

Desuric	Belgium, Italy, Netherlands, Switzerland
Desuric	France
Max-Uric	Argentina
Minuric	South Africa
Narcaricin	Germany
Normurat	Germany
Obason	Switzerland
Uricovac	Germany
Urinorm	Spain
Urinome	Japan

Allopurinol

Aloral	
Aluline	
Caplenel	
Cosuric	United Kingdom
Hamarin	
Zyloric	
Zyloric	Argentina, Belgium, Denmark, France, Germany, Italy, Netherlands, Norway, Spain, Switzerland
Uroquad	Argentina
Capurate	
Progout	Australia
Zyloprim	

Alloprin
Purinol   } Canada
Zyloprim

Apurin   Denmark

Bleminol
Cellidrin
Daprosan
Epidropal
Foligan   } Germany
Urbol-100
Urobenyl
Urosin
Xanturat

Milurit   Hungary

Allural
Allurit
Uricemil
Uriscel   } Italy
Urolit
Vedatan

Adenock
Allozym
Alositol
Anoprolin
Anzief
Aprinol
Ketanrift
Ketobun-A   } Japan
Masaton
Miniplanor
Monarch
Neufan
Riball
Takanarumin
Uric

Zyloprim   Mexico
Apurin   Norway
Zyloprim   New Zealand
Puricos   } South Africa
Zyloprim

Allopur
Foligan
Lysuran 300

} Switzerland

Lopurin
Zyloprim

} USA

Index